Multifunctional Marine Polysaccharides

Sougata Jana • Subrata Jana • John F. Kennedy
Editors

Multifunctional Marine Polysaccharides

Drug Delivery, Biomedicine and Food Technology Applications

Springer

Editors
Sougata Jana
Directorate of Health Services
Department of Health and Family Welfare
Kolkata, West Bengal, India

Subrata Jana
Department of Chemistry
Indira Gandhi National Tribal University
Amarkantak, Madhya Pradesh, India

John F. Kennedy
Advanced Science and Technology
Institute
Director of Chembiotech Research
Worcestershire, Worcestershire, UK

ISBN 978-981-95-4125-6 ISBN 978-981-95-4126-3 (eBook)
https://doi.org/10.1007/978-981-95-4126-3

This Springer imprint is published by the registered company Springer Nature Singapore Pte Ltd.
The registered company address is: 152 Beach Road, #21-01/04 Gateway East, Singapore 189721, Singapore

Preface

This book highlights on recent advances in various marine polysaccharides (MPs) and MP-based biological macromolecules with multifunctional approaches in biomedical engineering. MPs are eco-friendly, renewable, and derived from natural sources. Important biological properties of the MPs include biodegradability, biocompatibility, nontoxicity, low cost, and abundance. MPs exhibit a vast variety of structures and biological functions and should be considered as a novel resource of natural biomaterials for drug discovery. Generally MPs are classified into three categories such as marine plant polysaccharide, marine animal polysaccharide, and marine microbial polysaccharide.

This book is composed of three parts: Part I—Drug Delivery, Part II—Biomedical Applications, and Part III—Food Technology Applications. MPs are easily fabricated into nanoparticles, nanofibers, microparticles, hydrogels, patches, scaffolds, membranes, gels, beads, and sponge forms, and these forms have been used for various biomedical engineering applications in drug delivery, gene therapy, cancer therapy, nanotheranostic, tissue engineering, biosensors, wound dressing, and food technology.

This edited reference book is developed by a group of renowned scientists, chemists, biologists, and engineers from around the world. This book will be an important reference resource for scientists and researchers, who are working on marine polysaccharides (MPs) in the field of pharmaceuticals, biomedical science and engineering, nanotechnology, and material science for most updated findings and future research trends.

Chapter "Introduction of Marine Polysaccharides: Preparation, Characterization, Evaluation, and Applications" focuses on general overview of marine polysaccharides, sources, classification, extraction procedure, characterization techniques and their applications in the pharmaceutical field.

Chapter "Plant-Derived Marine Polysaccharides in Oral Drug Delivery" comprehensively addresses about the effective scenario of marine plant-derived polysaccharides for various flexible functionalities in oral delivery of various drugs/ molecules.

Marine polysaccharides have emerged as versatile and biocompatible materials for the development of injectable drug delivery systems, offering a sustainable alternative to synthetic polymers.

Chapter "Marine-Based Polysaccharides for Injectable Drug Delivery Approaches" highlights the current progress, challenges, and future directions in utilizing marine-based polysaccharides for injectable drug delivery systems, underscoring their role in the advancement of biocompatible and effective pharmaceutical platforms.

Chapter "Marine Seaweed Polysaccharide in Antiviral Activities" describes the most important marine seaweed polysaccharides with potential antiviral activities and uses in the treatment of various viral infections.

Chapter "Marine Animal Polysaccharide in Targeted Drug Delivery" emphasizes the importance of marine polysaccharides and studies their potential properties for targeted drug delivery. It also discusses the recent innovations related to drug delivery systems, including smart release systems and composite formulations that synergize marine polysaccharides with other materials. It also highlights future directions and perspectives in marine-based drug delivery technologies, outlining their role in the era of next generation of precision therapeutics and regenerative remedies.

Chapter "Marine-Based Polysaccharides in Nose-to-Brain Drug Delivery" explores the potential of marine-based polysaccharides in nose-to-brain drug delivery systems, focusing on their applications for treating central nervous system (CNS) disorders.

Chapter "Marine Algae Polysaccharides in Anticancer Drug Delivery" focuses on marine algae polysaccharide-based delivery systems and strategies to enhance the safety and efficiency of anticancer drug therapy, and their development avenues toward further integration in personalized medicine and the development of combination therapies.

Chapter "Marine Algal Polysaccharides in the Management of Liver Disease" highlights the role of marine algal polysaccharides in management of liver disease. Marine algal polysaccharides may lead to safe and effective agents for prevention and treatment of liver disease.

Chapter "Marine Polysaccharidic Matrix as Inhalational Drug Carrier" focuses on marine polysaccharide-based matrix as inhalational drug carrier for delivery of therapeutic agents into different regions of lungs through modulating particle size for inhalation and targeting the macrophages.

Chapter "Antioxidant Potentials from Marine-Derived Polysaccharides" highlights on antioxidant potentials from marine-derived polysaccharides.

Chapter "Marine Polysaccharides in Wound Healing" focuses on the structural properties of marine polysaccharides, particularly alginate and chitosan, their application in wound healing, various forms of alginate- and chitosan-based wound dressings, and their clinical applications.

Chapter "Marine Seaweed Polysaccharide-Based Scaffolds in Tissue Regenera tion" discusses on the current state of marine seaweed polysaccharide-based scaffolds in tissue regeneration and highlights their potential applications in various tissues, including bone, cartilage, skin, and nerve. It also discusses the advantages and challenges of using marine seaweed polysaccharides as scaffold materials, as well as the future directions for research and advances in this field.

Chapter "Marine Animal Polysaccharide Scaffolds in Tissue Engineering Applications" provides an overview of the recent advances in the development and application of marine animal polysaccharide-based scaffolds, focusing on their potential to treat various clinical conditions. It also highlights emerging trends and future directions, emphasizing the role of sustainable marine biomaterials in advancing tissue engineering and regenerative medicine.

Chapter "Multifunctional Marine Polysaccharides in Theranostic Applications" reveals the role of marine polysaccharides in theranostic applications along with their multifunctional capabilities, including therapeutic efficacy and diagnostic potential.

Chapter "3D Printed Marine Polysaccharides in Biological Applications" focuses on marine-sourced polysaccharide-based principles of 3D-printing technologies, material requirements, and significant biological applications, including drug delivery, tissue engineering (cartilage and bone tissue engineering), and antimicrobial and wound healing applications. Marine polysaccharides (e.g., chitosan, alginate, hyaluronic acid, fucoidan, laminarin, gelatin, and carrageenan) frequently employed for 3D printing are also included.

Chapter "Marine Polysaccharides in Food Processing and Preservation" explores the wide-ranging applications of marine-derived polysaccharides in food processing. This chapter describes the emerging trends and future perspectives, emphasizing sustainable extraction technologies and novel formulation strategies that position marine polysaccharides for health-focused and eco-friendly food innovations.

Chapter "Marine Polysaccharides in Delivery of Bioactive Molecules" provides an in-depth review of the structural and physicochemical properties and the use of most popular marine polysaccharides, including alginate, fucoidan, chitosan, carrageenan, and agar, as natural carriers for the entrapment and delivery of nutraceuticals and bioactive compounds in the field of pharmaceutical, food, and biomedical industries.

Chapter "Plant-Based Marine Polysaccharides in Food Applications" discusses on plant-based marine polysaccharides (alginate, carrageenan, fucoidan, ulvan, and agar) in food technology applications. Plant-based marine polysaccharides are widely used as food additives due to their stabilizing, gelling, thickening, fat replacement, and prebiotic properties in the industry and are also used in plastic packaging materials due to environmental and health concerns, as environmentally friendly, renewable, biodegradable, and nontoxic materials.

Chapter "Animal-Based Marine Polysaccharides in Food Packaging" highlights the potential of animal-based marine polysaccharides in transforming the food packaging industry by offering renewable, safe, and sustainable packaging alternatives.

Finally, Chapter "Marine-Based Polysaccharides in Food: Safety and Regulation" provides a comprehensive overview of the regulatory frameworks that oversee the usage of marine polysaccharides in major international regions, including the United States, the European Union, Japan, China, South Korea, Australia/New Zealand, India, and Canada with recent updates from authorities like the Food and Drug Administration (FDA), European Food Safety Authority (EFSA), Ministry of Health, Labour Welfare (MHLW), Food Standards Australia New Zealand (FSANZ), and Codex Alimentarius. The chapter also explores "Generally Recognized as Safe (GRAS)" materials based on toxicological data, historical dietary usage, and contemporary risk assessments, particularly emphasizing vulnerable groups such as infants.

We acknowledge that this book would not have been possible without the support and contribution of all the authors and their respective teams. Finally, the editors would also like to acknowledge the very efficient and friendly staff of Springer, Dr. Mei Hann Lee and other staff, for their support from the start to the course of the entire production process.

Kolkata, West Bengal, India — Sougata Jana
Amarkantak, Madhya Pradesh, India — Subrata Jana
Worcestershire, Worcestershire, UK — John F. Kennedy

Contents

Introduction of Marine Polysaccharides: Preparation, Characterization, Evaluation, and Applications 1
Bratati Ghosh, Olivia Sen, Sougata Jana, and Sreejan Manna

Part I Drug Delivery

Plant-Derived Marine Polysaccharides in Oral Drug Delivery 33
Vipul D. Prajapati, Aditya Shrivstav, Juhini Valand, Riddhi Dalal, Kavyasri Penemecha, and Shivani Gandhi

Marine-Based Polysaccharides for Injectable Drug Delivery Approaches 85
Mohamed Ashraf, Hossam S. El-Sawy, and Mona M. A. Abdel-Mottaleb

Marine Seaweed Polysaccharide in Antiviral Activities 103
Fatma Sa'eed El-Tokhy and Mona M. A. Abdel-Mottaleb

Marine Animal Polysaccharide in Targeted Drug Delivery 127
Sarra Akermi, Moufida Chaari, Khaoula Elhadef, Bouthaina Hadj Hmida, Gulzar Rather, Fakhreddine Ben Amara, Ashwani Sharma, and Slim Smaoui

Marine-Based Polysaccharides in Nose-to-Brain Drug Delivery 153
Shubhrat Maheshwari, Aditya Singh, Amita Verma, Vaseem A. Ansari, Juber Akhtar, and Bhupendra G. Prajapati

Marine Algae Polysaccharides in Anticancer Drug Delivery 173
Souad A. Elfeky, Gamal El-ghannam, Mostafa Zedan, and Nayer Qenawi

Marine Algal Polysaccharides in the Management of Liver Disease 207
Fatemeh Izadpanah Qeshmi, Saba Ghattavi, and Ahmad Homaei

Marine Polysaccharidic Matrix as Inhalational Drug Carrier 229
Muhammad Waseem Akram, Mohamed Effendi Mohamed Tenang, and Tin Wui Wong

Part II Biomedical Applications

Antioxidant Potentials of Marine-Derived Polysaccharides 255
Sowmiya Govindaragavan, Anandhi Anandaraj, and Rajasekar Thirunavukkarasu

Marine Polysaccharides in Wound Healing 293
M. R. Divya, Reshma Anns Raju, and M. R. Rekha

Marine Seaweed Polysaccharide-Based Scaffolds in Tissue Regeneration 339
Deepa Thomas and M. S. Latha

Marine Animal Polysaccharide Scaffolds in Tissue Engineering Applications 365
Krishnameera Sajayan and Kausik Kapat

Multifunctional Marine Polysaccharides in Theranostic Applications . . . 395
Kavipriya Murugaiyan, Sasvat Sayee Ram Ramesh, and Aravind Kumar Rengan

3D Printed Marine Polysaccharides in Biological Applications 423
Sujata Das, Upadhyayula Suryanarayana Murty, and Subham Banerjee

Part III Food Technology Applications

Marine Polysaccharides in Food Processing and Preservation 451
Vikramaditya Banerjee, Supriya Kumar Bose, Aparna Chaudhuri, Sabyasachi Ghosh, and Swarup Roy

Marine Polysaccharides in Delivery of Bioactive Molecules 473
Rassoul Kadkhodaee and Sara Keshvari Khojasteh

Plant-Based Marine Polysaccharides in Food Applications 503
Basak Ebru Ozcan

Animal-Based Marine Polysaccharides in Food Packaging 525
Bandana Padhan, Susrishta Mukherjee, Bidisha Ray, Samridhi Bhattacharjee, Rishita Rakshit, and Joyjyoti Das

Marine-Based Polysaccharides in Food: Safety and Regulation 549
Pottabathula Shyam Sundar, Veerachamy Alagarsamy, Subhash Chandra Bose, Arehalli S. Manjappa, Sunil T. Galatage, Potti Lakshmanarao, Kaipu Malli Karjun, and Viswas Raja Solomon

Contributors

Mona M. A. Abdel-Mottaleb Université de Franche-Comté, EFS, INSERM, UMR 1098 RIGHT, Besançon, France
Department of Pharmaceutics and industrial Pharmacy, Faculty of Pharmacy, Ain Shams University, Cairo, Egypt

Sarra Akermi Laboratory of Microbial Biotechnology, Enzymatic and Biomolecules, Centre of Biotechnology of Sfax, Sfax, Tunisia

Juber Akhtar Department of Pharmacy, Faculty of Pharmacy, Integral University, Lucknow, Uttar Pradesh, India

Muhammad Waseem Akram Non-Destructive Biomedical and Pharmaceutical Research Centre, Smart Manufacturing Research Institute, UniversitiTeknologi MARA Selangor, Puncak Alam, Malaysia
Particle Design Research Group, Faculty of Pharmacy, UniversitiTeknologi MARA Selangor, Puncak Alam, Malaysia

Veerachamy Alagarsamy Department of Medicinal Chemistry, MNR College of Pharmacy, Sangareddy, Telangana, India

Fakhreddine Ben Amara Laboratory of Microbial Biotechnology, Enzymatic and Biomolecules, Centre of Biotechnology of Sfax, Sfax, Tunisia

Anandhi Anandaraj Centre for Drug Discovery and Development, Sathyabama Institute of Science and Technology, Chennai, Tamil Nadu, India

Vaseem A. Ansari Department of Pharmacy, Faculty of Pharmacy, Integral University, Lucknow, Uttar Pradesh, India

Mohamed Ashraf Department of Pharmaceutics and Pharmaceutical Technology, Faculty of Pharmacy, Egyptian Russian University, Cairo, Egypt

Subham Banerjee Department of Pharmaceutics, National Institute of Pharmaceutical Education and Research (NIPER), Guwahati, Changsari, Assam, India

Vikramaditya Banerjee Department of Applied Biology, Maulana Abul Kalam Azad University of Technology, Haringhata Farm, West Bengal, India

Samridhi Bhattacharjee Department of Biotechnology, School of Life Science & Biotechnology, Adamas University, Kolkata, West Bengal, India

Subhash Chandra Bose Department of Pharmaceutics, MNR College of Pharmacy, Sangareddy, Telangana, India

Supriya Kumar Bose Department of Biotechnology, School of Life Science, Swami Vivekananda University, Barrackpore, West Bengal, India

Moufida Chaari Laboratory of Microbial Biotechnology, Enzymatic and Biomolecules, Centre of Biotechnology of Sfax, Sfax, Tunisia

Aparna Chaudhuri Department of Biotechnology, School of Life Science, Swami Vivekananda University, Barrackpore, West Bengal, India

Riddhi Dalal Department of Pharmaceutics, S.S.R. College of Pharmacy (Permanently Affiliated to Savitribai Phule Pune University), Sayli, Silvassa, Union Territory of Dadra Nagar Haveli & Daman Diu, India

Joyjyoti Das Department of Biotechnology, School of Life Science & Biotechnology, Adamas University, Kolkata, West Bengal, India

Sujata Das Department of Pharmaceutics, National Institute of Pharmaceutical Education and Research (NIPER), Guwahati, Changsari, Assam, India

M. R. Divya Division of Biosurface Technology, Biomedical Technology Wing, Sree Chitra Tirunal Institute for Medical Sciences and Technology, Thiruvananthapuram, Kerala, India

Souad A. Elfeky Department of Laser Applications in Metrology, Photochemistry, and Agriculture (LAMPA), National Institute of Laser Enhanced Science (NILES), Cairo University, Giza, Egypt

Gamal El-ghannam Department of Laser Applications in Metrology, Photochemistry, and Agriculture (LAMPA), National Institute of Laser Enhanced Science (NILES), Cairo University, Giza, Egypt

Khaoula Elhadef Laboratory of Microbial Biotechnology, Enzymatic and Biomolecules, Centre of Biotechnology of Sfax, Sfax, Tunisia

Hossam S. El-Sawy Department of Pharmaceutics and Pharmaceutical Technology, Faculty of Pharmacy, Egyptian Russian University, Cairo, Egypt
Department of Pharmaceutics, College of Pharmacy, University of Kut, Wasit, Iraq

Fatma Sa'eed El-Tokhy Department of Pharmaceutics and Industrial Pharmacy, Faculty of Pharmacy, Badr University in Cairo (BUC), Cairo, Egypt

Sunil T. Galatage Department of Pharmaceutics, Vasantidevi Patil Institute of Pharmacy, Kodoli, Maharashtra, India

Shivani Gandhi Department of Pharmaceutics, Faculty of Pharmacy, The Maharaja Sayajirao University of Baroda, Vadodara, Gujarat, India

Saba Ghattavi Persian Gulf and Oman Sea Ecological Research Center, Iranian Fisheries Sciences Research Institute, Agricultural Research Education and Extension Organization (AREEO), Bandar Abbas, Hormozgan, Iran

Bratati Ghosh Department of Pharmacy, Anand College of Education, Paschim Medinipur, West Bengal, India

Sabyasachi Ghosh Department of Biotechnology, School of Life Science, Swami Vivekananda University, Barrackpore, West Bengal, India

Sowmiya Govindaragavan Centre for Drug Discovery and Development, Sathyabama Institute of Science and Technology, Chennai, Tamil Nadu, India

Bouthaina Hadj Hmida Laboratory of Biochemistry and Enzymatic Engineering of Lipases, National Engineering School of Sfax (ENIS), Sfax, Tunisia

Ahmad Homaei Department of Marine Biology, Faculty of Marine Science and Technology, University of Hormozgan, Bandar Abbas, Iran

Sougata Jana Department of Health and Family Welfare, Directorate of Health Services, Kolkata, West Bengal, India

Rassoul Kadkhodaee Department of Food Physics, Research Institute of Food Science and Technology (RIFST), Mashhad, Iran

Kausik Kapat Department of Medical Devices, National Institute of Pharmaceutical Education and Research Kolkata, Kolkata, West Bengal, India

Kaipu Malli Karjun Department of Pharmacology, Vasantidevi Patil Institute of Pharmacy, Kodoli, Maharashtra, India

Sara Keshvari Khojasteh Department of Food Physics, Research Institute of Food Science and Technology (RIFST), Mashhad, Iran

Potti Lakshmanarao Department of Pharmaceutics, Vasantidevi Patil Institute of Pharmacy, Kodoli, Maharashtra, India

M. S. Latha Department of Chemistry, Sree Narayana College, Kollam, Kerala, India
Sree Narayana Guru College of Advanced Studies, Nangiarkulangara, Kerala, India

Shubhrat Maheshwari Bioorganic and Medicinal Chemistry Research Laboratory, Department of Pharmaceutical Sciences, Sam Higginbottom University of Agriculture, Technology and Sciences, Prayagraj, Uttar Pradesh, India

Arehalli S. Manjappa Department of Pharmaceutics, Vasantidevi Patil Institute of Pharmacy, Kodoli, Maharashtra, India

Sreejan Manna Department of Pharmaceutical Technology, Brainware University, Kolkata, West Bengal, India

Susrishta Mukherjee Department of Biotechnology, School of Life Science & Biotechnology, Adamas University, Kolkata, West Bengal, India

Upadhyayula Suryanarayana Murty Department of Pharmaceutics, National Institute of Pharmaceutical Education and Research (NIPER), Guwahati, Changsari, Assam, India

Kavipriya Murugaiyan Department of Biomedical Engineering, Indian Institute of Technology-Hyderabad, Sangareddy, Telangana, India

Basak Ebru Ozcan Department of Food Engineering, Faculty of Engineering, Kirklareli University, Kırklareli, Turkey

Bandana Padhan Department of Biotechnology, School of Life Science & Biotechnology, Adamas University, Kolkata, West Bengal, India

Kavyasri Penemecha Department of Pharmaceutics, S.S.R. College of Pharmacy (Permanently Affiliated to Savitribai Phule Pune University), Sayli, Silvassa, Union Territory of Dadra Nagar Haveli & Daman Diu, India

Bhupendra G. Prajapati Department of Pharmaceutics, Parul Institute of Pharmacy, Faculty of Pharmacy, Parul University, Vadodara, Gujarat, India

Vipul D. Prajapati Department of Pharmaceutics, S.S.R. College of Pharmacy (Permanently Affiliated to Savitribai Phule Pune University), Sayli, Silvassa, Union Territory of Dadra Nagar Haveli & Daman Diu, India

Nayer Qenawi Department of Laser Applications in Metrology, Photochemistry, and Agriculture (LAMPA), National Institute of Laser Enhanced Science (NILES), Cairo University, Giza, Egypt

Fatemeh Izadpanah Qeshmi Department of Marine Biology, Faculty of Marine Science and Technology, University of Hormozgan, Bandar Abbas, Iran

Reshma Anns Raju Division of Biosurface Technology, Biomedical Technology Wing, Sree Chitra Tirunal Institute for Medical Sciences and Technology, Thiruvananthapuram, Kerala, India

Rishita Rakshit Department of Biotechnology, School of Life Science & Biotechnology, Adamas University, Kolkata, West Bengal, India

Sasvat Sayee Ram Ramesh Department of Biomedical Engineering, Indian Institute of Technology-Hyderabad, Sangareddy, Telangana, India

Gulzar Rather AMR and Nanotherapeutics Lab, Department of Pharmacology, Saveetha Dental College and Hospital, Saveetha Institute of Medical and Technical Sciences, Chennai, India

Bidisha Ray Department of Biotechnology, School of Life Science & Biotechnology, Adamas University, Kolkata, West Bengal, India

M. R. Rekha Division of Biosurface Technology, Biomedical Technology Wing, Sree Chitra Tirunal Institute for Medical Sciences and Technology, Thiruvananthapuram, Kerala, India

Aravind Kumar Rengan Department of Biomedical Engineering, Indian Institute of Technology-Hyderabad, Sangareddy, Telangana, India

Swarup Roy Department of Food Technology and Nutrition, School of Agriculture, Lovely Professional University, Phagwara, India
Department of Food and Nutrition, Kyung Hee University, Seoul, Republic of Korea

Krishnameera Sajayan Department of Medical Devices, National Institute of Pharmaceutical Education and Research Kolkata, Kolkata, West Bengal, India

Olivia Sen Department of Pharmaceutical Technology, Brainware University, Kolkata, West Bengal, India

Ashwani Sharma Insight Biosolutions, Biopole Rennes, Rennes, France

Aditya Shrivstav Department of Pharmaceutics, S.S.R. College of Pharmacy (Permanently Affiliated to Savitribai Phule Pune University), Sayli, Silvassa, Union Territory of Dadra Nagar Haveli & Daman Diu, India

Aditya Singh Department of Pharmacy, Faculty of Pharmacy, Integral University, Lucknow, Uttar Pradesh, India

Slim Smaoui Laboratory of Microbial Biotechnology, Enzymatic and Biomolecules, Centre of Biotechnology of Sfax, Sfax, Tunisia

Viswas Raja Solomon Department of Medicinal Chemistry, MNR College of Pharmacy, Sangareddy, Telangana, India

Pottabathula Shyam Sundar Department of Pharmaceutical Chemistry, Vasantidevi Patil Institute of Pharmacy, Kodoli, Maharashtra, India

Mohamed Effendi Mohamed Tenang Tenang Pharma SdnBhd, Nilai, Negeri Sembilan, Malaysia

Rajasekar Thirunavukkarasu Centre for Drug Discovery and Development, Sathyabama Institute of Science and Technology, Chennai, Tamil Nadu, India

Deepa Thomas Research and Post Graduate Department of Chemistry, Bishop Moore College, Mavelikara, Kerala, India

Juhini Valand Department of Pharmaceutics, S.S.R. College of Pharmacy (Permanently Affiliated to Savitribai Phule Pune University), Sayli, Silvassa, Union Territory of Dadra Nagar Haveli & Daman Diu, India

Amita Verma Bioorganic and Medicinal Chemistry Research Laboratory, Department of Pharmaceutical Sciences, Sam Higginbottom University of Agriculture, Technology and Sciences, Prayagraj, Uttar Pradesh, India

Tin Wui Wong Non-Destructive Biomedical and Pharmaceutical Research Centre, Smart Manufacturing Research Institute, UniversitiTeknologi MARA Selangor, Puncak Alam, Malaysia
Particle Design Research Group, Faculty of Pharmacy, UniversitiTeknologi MARA Selangor, Puncak Alam, Malaysia
Department of Industrial Pharmacy, Faculty of Pharmacy, Silpakorn University, Nakhon Pathom, Thailand

Mostafa Zedan Department of Laser Applications in Metrology, Photochemistry, and Agriculture (LAMPA), National Institute of Laser Enhanced Science (NILES), Cairo University, Giza, Egypt

Introduction of Marine Polysaccharides: Preparation, Characterization, Evaluation, and Applications

Bratati Ghosh, Olivia Sen, Sougata Jana, and Sreejan Manna

Abstract Polysaccharides are the most important group of biopolymers with various roles in pharmaceutical, biomedical, and food industries. Marine polysaccharides are complex carbohydrates originated from marine organisms including algae, seaweeds, and bacteria. Structurally, the polymer molecules are connected by glycosidic bonds. A variety of chemical structures, source of organisms, and evolutionary history in different species of marine polysaccharide have contributed to their multifaceted applications in various sectors. This chapter would majorly focus on their sources, classification, extraction procedure, characterization techniques, and applications in the pharmaceutical field.

Keywords Marine polysaccharides · Chitosan · Alginate · Glycosaminoglycans · Carrageenan · Applications of marine polysaccharides

1 Introduction

Polysaccharides are widely used natural macromolecular polymers consisting of monosaccharides, alternating units of sugar connected with glycosidic linkage (Benalaya et al. 2024). Natural polysaccharides are isolated from different sources such as plant and marine sources. Polysaccharides are obtained from various natural sources including seaweeds, fungi, crustacean etc. The aqueous solubility of these polysaccharides also vary greatly depending on their physicochemical properties which may be soluble or insoluble in water or present in a semi-crystalline form (Kabir et al. 2022; Sen et al. 2025a). Marine polysaccharides are a large group of

B. Ghosh
Department of Pharmacy, Anand College of Education, Paschim Medinipur, West Bengal, India

O. Sen · S. Manna (✉)
Department of Pharmaceutical Technology, Brainware University, Kolkata, West Bengal, India

S. Jana
Department of Health and Family Welfare, Directorate of Health Services, Kolkata, West Bengal, India

S. Jana et al. (eds.), *Multifunctional Marine Polysaccharides*,
https://doi.org/10.1007/978-981-95-4126-3_1

complex macromolecular polymers with effective biological properties. Oceans are abundant with marine polysaccharides including alginate, carrageenan, laminarin, fucoidan (from seaweeds), and chitosan and hyaluronic acid (from marine animals). Marine polymers are biocompatible and biodegradable in nature with mucoadhesivity and diverse bioactivities such as anti-inflammatory, antioxidant, anticoagulant, antiviral, antimicrobial, and immunomodulatory effects (Lee et al. 2017; Chandika et al. 2022). Conventional drug delivery methods often face challenges such as poor solubility, rapid elimination, and low selectivity. To address these challenges, drug delivery systems (DDS) have been developed to increase bioavailability and reduce side effects (Adepu and Ramakrishna 2021). Marine polysaccharides have gained a considerable attention for developing DDS due to their non-toxicity, stability, low cost, ease of availability, and modulable features. Due to the biocompatibility of marine polysaccharides, it can be extensively used as bioresponsive DDS enabling them to detect environmental stimuli such as pH, ROS (e.g., OH^-, H_2O_2, O_2^-), GSH, light, heat, and magnetism (Sun et al. 2021; Geng et al.). These systems respond to pathological microenvironments to release drugs precisely, combining the bioactivity of polysaccharides with targeted delivery. Nowadays, marine polysaccharide-based DDS are being extensively investigated, and several marine polysaccharides have also used for industrial purposes. Key polysaccharides under investigation include alginate, chitosan, carrageenan, laminarin, fucoidan, and hyaluronic acid (Barbosa et al. 2019). This chapter explores the various marine polymers and their extraction, structural characteristics, and evaluation with their unique biological properties. Marine polysaccharides are abundantly used in tissue engineering, wound care, and disease diagnostics, offering a foundation for precision medicine.

2 Classification of Marine Polysaccharides

Marine polysaccharides (MPs) are complex carbohydrates derived from various marine organisms and categorized based on their biological sources and chemical structures as shown in Fig. 1. Depending on sources, marine polysaccharides are classified into three major types:

2.1 Algal Polysaccharides

These are complex carbohydrates extracted from various types of seaweed (marine algae) and are widely used in food, pharmaceutical, and biotechnology industries. They are valued for their natural gelling, thickening, and stabilizing properties (de Jesus Raposo et al. 2015). Key types include:

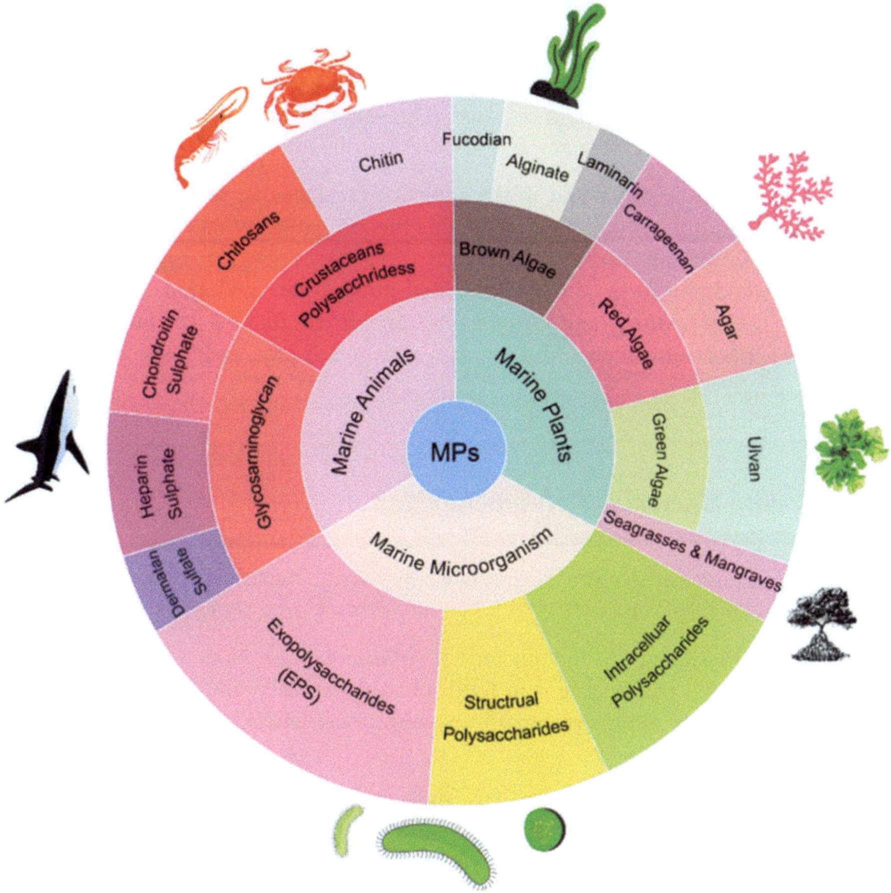

Fig. 1 Classification of marine polysaccharides. (Reprinted from open access article, Shen et al. 2021)

Agar: Sourced from red algae (e.g., *Gelidium*, *Gracilaria*), used as a gelling agent in food and microbiological media

Alginate: Extracted from brown seaweed (e.g., *Laminaria*, *Macrocystis*), used in wound dressings, food processing, and drug delivery systems

Carrageenan: Obtained from red seaweed (e.g., *Chondrus*, *Eucheuma*), used as a thickener and stabilizer in dairy and meat products

Ulvan: Derived from green seaweed (e.g., *Ulva*, *Enteromorpha*), known for its antioxidant and immune-boosting properties

These polysaccharides are biodegradable and biocompatible and support various biomedical applications, including tissue engineering and wound healing (Lomartire and Gonçalves 2023).

2.2 Crustacean-Derived Polysaccharides

These are complex carbohydrates extracted from the exoskeletons of marine arthropods such as shrimp, crabs, and lobsters (Ngasotter et al. 2023; Saravanan et al. 2023). The two primary types are:

Chitin: A natural polymer found in the shells of crustaceans, used in biomedicine, agriculture, and water treatment due to its biocompatibility and biodegradability (Elieh-Ali-Komi and Hamblin 2016).

Chitosan: A modified form of chitin obtained through deacetylation. It has *antimicrobial, wound-healing*, and *film-forming* properties, making it valuable in biomedical applications like *wound dressings*, drug delivery, and tissue engineering (Rossi et al. 2024).

2.3 Marine Bacterial Polysaccharides

These are complex carbohydrates produced by marine bacteria (Khan et al. 2022). They are mainly of two types:

Gellan Gum: Produced by the bacterium *Sphingomonas elodea*, gellan gum is widely used as a gelling agent in food, pharmaceuticals, and tissue engineering due to its stability and biocompatibility (AbdlAali and Al-Sahlany 2024; Bajaj et al. 2007).

These polysaccharides are valued for their biological activity, biodegradability, and potential in biomedical and industrial applications.

Sponge and tunicate polysaccharides are bioactive carbohydrates derived from marine animals such as sponges and tunicates. These polysaccharides are of special interest in biomedical research due to their unique structures and biological activities (Bharathi and Lee 2024; Romano et al. 2022). Key types include:

Glycosaminoglycans (GAGs): Heparin-like sulfated polysaccharides found in marine invertebrates, known for their anticoagulant and anti-inflammatory properties.

Fucoidan: A sulfated polysaccharide primarily from brown seaweed but also found in some tunicates, valued for its anti-inflammatory, anticancer, antiviral, and immune-modulating effects (Sasarman et al. 2016; Yamada et al. 2011).

These marine-derived polysaccharides are being explored for use in wound healing, drug delivery, and tissue engineering, due to their biocompatibility and therapeutic potential.

Exopolysaccharides (EPS): These polysaccharides are high-molecular-weight polymers produced by microorganisms, including bacteria, fungus, algae, and marine organisms, and are typically derived from fermentation processes. They are essential in microbial biofilm formation and protection while also providing various applications in medicine (as drug carriers and immunomodulators), business (as thickeners and stabilizers), and the environment (in bioremediation and soil structure enhancement) (Benhadda et al. 2023; Netrusov et al. 2023; Wang et al. 2023a).

3 Extraction Procedure of Marine Polysaccharides

3.1 Alginate

Alginate can be extracted from different seaweeds in multiple stages. At first, freshly collected seaweed is washed, dried, and grinded into powder. After that, the seaweed is immersed in water to rehydrate. Different chemicals are added to remove unwanted compounds from the seaweed. This is followed by an acid or alkali pretreatment to disrupt the plant cell wall. Subsequently, sodium carbonate is used to extract water-soluble alginate from the seaweed biomass. Alginate can then be recovered from the extract using one of the three precipitation methods: the sodium alginate route, the calcium alginate route, or the alginic acid route. The final product is most commonly isolated as sodium alginate (Manna et al. 2021, 2025; Trica et al. 2019).

3.2 Fucoidan

Fucoidan can be extracted through two following methods. It can be extracted using a chemical method that involves treating seaweed with hot dilute hydrochloric acid to break down cell structures. After acid treatment, the mixture is centrifuged and filtered to remove small molecules and impurities. Calcium chloride is then added to selectively precipitate and remove alginate, leaving fucoidan in solution. Finally, the fucoidan is recovered through freeze-drying. Alternatively, an enzymatic method of extraction utilizes specific enzymes, such as alginate lyases and Cellic® CTec2, to degrade cell wall components under controlled conditions. This process helps release fucoidan without the harsh effects of acid. The resulting mixture undergoes centrifugation and filtration to remove residues and small molecules, and alginate is again removed with calcium chloride. The purified fucoidan is then obtained by freeze-drying (Zhao et al. 2018; Chadwick et al. 2025).

3.3 *Carrageenan*

Carrageenan extraction methods involved direct aqueous extraction from seaweed, followed by filtration and drying. This approach, while effective, was more complex and costly due to the multiple processing steps required. Refined carrageenan is typically produced by treating seaweed with hot alkali, filtering the extract, concentrating it, and then precipitating the carrageenan using alcohol or gelation techniques before drying. In contrast, the production of semi-refined carrageenan (SRC), or seaweed flour, uses a simpler and more economical approach. The seaweed is washed with alkali and water to remove soluble components and then heated in a potassium hydroxide (KOH) solution, washed again, dried, and ground. This method omits the filtration and precipitation steps, yielding a product suitable for many industrial applications (Tarman et al. 2020; Rupert et al. 2022).

3.4 *Ulvan*

Ulvan is extracted from green algae (*Ulva* spp.) through a series of steps starting with pretreatment, which includes washing, drying, and grinding the biomass. The ground material is then solubilized in water with pH adjustment and heated to extract the polysaccharide. After extraction, the solution is filtered and ulvan is precipitated using alcohol, followed by washing. Finally, the product is dried by either freeze-drying or oven drying, with optional dialysis used for higher purity (Sari-Chmayssem et al. 2019; Malvis Romero et al. 2023).

3.5 *Chitosan*

Chitosan is typically extracted from crustacean shells through a series of chemical treatments. The process begins with deproteinization using sodium hydroxide (NaOH) to remove proteins, followed by demineralization with hydrochloric acid (HCl) to eliminate calcium carbonate. An optional decolorization step may be applied to improve purity. Finally, deacetylation with concentrated NaOH converts chitin to chitosan, which is then thoroughly washed and dried (Roy et al. 2024; Kozma et al. 2022).

4 Characterization of Marine Polysaccharides

Marine polysaccharides are complex carbohydrates derived from marine organisms like algae, bacteria, and other aquatic life. They are characterized by their unique structures, including sulfation patterns, monosaccharide composition, and branching, which influence their properties and applications. These properties include immunomodulatory effects, bioactivity, and potential for use in pharmaceuticals and other industries (Liu et al. 2025).

4.1 Alginate

Alginate is a type of anionic polysaccharide primarily extracted from brown seaweeds (*Laminaria, Macrocystis, Ascophyllum*). It has diverse applications in food, pharmaceuticals, and biotechnology due to its gel-forming and biocompatible properties. Alginate is a monosaccharide composed of β-D-mannuronic acid and α-L-guluronic acid. Molecular weight ranges from 10 kDa to over 500 kDa, influencing viscosity and gel strength (Shen et al. 2021). High-molecular-weight alginates often exhibit significant viscosity. Alginate is composed of two types of uronic acid residues such as β-D-mannuronate (M) and α-L-guluronate (G). These residues are linked in a linear chain, with varying arrangements that include blocks of pure M (poly-M), pure G (poly-G), and mixtures of both (poly-MG). Carboxyl ($-COO^-$) groups contribute to water-binding and gelation property of alginate (Abka-Khajouei et al. 2022; Xie et al. 2024).

Characterizations of Alginate

Spectroscopic Techniques:

FTIR and 1H NMR spectroscopy are used to identify the functional groups and monomer composition of alginate (Manna et al. 2023).

Dynamic Light Scattering (DLS):

DLS helps determine the particle size, polydispersity index, and scattering index of alginate (Stetefeld et al. 2016).

Thermogravimetric Analysis (TGA):

TGA is used to assess the thermal stability of alginate samples (Giri et al. 2023).

Alginate Lyases:

These enzymes can degrade alginate, providing insights into its structure and properties (Chen et al. 2024).

Molecular Weight Determination:

Techniques like gel permeation chromatography (GPC) are used to determine the molecular weight of alginate (Xing et al. 2017).

4.2 Fucoidan

Fucoidan is a sulfated marine polysaccharide primarily obtained from cell walls of brown seaweed (such as *Fucus vesiculosus*, *Undaria pinnatifida*, and *Laminaria japonica*) and some marine invertebrates. Fucoidan is a monosaccharide primarily composed of L-fucose with varying amounts of galactose, mannose, glucose, and xylose. Fucoidan contains sulfate groups ($–OSO_3^-$) that contribute to its biological activities. The molecular weight of fucoidan ranges from 10 kDa to over 1000 kDa, influencing its biological function. Fucoidan typically consists of (1 → 3)-linked and (1 → 4)-linked α-L-glucopyranose units (Zhao et al. 2018).

Characterization Methods

Monosaccharide Composition Analysis: Determines the types and ratios of monosaccharides present in the fucoidan (Zayed et al. 2020).

Degree of Sulfation (DS): Measures the amount of sulfate groups attached to the fucoidan structure (Kopplin et al. 2018).

Molecular Weight Determination: Identifies the size of the fucoidan molecules (Rajauria et al. 2023).

Spectroscopic Techniques: Methods like UV-visible, FTIR, and NMR spectroscopy are used to investigate the structure and composition of fucoidan (Zhao et al. 2021).

Mass Spectrometry: This spectrometry can identify and quantify the sulfate groups and other substituents on the fucoidan structure (Li et al. 2008).

Enzymatic Analysis: Fucoidanases, enzymes that degrade fucoidan, can be used to study the structure and specificity of the molecule (Kusaykin et al. 2006).

Bioactivity Assays: Assess the biological activities of fucoidan, such as anticoagulant, anti-inflammatory, and antioxidant properties (Wang et al. 2020).

4.3 Carrageenan

Carrageenan is an anionic polysaccharide because it contains 15–40% ester sulfate (Manna and Jana 2021).

Characterization Methods

FTIR Spectroscopy:

FTIR analysis identifies functional groups and molecular vibrations, helping to differentiate carrageenan types and assess modifications like carboxymethylation (Gieroba et al. 2023).

NMR Spectroscopy:

NMR, especially 1H NMR, provides detailed structural information about the glycosidic linkages and sulfate groups, aiding in identifying the specific carrageenan type (Van de Velde et al. 2002).

High-Performance Size Exclusion Chromatography (HPSEC):

HPSEC is used to determine the molecular weight distribution of carrageenan and its degradation products (Álvarez-Viñas et al. 2023).

Liquid Chromatography-Mass Spectrometry (LC-MS):

LC-MS is employed to analyze the degradation products of carrageenan, aiding in understanding the structure-activity relationships of oligosaccharides.

Viscosity and Gel Strength:

These measurements are important for assessing the gelling properties of carrageenan, especially for food applications.

Sulfur Content:

Measuring sulfate content is crucial for differentiating between carrageenan types, as it directly influences their gelling properties.

Ash Content and Moisture Content:

These analyses help determine the purity and stability of the carrageenan sample.

Scanning Electron Microscopy (SEM):

SEM provides information about the surface morphology and microstructure of carrageenan-based materials (Zhou et al. 2022).

4.4 Ulvan

Ulvan, a sulfated polysaccharide from the green algae *Ulva*, can be characterized using various methods including spectroscopic techniques like FTIR and NMR, as well as microscopy (Wahlström et al. 2020).

Characterization Methods

FTIR Spectroscopy:

Fourier transform infrared spectroscopy reveals the presence of characteristic absorption peaks for ulvan, indicating the presence of carboxyl and sulfate groups.

NMR Spectroscopy:

Proton NMR spectroscopy and carbon-13 NMR spectroscopy are used to identify the monosaccharide composition and structural features of ulvan, such as the presence of ulvanobiuronic acid and other disaccharides.

Electron Microscopy (SEM, TEM):

Scanning electron microscopy (SEM) and transmission electron microscopy (TEM) provide information about the morphology and surface structure of ulvan.

X-Ray Diffraction (XRD):

XRD helps determine the crystalline structure of ulvan, providing insights into its organization and ordering.

Gel Permeation Chromatography (GPC):

This method is used to determine the molecular weight distribution of ulvan, which can influence its properties.

Monosaccharide Analysis:

Ulvan is hydrolyzed to determine the composition of its constituent monosaccharides, and these are identified using techniques like GC-MS.

Other Methods:

Additionally, methods like differential scanning calorimetry (DSC) and thermogravimetric analysis (TGA) can be employed to characterize the thermal properties of ulvan (Tran et al. 2023).

4.5 Chitosan

Chitosan is a biopolymer derived from chitin through deacetylation. Its characterization is essential for understanding its physicochemical property, structural property, and various functions. Various analytical techniques are used to determine its molecular weight, degree of deacetylation, crystallinity, and thermal properties (Aranaz et al. 2021; Sen et al. 2025b).

Structural Characterization

Fourier Transform Infrared Spectroscopy (FTIR): Identifies functional groups and determines the degree of deacetylation (DD) by analyzing the absorption bands of amide and hydroxyl groups

X-Ray Diffraction (XRD): Examines crystallinity and amorphous regions, which affect solubility and mechanical properties

Nuclear Magnetic Resonance (NMR): Provides insights into molecular structure and deacetylation degree

Scanning Electron Microscopy (SEM): Analyzes the surface structure and porosity of chitosan films, membranes, or powders

Transmission Electron Microscopy (TEM): Offers a detailed view of nanoscale chitosan particles

Atomic Force Microscopy (AFM): Measures surface roughness and nanomechanical properties (Rupert et al. 2022)

Elemental Analysis (CHNS): Determines the composition of carbon, hydrogen, nitrogen, and sulfur

X-Ray Photoelectron Spectroscopy (XPS): Examines surface chemical composition and bonding states

Degree of Deacetylation (DD): Can be measured using FTIR, NMR, or acid-base titration, which is crucial for solubility and biological activity (Ma et al. 2019; Pacheco et al. 2011)

5 Application of Marine Polysaccharides

The applications of several marine polysaccharide-based drug deliveries are briefly discussed here as shown in Table 1.

5.1 Alginate-Based Drug Delivery

Alginate-based drug delivery systems have been extensively investigated to improve drug entrapment, controlled release, mucoadhesion, and oral bioavailability. A wide range of alginate-based floating beads and microspheres demonstrated great promise as mucoadhesive and gastroretentive drug delivery systems. Biswas and Sahoo developed metoprolol tartrate-based alginate containing floating beads using an ionotropic gelation method. Drug entrapment efficiency and prolonged release behavior have been demonstrated to significantly enhance with tapioca starch-containing beads. HPMC-coated beads showed that the drug's release extended for up to 11 h. Using a rabbit model for pharmacokinetic analysis, floating beads demonstrated a significantly greater oral bioavailability (Biswas and Sahoo 2016). Ghumman et al. developed metformin HCl-loaded *Linum usitatissimum* mucilage and alginate-based microspheres through the ionotropic gelation method. Different polymer ratios were used to analyze the drug's in vitro release and encapsulation efficiency during 12 h. The effectiveness of drug entrapment was sustained in all formulations. Analysis was also done using FTIR and SEM. The swelling behaviors of the formulations were influenced by the pH of the buffer medium. It was reported that these microspheres have good mucoadhesivity (Ghumman et al. 2020). Demitri et al. developed an encapsulating method to separate alginate-containing solution aerosols and facilitate cross-linking with *Lactobacillus kefiri* that contains $CaCl_2$ in order to produce alginate microbeads. The SEM micrographs distinctly identify the cross-linked microbeads, which exhibit porous surfaces, from the non-cross-linked microbeads, characterized by smooth surfaces. The study demonstrated that the inclusion of $CaCl_2$ in bead formulation can arrange the alginate molecules to form a surface with a rigid shell surrounding the microbeads (Demitri et al. 2017). Bera et al. developed oil-entrapped, risperidone-loaded alginate floating beads coated in a *Sterculia* gum gel membrane and alginate via ionic gelation method. Drug release and entrapment effectiveness were investigated for up to 8 h. The drug entrapment efficiency and cumulative drug release of the optimized formulations were $83.73 \pm 0.81\%$ and $70.84 \pm 0.27\%$, respectively, after 8 h. These beads

Table 1 Applications of several marine biopolymer-based drug deliveries

Sl. no.	Delivery strategy	Polymeric composition	Special features	Drug	References
1	Floating beads	Alginate, tapioca starch, HPMC	Improved entrapment efficiency, sustained release (up to 11 h), higher oral bioavailability, floating	Metoprolol tartrate	Biswas and Sahoo (2016)
2	Microspheres	*Linum usitatissimum* mucilage, alginate	Sustainable drug entrapment efficiency, pH-dependent swelling, good mucoadhesivity	Metformin HCl	Ghumman et al. (2020)
3	Microbeads	Alginate, carboxymethylcellulose	Excellent mucoadhesivity, porous/smooth surfaces depending on cross-linking, hard shell formation with $CaCl_2$	*Lactobacillus kefiri*	Demitri et al. (2017)
4	Floating beads	Alginate, *Sterculia* gum	Slow drug release, excellent buoyancy, good ex vivo mucoadhesion, Fickian diffusion release	Risperidone	Bera et al. (2015)
5	Microspheres	Alginate, *Bletilla striata*	Enhanced mucoadhesion, prolonged GIT retention, improved swelling ability, mucin adsorption capacity, flexibility	*Bletilla striata*	Wu et al. (2020)
6	Micelles	Octenyl succinic anhydride-grafted fucoidan (OSA-fucoidan)	Sustained drug release, exceptional physicochemical stability, enhanced cellular internalization, kidney-targeting, synergistic anti-inflammatory and antioxidant effects	Curcumin	Shu et al. (2021)
7	Nanocrystals (dry powder for inhalation)	Fucoidan	Uniform cubic-shaped amorphous nanocrystals, increased surface area and saturation solubility, enhanced dissolution, improved mucus permeation, excellent flowability, high aerosol performance	Bosutinib	Kumar et al. (2024)

8	Nanocarrier	Fucoidan, PLGA	Enhanced stability and dispersibility, smaller particle sizes, sustained drug release, low cytotoxicity, improved anticancer activity	Docetaxel (DTX)	Lai et al. (2020)
9	Nanoparticles	Fucoidan, polyethylenimine (PEI) (cross-linked)	Small size (<40 nm), strong hydrogen bonding, significant drug release at acidic pH, increased cytotoxicity, effective absorption by cancer cells, targeted delivery	Cytarabine	Geethakumari et al. (2024)
10	Multi-stimuli-responsive nanoparticles	Protamine, fucoidan	pH- and enzyme-responsive drug release, improved inhibition of metastatic breast cancer cells, P-selectin-mediated endocytosis, charge conversion	Doxorubicin	Lu et al. (2017)
11	Gelled beads	Carrageenan, chitosan	Good stability, pH-dependent swelling, sustained release	Echinochrome A	Yermak et al. (2021)
12	Nanoparticles	Carboxymethylated iota-carrageenan, chitosan	Improved delivery efficiency, pH-responsive release (low in gastric, high in intestinal fluid)	Insulin	Sahoo et al. (2017)
13	Nanoparticles (polymer complex)	Chitosan, carboxymethylated iota-carrageenan	Good mucoadhesiveness, stable and biologically active in simulated GI environment, increased bioavailability, prolonged blood glucose-lowering effect	Insulin	Sahoo et al. (2019)
14	In situ mucoadhesive gel	κ-Carrageenan, hydroxypropyl cellulose	Gelling capacity, enhanced mucoadhesion, validated capacity to create gel with saliva ion interaction and biological substrate adhesion	Therapeutic use in oral mucositis and esophagitis	Vigani et al. (2019a)

(continued)

Table 1 (continued)

Sl. no.	Delivery strategy	Polymeric composition	Special features	Drug	References
15	In situ mucoadhesive gel	κ-Carrageenan, hydroxypropyl cellulose, *Hibiscus sabdariffa* hydroalcoholic extract	Pronounced elastic and mucoadhesive at 37 °C, low viscosity at 25 °C for convenient administration, biocompatibility, and proliferative, antioxidant, and anti-inflammatory effects	*Hibiscus sabdariffa* hydroalcoholic extract (for oral mucositis and esophagitis treatment)	Vigani et al. (2019b)
16	Liposomes	Ulvan	Interactions with polar groups and lipid chains in liposomal bilayer, improved stability and physicochemical characteristics	Fusidic acid	Tziveleka et al. (2022)
17	Targeted drug delivery system	Graphene oxide functionalized with chitosan, *Ulva lactuca*	D-Mannose-mediated targeting, high ulvan entrapment efficiency, biocompatibility, pH-dependent controlled drug release	For glioblastoma	Kesavan et al. (2021)
18	Dissolving microneedles (DMNs)	Ulvan	Rapid disintegration and skin penetration, effective delivery of model medications into skin tissue, good biocompatibility	FITC-BSA, R6G	Don et al. (2022)
19	Microcapsules	Chitosan, alginate, resistant starch	Spherical shape, good mucoadhesive behavior (chitosan-containing), increased size with chitosan coating	Probiotics	Ta et al. (2021)
20	Beads	Chitosan, nanomicelles (containing emodin)	No cytotoxicity of blank nanomicelles, better antitumor activity, good mucoadhesion, in vitro floating behavior, swelling, prolonged gastric retention (8 h), local drug release, inhibition of gastric cancer cells	Emodin	Chen et al. (2019)

21	Mucoadhesive films	Chitosan, ascorbic acid	Acidic pH to formulation, good mucoadhesion force, improved permeability	Ascorbic acid	Kristó et al. (2022)
22	Mucoadhesive matrix tablets	Chitosan, polycaprolactone	Sustained release, improved adhesion time (12 h), longer elimination half-life, increased bioavailability	Milnacipran HCl	Hussain et al. (2020)
23	Mucoadhesive tablets	Chitosan, Carbopol 934, HPMC K4M	Faster drug release, high swelling, good mucoadhesion	Tranexamic acid	Agarwal and Murthy (2015)
24	Nanoparticles	Chitosan, thiolated chitosan, genipin, Eudragit® L100	Slightly oblong shape, increased drug loading, limited release in upper GIT, enhanced colonic delivery, strong mucoadhesion to colon mucosa, antitumor action	α-Mangostin	Samprasit et al. (2021)

demonstrated good ex vivo mucoadhesion, delayed drug release, and outstanding buoyancy. For both coated and uncoated risperidone beads, the drug release occurred in accordance with Korsmeyer-Peppas Fickian diffusion. SEM, FTIR, and P-XRD were used to evaluate the surface morphology, drug-excipient compatibility, and drug crystallinity of optimized beads, respectively (Bẹra et al. 2015). Wu et al. developed alginate-based microspheres loaded with *Bletilla striata* to improve mucoadhesion and remain in the GIT for a long time. The prepared microspheres were distinctive and spherical in shape. Swelling capacity, mucin adsorption capacity, and retention rate on the stomach mucosa of sodium alginate matrix were all enhanced after combining with *Bletilla striata*. According to a mucoadhesion test, alginate microspheres and *Bletilla striata* stayed in rats' stomachs longer than the alginate microspheres. In the development of the gastroretentive drug delivery system, the *Bletilla striata* and alginate-based microspheres with the enhanced mucoadhesion are highly recommended as a potential drug carrier (Wu et al. 2020).

5.2 *Fucoidan-Based Drug Delivery*

Fucoidan-based systems for drug delivery have been developed in several types, such as micelles, nanocrystals, and nanoparticles, to improve therapeutic efficacy. Numerous formulations, including fucoidan/curcumin micelles, fucoidan-bosutinib nanocrystals, fucoidan-PLGA nanoparticles, and fucoidan-PEI nanoparticles, showed better cytotoxic or anti-inflammatory effects, increased cellular uptake through P-selectin interactions, and superior bioavailability when compared to conventional systems. Further improving the efficacy of cancer treatment, pH- and enzyme-triggered medication release was made possible by multi-stimuli-responsive fucoidan nanoparticles. Fucoidan provides an adaptable basis to develop drug delivery systems that are highly efficient, specific, and biocompatible. Shu et al. developed octenyl succinic anhydride-grafted fucoidan (OSA-fucoidan) incorporating curcumin-loaded micelles for the treatment of acute kidney injury. Cellular uptake studies revealed that the specific interaction between fucoidan and P-selectin, which is amplified on H_2O_2-stimulated HUVECs, significantly enhanced the internalization of OSA-fucoidan/curcumin micelles by the cells. In vivo experiments further showed that the combination of curcumin and OSA-fucoidan imparted synergistic anti-inflammatory and antioxidant effects to the micelles, thereby substantially improving their therapeutic efficacy against acute kidney injury (Shu et al. 2021). Kumar et al. formulated fucoidan-based bosutinib nanocrystals (FBNCs) into a dry powder to be used for inhalation (DPI). In vitro drug release in simulated lung fluid showed over a fivefold enhancement in dissolution compared to the coarse drug, along with significantly improved mucus permeation. Flow property and aerosolization studies demonstrated excellent flowability and high aerosol performance (ED, 70–80%; FPD, 40–60%), supporting the potential of FBNCs as an effective DPI formulation for targeted pulmonary drug delivery (Kumar et al. 2024). Fucoidan-PLGA nanoparticles (FPNs-DTX), created by Lai et al., have better stability, dispersibility, reduced size, and prolonged drug release than PLGA-DTX. There was a good encapsulation efficiency at the ideal 10:3 Fu/PLGA ratio. FPNs-DTX demonstrated more anticancer efficacy against MDA-MB-231 cells with less toxicity when drug-free, indicating its therapeutic potential, but exhibiting lesser absorption because of its hydrophilicity (Lai et al. 2020). Geethakumari et al. synthesized fucoidan nanoparticles cross-linked with polyethylenimine (PEI) to more effectively distribute cytarabine. These nanoparticles, which were smaller than 40 nm, demonstrated strong hydrogen bonding and significant drug release at acidic pH. They showed more cytotoxicity than free cytarabine and were effectively absorbed by MCF-7 breast cancer cells. Fucoidan nanoparticles improve the therapeutic efficacy of cytarabine and show potential as a targeted drug delivery strategy, following gene and apoptosis analyses that demonstrated increased cancer cell death (Geethakumari et al. 2024). Lu et al. prepared multi-stimuli-responsive nanoparticles by using the cationic polypeptide protamine and fucoidan. Using zeta potential analysis, dynamic light scattering (DLS), and circular dichroism (CD) spectroscopy, their sensitivity to pH and enzymes was assessed. In reaction to enzymatic destruction and the acidic intracellular milieu (pH 4.5–5.5) found in cancer cells, these nanoparticles released the drug doxorubicin. The protamine/fucoidan nanoparticles showed improved inhibition of the metastatic breast cancer cell line (MDA-MB-231) by P-selectin-mediated endocytosis, charge conversion, and stimuli-responsive drug release (Lu et al. 2017).

5.3 Carrageenan-Based Drug Delivery

Drug delivery strategies based on carrageenan have shown great potential for increasing mucoadhesion, stability, and controlled drug release. Carrageenan-chitosan matrix demonstrated pH-responsive behavior, sustained release, and enhanced bioavailability, particularly for insulin nanoparticles. Furthermore, κ-carrageenan-based in situ gels incorporated with polymers such hydroxypropyl cellulose showed good mucoadhesive properties and protective action for mucosal injuries such as oral mucositis and esophagitis. These results significantly indicated the adaptability of carrageenan as a potential polymer for mucosal and oral drug delivery. Yermak et al. developed gelled echinochrome A beads by combining chitosan and carrageenan. The stability of the produced mucoadhesive beads was determined to be good. Chitosan was used to shield the carrageenan beads in layers. According to the swelling study, swelling behavior is pH-dependent. The prolonged release of echinochrome A from the polymer matrix has been demonstrated by the in vitro dissolution study (Yermak et al. 2021). Sahoo et al. used a response surface approach to develop insulin-containing nanoparticles loaded with carboxymethylated iota-carrageenan and chitosan for oral administration in order to increase drug delivery efficiency. The drug release from the nanoparticles was modest in an artificially acidic gastric environment, but it was high within 12 h of the trial in a condition that resembled intestinal fluid. The drug release exhibited pH-responsive release characteristics in simulated intestinal fluid (Sahoo et al. 2017). In another study, Sahoo et al. formulated insulin nanoparticles employing chitosan-carboxymethylated iota-carrageenan, demonstrating significant stability, mucoadhesiveness, and the capacity to open tight junctions for enhanced absorption. In vivo, they exhibited around 16.1% bioavailability with sustained glucose-lowering effects for 36 h at a dosage of 100 IU/kg. The estimated human bioavailability was 44.7–46.9%, approximately three times greater than that observed in rats, underscoring significant potential for oral insulin administration (Sahoo et al. 2019). Vigani et al. developed in situ mucoadhesive gel formulations with κ-carrageenan and hydroxypropyl cellulose for therapeutic use in esophagitis and oral mucositis. In order to maintain the gelling ability, κ-carrageenan was used as a polymer, and hydroxypropyl cellulose was employed to improve the mucoadhesion properties. The pig esophagus mucosa was used for the washability investigation, which confirmed the formulations' ability to form a gel with biological substrate adherence and saliva ion interaction. The overall results indicate that these formulations are potential therapeutics for the treatment of esophagitis and oral mucositis caused by chemotherapy and radiation therapy (Vigani et al. 2019a). In another study, Vigani et al. formulated an in situ mucoadhesive gel utilizing κ-carrageenan, hydroxypropyl cellulose, and *Hibiscus sabdariffa* extract for the treatment of oral mucositis and esophagitis. These formulations exhibited significant elasticity and mucoadhesiveness at 37 °C, providing a protective role for the injured mucosa while maintaining low viscosity at 25 °C to facilitate convenient administration (Vigani et al. 2019b).

5.4 Ulvan-Based Drug Delivery

Ulvan-based drug delivery methods have demonstrated great drug entrapment, pH-responsive release, and exceptional biocompatibility in liposomal, nanocarrier, and microneedle formulations. These approaches showed promising transdermal application and antibacterial and anticancer properties, highlighting ulvan's versatility as a natural polymer with potential for tailored therapy. Tziveleka et al. developed the associated neutral and charged liposomes with ulvan, which interacts with the polar groups and lipid chains in the liposomal bilayer. The antibacterial activity of fusidic acid, a model antibacterial drug, against *Staphylococcus aureus* was assessed in a different study phase after it was encapsulated in liposomes. The developed liposomal formulations were evaluated for entrapment efficiency, stability, structure, and physicochemical characteristics (size and ζ-potential) (Tziveleka et al. 2022). Kesavan et al. prepared a D-mannose-mediated targeted drug delivery system (GO–CH–Ma) that loads *Ulva lactuca* onto graphene oxide functionalized with chitosan to treat glioblastoma. UV-Vis, FTIR, XRD, and zeta-potential were used to characterize the physicochemical properties, while surface morphology was disclosed by SEM and TEM. The efficacy of ulvan entrapment was 88%. Biocompatibility was verified using anti-inflammatory and hemolysis tests. A pH-dependent, regulated drug release was revealed by UV-Vis examination. The approach showed promise as a successful targeted treatment when tested for cytotoxicity against U87 glioblastoma cells in vitro (Kesavan et al. 2021). Don et al. prepared a two-step casting method for ulvan dissolving microneedles (DMNs). A 4% ulvan solution was used to prepare the pyramid-shaped ulvan microneedles (UMNs), which had an aspect ratio of 2.63 and an average height of 655 μm. In vitro studies demonstrated that the UMNs could quickly disintegrate and penetrate pig skin completely, losing 90.3% of their height in just 2 min after implantation. This made it possible to distribute model medications (FITC-BSA and R6G) into skin tissue effectively. As demonstrated by biocompatibility tests, UMNs were not harmful to NIH3T3 and HaCaT cells, and drug release experiments validated improved transdermal delivery (Don et al. 2022).

5.5 Chitosan-Based Mucoadhesive Drug Delivery

The potential of chitosan-based mucoadhesive systems to enhance stomach retention, prolonged release, and targeted administration of drugs and probiotics has been extensively investigated. In comparison to conventional approaches, various formulations, including chitosan-coated alginate microparticles, nanomicelles, floating beads, mucoadhesive films, and gastroretentive tablets, showed improved mucoadhesion, swelling, and bioavailability. Various researches demonstrated the versatility of chitosan by combining it with polymers such as carbopol, alginate, PCL, HPMC, or thiolated derivatives to provide better stability, controlled release, and increased therapeutic efficacy. In general, chitosan-based carriers exhibit significant potential for efficient oral administration in treatments involving the colon and stomach. Ta et al. prepared chitosan-coated alginate microparticles via electrospray for mucoadhesive probiotic delivery. A low-cost in vitro wash-off test using USB microscopy validated mucoadhesion, with chitosan showing the highest retention. The study revealed that the alginate-resistant starch microparticles (negative control) were the least retentive on a gastric mucosa, whereas pure chitosan microparticles (positive control) had the most mucoadhesive activity. These spherically shaped electrosprayed formulations ranged in size from 30 to 600 μm (60–1300 μm when coated with chitosan). *Lactobacillus plantarum* showed improved gastric protection in alginate-starch formulations, with chitosan-coated offering superior protection (Ta et al. 2021). Chen et al. formulated emodin-loaded nanomicelles coated with chitosan, which showed superior antitumor efficacy compared to emodin suspensions, although blank nanomicelles exhibited no toxicity. NFM beads (floating mucoadhesive beads) show good mucoadhesion, swelling, and floating capabilities, with an unusual mechanism for drug release. In in vivo studies of chitosan-coated emodin-loaded nanomicelles demonstrated 8 h of stomach retention and potential effectivity for gastric cancer (Chen et al. 2019). Kristó et al. formulated ascorbic acid-loaded chitosan mucoadhesive films were by solvent casting and evaluated for physical properties, mucoadhesive force, surface energy, and strength. Structural analysis was done using AFM, PALS, XRPD, and FTIR. Optimized films showed good applicability with active ingredients, where ascorbic acid acted as a permeation enhancer and biodegradable component and was effective at 2% concentration (Kristó et al. 2022). Hussain et al. formulated milnacipran HCl (MCN) incorporated chitosan (low and medium molecular weight) and polycaprolactone added gastro-retentive, mucoadhesive sustained-release tablets through a modified wet granulation method, optimized by DoE. The formulations had significant swelling and controlled-release characteristics and no drug-polymer interactions (DSC, FTIR). Stomach retention for 12 h for optimized batches (MOPT3, MOPT4) was validated by mucoadhesion experiments. Longer elimination half-life, greater bioavailability (272.20 ± 48.11%), decreased C_{max}, and increased T_{max} from 2 h (solution) to 12 ± 1.63 h (MOPT4) have been shown in in vivo studies in dogs. These results demonstrate that the method can provide MCN orally in a consistent effective manner (Hussain et al. 2020). Agarwal et al. developed tranexamic acid-incorporated chitosan-based gastroretentive mucoadhesive tablets containing carbopol 934 and hydroxypropyl methylcellulose K4M by employing wet granulation method. By varying the amounts of chitosan and hydroxypropyl methylcellulose K4M (HPMC K4M), several batches were formulated. Formulations with a higher chitosan content showed faster drug release, decreased mucoadhesion, increased erosion, and increased edema. Batches with a higher percentage of HPMC K4M, on the other hand, had delayed drug release, less erosion, better mucoadhesion, and less edema (Agarwal and Murthy 2015). Samprasit et al. formulated α-mangostin-incorporated mucoadhesive nanoparticles containing chitosan (CS), thiolated chitosan (TCS), genipin (GP) cross-linking, and Eudragit® L100 coating for colon-targeted delivery. The nanoparticles (NPs) ranged in size from 300 to 900 nm and were slightly oblong. TCS developed smaller particles, whereas GP and L100 formed larger ones. GP and L100 boosted colon delivery, limited its release in the upper GI tract, and enhanced α-mangostin loading. Compared to uncoated or CS-based NPs, TCS-based NPs containing GP and L100 exhibited greater colon mucoadhesion and antitumor action, suggesting that they could be used as controlled-release carriers of α-mangostin to the colon (Samprasit et al. 2021).

6 Evaluation of Marine Polysaccharides

Marine polysaccharides, derived from marine organisms such as algae, crustaceans, and microbes, have gained significant attention due to their diverse biological properties and applications in pharmaceuticals, biotechnology, and food industries. To ensure their efficacy, safety, and applicability, these biopolymers undergo various evaluations. The major evaluation parameters include physicochemical characterization, structural analysis, biological activity assessments, and biocompatibility testing as shown in Table 2 (Paul et al. 2022; Manna and Jana 2022).

Table 2 Major evaluation parameters of marine polysaccharides

Evaluations	Evaluation parameters	Analytical or characterization methods
Physicochemical evaluation	Molecular weight and viscosity	Assessed via gel permeation chromatography (GPC) and viscometry; influence solubility, mechanical properties, and biological activity
	Solubility and pH stability	Evaluated under varying pH and ionic conditions; critical for formulation and drug delivery
	Thermal properties	Assessed by differential scanning calorimetry (DSC) and thermogravimetric analysis (TGA); essential for processing and storage
Structural characterization	Functional group identification	Fourier transform infrared spectroscopy (FTIR)
	Sugar units and linkages	Nuclear magnetic resonance (NMR) spectroscopy
	Crystalline nature	X-ray diffraction (XRD)
	Morphology and porosity	Scanning electron microscopy (SEM) and atomic force microscopy (AFM)
Biological activity evaluation	Antimicrobial activity	Especially chitosan and fucoidan; tested via diffusion or dilution methods
	Antioxidant activity	Assessed using DPPH, ABTS, and FRAP assays; common in red algae polysaccharides
	Anti-inflammatory and immunomodulatory	Measured by cytokine analysis (e.g., TNF-α, IL-6)
	Anticancer potential	Evaluated through cytotoxicity and apoptosis assays in cancer cell lines
Pharmacokinetic and biocompatibility evaluation	In vitro cytotoxicity	Tests cell compatibility
	Hemocompatibility	Assesses safe interaction with blood
	In vivo pharmacokinetics	Studies absorption and distribution
	Mucoadhesion and gel formation	Important for controlled drug delivery (e.g., chitosan, alginate)
Toxicological evaluation	Acute toxicity	Single high-dose administration; determines LD_{50}; follows OECD guidelines
	Subacute toxicity	Repeated dosing over 14–28 days; evaluates organ function and blood parameters
	Chronic toxicity	Long-term studies (months); examines cumulative effects and carcinogenicity
	Safety profile considerations	Generally low toxicity (e.g., chitosan, alginate), but structural modifications (e.g., sulfation) or high doses may cause cytotoxicity or immune reactions

6.1 Physicochemical Evaluation

The physicochemical evaluation of marine polysaccharides involves analyzing their molecular weight, solubility, and thermal stability. Molecular weight and viscosity are measured using gel permeation chromatography (GPC) and viscometry. Molecular weight influences solubility, mechanical properties, and biological activity. Solubility and pH stability are assessed under various pH and ionic strength conditions to determine formulation compatibility, especially for drug delivery applications. Differential scanning calorimetry (DSC) and thermogravimetric analysis (TGA) are used to evaluate thermal properties, essential for processing and storage (Michael et al. 2021).

6.2 Structural Characterization

Structural characterization is essential to understand how the molecular structure of marine polysaccharides influences their properties and functions. Techniques like FTIR help identify functional groups, NMR determines sugar units and linkages, XRD reveals crystalline structure, and SEM/AFM examines surface morphology and porosity. Together, these methods provide a comprehensive picture of the polymer's structural features (Zhou et al. 2024).

6.3 Biological Activity Evaluation

Marine polysaccharides exhibit diverse biological activities. They show antimicrobial effects, especially chitosan and fucoidan, tested via diffusion or dilution methods. Their antioxidant capacity, particularly from sulfated red algae polysaccharides, is measured using DPPH, ABTS, and FRAP assays. Anti-inflammatory and immunomodulatory actions are evaluated by monitoring cytokines like TNF-α and IL-6. Additionally, they demonstrate anticancer potential through cytotoxicity and apoptosis assays in cancer cell lines (Geng et al. 2024).

6.4 Pharmacokinetic and Biocompatibility Evaluation

Pharmacokinetic and biocompatibility evaluation of marine polysaccharides involves assessing their safety and suitability for therapeutic use. This includes in vitro cytotoxicity tests to check cell compatibility, hemocompatibility tests for safe blood interactions, and in vivo studies to determine how the body absorbs and distributes them. Additionally, their mucoadhesive and gel-forming abilities, especially in alginate and chitosan, are crucial for effective controlled drug delivery systems (Yin et al. 2018).

6.5 Toxicological Evaluation

Toxicological evaluation is a critical component in assessing the safety of marine polysaccharides, especially for biomedical and pharmaceutical applications. These studies help determine potential adverse effects, dosage safety limits, and long-term implications of use (Ju et al. 2023). Marine polysaccharides typically undergo acute, subacute, and chronic toxicity studies, primarily in animal models, following OECD (Organisation for Economic Co-operation and Development) guidelines. Acute toxicity assesses the effects of a single high dose to identify immediate toxic symptoms or mortality, determining the LD_{50} (lethal dose for 50% of subjects). Subacute toxicity involves repeated administration over a short duration (14–28 days) to monitor effects on organs, blood parameters, and behavior (Rameshwar et al. 2023; Negreanu-Pirjol et al. 2022). Chronic toxicity studies extend over several months to evaluate long-term effects, carcinogenicity, or cumulative toxicity. Most marine polysaccharides such as chitosan, alginate, fucoidan, and carrageenan are biocompatible and exhibit low toxicity, making them suitable for medical use (Kumar et al. 2023; Wang et al. 2023b). However, structural modifications (e.g., sulfation, carboxymethylation) or high concentrations can potentially alter their safety profile, sometimes triggering immune responses or cytotoxicity (Zhong et al. 2019; Xu et al. 2017).

7 Conclusions

Various properties of marine polysaccharides have a wide range of applications in therapeutics and biomedical area. Specifically, alginate, carrageenan, chitosan, ulvan, and fucoidan have several therapeutic benefits including antiviral, anti-inflammatory, anticancer, antioxidant, and antitumor activity. They are also explored as additives in pharmaceutical formulations due to their suitable biological and physicochemical characteristics. More researches need to be performed to understand the degradation pathways and metabolic products of marine polysaccharides. The diverse properties of marine polysaccharides may help us to achieve alternative and sustainable resources in pharmaceutical industries.

References

Benalaya I, Alves G, Lopes J, Silva LR. A review of natural polysaccharides: sources, characteristics, properties, food, and pharmaceutical applications. International Journal of Molecular Sciences. 2024 Jan 22;25(2):1322.

Kabir SF, Rahman A, Yeasmin F, Sultana S, Masud RA, Kanak NA, Haque P. Occurrence, distribution, and structure of natural polysaccharides. In Radiation-processed polysaccharides 2022 Jan 1 (pp. 1–27). Academic Press.

Sen O, Manna S, Jana S. Marine Biopolymer-Based Gastro-Intestinal Mucoadhesive Drug Delivery Systems. In Handbook of Research in Marine Pharmaceutics 2025a Feb 3 (pp. 299–328). Apple Academic Press.

Lee YE, Kim H, Seo C, Park T, Lee KB, Yoo SY, Hong SC, Kim JT, Lee J. Marine polysaccharides: therapeutic efficacy and biomedical applications. Archives of Pharmacal Research. 2017 Sep;40:1006–20.

Chandika P, Tennakoon P, Kim TH, Kim SC, Je JY, Kim JI, Lee B, Ryu B, Kang HW, Kim HW, Kim YM. Marine biological macromolecules and chemically modified macromolecules; potential anticoagulants. Marine Drugs. 2022 Oct 21;20(10):654.

Adepu S, Ramakrishna S. Controlled drug delivery systems: current status and future directions. Molecules. 2021 Sep 29;26(19):5905.

Sun Y, Ma X, Hu H. Marine polysaccharides as a versatile biomass for the construction of nano drug delivery systems. Marine Drugs. 2021 Jun 16;19(6):345.

Geng H, Guo C, Wang W, Chen D. Marine Polysaccharides: Biological Activity and Drug Delivery. Available at SSRN 4673644.

Barbosa AI, Coutinho AJ, Costa Lima SA, Reis S. Marine polysaccharides in pharmaceutical applications: Fucoidan and chitosan as key players in the drug delivery match field. Marine Drugs. 2019 Nov 21;17(12):654.

de Jesus Raposo MF, De Morais AM, De Morais RM. Marine polysaccharides from algae with potential biomedical applications. Marine drugs. 2015 May 15;13(5):2967–3028.

Lomartire S, Gonçalves AM. Algal phycocolloids: Bioactivities and pharmaceutical applications. Marine drugs. 2023 Jun 28;21(7):384.

Ngasotter S, Xavier KM, Meitei MM, Waikhom D, Pathak J, Singh SK. Crustacean shell waste derived chitin and chitin nanomaterials for application in agriculture, food, and health–A review. Carbohydrate Polymer Technologies and Applications. 2023 Dec 1;6:100349.

Saravanan A, Kumar PS, Yuvaraj D, Jeevanantham S, Aishwaria P, Gnanasri PB, Gopinath M, Rangasamy G. A review on extraction of polysaccharides from crustacean wastes and their environmental applications. Environmental Research. 2023 Mar 15;221:115306.

Elieh-Ali-Komi D, Hamblin MR. Chitin and chitosan: production and application of versatile biomedical nanomaterials. International journal of advanced research. 2016 Mar 1;4(3):411.

Rossi N, Grosso C, Delerue-Matos C. Shrimp waste upcycling: unveiling the potential of polysaccharides, proteins, carotenoids, and fatty acids with emphasis on extraction techniques and bioactive properties. Marine Drugs. 2024 Mar 28;22(4):153.

Khan R, Shah MD, Shah L, Lee PC, Khan I. Bacterial polysaccharides—A big source for prebiotics and therapeutics. Frontiers in Nutrition. 2022 Nov 3;9:1031935.

AbdlAali RA, Al-Sahlany ST. Gellan gum as a unique microbial polysaccharide: Its characteristics, synthesis, and current application trends. Gels. 2024 Mar 6;10(3):183.

Bajaj IB, Survase SA, Saudagar PS, Singhal RS. Gellan gum: fermentative production, downstream processing and applications. Food Technology and Biotechnology. 2007 Dec 13;45(4):341–54.

Bharathi D, Lee J. Recent Advances in Marine-Derived Compounds as Potent Antibacterial and Antifungal Agents: A Comprehensive Review. Marine Drugs. 2024 Jul 29;22(8):348.

Romano G, Almeida M, Varela Coelho A, Cutignano A, Gonçalves LG, Hansen E, Khnykin D, Mass T, Ramšak A, Rocha MS, Silva TH. Biomaterials and bioactive natural products from marine invertebrates: From basic research to innovative applications. Marine Drugs. 2022 Mar 22;20(4):219.

Sasarman F, Maftei C, Campeau PM, Brunel-Guitton C, Mitchell GA, Allard P. Biosynthesis of glycosaminoglycans: associated disorders and biochemical tests. Journal of inherited metabolic disease. 2016 Mar;39(2):173–88.

Yamada S, Sugahara K, Özbek S. Evolution of glycosaminoglycans: Comparative biochemical study. Communicative & integrative biology. 2011 Mar 1;4(2):150–8.

Benhadda F, Zykwinska A, Colliec-Jouault S, Sinquin C, Thollas B, Courtois A, Fuzzati N, Toribio A, Delbarre-Ladrat C. Marine versus non-marine bacterial exopolysaccharides and their skincare applications. Marine drugs. 2023 Nov 7;21(11):582.

Netrusov AI, Liyaskina EV, Kurgaeva IV, Liyaskina AU, Yang G, Revin VV. Exopolysaccharides producing Bacteria: a review. Microorganisms. 2023 Jun 9;11(6):1541.

Wang W, Ju Y, Liu N, Shi S, Hao L. Structural characteristics of microbial exopolysaccharides in association with their biological activities: A review. Chemical and Biological Technologies in Agriculture. 2023a Nov 28;10(1):137.

Shen S, Chen X, Shen Z, Chen H. Marine polysaccharides for wound dressings application: An overview. Pharmaceutics. 2021 Oct 12;13(10):1666.

Manna S, Nath NC, Sarkar P, Karmakar S, Gupta P, Jana S, Nandi G, Sen O. Alginate-based target specific bioadhesive drug delivery systems: a review. International Journal of Polymeric Materials and Polymeric Biomaterials. 2025 Jun 24:1–27.

Trica B, Delattre C, Gros F, Ursu AV, Dobre T, Djelveh G, Michaud P, Oancea F. Extraction and characterization of alginate from an edible brown seaweed (Cystoseira barbata) harvested in the Romanian Black Sea. Marine drugs. 2019 Jul 8;17(7):405.

Manna S, Mal M, Das S, Mandal D, Bhowmik M. Ionically gelled alginates in drug delivery. Ionically Gelled Biopolysaccharide Based Systems in Drug Delivery. 2021:29–53.

Zhao Y, Zheng Y, Wang J, Ma S, Yu Y, White WL, Yang S, Yang F, Lu J. Fucoidan extracted from Undaria pinnatifida: Source for nutraceuticals/functional foods. Marine drugs. 2018 Sep 9;16 (9):321.

Chadwick M, Carvalho LG, Vanegas C, Dimartino S. A Comparative Review of Alternative Fucoidan Extraction Techniques from Seaweed. Marine Drugs. 2025 Jan 7;23(1):27.

Tarman K, Sadi U, Santoso J, Hardjito L. Carrageenan and its enzymatic extraction. Encyclopedia of Marine Biotechnology. 2020 Aug 11;1:147–59.

Rupert R, Rodrigues KF, Thien VY, Yong WT. Carrageenan from Kappaphycus alvarezii (Rhodophyta, Solieriaceae): Metabolism, structure, production, and application. Frontiers in Plant Science. 2022 May 10;13:859635.

Sari-Chmayssem N, Taha S, Mawlawi H, Guégan JP, Jeftić J, Benvegnu T. Extracted ulvans from green algae Ulva linza of Lebanese origin and amphiphilic derivatives: evaluation of their physico-chemical and rheological properties. Journal of Applied Phycology. 2019 Jun 15;31: 1931–46.

Malvis Romero A, Picado Morales JJ, Klose L, Liese A. Enzyme-assisted extraction of ulvan from the green macroalgae Ulva fenestrata. Molecules. 2023 Sep 23;28(19):6781.

Roy C, Gandhi A, Manna S, Jana S. Fabrication and evaluation of carboxymethyl guar gum-chitosan interpenetrating polymer network (IPN) nanoparticles for controlled drug delivery. Medicine in Novel Technology and Devices. 2024 Jun 1;22:100300.

Kozma M, Acharya B, Bissessur R. Chitin, chitosan, and nanochitin: extraction, synthesis, and applications. Polymers. 2022 Sep 23;14(19):3989.

Liu B, Zhang L, Zhu T, Liu Y, Chu J, Chen N. Structural characterization of polysaccharides of marine origin: A review. International Journal of Biological Macromolecules. 2025 May 30: 144797.

Abka-Khajouei R, Tounsi L, Shahabi N, Patel AK, Abdelkafi S, Michaud P. Structures, properties and applications of alginates. Marine drugs. 2022 May 29;20(6):364.

Xie F, Gao C, Avérous L. Alginate-based materials: Enhancing properties through multiphase formulation design and processing innovation. Materials Science and Engineering: R: Reports. 2024 Jun 1;159:100799.

Manna S, Gupta P, Nandi G, Jana S. Recent update on alginate based promising transdermal drug delivery systems. Journal of Biomaterials science, Polymer edition. 2023 Nov 2;34(16): 2291–318.

Stetefeld J, McKenna SA, Patel TR. Dynamic light scattering: a practical guide and applications in biomedical sciences. Biophysical reviews. 2016 Dec;8:409–27.

Giri S, Markandeywar TS, Irfan Z, Manna S. Gellan gum and sodium alginate in-situ gel of monocaprin for effective corneal permeation. Food Hydrocolloids for Health. 2023 Dec 15;4: 100156.

Chen C, Li X, Lu C, Zhou X, Chen L, Qiu C, Jin Z, Long J. Advances in alginate lyases and the potential application of enzymatic prepared alginate oligosaccharides: A mini review. International Journal of Biological Macromolecules. 2024 Mar 1;260:129506.

Xing H, Lu M, Xian L, Zhang J, Yang T, Yang L, Ding P. Molecular weight determination of a newly synthesized guanidinylateddisulfide-containing poly(amido amine) by gel permeation chromatography. Asian journal of pharmaceutical sciences. 2017 May 1;12(3):292–8.

Zayed A, El-Aasr M, Ibrahim AR, Ulber R. Fucoidan characterization: Determination of purity and physicochemical and chemical properties. Marine Drugs. 2020 Nov 19;18(11):571.

Kopplin G, Rokstad AM, Mélida H, Bulone V, Skjåk-Bræk G, Aachmann FL. Structural characterization of fucoidan from Laminaria hyperborea: Assessment of coagulation and inflammatory properties and their structure–function relationship. ACS Applied Bio Materials. 2018 Nov 15;1 (6):1880–92.

Rajauria G, Ravindran R, Garcia-Vaquero M, Rai DK, Sweeney T, O'Doherty J. Purification and molecular characterization of fucoidan isolated from Ascophyllum nodosum brown seaweed grown in Ireland. Marine drugs. 2023 May 21;21(5):315.

Zhao M, Garcia-Vaquero M, Przyborska J, Sivagnanam SP, Tiwari B. The development of analytical methods for the purity determination of fucoidan extracted from brown seaweed species. International Journal of Biological Macromolecules. 2021 Mar 15;173:90–8.

Li B, Lu F, Wei X, Zhao R. Fucoidan: structure and bioactivity. Molecules. 2008 Aug 12;13(8): 1671–95.

Kusaykin MI, Chizhov AO, Grachev AA, Alekseeva SA, Bakunina IY, Nedashkovskaya OI, Sova VV, Zvyagintseva TN. A comparative study of specificity of fucoidanases from marine microorganisms and invertebrates. Journal of Applied Phycology. 2006 Oct;18:369–73.

Wang SH, Huang CY, Chen CY, Chang CC, Huang CY, Dong CD, Chang JS. Structure and biological activity analysis of fucoidan isolated from Sargassum siliquosum. ACS omega. 2020 Dec 12;5(50):32447–55.

Manna S, Jana S. Carrageenan-based nanomaterials in drug delivery applications. In Biopolymer-Based Nanomaterials in Drug Delivery and Biomedical Applications 2021 Jan 1 (pp. 365–382). Academic Press.

Gieroba B, Kalisz G, Krysa M, Khalavka M, Przekora A. Application of vibrational spectroscopic techniques in the study of the natural polysaccharides and their cross-linking process. International journal of molecular sciences. 2023 Jan 30;24(3):2630.

Van de Velde F, Knutsen SH, Usov AI, Rollema HS, Cerezo AS. 1H and 13C high resolution NMR spectroscopy of carrageenans: application in research and industry. Trends in Food Science & Technology. 2002 Mar 1;13(3):73–92.

Álvarez-Viñas M, Rivas S, Torres MD, Domínguez H. Microwave-assisted extraction of carrageenan from Sarcopeltis skottsbergii. Marine Drugs. 2023 Jan 25;21(2):83.

Zhou F, Wang D, Zhang J, Li J, Lai D, Lin S, Hu J. Preparation and characterization of biodegradable κ-carrageenan based anti-bacterial film functionalized with Wells-Dawson polyoxometalate. Foods. 2022 Feb 18;11(4):586.

Wahlström N, Nylander F, Malmhäll-Bah E, Sjövold K, Edlund U, Westman G, Albers E. Composition and structure of cell wall ulvans recovered from Ulva spp. along the Swedish west coast. Carbohydrate polymers. 2020 Apr 1;233:115852.

Tran VH, Mikkelsen MD, Truong HB, Vo HN, Pham TD, Cao HT, Nguyen TT, Meyer AS, Thanh TT, Van TT. Structural characterization and cytotoxic activity evaluation of ulvan polysaccharides extracted from the green algae Ulva papenfussii. Marine Drugs. 2023 Oct 25;21(11):556.

Aranaz I, Alcántara AR, Civera MC, Arias C, Elorza B, Heras Caballero A, Acosta N. Chitosan: An overview of its properties and applications. Polymers. 2021 Sep 24;13(19):3256.

Sen O, Jana S, Nandi G, Manna S. Recent progress in chitosan-based nanofibers as potential drug carriers in cancer therapy. International Journal of Polymeric Materials and Polymeric Biomaterials. 2025b Apr 13;74(6):555–73.

Ma X, Qiao C, Wang X, Yao J, Xu J. Structural characterization and properties of polyols plasticized chitosan films. International journal of biological macromolecules. 2019 Aug 15;135:240–5.

Pacheco N, Garnica-Gonzalez M, Gimeno M, Bárzana E, Trombotto S, David L, Shirai K. Structural characterization of chitin and chitosan obtained by biological and chemical methods. Biomacromolecules. 2011 Sep 12;12(9):3285–90.

Biswas, N.; Sahoo, R. K. Tapioca starch blended alginate mucoadhesive-floating beads for intragastric delivery of metoprolol tartrate. *Int j biolmacromol.***2016**, 83, 61–70.

Ghumman, S. A.; Noreen, S.; tul Muntaha, S. Linum usitatissimum seed mucilage-alginate mucoadhesive microspheres of metformin HCl: Fabrication, characterization and evaluation. *Int. J. Biol. Macromol.* **2020**, 155, 358–368.

Demitri, C.; Lamanna, L.; De Benedetto, E.; Damiano, F.; Cappello, M. S.; Siculella, L.; Sannino, A. Encapsulation of Lactobacillus kefiri in alginate microbeads using a double novel aerosol technique. *Mater SciEng C Mater Biol Appl.* **2017**, 77, 548–555.

Bera, H.; Kandukuri, S. G.; Nayak, A. K.; Boddupalli, S. Alginate-sterculia gum gel-coated oil-entrapped alginate beads for gastroretentive risperidone delivery. *Carbohydr. Polym.***2015**, 120, 74–84.

Wu, Y.; Zhang, W.; Huang, J.; Luo, Z.; Li, J.; Wang, L.; Di, L. Mucoadhesive improvement of alginate microspheres as potential gastroretentive delivery carrier by blending with Bletilla striata polysaccharide. *Int. J. Biol. Macromol.***2020**, 156, 1191–1201.

Shu G, Lu C, Wang Z, Du Y, Xu X, Xu M, Zhao Z, Chen M, Dai Y, Weng Q, Fang S, Fan K, Liu D, Du Y, Ji J. Fucoidan-based micelles as P-selectin targeted carriers for synergistic treatment of acute kidney injury. Nanomedicine. 2021 Feb;32:102342. https://doi.org/10.1016/j.nano.2020.102342. Epub 2020 Nov 27. PMID: 33253922.

Kumar M, Jha A, Bharti K, Mishra B. Fucoidan-based bosutinib nanocrystals for pulmonary drug delivery: Solid state characterization and in-vitro assessment. Chemical Physics Impact. 2024 Jun 1;8:100644.

Lai YH, Chiang CS, Hsu CH, Cheng HW, Chen SY. Development and Characterization of a Fucoidan-Based Drug Delivery System by Using Hydrophilic Anticancer Polysaccharides to Simultaneously Deliver Hydrophobic Anticancer Drugs. Biomolecules. 2020 Jun 28;10(7):970. https://doi.org/10.3390/biom10070970. PMID: 32605162; PMCID: PMC7408464.

Geethakumari D, Veettil SP, Chandrika SK, Sathyabhama AB, Joseph R, Padmini SS, Somasekharan JV, Puthiyedathu ST. Development of polyethyleneimine cross-linked fucoidan nanoparticles as delivery systems for improved anticancer efficiency of cytarabine in breast adenocarcinoma cell lines. RSC Pharmaceutics. 2024;1(2):305–16.

Lu KY, Li R, Hsu CH, Lin CW, Chou SC, Tsai ML, Mi FL. Development of a new type of multifunctional fucoidan-based nanoparticles for anticancer drug delivery. Carbohydrate polymers. 2017 Jun 1;165:410–20.

Yermak, I. M.; Gorbach, V. I.; Karnakov, I. A.; Davydova, V. N.; Pimenova, E. A.; Chistyulin, D. A.; Isakov, V. V.; Glazunov, V. P. Carrageenan gel beads for echinochrome inclusion: Influence of structural features of carrageenan. *Carbohydr. Polym.***2021**, 272, 118479.

Sahoo, P.; Leong, K. H.; Nyamathulla, S.; Onuki, Y.; Takayama, K.; Chung, L. Y. Optimization of pH-responsive carboxymethylated iota-carrageenan/chitosan nanoparticles for oral insulin delivery using response surface methodology. *React FunctPolym.***2017**, 119, 145–155.

Sahoo, P.; Leong, K. H.; Nyamathulla, S.; Onuki, Y.; Takayama, K.; Chung, L. Y. Chitosan complexed carboxymethylated iota-carrageenan oral insulin particles: Stability, permeability and in vivo evaluation. *Mater. Today Commun.* **2019**, 20, 100557.

Vigani, B.; Faccendini, A.; Rossi, S.; Sandri, G.; Bonferoni, M. C.; Gentile, M.; Ferrari, F. Development of a Mucoadhesive and In Situ Gelling Formulation Based on κ-Carrageenan for Application on Oral Mucosa and Esophagus Walls. I. A Functional In Vitro Characterization. *Mar. Drugs* **2019a**, 17, 112.

Vigani, B.; Rossi, S.; Gentile, M.; Sandri, G.; Bonferoni, M. C.; Cavalloro, V.; Martino, E.; Collina, S.; Ferrari, F. Development of a Mucoadhesive and an in Situ Gelling Formulation Based on κ-Carrageenan for Application on Oral Mucosa and Esophagus Walls. II. Loading of a Bioactive Hydroalcoholic Extract. *Mar Drugs* **2019b**, 17, 153.

Tziveleka LA, Pippa N, Ioannou E, Demetzos C, Roussis V. Development of ulvan-containing liposomes as antibacterial drug delivery platforms. Journal of Functional Biomaterials. 2022 Oct 13;13(4):186.

Kesavan S, Meena KS, Sharmili SA, Govindarajan M, Alharbi NS, Kadaikunnan S, Khaled JM, Alobaidi AS, Alanzi KF, Vaseeharan B. Ulvan loaded graphene oxide nanoparticle fabricated with chitosan and d-mannose for targeted anticancer drug delivery. Journal of Drug Delivery Science and Technology. 2021 Oct 1;65:102760.

Don TM, Chen M, Lee IC, Huang YC. Preparation and characterization of fast dissolving ulvan microneedles for transdermal drug delivery system. International Journal of Biological Macromolecules. 2022 May 15;207:90-9.

Ta LP, Bujna E, Kun S, Charalampopoulos D, Khutoryanskiy VV. Electrosprayed mucoadhesive alginate-chitosan microcapsules for gastrointestinal delivery of probiotics. International Journal of Pharmaceutics. 2021 Mar 15;597:120342.

Chen, N.; Li, Q.; Li, J.; Ren, Y.; Wu, G.; Liu, Y.; Shi, Y. Development and evaluation of a new gastroretentive drug delivery system: Nanomicelles-loaded floating mucoadhesive beads. *J Drug Deliv Sci Technol.* **2019**, 51, 485–492.

Kristó, K.; Módra, S.; Hornok, V.; Süvegh, K.; Ludasi, K.; Aigner, Z.; Kelemen, A.; Sovány, T.; Pintye-Hódi, K.; Regdon, G Jr. Investigation of Surface Properties and Free Volumes of Chitosan-Based Buccal Mucoadhesive Drug Delivery Films Containing Ascorbic Acid. *Pharmaceutics* **2022**, 14, 345.

Hussain T, Ijaz M, Shamim R, Hussain K, Abbas N, Hussain A, Griessinger JA, Bukhari NI. In Vivo Evaluation of a Novel Chitosan-Polycaprolactone Based Mucoadhesive Gastro-Retentive Sustained Release Drug Delivery System for Milnacipran HCl. AAPS PharmSciTech. **2020** Jan 7;21(2):58. https://doi.org/10.1208/s12249-019-1606-6. PMID: 31912249.

Agarwal, S.; Murthy, R. S. Effect of Different Polymer Concentration on Drug Release Rate and Physicochemical Properties of Mucoadhesive Gastroretentive Tablets. *Indian J Pharm Sci.* **2015**, 77, 705–714.

Samprasit, W.; Opanasopit, P.; Chamsai, B. Mucoadhesive chitosan and thiolated chitosan nanoparticles containing alpha mangostin for possible Colon-targeted delivery. *Pharm Dev Technol.* **2021**, 26, 362–372.

Paul R, Kabiraj S, Manna S, Jana S. Marine polysaccharides in pharmaceutical applications. In Marine Biochemistry **2022** Oct 12 (pp. 111–136). CRC Press.

Manna S, Jana S. Marine polysaccharides in tailor-made drug delivery. Current pharmaceutical design. **2022** Apr 1;28(13):1046–66.

Michael OS, Adetunji CO, Ayeni AE, Akram M, Inamuddin, Adetunji JB, Olaniyan M, Muhibi MA. Marine polysaccharides: Properties and applications. Polysaccharides: Properties and Applications. **2021** May 17:423–39.

Zhou QL, Wang Z, Chen WT, Liu XF, Cheong KL, Zou YX, Zhong SY, Li R. The structural characteristics, biological activities and mechanisms of bioactive brown seaweed polysaccharides: A review. Journal of Functional Foods. **2024** Aug 1;119:106303.

Geng H, Chen M, Guo C, Wang W, Chen D. Marine polysaccharides: Biological activities and applications in drug delivery systems. Carbohydrate research. **2024** Apr 1;538:109071.

Yin J, Wang W, Xu X, Li H, Cong M, Zhao X, Wang C. Preparation, characterization and pharmacokinetics of extended-release tablets of marine polysaccharide drug. Journal of Drug Delivery Science and Technology. **2018** Feb 1;43:353–61.

Ju H, Yu C, Liu W, Li HH, Fu Z, Wu YC, Gong PX, Li HJ. Polysaccharides from marine resources exhibit great potential in the treatment of tumor: A review. Carbohydrate Polymer Technologies and Applications. **2023** Jun 1;5:100308.

Rameshwar GS, Venkatrao PU, Vithalrao NA, Pramodrao AM. OECD Guidelines for Acute Oral Toxicity Studies: An Overview. Int. J. Res. Ayurveda Pharm. **2023**;14:137–40.

Negreanu-Pirjol BS, Negreanu-Pirjol T, Popoviciu DR, Anton RE, Prelipcean AM. Marine bioactive compounds derived from macroalgae as new potential players in drug delivery systems: a review. Pharmaceutics. **2022** Aug 25;14(9):1781.

Kumar M, Kumar D, Garg Y, Mahmood S, Chopra S, Bhatia A. Marine-derived polysaccharides and their therapeutic potential in wound healing application-A review. International Journal of Biological Macromolecules. **2023** Dec 31;253:127331.

Wang Y, Chen L, Wang Y, Wang X, Qian D, Yan J, Sun Z, Cui P, Yu L, Wu J, He Z. Marine biomaterials in biomedical nano/micro-systems. Journal of Nanobiotechnology. **2023b** Nov 5;21(1):408.

Zhong Q, Wei B, Wang S, Ke S, Chen J, Zhang H, Wang H. The antioxidant activity of polysaccharides derived from marine organisms: An overview. Marine drugs. **2019** Nov 29;17(12): 674.

Xu SY, Huang X, Cheong KL. Recent advances in marine algae polysaccharides: Isolation, structure, and activities. Marine Drugs. **2017** Dec 13;15(12):388.

Part I
Drug Delivery

Plant-Derived Marine Polysaccharides in Oral Drug Delivery

Vipul D. Prajapati, Aditya Shrivstav, Juhini Valand, Riddhi Dalal, Kavyasri Penemecha, and Shivani Gandhi

Abstract Marine plant polysaccharides (MPPs), which are purified from the major marine plants, namely, seaweeds (algae) and kelp, have gained significant attention owing to their multifunctional uses in biomedical and pharmaceutical applications through various routes. The major MPPs are alginate, carrageenans, agar, fucoidan, laminarin, and ulvan that have extensively used for oral delivery systems (ODSs) to impart needful functionalities in development of therapeutic dosage forms via their flexible unique features such as ease of tolerability, biodegradability, gelation ability, and responsiveness to environmental stimuli. Their structural heterogeneity allows them to exhibit antimicrobial, antioxidant, anti-inflammatory, and anticancer types of therapeutic activities. Such characteristics are widely explored in marine polysaccharides for conventional and novel DSs for various molecules via oral route. Furthermore, they find themselves to be key players in emerging platforms such as hydrogels, nanoparticles, microspheres, and implants that are enhancing controlled release of drugs, tissue healing, and target disease specificity. Hopeful opportunities notwithstanding, complications remain to check standardization, structural variety, stability, and approval by regulating bodies. Further research and development of extraction methods, functional amendment, and sea biology are indispensable in maximizing their potential for drug delivery. This chapter comprehensively addresses about the effective scenario of marine plant-derived polysaccharides for various flexible functionalities in oral delivery of various molecules as per rationale of the required dosage form preparations.

Keywords Marine plant polysaccharides · Oral drug delivery · Alginate · Carrageenan · Fucoidan · Nanoparticles · Hydrogels · Pharmaceutical applications

---

V. D. Prajapati (✉) · A. Shrivstav · J. Valand · R. Dalal · K. Penemecha
Department of Pharmaceutics, S.S.R. College of Pharmacy (Permanently Affiliated to Savitribai Phule Pune University), Sayli, Silvassa, Union Territory of Dadra Nagar Haveli & Daman Diu, India

S. Gandhi
Department of Pharmaceutics, Faculty of Pharmacy, The Maharaja Sayajirao University of Baroda, Vadodara, Gujarat, India

S. Jana et al. (eds.), *Multifunctional Marine Polysaccharides*,
https://doi.org/10.1007/978-981-95-4126-3_2

Abbreviations

MPPs	Marine plant polysaccharides
FDA	Food and Drug Administration
EMA	European Medicines Agency
PMDA	Pharmaceuticals and Medical Devices Agency
CDSCO	Central Drugs Standard Control Organization
TGA	Therapeutic Goods Administration
DDS	Drug delivery system

1 Introduction

The pharmaceutical and drug formulation industries are increasingly utilizing natural materials to develop safer and more effective delivery systems (DSs) for medications. Polysaccharides are a primary natural biomaterial of interest because of their versatility, biocompatibility, and diversity in structure (Benalaya et al. 2024). These complex carbohydrates are sourced from plant, animal, or marine sources, are characterized by their extended sugar units, and have unique functional characteristics such as gelling, swelling, or mucoadhesion. Within the last few years, marine polysaccharides, including those that could potentially be produced or mimicked through the use of plant-based systems, have emerging possibilities for use as components in oral drug delivery formulations. Their natural abundance and versatility in terms of physicochemical properties make them excellent candidates for improving the stability, availability, and controlled release properties of medicines (Prasher et al. 2021).

The ability of these natural polymers to overcome several of the challenges via oral passage including poor solubility, enzymatic digestion, and discrepancy in absorption. These also make them viable candidates for the evolution of next-generation oral pharmaceuticals (Homayun et al. 2019).

1.1 Summary of Polysaccharides in Pharmaceutical Delivery

Polysaccharides are the long chain padded molecules formed by the repeating units of monosaccharides, which are joined via glycosidic linkages. They are, in general, classified as either homopolysaccharides (a single type of sugar) or heteropolysaccharides (multiple types of sugars) (Chaudhary et al. 2022). They are in general utilized in the creation of flexible delivery of various molecules mostly via oral route. The varieties of marine plant polysaccharides (MPPs), in general, are nontoxic, easily tolerable, biologically degradable, and capable to form desired gels/films making them suitable for tailored release formulations. They can serve a multitude of functions in suitable types of platforms of deliveries of compatible molecules. They may function as active ingredient's carriers, entrapping/matrix/coating agent for varieties of active pharmaceutical ingredients (APIs) from premature degradation. Any polysaccharides can change the incorporated drug release rates, extending the duration time of therapeutic effect while reducing frequency of doses. Many polysaccharides contain structural functional groups lending themselves to chemical modification, opening avenues for producing targeted drug delivery systems or stimulus-responsive drug delivery systems (Vieira et al. 2022).

Since decades, marine polysaccharide materials (MPPs), which include alginates, agar, agarose, carrageenan, and fucoidan, are primarily derived from algae and various seaweeds. Researchers are active in exploring some of the potential plant-based, sustainable, or scalable alternatives by making the so-called marine-like polysaccharides or by developing structural analogues. Their pharmaceutical efficacy is currently being realized as they compete with some of the characteristics presented by synthetic polymers, thus representing a natural alternative to creating innovation in new oral drug delivery systems (ODDSs) (Teixeira et al. 2022).

1.2 Importance of ODDSs

ODD is the most popular delivery method due primarily to its non-invasive characteristics, ease of administration, and cost-effectiveness. Patients of all ages highly accept ODD, which greatly enhances compliance with therapeutic regimens. From a manufacturing perspective, oral formulations, namely, powders, tablets, or capsules, are less expensive to manufacture, ship, and store than injectable delivery methods or transdermal deliveries. While there are advantages to ODDSs, there are few physiological and physicochemical barriers to ODD. Many drugs have poor aqueous solubility, poor stability in the acidic gastric environment, or poor permeability through intestinal membranes. Because of hepatic metabolism, bioavailability may also be very limited for certain compounds. These limitations highlight the need for the generation of more advanced DDSs using suitable MPPs that can protect the active component, increase absorption, and provide tailored release (Maheshwari et al. 2024).

Polysaccharides from marine plants may be able to meet these challenges. These materials are hydrophilic enough to solubilize the drug, and they have gel-forming and mucoadhesive properties that can help with localization at the area of absorption and with the tailor-made delivery of the compatible molecules. Also, many polysaccharides are resistant to enzymatic degradation in the upper GIT as the requirement for colonic DDSs (Luo and Wang 2014).

1.3 Potential of Plant-Derived Marine Polysaccharides

The study of plant-derived marine polysaccharides presents a reflection of two integrated concepts in the pharmaceutical sciences as the transition to natural, sustainable excipients and a desire for better ODDSs. Marine polysaccharides tend to come from marine animals, although there are efforts to derive similar structures from plants. This may entail extracting from species of marine plant analogues like algae raised in controlled environments or culturing marine-type polysaccharides using genetic engineered plant systems. The plant counterparts offer a number of advantages (Beneke et al. 2009). Most importantly, they lessen reliance on wild marine biomass, positively impacting conservation and scalability, plus they may offer better biosynthetic pathways that can be possibly more regulated and standardized, thereby reducing the variability seen with naturally derived marine polysaccharides (Jansen et al. 2021).

These polysaccharides also have very good potential in oral DD. They may entrap drugs within matrices that protect against gastric degradation and exhibit either sustained or target release in the gut or colonic region (Baranov et al. 2021). Additionally, their mucoadhesive properties may enhance the absorption of API by prolonging the residence duration in the GIT. Newer technologies have also been developed to incorporate these polysaccharides into nanoparticles, films, and hydrogels, which can provide novel DD forms, such as buccal strips, rapid dissolve tablets, and colon-targeted microparticles. Some plant-based marine polysaccharides exhibit biological activity (e.g. antioxidant, antibacterial, or immunomodulatory potential), which can also improve or augment the effect of the drug. This ability for dual functionality will also make these polysaccharides unique options for nutraceuticals and functional food use, in addition to conventional drug use (Di Sotto et al. 2020).

The possibilities of plant-based marine polysaccharides for oral administration of medications are exciting and developing. With further improvements in the characterization, functionalization, and formulation of these natural polymers, they are expected to advance the next wave of drug delivery technologies (Sekinat Olayem et al. 2024).

2 Origins of Marine Polysaccharides Derived from Plants

Numerous physiologically active materials can be found in marine environments, including polysaccharides from various algae, which play versatile role in the pharmaceutical industry (Laurienzo 2010). These biopolymers have been attractive to researchers for their structural complexity and nature-derived biocompatibility, and they are also obtainable from sustainable plant-based marine resources, namely, algae. Algae do not come from terrestrial plants, but they provide a form of plant-based marine resource, some of which can be sustainably cultivated and/or harvested. MPPs generated from the green-, red-, and brown-coloured algae have different chemical compositions and physicochemical properties and, therefore, have a number of functions for drug delivery purposes (Nickerson and Paulson 2004a).

2.1 Marine Algae: Chlorophyta, Rhodophyta, *and* Phaeophyta

Marine algae are broadly categorized into three major groups such as Chlorophyta, Rhodophyta, and Phaeophytaaccording to the differences in the composition of pigments, cellular development, and biochemical composition. These groups have been recognized for their production of specific polysaccharides with potential as carriers to deliver oral medicines (Lee et al. 2017).

2.1.1 *Chlorophyta* (Green Algae)

Green algae, such as *Ulva* and *Enteromorpha*, are a source of sulfated polysaccharides known as ulvan containing large amount of rhamnose, glucuronic acid, iduronic acid, and xylose. It exhibits antioxidant, immunomodulatory, and anti-inflammatory properties. It is highly hydrophilic, which, coupled with its ability to form highly viscous solutions, makes ulvan a compelling option for oral formulations that support gut health or that produce a controlled release of a drug (Drew 1955).

2.1.2 *Rhodophyta* (Red Algae)

Red algae include *Chondrus crispus*, *Gracilaria*, and *Gigartina* and produce agar and carrageenan. Agar is mainly agarose and agaropectin—it is useful because it has thermoreversible gelation ability, which is useful in controlled release therapeutic systems. Carrageenan appears in several forms (*kappa*, *iota*, *lambda*)—they differ from one another in sulfation and gelling. *Kappa*-carrageenan produces strong, inflexible gels and is commonly used in matrix tablets for sustained release (Alves et al. 2013).

2.1.3 *Phaeophyta*

Brown algae include *Laminaria*, *Fucus*, and *Ascophyllum*—they produce polysaccharides such as alginic acid and fucoidan. Alginate/alginic acid is a linear copolymer of β-D-mannuronic acid and α-L-guluronic acid. Alginate forms hydrogels via ionic transformation with a divalent cation (e.g. Ca^{+2} or Ba^{+2}), which makes it a unique auxiliary for drug as the hydrogel entrapments. Fucoidan, a sulfated polysaccharide, is obtained from brown algae that has significant bioactivities especially as anticoagulant, antiviral, and anti-inflammatory actions and is being researched for its delivery mechanisms and therapeutic applications (Gabrielson et al. 1986).

2.2 *Types of Marine Plants*

In addition to supplying food and shelter, naturally available materials' relevant formulations have long been used in traditional medicated formulation to find cures for illnesses and to prolong and enhance human life. Since the oceans cover most of the planet's surface, a wide variety of species, most of which are unnamed, are found in its huge ecosystem. In order to ease of learning the diversity of sea life, many scientists calculated that there are between 0.7 and 1.0 million aqua species, of which about 226,000 are eukaryotic (Kraan 2012).

With its vast ecology and highly varied biodiversity, the marine living things are thought to be the significant source of naturally occurring biologically active components. Saltwater makes up the majority of the oceans, covering over 71% of the Earth's surface. The growth of such system containing the broad range of biotechnological and therapeutic agents benefits from sea reconnaissance, which is the primary source of various natural components (Hahn et al. 2012). Marine species are the significant source of structurally and physiologically active secondary metabolites because marine biomaterials show a higher degree of biological activity and chemical innovation than the biologically active components obtained from terrestrial life forms (Hanisak 1998). At least eight related medications have been licenced by the USFDA and the EMA as a result of the significant surge in the development of marine-based medications over the last few years (Harding et al. 2017a). Marine algae have high biological diversity and are simple in extraction and purification to get different marinechemicals, which attracts their use in various scientific fields. Some of the marine plant species are phytoplankton, pigmented algae, kelp, and seaweeds.

2.2.1 Phytoplankton

Microalgae, also known as phytoplankton, are living plants that need sunlight to exist and grow and contain suitable proportion of chlorophyll. Their buoyancy property makes them to float in the ocean's upper regions, where natural light may reach the surface water (Imeson 2009). Small, unicellular photosynthetic organisms that live suspended in water make up the majority of phytoplankton. They are the main producers in the water and the base of the food chain because, like land plants, they take carbon dioxide, use light energy to make carbohydrates, and release oxygen. Phytoplankton thrives at or near the ocean's surface whenever sunlight can penetrate the water and fuel photosynthesis. Phytoplankton is a broad term that includes a variety of creatures. The larger group includes single-celled algae and sophisticated eukaryotic cells known as protists, which share many characteristics with protozoans. These minuscule cells, as little as a micron and thus invisible in marine waters containing hundreds of thousands of cells per tablespoon, were deemed untraceable by any type of net. It wasn't until the 1970s that innovative technology made them visible. Scientists have since discovered that these bacteria account for half of the ocean's primary productivity and are the most abundant species in the water (Jacob et al. 2018a).

2.2.2 Algae

The word "algae" is the plural of the Latin word "alga", which signifies seaweed, and dates back to the sixteenth century. The word is thought to have originated from the Latin alliga, meaning "binding" or "entwining". The taxonomic definition of "algae" is unclear.

The earliest photosynthetic creature, a coccoid cyanobacterium, is estimated to have been consumed by a heterotrophic eukaryote some 1.6 billion years ago. The cyanobacterium was preserved rather than digested. The evolution of the cyanobacterium resulted in a primary alga, or unicellular red or green algae, by reducing the size of its genome significantly, transferring many of its gene activities to and from the host nucleus, and losing its cell wall. When another eukaryote ate a primary red or green alga, it is believed that subsequent endosymbiotic processes took place, producing new plastid-based organelles and structures as well as extra membrane layers. Green algae eventually gave rise to land plants, but red, green, and brown algae went on to develop unique plastids, structures, and functions that made it possible for water to exist (Kadam et al. 2015; Keeling 2004).

There are currently 144,393 species and infraspecific names for algae and marine plants in AlgaBase, a database of data on various types of algae (Kidgell et al. 2019a). There are 38 groups of marine algae and 11 phyla—*Cyanophyta*, *Glaucophyta*, *Rhodophyta*, *Cryptophyta*, *Dinophyta*, *Haptophyta*, *Ochrophyta*, *Euglenophyta*, *Chlorarachniophyta*, *Chlorophyta*, and *Charophyta*—as well.

Green Algae

With their wide range of shapes, sizes, and behaviours, green algae are the most varied group of photoautotrophic Protoctista in the biosphere. The significance of green algae and rainforests as the Earth's primary producers is comparable. From a taxonomical standpoint, these species can be classified as a paraphyletic group that is closely related to terrestrial plants. They are a diverse cluster of organisms belonging to the Archaeplastida's green lineage (Chloroplastida). These algae, which have existed for more than a billion years, now occupy the majority of the planet's photic environment and play important roles in regulating atmospheric dynamics, biogeochemistry, and food chains. They are the important fundamental organisms in freshwater, marine, and terrestrial environments. They can produce eye-catching blooms, are frequently found in aquatic biofilms, and can form special partnerships with other invertebrate organisms or fungi, such as lichens (Kong et al. 2010).

Red Algae

With more than 5000 species, red algae represent the earliest division of lower plants. Macrophytes, or marine multicellular organisms, make up the majority of them. They differ from all other plants due to the polysaccharide composition of their intercellular matrix and cell walls. Two polysaccharides, agars and carrageenan, are produced locally from algae and are commonly used as potent gel-forming agent and stabilizer. The majority of them contain special sulfated galactan (Martins et al. 2014; McHugh 2003). Red algae (*Rhodophyta*) are a large category of aquatic photoautotrophic plants that range from unicellular to multicellular.

Red algae species produce valuable commercial goods such as phycocolloids (gel-forming agent, thickener, emulsifier, binder, stabilizer, clarifier, and protector), soil excipients, fertilizers, animal feed, medicines, nutraceuticals, cosmeceuticals, and cosmetics (Misiurova et al. 2014; Molinski et al. 2009).

Brown Algae

They are most typically found as seaweeds in the cooler waters of the Northern Hemisphere. Brown algae are the most common seaweeds found in temperate and polar climates. The members of the Fucales order of this variety thrive in stony seashores; nevertheless, the majority of brown algae are marine and provide important food and habitat functions. Brown algae, which belong to the Phaeophyceae class and include over 1500 algae species classified as Chromophyta, are prevalent in cold seas along continental coasts. Depending on the ratio of colour brown (fucoxanthin) to green (chlorophyll), their hue can range from dark brown to olive green. From tiny filaments epiphytes (*Ectocarpus*) to enormous kelps that range between 1 and over 100 m (3.3–330 ft; *Laminaria*, *Macrocystis*, *Nereocystis*), these algae are available in various shapes and sizes.

In temperate regions, other brown algae like *Sargassum* or *Fucus* and *Ascophyllum* flourish on rocky shorelines. There aren't many freshwater species. Both asexual and sexual reproductions are used by brown algae, which produce gametes with two unequal flagella and motile zoospores. The photosynthetic portions of the algal thallus of certain seaweed species remain afloat on or close to the water's surface thanks to gas-filled bladders called pneumatocysts.

Once a significant provider of potash and iodine, brown algae are currently utilized as a stabilizing agent in the ice cream and baking sectors. In East Asia and beyond, some species—like *Laminaria*—are consumed as vegetables, while others serve as fertilizers (Mortensen et al. 2016).

They contain various biologically active components, namely, proteins, amino acids, polysaccharides, fatty acids, vitamins, minerals, dietary fibre, sterols, pigments, and polyphenols. These molecules exhibited the activities, namely, anticoagulant, antithrombotic, antiviral, anticancer, anti-inflammatory, and antibacterial values (Muhammad et al. 2019). Components of these algae, therefore, have great medicinal promise. These include the therapy of skin problems, rheumatic problem, hypertension, goitre, ulcers, asthma, menstrual irregularities, syphilis, and arteriosclerosis.

Polysaccharides, the essential biologically active ingredients, contribute significantly to brown algae's biological value. Brown algal cell wall polysaccharides, including laminarins, alginates, and fucoidans, have created an attention for research because of their possible biological utilization in medications, cosmeceuticals, and functional foods (Munro et al. 1999; National Oceanic and Atmospheric Administration 2025; Ngo and Kim 2013).

2.2.3 Kelp

About 30 kinds of brown algae, known as kelp (order Laminariales), grow into enormous coastal seaweeds in colder waters. For a wide variety of coastal creatures, such as fish and crustaceans, kelps offer essential shelter and food.

Kelps of the genus *Laminaria* have exceptionally long flat blades and are typically found on the Atlantic and Pacific Oceans' northern coasts. These prolific kelps can grow to be 1–3 m long (3.3–9.8 ft) and have a stipe that superficially resembles a terrestrial plant's stem. Growth extension occurs in the meristematic zone between the stipe (perennial) and the blade (shedding yearly). A commercially and environmentally important category of seaweeds, kelps are mostly used as food for humans and as a source of alginate for a number of industries, including food, paper, cosmetics, medicines, and textiles. Conversely, kelps have a variety of commercial uses, such as feed for aquaculture and animal husbandry, fertilizers for agriculture, feedstock for biofuel, and medicinal uses (Nussinovitch 1997).

2.2.4 Seaweeds

Seaweeds are an important biological resource in the ocean, having both culinary and therapeutic properties. The main source of organic matter in the oceans, seaweeds also carry out photosynthesis and contain chlorophyll. Data indicates that there are about 100 varieties that are edible worldwide, such as spirulina from the phylum *Cyanophyta*, laver and cauliflower from the phylum *Rhodophyta*, and kelp and *Undaria pinnatifida* from the phylum *Phaeophyta*. Seaweeds can also be processed to extract polysaccharides, proteins, carotenoids, and other beneficial compounds. Seaweed polysaccharides are the popular name for a variety of big molecular carbohydrates found in seaweeds. They are made up of a number of monosaccharide groups bound together by glycosidic linkages. These polysaccharides can be combined to create multi-component mixtures, which typically have a high viscosity or coagulation ability and are soluble in water.

Marine natural resources are a major source of knowledge for agricultural and pharmaceutical applications. Recent research has shown that chemically modified marine compounds and bioactive secondary metabolites obtained from marine seaweeds have pharmacological utility in the treatment and prevention of a range of illnesses. The presence of numerous bioactive metabolites in natural seaweeds endowed with pharmacological qualities makes them unique and helpful in drug lead identification for drug development due to their diverse chemical ecologies (Pangestuti and Kim 2014).

2.3 *Techniques for Classification and Extraction of MPPs*

Polysaccharides obtained from marine algae are complex biopolymers that can be classified based on their monosaccharide composition, structural properties, and solubility. The classification method impacts extraction, purification, and applications for oral drug delivery (Pereira 2018).

2.3.1 Classification of Marine Plant Polysaccharides (MPPs)

Based on Monomer Composition

(a) **Homopolysaccharides:** These contain one type of monosaccharide (e.g. agarose—galactose units).
(b) **Heteropolysaccharides:** These contain two or more different types of sugar monomers (e.g. ulvan—rhamnose, glucuronic acid, xylose) (Peteiro et al. 2016).

Based on Sulfation Level

(a) **Neutral polysaccharides** (e.g. agarose).
(b) **Sulfated polysaccharides:** These demonstrate greater bioactivity and mucoadhesiveness (e.g. carrageenan, fucoidan, ulvan) (Xu et al. 2017).

Based on Source and Functionality

(a) **Structural polysaccharides:** These serve as components of cell wall matrices (cellulose-like polymers in algae).
(b) **Storage polysaccharides:** These serve as energy stores, like laminarin in brown algae (Notararigo et al. 2013).

2.3.2 Extraction Methods

Extraction is a vital part of determining the purity, functionality, and use of the polysaccharide obtained via dried varieties of the algae in Fig. 1. The most common methods for their extractions are as follows:

Aqueous Extraction

This is a standard practice, in which dried algae are boiled or soaked in water, which is maintained at a specific pH and temperature, to solubilize polysaccharides. Some polysaccharides are only lost at specific temperatures, which can affect the specificity of the extraction (e.g. agar 85–95 °C) (Nagahawatta et al. 2023).

Alkaline Extraction

Alkaline extraction employs dilute sodium hydroxide to extract certain polysaccharides, including alginates. Alkaline conditions degrade cell membranes and release polysaccharides from the cell into solution (Harding et al. 2017b).

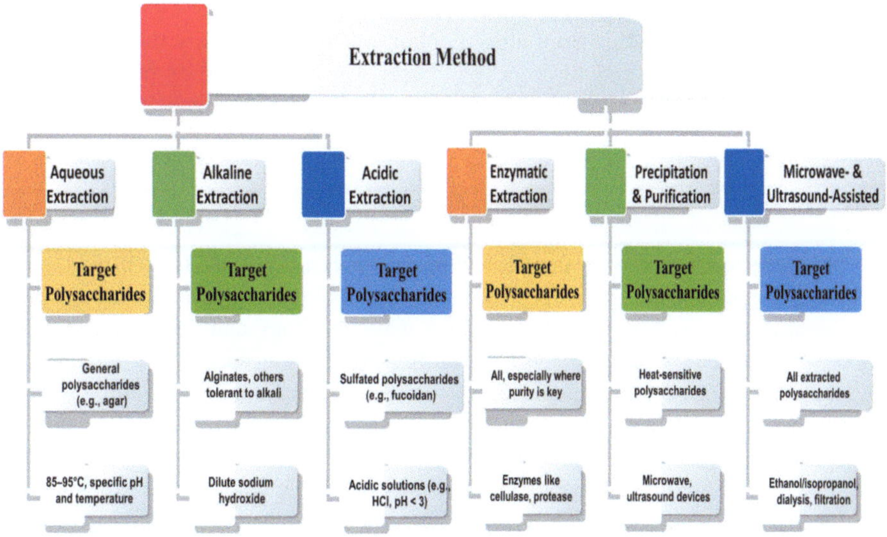

Fig. 1 A diagrammatic image showing the reported extraction methods of various MPPs

Acidic Extraction

It is typically used for sulfated polysaccharides, such as fucoidan. Acid hydrolysis helps break down non-polysaccharide components, hence increasing yields (Jönsson et al. 2020).

Enzymatic Extraction

This method uses enzymes such as cellulases or proteases to break down unwanted proteins and cellulose to yield a purer polysaccharide fraction (Sun et al. 2018).

Microwave- and Ultrasound-Assisted Extraction

These advanced methods utilize physical energy to promote cell wall disruptions and improve extraction efficiencies at low temperatures, conserving polysaccharide bioactivity (Dobrinčić et al. 2020).

Precipitation and Purification Following extraction, polysaccharides are typically precipitated using alcohols, such as ethanol or isopropanol. The purification process may involve dialysis, filtration, and lyophilization to remove salts and small molecules (Fleurence et al. 1995).

2.4 *Phytochemical Composition and Variability*

The marine polysaccharides from algae contain inherent variability through a spectrum of environmental and biological impacts. Understanding its phytochemical composition is critical for trustworthy pharmacological use (Mirzadeh et al. 2020).

2.4.1 Key Phytochemical Components

The phytochemical profile of plant-based marine polysaccharides is highly dynamic and complex with many bioactive elements that have a strong influence on their functional properties based on the different ways that they can be applied in drug delivery systems. The main aspects include the various monosaccharide units, which include glucose, galactose, mannose, xylose, fucose, and rhamnose, among many others (Shi 2016). The type and relative amount of sugars will determine critical properties of the polysaccharide, such as the solution properties, viscosity, and gel strength. Uronic acids, such as glucuronic and guluronic acid, which are found in polysaccharides like alginate and ulvan, add to chelating capacity of the polymer for divalent ions, which enhances the gelling just like sulfate groups. The polysaccharides gain sulfate status, which also provides the polysaccharide chains with negative charges, further enhancing their solubility and biological activity (Stengel et al. 2011). Therefore, polysaccharides having sulfate groups, such as carrageenan and fucoidan, through their antiretroviral, anticoagulant, and immunomodulatory properties, are highly useful when applied as an oral agent. For many marine polysaccharides, their molecular weights can vary widely and can have effects on viscosity of the polysaccharides, encapsulation characteristics, and degradation activities. Structural characteristics, such as branching and acetylation of fucoidan, can influence many properties, such as water absorption capability, mucoadhesiveness, and certain enzyme stability, which are necessary for drug delivery applications in the gut (Stevanović and Filipović 2024).

The structural and functional uniformity of these marine polysaccharides has been affected by a number of intrinsic and extrinsic factors. The species of algae is probably the most significant factor since different species produce various polysaccharides, which differ in structure and functionality (Silva et al. 2012). For example, *Gracilaria* species are known to produce softer agar, while the gels produced by *Gelidium* are firmer. The geographical origins affect the biochemical composition of algae collected, as extrinsic environmental factors (e.g. water temperature, salinity, light, and nutrients) alter the biochemical composition (Zayed et al. 2020). In addition, seasonal variations may cause differences in outcomes and quality due to the metabolic adjustments made by algae when spiralling through their phase of development. Lastly, very importantly, the conditions inherent during harvesting as well as post-harvest processing (e.g. method and time of drying, exposure to heat, air, and/or light) can sometimes destroy and/or lose sensitive bioactive compounds. These differences must be characterized and have standardization procedures applied to ensure consistency in pharmaceutical development and outcomes (Silva and Fabi 2022).

3 Physicochemical Characteristics of MPPs

Such properties of MPPs are essential to evaluating their suitability and functionality within ODDSs. These properties control polymers' interactions with biological environments, modulate the encapsulation and release of drugs, and ultimately influence therapeutic efficacy. The key properties of polysaccharides include their solubility, rate of swelling, mucoadhesion, gel-forming ability, and stability over stomach pH levels. Understanding these properties is vital to the rational design and utilizing therapeutic potential of polysaccharide-based DDs (Juneja et al. 2013).

3.1 Solubility and Swelling Properties

Solubility is a fundamental physicochemical property of marine polysaccharides that influences their practical use in oral applications. These biopolymers, like other polysaccharides, are generally hydrophilic because of the hydroxyl, carboxyl, and sulfate groups in their structure. Solubility characteristics are variably dependent upon the type of polysaccharide, molecular weight, degree of branching, and functional substituents such as sulfate or uronic acid groups (Feng et al. 2024).

Alginate is generally an anionic polymeric substance isolated from the cellular membrane of brown algae, which is soluble in water but forms hydrogels in the presence of two-valent cations (either Ca^{+2}, Ba^{+2}, Sr^{+2}, etc.). Solubility depends on the ratio of the alternating mannuronic acid (M) and guluronic acid (G) units, such that more guluronic acid means firmer gels. Carrageenan, from red algae, is also soluble, but the gel characteristics depend on the levels of sulfate and whether it is kappa-, iota-, or lambda-carrageenan; kappa has slightly higher hydrophilicity than iota, which is hydrophilic than lambda. Ulvan is a water-soluble sulfated polysaccharide derived from green algae and has a high swelling capacity (Domozych et al. 2023). This ability makes ulvan useful for swelling-controlled release systems (Cardoso et al. 2016).

Swelling is closely related to solubility, as it is indicative of how much water a polymer can absorb and swell without dissolving. Swelling is important for controlled release of drugs, as swelling will greatly influence the diffusion of the drug from the polymeric network. Swelling often occurs in a very loose network polymer and with a high proportion of hydrophilicity, for example, fucoidan and ulvan. Swelling characteristics of the polymers could be modified by cross-linkage or chemical modification to develop the most desirable drug release characteristics (Barbosa et al. 2019a).

3.2 *Mucoadhesive and Gel-Forming Properties*

A distinctive property of marine polysaccharides in oral drugs is their mucoadhesive property. This characteristic allows them to adhere to the mucosal lining of the GIT. This property has a significant advantage since it extends the retaining time of the drug at the absorption site, thereby increasing bioavailability, especially for insoluble and/or unstable drugs (Lin et al. 2022). Mucoadhesion mainly occurs through hydrogen bonding, electrostatic interactions, and Van der Waals forces between polysaccharide chains and mucin glycoproteins on the mucosal surface. Furthermore, functional groups on polysaccharides such as $–OH^-$, $–COOH^-$, and $–SO_4{}^{-2}$ groups increase the interactions of the polysaccharides. Polysaccharides such as alginate, carrageenan, and fucoidan exhibit excellent mucoadhesivity and could potentially have greater mucoadhesive properties through simple physical mixing or forming a chemical conjugate with a different polymer (e.g. chitosan) (Colombo et al. 1996).

In addition to mucoadhesion, many marine polysaccharides have excellent gel-forming capabilities for drug protection and tailored release. There are various gelation mechanisms, including alginate gels that rely on ionic cross-linking (often with calcium) in the presence of divalent cations. This process yields a robust hydrogel matrix that is ideal for encapsulating sensitive formats such as peptides or probiotics (Lukova and Katsarov 2023). Moreover, carrageenan is capable of generating thermo-reversible gels upon cooling, primarily kappa-carrageenan (with potassium ions) that forms stiff networks appropriate to the creation of tablet matrices or film formats. Finally, ulvan and agar can also form viscous or gel-like solutions that can have a variety of uses depending on conditions. The unique properties of mucoadhesion and gelation provide marine polysaccharides a prime place in developing sustained-release oral medication delivery systems. These properties not only help protect medications from degradation but also control their release at different areas of the GI system (Bayer 2022).

3.3 Stability at Gastrointestinal pH of MPPs

The gastrointestinal system presents a complicated and challenging environment for orally delivered medications due to fluctuation in pH, enzymatic activity, and mechanical motion. To be useful, a polysaccharide-based drug carrier should be stable in these conditions or provide a responsive release of the medication at a specific location. Marine polysaccharides exhibit different stability in the pH range of the GIT, which is pH 1.5 in the stomach to pH 7.5 in the intestines. For example, alginate is relatively stable under low stomach pH (1.5), where it forms an insoluble alginic acid gel to protect the encapsulated medication from acid destruction. When the pH of the intestinal environment increases, the gel expands and starts to dissolve, thus allowing drug release. This pH-responsive solubility property is advantageous for targeted intestinal delivery (Makarova et al. 2023).

Carrageenan shows good pH stability, although its properties vary by type, since kappa and iota types form strong gels at neutral to slightly alkaline pH and are therefore well suited for drug delivery to the intestinal tract (Kraithong et al. 2024). Fucoidan, on the other hand, is soluble over a very large pH range and is relatively resistant to enzyme digestion in the upper GIT, making it a model for initiating sustained systemic effects when delivered with an appropriate pharmaceutical compound (Liu et al. 2017). In addition, the extensive range of potential chemical modifications of marine polysaccharides may improve their pH stability. For example, sulfating, acetylating, and copolymerizing with synthetic polymers might improve their resistance to acid or enzymatic digestion. Cross-linked alginate beads or interpolymer complexes with chitosan may hold their integrity for longer in the gastric region and selectively release their contents in the intestine (Pacheco-Quito et al. 2020).

4 Common Uses of MPPs

The polysaccharides of marine algae have many different physicochemical and biological properties applicable for oral delivery of pharmaceuticals. Alginate, carrageenan, agar/agarose, ulvan, and fucoidan are polysaccharides that are widely researched and exploited for many properties in the marshmallow pharmacological area including biocompatibility, gel strength, mucoadhesiveness, and response to pH and ions (Citkowska et al. 2019).

4.1 Alginate

Alginate is a linear, anionic polymeric material primarily available from brown seaweeds such as *Laminaria* and *Ascophyllum*. It contains two uronic acid residues, namely, β-D-mannuronic acid (M) and α-L-guluronic acid (G), and can consist of blocks that are homopolymeric (M-M or G-G) or heteropolymeric (M-G). The amount and arrangement of these blocks affect its gelling properties and subsequent drug release properties. The common feature of alginate is its ability to creating hydrogels against the divalent cations, e.g. calcium ions, in an "egg-box" model of cross-linking. This property allows the formation of calcium alginate beads or hydrogels to encapsulate a variety of pharmaceuticals. These gels may protect sensitive pharmaceuticals from destruction in the stomach and provide pH-dependent or sustained release of pharmaceuticals in the intestine. Alginate is also non-toxic and biodegradable and has good mucoadhesive properties that prolong drug residency time at the absorption site (George and Abraham 2006).

4.2 Carrageenan

It is a group of sulfated galactans isolated from red algae species, including *Kappaphycus alvarezii* and *Chondrus crispus*. It consists of recurring disaccharide units of D-galactose and 3,6-anhydro-D-galactose, exhibiting variable degrees and locations of sulfation, resulting in three principal types: kappa (κ), iota (ι), and lambda (λ). Kappa-carrageenan generates robust, brittle gels against K^{+1} ions, whereas iota-carrageenan yields soft, elastic gels with Ca^{+2} ions. Lambda-carrageenan, characterized by its elevated sulfation, remains non-gelling but very viscous, making it appropriate for liquid formulations. The gel-forming characteristics are used to create controlled release tablets, films, and microparticles for oral medication administration. Furthermore, sulfate groups impart biological properties, including antiviral, anticoagulant, and immunomodulatory actions, rendering carrageenan both a structural carrier and a bioactive element in therapeutic systems (Sutapa et al. 2017).

4.3 *Agar and Agarose*

Agar is an example of a heterogeneous MPP isolated from red algae, specifically *Gelidium* and *Gracilaria*. Agar consists of two main components: the gel-forming agarose and the non-gelling agaropectin. Agarose, isolated from agar, is composed of alternating D-galactose and 3,6-anhydro-L-galactopyranose units arranged in a linear fashion, while agaropectin has sulfated and pyruvated side chains, which impart certain solubility and functionality properties. Agar gels are strong, thermoreversible gels, which form upon cooling from a heated aqueous solution. They were engineered into matrix tablets, beads, and films allowing sustained or controlled drug release for extended periods of time. The inertness of agar, the strength of its gel, and its low toxicity make agar ideal to encapsulate sensitive chemicals, probiotics, and proteins. Similarly, agarose is also a pure material and does not contain any charge groups making it excellent for producing uniform drug-loaded microspheres and biocompatible scaffolds for oral administration systems (Zhang et al. 2023).

4.4 *Ulvan*

Ulvan is a water-soluble and sulfated polysaccharide isolated from green algae, primarily *Ulva* and *Enteromorpha*. Ulvan is unique in composition, consisting of rhamnose, xylose, glucuronic acid, and iduronic acid, often in repeat disaccharide form called ulvanobiuronic acids. The inclusion of sulfate and uronic acid groups gives ulvan polyanionic properties and bioactivity. Ulvan is stated to be gel-forming and mucoadhesive. However, ulvan is not as gel-forming as alginate or carrageenan. Ulvan can form viscous hydrogels and films alone or with other polymers such as chitosan or gelatin. In terms of oral drug delivery, ulvan must be addressed for sustained drug release and targeting the intestine for drugs of anti-inflammatory and antioxidant class. Additionally, ulvan is immunostimulatory, antiviral, and prebiotic, which makes it appropriate as a nutraceutical and medicinal polysaccharide (Kumar et al. 2021).

4.5 *Fucoidan*

It is a complex sulfated polysaccharide found in brown algae such as *Fucus vesiculosus* and *Undaria pinnatifida*. The structure predominantly consists of L-fucose units, with the possibility of being bound with sulfate groups, and may have small amounts of galactose, xylose, and uronic acids. The specific composition and branching structures depend on the algal source and method of extraction. Fucoidan has remarkable bioactivity, including anticancer, anti-inflammatory, anti-coagulant, and antiviral activities. As both an active ingredient in topical and hydrophilic formulation as a medicine and a functional excipient in an oral dosage form, fucoidan contributes its mucoadhesive properties provide extended gastrointestinal retention, and its anti-tumour and anti-immunity activity mean that fucoidan will not be destroyed by digestion until the necessary release occurs. In fact, fucoidan-based nanoparticles, films, and hydrogel-based materials have been created to deliver proteins, peptides, and/or anticancer agents orally, with evidence demonstrating positive effects to increase bioavailability with reduced toxicity (Lee et al. 2022).

4.6 *Laminarin*

In 1885, Oswald Schmiedeberg discovered laminarin, also called laminaran, in the brown macroalgae family Laminariaceae (Madany et al. 2021). Depending on the degree of polymerization, its molecular weight (MW) is approximately 5 kDa, and it is found in seaweed vacuoles. Likewise, solubility may be impacted by the extent of branching. A laminarin with numerous branches dissolves in cold water, whereas one with fewer branches is only soluble in hot water (January et al. 2019). Laminarin is composed of glucose units joined by β-(1,3) connections with β-(1,6)-linked side chains (Pomponi 1999). At the end of the chain of this polysaccharide, there could additionally be a mannitol residue. The type of seaweed and environmental elements including depth, sea current, salinity, and water temperature determine how common this residue is in the laminarin structure (Sithranga Boopathy and Kathiresan 2010). Laminarin, which makes up 22–49% of the dry matter in seaweed, is the primary energy source in macroalgae. After building up polysaccharides throughout the hot months, seaweed mostly uses it in the winter. Because the human body cannot digest it, this compound's capacity to function as dietary fibre is one of its most pertinent advantages (Skják-Bræk and Draget 2012). However, because laminarin can efficiently support cell activities and stimulate tissue regeneration—both of which are crucial for the healing process—it has been discovered to be a significant asset in the fields of therapeutic administration and tissue engineering (Urbán-Morlán et al. 2020).

5 Mechanism of Oral Pharmaceutical Formulations Containing MPPs

Oral medication administration remains one of the preferred ways of medicine administration due to convenience, safety, and patient compliance. The gastrointestinal (GI) tract is not straightforward; there is uncertainty in pH, enzyme activity, and mucosal barriers, each of which creates issues with stability and absorption. Marine polysaccharides offer interesting new approaches and opportunities given their unique structural and functional properties. It is essential to study the nature of marine polysaccharides in the release and absorption of encapsulated drug, as well as interactions with the GI mucus for their potentiality in semisustainable, regulated and targeted drug delivery systems (Zhu et al. 2021).

5.1 Mechanisms of Drug Release and Absorption

The release of pharmaceuticals from marine polysaccharide-based formulations is governed by an intricate set of interactions, which include swelling of the polymer, degradation of the matrix, molecular diffusion, and environmental effects with regard to physiological stimuli like pH and ionic strength. Typically, these systems work concurrently, influencing the rate and location of drug release, as with diffusion-controlled release, for pharmaceuticals traversing a hydrated gel matrix of polysaccharide materials such as alginate or agar. These polysaccharide materials form large viscous, viscoelastic networks that impede the transport of the drug and promote prolonged release. Swelling-controlled systems utilize polysaccharides such as ulvan and fucoidan to imbibe gastrointestinal fluid and swell, creating voids in the matrix that facilitate the stepwise release of drug molecules. An important mechanism of drug release is erosion or degradation release, where polymer erosion occurs as a result of hydrolysis or enzyme action. Marine polysaccharides are generally resistant to degradation by gastric enzymes but are partially degraded by colonic bacteria making them ideal candidates for oral colon delivery systems. Stimuli-responsive systems take advantage of pH changes that occur in the GIT for site-specific drug release. Alginate is stable in acid and, therefore, cannot be degraded by stomach enzymes until the changes in pH occur in the alkaline conditions of the small intestine allowing it to dissolve. The acid-sensitive drug is protected, and the resulting drug release can be targeted to specific regions of the GIT while allowing for absorption of the active drug. Both of these strategies improve drug therapeutic efficacy and bioavailability when administered orally, especially for drugs that have been developed exploiting the unique physicochemical properties of each marine-derived polysaccharide (Fernando et al. 2020).

5.2 Targeted and Controlled Release Mechanisms

Controlled and targeted systems of DDs are designed to improve the therapy by delivering the drug to a precise area and over a specific time frame. Marine polysaccharides, because of their vast structural diversity, biocompatibility, and ability to form hydrogels, are well suited to serve as carriers for these advanced delivery methods. Modified release systems are designed to maintain steady-state concentrations of the medication by providing a slow and prolonged release, over much longer time periods. Hydrogels, microspheres, and tablets based on polysaccharides derived from carrageenan, alginate, or agar can be formulated to deliver pharmaceuticals over time frames extending from a few hours up to several days (Shahiwala 2011). Regulated delivery depends on different variables—cross-linking density, polymer concentration, and interactions with ions or pH in the gastrointestinal environment. Targeted delivery systems are based on delivering the medicine to a targeted physiologic site. An example of a marine polysaccharide with pH-sensitive properties is alginate, which is stable in the gastric region but will dissolve in the alkaline region of the intestine to protect acid-labile pharmaceuticals and allow for targeted release. Fucoidan and ulvan cannot be enzymatically degraded in the upper GIT, although they can be metabolized by the microbes in the colon, making them particularly appropriate for targeting the colon, which can include inflammatory bowel disease therapy (Atmaca et al. 2022).

Moreover, mucoadhesive targeting enhances local drug retention and absorption by enhancing the ability of the polysaccharide to adhere to a mucosal barrier, specifically the duodenum and jejunum. Polymers such as carrageenan and alginate adhere to mucus via electrostatic and hydrogen bonding interactions, which would lengthen the amount of time that the formulation resides in the intestine. In addition, ligand-based targeting is emerging as a powerful tool in targeted delivery in which polysaccharides such as fucoidan are chemically modified with ligands such as peptide or folic acid to facilitate receptor-mediated endocytosis for the target cell, particularly for cancer or infection-based applications. Altogether, these properties make marine polysaccharides very useful for the modulation of next-generation ODDSs that are both effective and easy to administer (Zhong et al. 2020).

5.3 Interaction with Gastrointestinal (GI) Mucosa

The GI mucosa serves as the primary interface through which we absorb nutrients from food and uptake of orally administered drugs. The GI mucosa is composed of two major layers, a reconcilable mucus layer that is rich in mucins and a unique barrier of epithelial cells immediately below. The appropriateness of polysaccharide-based oral drug delivery systems depends almost exclusively on their interaction with this complex environment (Negreanu-Pirjol et al. 2022). Alginates, carrageenans, and fucoidans, all marine polysaccharides, have considerable mucoadhesive properties that allow for their efficient engagement with mucin glycoproteins via H^+ bonding, electrostatic, and van der Waals interactions. This adherence increases the time of the drug molecule to retain at the absorption site, which will improve bioavailability because the duration of contact is improved with the epithelial surface, and is also susceptible to reduced clearance by the activity of peristalsis. In addition, some marine polysaccharides can (in an otherwise non-permanent manner) alter the tight junction protein of epithelial cells, therefore increasing paracellular permeability, and facilitating the absorption of macromolecules (peptides and proteins) that typically have a poor oral bioavailability. In addition to supporting absorption, these polysaccharides also act as a protective coating on the mucosal surface. They create biocompatible barriers to protect the epithelium from irritants while reducing mucosal injury, especially with medications that harm the gastrointestinal lining, or in the case of ulcers and inflammatory bowel disease (IBD). Some polysaccharides including fucoidan and ulvan may even have a baseline biological activity at the mucosal interface, and their anti-inflammatory and immunomodulatory abilities can assist in mucosal repair and have the potential to treat inflammatory gastrointestinal conditions. These multifunctional interactions speak to the importance of marine polysaccharides as both passive carriers of drugs and biologically active agents that can enhance the therapy and safety of ODDSs (Subramanian et al. 2022).

6 Strategies for Formulation Using MPPs for Oral Route

Marine polysaccharides have enormous potential for the fabrication of numerous ODDSs, due to their gelling capacity, mucoadhesive nature, pH responsiveness, and biodegradability. These natural polymers can be formulated into several dosage forms to achieve various therapeutic goals, whether it is sustained release, targeted delivery, or protection from stomach degradation. This section outlines formulation approaches using marine-derived plant polysaccharides and focuses on tablets, capsules, hydrogels, films, nanoparticles, microparticles, and coatings for colon targeting (Azman et al. 2022).

Any delivery system is a formulation or device that allows the entry of a therapeutic molecule into the living thing and improves its safety and efficacy by maintaining the rate, timing, and location of drug release into the body (Yermak et al. 2022). Numerous organisms, particularly plants, have been made useful in the advancement of medicine and DD methods by nature (Yuan et al. 2023). Marine algae have many components that can be employed as medications and pharmaceuticals (Toumi et al. 2021; Ganesan et al. 2020). Figure 2 depicts an outlook illustration of various strategies used for the formulation of oral dosage forms using various types of MPPs and their purpose.

6.1 *Types of Forms Used for Oral Route*

They are divided into two major forms as the conventional and the novel or advanced DDSs. Figure 3 depicts various types of MPPs for specific functionalities in various types of dosage forms retaining in oral cavity as well as swallowing via oral route for specific purposes.

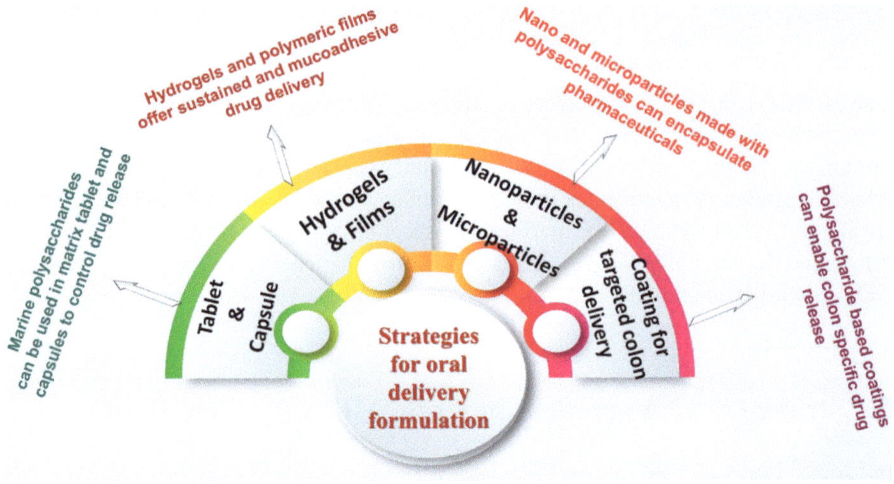

Fig. 2 An outlook illustration depicting the formulation strategies of various MPPs for ODDSs

6.1.1 Conventional DDSs

The traditional approach to delivering medications into the body is known as a conventional drug delivery system; typical examples of these systems are oral and sublingual and buccal.

These include tablets and capsules, system for oral drug delivery, mucoadhesive DDS, and sublingual and buccal.

Tablets and Capsules

The safety and acceptance of tablets and capsules continue to make these popular oral dosage forms due to their uncomplex administration and patient adherence in Fig. 2. Marine polysaccharides, including alginates, carrageenan, and agars, have typically been used as a matrix-forming agent, binder, and/or disintegrants in tablet and capsule formulation (Grewal et al. 2021). The drug incorporated within a matrix tablet is entrapped within a polymeric collation of one or several marine polysaccharides. The release time may be modulated by the slow hydration and gelation of the alginate or carrageenan polymeric frameworks, allowing drug release to occur over an extended period. Calcium alginate matrices, for example, form robust gels, which may not readily dissolve in the stomach, but allow the drug to be released in the intestine. In case of capsules, the marine polysaccharides may be used as either drug-loaded carriers or drug loaded granulates and can be filled into either animal or plant-based shells of capsules. Enteric-coated capsules made with polysaccharides sensitive to pH can shield the drug from gastric acid and will release it in the small intestine or colon (Iliou et al. 2022).

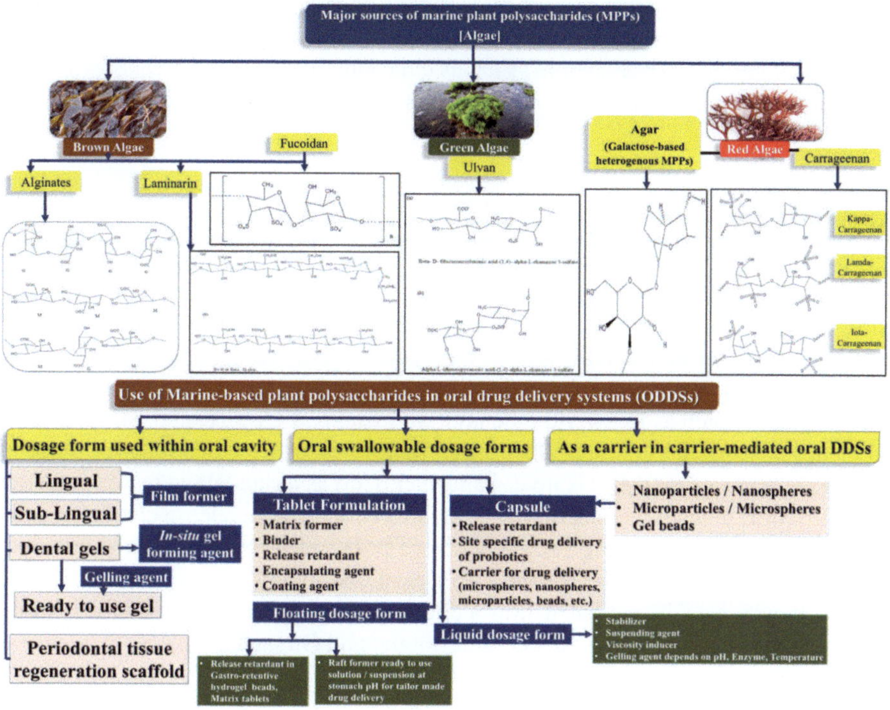

Fig. 3 An outlook chart exhibiting various types of MPPs and their specific functionalities for various dosage forms for use either in oral cavity or swallowed through oral route for specific rationale in the gastrointestinal tract

System for Oral DD

Because of their special qualities, such as low toxicity, biocompatibility, and biodegradability, marine plant polysaccharides are receiving a lot of attention in the biomedical area, especially for ODDSs (Ahmed et al. 2024; Santhanes et al. 2018).

Alginate in Oral DDSs

Alginate is frequently utilized as an excipient in both conventional and cutting-edge medication delivery techniques. Alginate is utilized as a thickening and stabilizing ingredient in oral liquid formulations for conventional drug delivery. Compared to tablets containing alginate, those containing the conjugated polymer showed a much longer residence length (Jacob et al. 2018b). Alginates' chemical changes to regulate drug release from polymeric network systems determine their tableting behaviour (Dhamecha et al. 2019). Alginate microsphere swelling was reduced by glutaraldehyde cross-linking, which also increased the loading of the hydrophilic nimesulide.

Iron-cross-linked hydroxamated alginate has been demonstrated to be beneficial for a number of medications' delayed release. Alginate produces powerful compounds that are rich in polycations, such as chitosan. To lessen the breakdown of the gel matrix, alginate beads treated with chitosan have been developed (Abasalizadeh et al. 2020).

Carrageenan in Oral DDSs

Carrageenan's gelling, thickening, and stabilizing properties make it a popular excipient in medicated dosage forms. It is frequently used in conventional drug administration techniques to control drug release and improve dosage form stability (Bulut 2021). Proteins and small molecule drugs can be delivered using nanocomposites made from three different forms of carrageenans. Carrageenan's characteristics, such as its swelling behaviour, mean particle size, and encapsulation efficiency that results in water absorption, help to protect medications for delayed release (Tomić et al. 2023). Using carrageenan (CG) as a standalone matrix material to control drug release can occasionally result in undesirable release characteristics, such as pH-independent drug release and zero-order release. It has been shown that λ-CG and HPMC together lessen the variance in dissolving behaviour at various pH values. It was also investigated how cellulose ethers and CGs affected the way ibuprofen was released from tablets (Aderibigbe and Buyana 2018).

Mucoadhesive DDSs

Marine plant-based polysaccharides are gaining prominence in drug delivery, particularly for mucoadhesive systems that improve drug retention and absorption. Conventional drug delivery systems often lack site specificity and can result in rapid drug release and clearance. Mucoadhesive drug delivery systems, however, enhance the interaction between the drug carrier and the mucosal surface, prolonging residence time and improving bioavailability. Wan et al. (2021) in *Bioactive Materials* discuss the applications of marine polysaccharides in drug delivery, highlighting their biocompatibility and biodegradability (Bui et al. 2019). Bose et al. (2023a, b) in *Materials* review various mucoadhesive materials and their applications, including marine polysaccharides (Stenner et al. 2016). Alginate, carrageenan, and chitosan can be used in various mucoadhesive formulations, including hydrogels, microparticles, and nanoparticles, for targeted drug delivery.

Sublingual and Buccal DDSs

Alginate, carrageenan, fucoidan, and chitosan have emerged as promising biomaterials for ODDSs, particularly in sublingual and buccal applications. Due to their inherent features of biocompatibility, biodegradability, non-toxicity, and strong mucoadhesivity, they are essential for effective DD through the oral mucosal membrane (Thakur et al. 2016).

Buccal and sublingual DDSs provide several advantages over traditional oral administration. By delivering drugs directly through the mucosal tissues of the mouth, these systems bypass the harsh GI layer and hepatic first-pass metabolism, resulting in extending bioavailability and a rapid onset of action. Marine polysaccharides are particularly suited for these applications because their hydrophilic nature allows them to swell and adhere to the moist mucosal surfaces, ensuring prolonged residence time and controlled drug release (Zhu et al. 2017).

Various dosage forms have been developed using marine polysaccharides for buccal and sublingual delivery, including tablets, gels, films, patches, and micro-/nanoparticles. For example, mucoadhesive buccal tablets and films made from alginate, chitosan, and other marine polysaccharides provide sustained release and improved drug absorption. Recent advances include the development of protein-loaded mucoadhesive buccal patches using chitosan and hyaluronic acid multilayers, which demonstrated effective sublingual delivery and prolonged retention in preclinical models (Barbosa et al. 2019b). The use of MPPs in these delivery systems not only enhances drug stability and absorption but also allows for encapsulating various therapeutic agents, including peptides, proteins, and poorly soluble drugs (Pelin and Suflet 2020).

Targeted DDSs

Conventional drug delivery systems involve immediate or bolus release, often leading to systemic exposure and potential toxicity, whereas targeted drug delivery (TDD) aims for site-specific drug release, enhancing therapy and reducing side effects. Marine plant-based polysaccharides are gaining prominence in TDD due to their good tolerability and biodegradability (Dubashynskaya et al. 2024). MPPs also plays the significant role in desired DDSs including stimuli-responsive systems either for controlled or targeted release. The use of alginate and carrageenan for targeted cancer therapy, showcasing their potential in nanoparticle-based drug carriers (Sacramento et al. 2022).

Wipes

Wipe is a three-layered, porous material that can be used to transport medications. They have many benefits over conventional DDSs, including a large surface area, biodegradability, and biocompatibility. Alginate and chitosan are two examples of marine biopolymers that have been studied as permeable drug delivery vehicles. Alginate wipes have been used to transfer development factors and anticancer drugs, whereas chitosan wipes have been used to transfer compatible proteins and peptides (Yuan et al. 2005; Aparna et al. 2018).

6.2 Novel/Advanced DDSs

It combines cutting-edge methodology with novel dosage forms that are superior to traditional dosage forms and incorporate medical devices. It increases a medication's potency, regulates its release to produce a long-lasting therapeutic impact, increases safety, and precisely targets a drug to a target region (Mihaila et al. 2013). Typical instances of these systems are hydrogels, nanoparticles, microspheres, and implants.

6.2.1 Hydrogels

Because of their many uses and intrinsic benefits, marine-derived polysaccharide hydrogels are an intriguing development in material science. They are especially useful in the biomedical industry, where they are employed as medication delivery systems and in wound dressings (Varghese et al. 2014). They create an environment that encourages cell growth, tissue regeneration, and healing because of their high water content and biocompatibility, which make them ideal mimics of natural tissue (Liu et al. 2015).

Hydrogels and Films

Hydrogels and polymeric films are advanced formulation technologies that can deliver pharmaceuticals in a controlled and targeted manner. Various grades of alginates, agarose, ulvan, and carrageenans have been utilized in hydrogel formulations via either ionic cross-linking or heat gelation techniques. Hydrogels made from alginate or carrageenan can expand in the presence of gastrointestinal fluids to create a gelled matrix, which encapsulates the drug. Hydrogels made from these polysaccharides are ideal for sustained DDSs, mucoadhesiveness, and targeting the colon (Keppeler et al. 2009). Drug released from hydrogel formulations is controlled via diffusion, swelling, and sometimes erosion. Cross-linkers like calcium ions (for alginate) or potassium ions (for carrageenan) are used to modify gel strength and drug release rate (Santo et al. 2009).

Polymeric films are thin, flexible layers obtained by casting an aqueous polysaccharide solution, allowing the solution to gel and solidify into a matrix. These films can be loaded with drugs and applied for oral transmucosal delivery (e.g. buccal or sublingual dosing) with advantages such as avoiding hepatic metabolism and faster onset of action. Polysaccharide films can serve as protective coat for tablets or capsules, providing a better mucoadhesive delivery and localized action. By manipulating the polymer concentration, the degree of cross-linking, and the polymer-drug interactions, hydrogels and films made from marine polysaccharides can provide custom-made drug delivery profiles, along with superior biocompatibility (Frederiksen et al. 2015).

Alginate-Based Hydrogel Beads for Oral DDSs

A complex hydrogel containing divalent ions, especially calcium, is produced by alginate. Microencapsulation technology is the outcome of using this characteristic to collect bioactive substances. Alginate microencapsulation involves creating tiny microspheres that contain the targeted active ingredient. It is possible to use these microspheres to regulate the release of bioactive substances such as vitamins, probiotics, and medications (Nickerson and Paulson 2004b). Because of this, several researchers are looking into other cross-linking technologies, such as interpenetrating network technology and chemical cross-linking (Xie et al. 2024). Because of its nature and specific functional groups, alginate can easily be combined with the biopolymers, namely, collagen, hyaluronic acid, agarose, and chitosan, to generate hydrogels for desired usage at oral and other area as wound healing scaffold/films/sponges (Jiang et al. 2023). In the realm of antibacterial materials, alginate-based solutions are very beneficial due to their absorptivity of liquids and keep the wound surface dry (Khodadadi Yazdi et al. 2020). Hydrogels based on alginate have been used extensively to distribute natural chemicals, proving their adaptability and efficiency in a range of applications (Guastaferro et al. 2021).

Carrageenan-Based Gel

Carrageenan is often used in the manufacturing of hydrogel because of its well-known rheological characteristics. The resulting gels can be reversed both thermally and ionically. Potassium ions and other carrageenan cations are crucial to the gel's formation. Additionally, the ability to produce gels is improved by the addition of sugars and polyols (Ninan et al. 2016). Because of their high swelling ratio, gels based on carrageenan are mechanically unstable and brittle in physiological conditions (Kolanthai et al. 2017). It is also widely utilized as a gel former, stabilizer, and thickener in the industrial and pharmaceutical sectors. It is also utilized as a vehicle for the controlled administration of medications and bioactive substances (Ajmal et al. 2019). Alginate/carrageenan microgels actually increase the amount of immunoglobulin released, loading efficiency, and retention.

Agarose-Based Hydrogel

The manufacturing of particles, hydrogels, microcapsules, and microspheres all make extensive use of agarose. In fact, agarose hydrogels are used to construct drug delivery systems because of their hemocompatibility and biocompatibility (Bairagi et al. 2018). Additionally, agarose hydrogels are perfect for loading and controlling drug release in response to different environmental conditions because they are electrically conductive, pH-sensitive, and thermally reversible. This diminishes the adverse effects of the medicine, decreases the need for frequent dosage, and extends the duration of the drug's residence in the body (Bansal et al. 2022).

Furthermore, the ability to modify the features of agarose gelation by chemical modifications allows for the creation of hydrogels with various mechanical and bioactive properties for a range of applications. In biomedical utilizations like tissue engineering, cell therapy, and targeted medication administration of natural substances, agarose is widely utilized. The rheological qualities of AGR gels are intimately linked to the diffusion characteristics of natural chemicals from the gels. Because the double helicoidal structure that forms during gelation is decreased, AGR derivatives with low gelation temperatures allow for faster material administration and a lower storage modulus (Bonde et al. 2018). Drug loading can be achieved by immersing agarose gels in water solutions, which causes them to swell. Once the maximum quantity of drug diffusion has occurred, the swollen hydrogel can be collected.

6.2.2 Nanoparticle

Submicroscopic particles known as nanoparticles can be used as drug delivery vehicles. Better medication dissolvability, regulated discharge, and designated conveyance are some advantages they provide over standard medication conveyance frameworks. Examples of marine biotoxins that have been employed as drug delivery nanoparticles include fucoidan, carrageenan, and agarose. While marine plant polysaccharide nanoparticles have been employed for quality exchange, anti-infective medications, and malignant growth drugs, chitin nanoparticles have been used for the transportation of proteins and peptides (Lira et al. 2011).

Fucoidan-Based Nanoparticles

Researchers have reported utilizing carboxymethylated fucoidan to produce silver nanoparticles (AgNPs) for in vitro anticancer activity. In 2020, Etman and associates assessed *Undaria pinnatifida* fucoidan's ability to inhibit PANC-1 cells. The nanoparticles were created using the ionic interaction technique, and the outcomes showed that they had successfully halted the migration of cancerous cells. Alginate, chitosan, and fucoidan were combined in a similar but complementary way by various scientists to construct bio-multifunctional sponges that promote angiogenesis, hair follicle regeneration, and wound healing (Etman et al. 2020).

Carrageenan-Based Nanoparticle

Shuai Chen and associates developed a co-delivery system combining nanoparticles with a hydrogel shell. The curcumin- and piperine-loaded nanoparticles show efficacy in thermal and photodegradation. Core-shell nanoparticles were summed up as a potential carrier system (Chen et al. 2020).

Agarose-Based Nanoparticle

In 2020, AB Bonhome-Espinosa and colleagues created hydrogel and enclosed new magnetic nanoparticles in fibrin-agarose for cartilage tissue engineering medications. When cultivated on agarose gels, magnetic particles produced better mechanical characteristics. The significant potential of magnetic hydrogel for cartilage tissue engineering was demonstrated (Bonhome-Espinosa et al. 2020).

6.2.3 Microspheres

Round particles, microspheres range in width from a few microns to a few millimetres. Because of their unique qualities, including regulated distribution, biodegradability, and biocompatibility, they have been used as DD media (Cheba 2011). Alginate and chitosan are two marine biotoxins that have been studied as drug delivery microsphere transporters. Alginate microspheres have been used for protein transport, malignant growth drugs, and the transportation of chitosan and insulin particles (Fathiraja et al. 2022).

Alginate-Based Microspheres

Scientists observed that adjusting the amounts of sodium alginate and sodium carboxymethyl cellulose polymers was necessary in order to produce mucoadhesive microspheres through the ionic gelation process (Pushpamalar et al. 2021; Essa et al. 2021). Ibuprofen-containing mucoadhesive microspheres were examined for their drug content, manufacturing yield, particle size distribution, entrapment effectiveness, and in vitro drug release (Hariyadi et al. 2019). All batches of mucoadhesive microspheres showed delayed drug release, in accordance with the findings obtained from the in vitro drug release profiles of ibuprofen (Muhamad et al. 2019).

Carrageenan-Based Microspheres

They are frequently used in oral DDSs because of their biocompatibility and thermoresponsive gelling qualities. Derived from red algae (e.g. *Chondrus crispus* and *Kappaphycus alvarezii*), carrageenan forms microspheres through ionic cross-linking with cations like K^+ or Ca^{2+}, enabling pH- and temperature-sensitive drug release. These microspheres exhibit mucoadhesive properties, enhancing gastrointestinal retention for sustained delivery of proteins, peptides, and hydrophobic drugs. Their porous structure allows high drug-loading efficiency, while sulfated groups enable functionalization for targeted therapies, such as folate-conjugated systems for cancer treatment (Chiang et al. 2021). Recent advances include hybrid carrageenan-chitosan microspheres that improve mechanical stability and controlled release kinetics for NSAIDs like indomethacin. Challenges include batch-to-batch variability in algal sources, addressed through standardized extraction protocols. Applications span oral vaccines, wound healing dressings, and localized chemotherapy, with studies demonstrating 72-h sustained release profiles for doxorubicin in breast cancer models (Du et al. 2022).

Fucoidan-Based Microspheres

Fucoidan-based microspheres have gained prominence in drug delivery due to fucoidan's inherent bioactivities, such as anticoagulant and antitumor properties, which can synergize with encapsulated drugs. These microspheres, derived from marine algae, offer biocompatibility and tuneable release, making them suitable for various therapeutic applications (Kidgell et al. 2019b). For instance, fucoidan microspheres can be designed for targeted drug delivery in cancer treatment, enhancing therapeutic outcomes while reducing systemic toxicity. The extraction and processing of fucoidan into microspheres often involve green chemistry approaches to maintain its structural integrity and bioactivity. Ongoing research emphasizes optimizing these microspheres for improved stability and targeted delivery (Wan et al. 2021).

Ulvan-Based Microspheres

Ulvan, a sulfated polysaccharide extracted from green seaweeds, presents a promising material for microsphere fabrication due to its biocompatibility and potential for drug delivery. Kidgell et al. (2019a, b, c) in *Algal Research* reviewed ulvan's extraction, composition, and function, highlighting its versatility (Bose et al. 2023a). Marine polysaccharides, including ulvan, are detailed regarding their food applications by Venugopal (2011) in *Marine Polysaccharides: Food Applications*. These microspheres can be tailored for controlled release and various biomedical applications, leveraging ulvan's unique structural and biological properties.

6.2.4 Dental Treatment Gels

Marine plant polysaccharides—including alginate, chitosan, agarose, and carrageenan—are increasingly recognized as valuable components in dental treatment gels for oral drug delivery. Their widespread use is attributed to their excellent biocompatibility, mucoadhesive properties, and ability to provide controlled and sustained drug release, making them particularly effective in addressing a variety of oral health challenges.

Alginate, derived from brown algae, is a staple in dental gels due to its stability, viscosity, and safety profile. Its polyanionic nature enables strong adhesion to the oral mucosa, facilitating effective drug retention and prolonged therapeutic action. For example, sodium alginate gels have been shown to alleviate pain and accelerate healing in recurrent aphthous ulcers by maintaining drug presence at the lesion site. Alginate hydrogels also serve as scaffolds for biomimetic mineralization, inducing hydroxyapatite formation that occludes dentinal tubules and reduces dentin hypersensitivity. Moreover, alginate's fluidity and plasticity make it the material of choice for dental impression gels in prosthodontics and orthodontics, providing accurate oral models for treatment planning (Karthikeyan et al. 2022).

Agarose, extracted from red algae, is a linear polymer known for its thermoresponsive gelation and biocompatibility. In dental applications, agarose hydrogels are used to induce hydroxyapatite deposition on demineralized dentin, offering a novel approach to remineralization and hypersensitivity treatment. Agarose's porous structure also makes it suitable as a matrix for the sustained release of antimicrobial or anti-inflammatory agents in periodontal pockets, ensuring prolonged therapeutic action at the site of disease.

Carrageenan, another red algae-derived polysaccharide, is prized for its gel-forming capacity and is used in dental gels and mucoadhesive films to enhance drug retention, especially in conditions like oral mucositis. Carrageenan gels have also demonstrated potential as antiviral agents, capable of inhibiting pathogens such as herpes simplex virus within the oral cavity. Furthermore, ι-carrageenan-based gels have been formulated for the sustained oral delivery of drugs like acetaminophen, offering both ease of administration and prolonged therapeutic effects for patients with swallowing difficulties (Li and Li 2021).

6.2.5 Carriers for DDSs

Polysaccharide-based multi-particulates can act as the carriers for controlled drug release at targeted sites, responding to stimuli such as pH or temperature. Fucoidans have been integrated into nanostructures for therapeutic applications like cancer treatment and inflammation control (Yang et al. 2022). Carrageenan, extracted from red algae, exhibits thermoresponsive gelation, forming gels at body temperature. This property is exploited in the development of in situ gelling systems for oral, nasal, or buccal drug administration, where the formulation remains liquid at room temperature and gels upon contact with mucosal surfaces, thereby prolonging drug residence time and enhancing absorption (Miyazaki et al. 2011).

6.2.6 Neurodegenerative Disease Applications

Because of their anti-inflammatory and antioxidant qualities, polysaccharides like fucoidan have demonstrated promise in the treatment of neurodegenerative illnesses (Venugopal 2011; Syed et al. 2022).

6.2.7 Coatings for Targeted Delivery at Colonic Region

The delivery of medications to specifically target the colon is vital for the treatment of localized gastrointestinal diseases such as ulcerative colitis, Crohn's disease, and colorectal cancer. Marine polysaccharides contain properties that make them ideally suited for the development of advanced coating systems that achieve targeted drug release in the colon via ODDSs. These polymers can be used to design pH-sensitive, enzyme-sensitive, or time-dependent coatings that provide protection to the active drug as it moves through the upper gastrointestinal tract. In the pH-sensitive case, polysaccharides, such as alginate and carrageenan, maintain stability in the acidic stomach but dissolve or swell in the alkaline pH of the colon, resulting in release only when desired. On the other hand, enzyme-sensitive coatings use the unique enzymatic action of intestinal bacteria. Polysaccharides like fucoidan and ulvan are not digested in the upper GI tract, but rather digested by gut microbiota-generated enzymes and can release drug in the colon (D'Ayala et al. 2008). This is particularly useful in targeted therapy of inflammation or cancer in the lower intestine. Time-controlled delivery methods are more ubiquitous for these systems and are based on expected passage time through the stomach and small intestine. These systems, similar to the previously described types, also use polysaccharide coatings that slowly disintegrate and provide a period of lag before delivery occurs to coincide with expected arrival to the colon. Since marine polysaccharides are biocompatible, biodegradable, and versatile, they are ideal candidates for development of safe and effective colon-targeted drug delivery systems (Zhu et al. 2024).

7 Benefits of MPPs in Oral Delivery of Formulations

The oral route of therapeutic administration is the most popular and widely accepted method because it is simple and economical and results in high patient compliance. Polysaccharides derived from marine plants are of interest as components of oral dosage forms because they have unique physicochemical and biological properties. One of the most important features of the natural polymers is biocompatibility and lack of toxicity. Polysaccharides including alginate, carrageenan, agar, ulvan, and fucoidan sourced from edible marine algae present little safety risk because they are considered generally recognized as safe (GRAS) by regulatory agencies and have little risk of adverse immunological reactions to toxicity. Their gentle interaction with biological tissues makes them suitable for long-term therapeutic use and in patients who are immunologically weakened or have sensitive gastrointestinal conditions (De Anda-Flores et al. 2021). Aside from safety, marine polysaccharides demonstrate excellent biodegradability. Once ingested, they slowly degrade to harmless monosaccharides (or are metabolized by natural mechanisms, in the human body or by intestinal bacteria)—ensuring minimal accumulation or environmental harm. They have the additional advantage of being obtained from renewable marine resources, like seaweeds, which are an eco-favourable alternative to synthetic polymers (Lai et al. 2009). Algal cultivation has a minor environmental impact, as it requires no natural habitat or freshwater—so it is regarded as a sustainable source of biopolymers. Another major benefit is the ability of marine polysaccharides to increase bioavailability of orally administered drugs. Many marine polysaccharides not only improve drug solubility but also protect drugs from being degraded in the stomach early and promote absorption in the intestine. Some components such as fucoidan and alginate can exhibit mucoadhesive properties, which allow them to stay longer at the site of absorption, therefore improving therapeutic effect. These polymers can also form hydrogels or nanoparticles that permit sustained and targeted release, thereby improving the amount of drug that actually reaches systemic circulation and reducing the frequency of doses and side effects. Overall, these characteristics make plant-based marine polysaccharides extremely useful for improving the efficacy and sustainability of oral drug delivery systems (Cui et al. 2021).

8 Obstacles and Constraints

Although plant-derived marine polysaccharides show great potential as oral drug delivery systems, there are significant challenges and limitations that must be resolved to allow for widespread use and commercialization. These challenges are largely related to stability, standardization, and regulatory issues that can impact the efficacy, consistency, and safety of polysaccharide-based drug delivery systems (Kurl et al. 2023).

8.1 Stability and Shelf-Life Issues

One of the major challenges involved with utilizing marine polysaccharides for oral drug delivery remains stability over time. These natural biopolymers are often hygroscopic, particularly polysaccharides derived from marine sources, in that they are capable of absorbing moisture from the surrounding environment. This property can influence the physical properties of the polysaccharide, influencing viscosity, gelling characteristics, and the released profile and bioavailability of the drug being encapsulated in the polymer (Wen et al. 2015). Due to exposure to the external environment, while also considering specific external variables such as temperature, humidity, light, and oxygen, the shelf-life of polysaccharide formulations can also be exigent, since the external environment can engage degradation/deterioration of the polymer structure limiting their functionality, consistency, and drug release over time (Lindequist 2016).

Furthermore, many marine polysaccharides, especially those with high levels of sulfate like carrageenan or fucoidan, are at risk of microbial contamination during processing or storage, which diminishes their shelf-life (Cockburn and Koropatkin 2016). Many manufacturers strictly adhere to a diligent formulation process when using stabilizers or protective packaging and temperature control to improve their formulations' stability and storage life. It is critical to understand and control the environmental factors affecting stability to create reliable drug delivery systems based on marine polysaccharides with consistent efficacy throughout their shelf-life (Anisha et al. 2022).

8.2 Standardization and Quality Assurance

The standardization of marine polysaccharides presents a great challenge. In terms of biochemical composition, polysaccharides demonstrate heterogeneity, which can be dependent on a variety of factors, for example, algal species, geographical origin, and harvesting time. Oceanic polysaccharides can thus manifest significant differences in molecular weight, degree of branching, and sulfation as a result of various chemical changes affecting properties like gelation, swelling, and drug release. The unpredictability involved with the standardization of marine polysaccharides means that reproducible and consistently high-quality formulations can be difficult to develop (Jiang et al. 2024).

In pharmaceutical settings, specifically for oral drug delivery, it is critical to achieve consistent characteristics in polysaccharide material between and among many production batches. These actions require development of robust methods for characterization and/or quantification of the relevant chemical and physical characteristics of marine polysaccharides, including molecular weight distributions, degree of sulfation, and gel strength. Quality control procedures must be established to ensure compliance of each batch with required purity and performance specifications. These procedures are matched with standardized extraction and processing methods to minimize variability and ensure that final dosage forms demonstrate consistency and reliability in their performance. A major element for ensuring batch consistency is evaluating the consistency between production batches of marine polysaccharide-based drug delivery systems, thus ensuring that they meet rigorous requirements for clinical applications (Szymańska and Winnicka 2015).

8.3 Regulatory and Safety Issues

Regulatory and safety issues are a challenging barrier to the continued development and commercialization of marine polysaccharide-mediated drug delivery systems. Even though many marine polysaccharides, such as alginate and carrageenan, are recognized as safe (GRAS) or generally safe for many products, they still have to go through an industry process to get regulatory approval when they are included in a pharmaceutical formulation. The regulatory process for new drug delivery systems is complex and varies from country to country and region to region, with local regulatory requirements and international regulations to follow (Bose et al. 2023b).

A major challenge is the lack of in-depth toxicology data for some of the marine polysaccharides, particularly those that have not been studied in clinical settings. Regulatory bodies will require detailed preclinical studies, including acute and chronic toxicity, genotoxicity, and longer-term safety studies before allowing the use of drug formulation using these components. The biocompatibility of these materials must be well-studied to show they do not evoke a negative immune response or irritate the gastrointestinal tract when used as a drug carrier (Quitério et al. 2021).

There has been a lot of interest in the field of varied drug delivery systems due to the special properties of marine plant-based polysaccharides, such as their biocompatibility, biodegradability, and ability to form a range of forms that can improve medicine absorption and efficacy (Long et al. 2016). A summary of the several marine polysaccharides, their sources, the regulatory bodies that regulate their usage, acceptance standards, and drug delivery applications are depicted in Table 1.

A wide variety of marine polysaccharides on the above list demonstrate how they may be used in different medication delivery strategies. Because of its distinct qualities, each polysaccharide is appropriate for a certain use. Alginate, for example, is well known for its capacity to create hydrogels that efficiently encapsulate medications. Furthermore, the regulatory environment pertaining to these polysaccharides is essential to guaranteeing their safe application. Acceptance criteria that emphasize biocompatibility, biodegradability, safety evaluations, and adherence to good manufacturing procedures have been set by regulatory bodies including the FDA and EMA. These standards maximize therapeutic efficacy while preserving the integrity of pharmaceutical products. Utilizing marine-derived polysaccharides has several benefits, such as their non-toxicity, affordability because of their wide availability, and formulation flexibility. They are perfect candidates for creating cutting-edge drug delivery systems that can increase bioavailability while reducing negative effects because of these qualities.

Additionally, many of the marine polysaccharides do not have enough regulatory documentation for their use in drug delivery systems, which could add additional time to their approval. The use of new delivery systems that use marine biopolymers will necessitate the completing of clinical studies to determine safety, efficacy, and bioavailability in humans. Besides safety concerns, the regulatory aspects for quality assurance and traceability of the marine polysaccharides will need to demonstrate thorough documentation of their source and methods of extraction to fulfil the requirements of regulatory agency standards. In order to establish the safety and efficacy of marine polysaccharides for drug delivery applications and to address the regulatory and safety concerns regarding marine polysaccharides, further research and clinical trials are needed to demonstrate the long-term safety and efficacy of developing marine polysaccharides. Furthermore, engaging with relevant regulatory agencies to develop clear guidelines and standardized testing methods for marine polysaccharides would allow for the potential translations into clinical practice (Lahaye et al. 2007).

Table 1 The regulatory body that sets acceptable standards for marine plant-based polysaccharides in medicine delivery

Marine plant-based polysaccharide	Source	Regulatory authority	Acceptance criteria	Applications in drug delivery	References
Alginate	Brown algae (Phaeophyceae)	FDA, EMA, PMDA, CDSCO	Biocompatibility and biodegradability Quality control measures required	Used in hydrogels and controlled release systems Effective for encapsulating drugs and proteins	Choudhury et al. (2025)
Carrageenan	Red algae (*Rhodophyta*)	FDA, EMA, TGA	Safety assessments including allergenicity Compliance with GMP	Utilized in oral drug delivery and as a thickening agent in formulations	Wang et al. (2024)
Fucoidan	Brown seaweeds	FDA, EMA, CDSCO	Evaluation of safety and efficacy Must meet specific quality standards for human use	Applications in cancer therapy and as an immunomodulator; enhances drug absorption	Lee and Mooney (2011)
Agarose	Red algae	FDA, EMA	Free from contaminants Quality control measures required for gel formation	Widely used in gel electrophoresis and as a matrix for drug delivery systems	Geng et al. (2024)
Ulvan	Green algae (*Ulva* spp.)	FDA, EMA	Safety evaluations required Must meet specific quality standards	Applications include drug delivery systems due to its gel-forming properties	Barbosa et al. (2019c)
Sulfated fucans	Brown algae	FDA, EMA	Must demonstrate low toxicity Compliance with GMP standards	Used for targeted drug delivery and as anticoagulants	Da Silva et al. (2018)
Kappa-carrageenan	Red algae	FDA, EMA	Must demonstrate safety for human use Quality control measures needed	Commonly used as a thickener and stabilizer in various types of pharmaceutical formulations	Hafiza et al. (2023)

Lambda-carrageenan	Red algae	FDA, EMA	Safety assessments required Compliance with GMP	Utilized in gel formulations for sustained release of various drugs using suitable cross-linkers	FDA (2018)
Sodium alginate	Brown seaweed	FDA, EMA	Must meet safety regulations for food additives Quality checks required	Used for encapsulating live cells, compatible probiotics, and various drugs via oral administration	Boychenko et al. (2024)
Agar	Red algae	FDA, EMA	Must be free from contaminants Quality control measures required	Utilized as the nutritive component in microbiological culture media and polymeric substance for oral delivery of various molecules	Hathcock and Shao (2006)

9 Recent Developments and Case Analyses

Recent advancements in marine polysaccharides from plants for oral drug delivery have brought cutting-edge new delivery systems such as stimuli-responsive hydrogels, mucoadhesive nanocarriers, and smart biopolymer-based systems that can respond to pH, enzymes, or ionic triggers in the gastrointestinal tract. These innovative formulations not only offer more targeted delivery and better bioavailability but also they may allow for a lower dosing frequency, an important consideration for patients. Clinical studies of marine polysaccharide formulations are in the rise for delivery systems evaluating everything from colonic inflammation treatments to therapeutics for cancer treatment. Results from early-phase clinical studies are promising, indicating an improvement in patient outcomes and tolerance with marine polysaccharide formulations showing reduced unwanted side effects compared to existing pharmaceuticals on the market today (Pomin et al. 2008). With increased interest in using marine polysaccharides in both nutraceutical and pharmaceutical applications, there has also been an increase in intellectual property activity associated with these developments with new patents being filed not only for employing marine polysaccharides in drug formulations but also new polysaccharide derivatives, modified release systems, and hybrid composites with synthetic polymers. With the growing interest in using polysaccharides, there has also been an increase in companies both nutraceutical and pharmaceutical that are using marine polysaccharides in system products such as functional capsules, matrix tablets, and oral films. Furthermore, the natural origin, safety, and sustainability of marine polysaccharides are all attractive elements from an industry perspective for developing new health products for consumers (Cotas et al. 2024).

10 Challenges and Future Prospects

10.1 Challenges in Marine Plant-Based Polysaccharides for ODDs

The biocompatibility and natural availability of marine-based polysaccharides make them very promising for drug delivery applications; yet, a number of obstacles prevent their widespread use. Due to variations in species, ambient conditions, and extraction methods, one of the main problems is their structural variability and batch-to-batch inconsistency. These discrepancies can have a major effect on the molecular weight and composition of the functional groups, which can cause problems with formulation scalability and repeatability. Furthermore, the mechanical strength and stability of many marine polysaccharide-based hydrogels under physiological settings are insufficient, which restricts their use in load-bearing or long-term drug release systems. These materials' hydrophilicity makes it more difficult to construct controlled release systems and frequently leads to early medication leakage. Furthermore, the presence of environmental pollutants or impurities in marine sources might cause hazardous or immunogenic reactions, requiring strict purification procedures. Lastly, inconsistent product development and regulatory approval are hampered by the lack of standardized extraction, characterization, and quality control procedures; further difficulties are listed in Table 2. Successful integration of marine polysaccharides into contemporary drug delivery systems will depend on addressing these complex issues through focused research, strict standardization, and improved material engineering.

10.2 Future Prospects and Opportunities

The future for marine polysaccharides from plants in oral drug delivery is very bright, due to the ongoing advancements in biopolymer engineering, structure modification, and functionalization techniques to enhance performance and flexibility. Additionally, developments in nanotechnology are helping produce nanoparticles and nanogels, based on marine polysaccharides, with drug loading and targeted delivery capabilities. With artificial intelligence (AI) being employed to advance formulation development, predict drug release rates, and customize therapy for individual patients, it's certainly an exciting time for the field.

Marine plant-based polysaccharides have a bright future in medication delivery methods, with several creative avenues influencing their development. Sulfation and acetylation are two examples of chemical modification and functionalization processes that are increasing their physicochemical properties, which in turn improve stability, controlled release behaviour, and drug loading efficiency. Another revolutionary development is the incorporation of nanotechnology, which makes it possible to use these biopolymers in the creation of nanocarriers such as nanoparticles and nanogels. Table 3 depicts the future prospects of various types of MPPs in suitable ODDSs of various molecules based on their compatibilities and desire functionalities. These formulations can greatly increase bioavailability and facilitate targeted delivery. Additionally, accurate, site-specific, and on-demand medication release in response to environmental triggers like pH, temperature, or enzyme activity is made possible by the invention of stimuli-responsive systems using marine polysaccharides. In tissue engineering and regenerative medicine, these polysaccharides are also becoming more popular because they operate as biocompatible scaffolds that promote tissue healing and cell proliferation. Furthermore, because they are renewable and biodegradable, they may be used as environmentally benign substitutes for synthetic polymers, supporting sustainable pharmaceutical development and green chemistry. The enormous potential of marine polysaccharides in next-generation biological applications is highlighted by these developments taken together.

Also, the inherently renewable and biodegradable nature of marine polysaccharides aligns well with the global drive for sustainable healthcare. As eco-sustainable approaches increase, the pharmaceutical industry is steadily integrating marine polysaccharides as sustainable substitutes for synthetic excipients, facilitating an eco-sustainable drug delivery system that reduces ecological consequence while maintaining therapeutic activity.

Table 2 Various challenges in marine plant-based polysaccharides for ODDSs

Category	Challenges	References
Extraction and purity	Variation in quality depending on the source and season Need for standardized and scalable purification processes Presence of impurities that may affect biocompatibility	Alharbi (2024)
Structural variability	Heterogeneity in molecular weight and composition Batch-to-batch inconsistency, impacting reproducibility Complexity in understanding structure-activity relationships	Alsaikhan and Farhood (2024)
Mechanical limitations	Poor mechanical strength (in hydrogels or films) Limited elasticity for injectable or load-bearing applications Need for blending with other polymers	Kidgell et al. (2019c)
Drug loading and release	Uncontrolled drug release (burst effect) Limited encapsulation efficiency for hydrophobic drugs Difficulty in tuning release profiles for sustained delivery	Samalens et al. (2022)
Regulatory and safety	Lack of global harmonization in regulatory approvals Need for extensive toxicity and immunogenicity data Limited number of marine polysaccharides with GRAS status	Jacob et al. (2018c)
Stability and storage	Susceptibility to degradation under physiological conditions Requirement for cold storage or protective formulations pH- or ion-sensitive behaviour affecting stability	Martins et al. (2014b)
Cost and sustainability	High production costs of marine polysaccharide-based systems Environmental impact of large-scale harvesting Limited commercial supply chain infrastructure	https://www.fda.gov/science-research/fda-stem-outreach-education-and-engagement

Table 3 Details of the future prospects and opportunities of MPPs for ODDSs

Various areas	Prospective advances	References
Nanotechnology integration	Design of marine polysaccharide-based nanoparticles and nanogels Targeted and responsive drug delivery systems Co-delivery of multiple therapeutics (e.g. drugs + siRNA)	Atanase et al. (2017)
Stimuli-responsive systems	Smart hydrogels responding to pH, enzymes, or temperature Site-specific drug release (e.g. tumour, colon) Integration with biosensors for theragnostics	Bai et al. (2022)
3D bioprinting and injectable hydrogels	Marine polysaccharides as bioinks for tissue engineering Injectable formulations for wound healing or joint therapy Personalized DDS via additive manufacturing	Khrunyk et al. (2020)
Hybrid materials	Blending with chitosan, synthetic polymers, or peptides Improved mechanical, mucoadhesive, and release properties Use in transdermal, nasal, ocular, and oral DDS	Oyervides-Muñoz et al. (2022)
Regulatory advancement	Development of region-specific pharmacopeial monographs Expanded GRAS and pharmaceutically approved lists Enhanced collaboration with FDA, EMA, and WHO	Singh and Lillard (2009)
Marine biotechnology and sustainability	Cultivation of seaweeds in eco-friendly systems Genetic engineering of marine algae for high-yield production Circular bioeconomy models for marine biomass use	Riess (2003)

References

Benalaya I, Alves G, Lopes J, Silva LR (2024) A Review of Natural Polysaccharides: Sources, Characteristics, Properties, Food, and Pharmaceutical Applications. Int J Mol Sci 25(2):1322. https://doi.org/10.3390/ijms25021322.

Prasher P, Sharma M, Mehta M, Satija S, Aljabali AA, Tambuwala MM, et al (2021) Current-status and applications of polysaccharides in drug delivery systems. Colloid Interface Sci Commun 42: 100418. https://doi.org/10.1016/j.colcom.2021.100418

Homayun B, Lin X, Choi HJ (2019) Challenges and Recent Progress in Oral Drug Delivery Systems for Biopharmaceuticals. Pharmaceutics 11(3):129. https://doi.org/10.3390/pharmaceutics11030129

Chaudhary S, Jain VP, Jaiswar G (2022) The composition of polysaccharides: monosaccharides and binding, group decorating, polysaccharides chains. In: Innovation in Nano-Polysaccharides for Eco-sustainability. p. 83–118. https://doi.org/10.1016/B978-0-12-823439-6.00005-2

Vieira WT, Nicollini MVS, Da Silva MGC, De Oliveira Nascimento L, Vieira MGA (2022) Natural polysaccharides and proteins applied to the development of gastroresistant multiparticulate systems for anti-inflammatory drug delivery—a systematic review. EurPolym J172:111205.. https://doi.org/10.1016/j.eurpolymj.2022.111205

Teixeira MC, Lameirinhas NS, Carvalho JPF, Silvestre AJD, Vilela C, Freire CSR (2022) A Guide to Polysaccharide-Based Hydrogel Bioinks for 3D Bioprinting Applications. Int J Mol Sci 23(12):6564. https://doi.org/10.3390/ijms23126564

Maheshwari S, Singh A, Varshney AP, Sharma A (2024) Advancing oral drug delivery: The science of fast dissolving tablets (FDTs). Intell Pharm 2(4):580–7. https://doi.org/10.1016/j.ipha.2024.01.011

Luo Y, Wang Q (2014) Recent development of chitosan-based polyelectrolyte complexes with natural polysaccharides for drug delivery. Int J Biol Macromol 64:353–67. https://doi.org/10.1016/j.ijbiomac.2013.12.017

Beneke CE, Viljoen AM, Hamman JH (2009) Polymeric Plant-derived Excipients in Drug Delivery. Molecules 14(7):2602–20. https://doi.org/10.3390/molecules14072602

Jansen C, Baker JD, Kodaira E, Ang L, Bacani AJ, Aldan JT, et al (2021) Medicine in motion: Opportunities, challenges and data analytics-based solutions for traditional medicine integration into western medical practice. J Ethnopharmacol 267:113477. https://doi.org/10.1016/j.jep.2020.113477

Baranov N, Popa M, Atanase LI, Ichim DL (2021) Polysaccharide-Based Drug Delivery Systems for the Treatment of Periodontitis. Molecules 26(9):2735. https://doi.org/10.3390/molecules26092735

Di Sotto A, Vitalone A, Di Giacomo S (2020) Plant-Derived Nutraceuticals and Immune System Modulation: An Evidence-Based Overview. Vaccines 8(3):468. https://doi.org/10.3390/vaccines8030468

Sekinat Olayem B, Babawande Olaitan O, Badiu Akinola A (2024) Immunomodulatory Plant Based Foods, It's Chemical, Biochemical and Pharmacological Approaches. In: Santana De Oliveira M, Helena De Aguiar Andrade E, Kumar R, N. Mali S, editors. J. Med. Plant Res. and J. Herb. https://doi.org/10.5772/intechopen.112406

Laurienzo P (2010) Marine Polysaccharides in Pharmaceutical Applications: An Overview. Mar. Drugs 8(9):2435–65. https://doi.org/10.3390/md8092435

Nickerson MT, Paulson AT. Rheological properties of gellan, κ-carrageenan and alginate polysaccharides: effect of potassium and calcium ions on macrostructure assemblages. CarbohydrPolym. 2004a;58(1):15–24. https://doi.org/10.1016/j.carbpol.2004.02.003

Lee YE, Kim H, Seo C, Park T, Lee KB, Yoo SY, et al (2017) Marine polysaccharides: therapeutic efficacy and biomedical applications. Arch Pharm Res 40(9):1006–20.

Drew Km (1955) Life histories in the algae with special reference to the Chlorophyta, Phaeophyta and Rhodophyta. Biological Reviews, 30(4), 343–387. https://doi.org/10.1111/j.1469-185X.1955.tb01544.x

Alves A, Sousa RA, Reis RL (2013) A practical perspective on ulvan extracted from green algae. J Appl Phycol 25(2):407–24. https://doi.org/10.1007/s10811-012-9875-4

Gabrielson PW, Garbary D, Hommersand MH (1986) Systematics of red algae (Rhodophyta). Crit Rev Plant Sci 3(4):325–66. https://doi.org/10.1080/07352688609382215

Kraan S (2012) Algal Polysaccharides, Novel Applications and Outlook. In: Chang CF, editor. Carbohydrates—Comprehensive Studies on Glycobiology and Glycotechnology. Available from: http://www.intechopen.com/books/carbohydrates-comprehensive-studies-on-glycobiology-and-glycotechnology/algal-polysaccharides-novel-applications-and-outlook

Hahn, T., Lang, S., Ulber, R., & Muffler, K (2012) Novel procedures for the extraction of fucoidan from brown algae. Process Biochemistry, 47(12), 1691–1698. https://doi.org/10.1016/j.procbio.2012.06.016

Hanisak, M. D(1998) Seaweed cultivation: Global trends. World Aquaculture, 29(2), 18–21. https://doi.org/10.1023/A:1008114112852

Harding SE, Tombs MP, Adams GG, Paulsen BS, Inngjerdingen KT, Barsett H. An Introduction to Polysaccharide Biotechnology [Internet]. 2nd ed. Second edition / Stephen E. Harding [and five others]. | Boca: CRC Press; 2017a [cited 2025 May 7]. Available from: https://www.taylorfrancis.com/books/9781482248326

Imeson, A. (2009) Agar. In A. Imeson (Ed.), Food stabilisers, thickeners and gelling agent. Wiley-Blackwell pp.31–49. https://doi.org/10.1002/9781444314724.ch3

Jacob, J., Haponiuk, J. T., Thomas, S., & Gopi, S. (2018a) Biopolymer based nanomaterials in drug delivery systems: A review. Materials Today Chemistry, 9, 43–55. https://doi.org/10.1016/j.mtchem.2018.05.002

Kadam, S. U., Tiwari, B. K., & O'Donnell, C. P. (2015) Extraction, structure and biofunctional activities of laminarin from brown algae. International Journal of Food Science & Technology, 50(1), 24–31. https://doi.org/10.1111/ijfs.12692

Keeling, P. J. (2004) Diversity and evolutionary history of plastids and their hosts. American Journal of Botany, 91(10), 1481–1493. https://doi.org/10.3732/ajb.91.10.1481

Kidgell, J. T., Magnusson, M., De Nys, R., & Glasson, C. R. (2019a) Ulvan: A systematic review of extraction, composition and function. Algal Research, 39, 101422. https://doi.org/10.1016/j.algal.2019.101422

Kong, D. X., Jiang, Y. Y., & Zhang, H. Y. (2010) Marine natural products as sources of novel scaffolds: Achievement and concern. Drug Discovery Today, 15(19–20), 884–886. https://doi.org/10.1016/j.drudis.2010.09.002

Martins, A., Vieira, H., Gaspar, H., & Santos, S. (2014) Marketed marine natural products in the pharmaceutical and cosmeceutical industries: Tips for success. Marine Drugs, 12(2), 1066–1101. https://doi.org/10.3390/md12021066

McHugh, D. J. (2003) A guide to the seaweed industry (FAO Fisheries Technical Paper No. 441). Food and Agriculture Organization of the United Nations.

Misiurova, L., Orsavova, J., & Ambrozova, J. V. (2014) Algal polysaccharides and health. In Polysaccharides (pp. 1–29). Springer. https://doi.org/10.1007/978-3-319-16298-0_24

Molinski, T. F., Dalisay, D. S., Lievens, S. L., & Saludes, J. P. (2009) Drug development from marine natural products. Nature Reviews Drug Discovery, 8(1), 69–85. https://doi.org/10.1038/nrd2487

Mortensen, A., Aguilar, F., Crebelli, R., Di Domenico, A., Frutos, M. J., Galtier, P., Gott, D., Gundert-Remy, U., Lambré, C., Leblanc, J. C., et al. (2016) Re-evaluation of agar (E 406) as a food additive. EFSA Journal, 14(4), e04645. https://doi.org/10.2903/j.efsa.2016.4645

Muhammad, I. I., Zulkifli, N., Selvakumaran, S. A., & Lazim, N. A. M. (2019) Marine-derived bioactive compounds as potential anticancer agents. Current Pharmaceutical Design, 25(11), 1147–1162. https://doi.org/10.2174/1381612825666190618152133

Munro, M. H., Blunt, J. W., Dumdei, E. J., Hickford, S. J., Lill, R. E., Li, S., Battershill, C. N., & Duckworth, A. R. (1999) The discovery and development of marine compounds with pharmaceutical potential. Journal of Biotechnology, 70(1–3), 15–25. https://doi.org/10.1016/S0168-1656(99)00054-0

National Oceanic and Atmospheric Administration. (2025) What are phytoplankton? https://oceanservice.noaa.gov/facts/phytoplankton.html

Ngo, D. H., & Kim, S. K. (2013) Sulfated polysaccharides as bioactive agents from marine algae. International Journal of Biological Macromolecules, 62, 70–75. https://doi.org/10.1016/j.ijbiomac.2013.08.036

Nussinovitch, A. (1997) Hydrocolloid applications: Gum technology in the food and other industries. Springer. https://doi.org/10.1007/978-1-4615-6385-3

Pangestuti, R., & Kim, S. K. (2014) Biological activities of carrageenan. Advances in Food and Nutrition Research, 72, 113–124. https://doi.org/10.1016/B978-0-12-800269-8.00007-5

Pereira, L. (2018) Seaweeds as source of bioactive substances and skin care therapy—Cosmeceuticals, algotherapy, and thalassotherapy. Cosmetics, 5(4), 68. https://doi.org/10.3390/cosmetics5040068

Peteiro, C., Sánchez, N., & Martínez, B. (2016) Mariculture of the Asian kelp Undaria pinnatifida and the native kelp Saccharina latissima along the Atlantic coast of southern Europe: An overview. Algal Research, 15, 9–23. https://doi.org/10.1016/j.algal.2016.01.012

Xu SY, Huang X, Cheong KL (2017) Recent Advances in Marine Algae Polysaccharides: Isolation, Structure, and Activities. Mar Drugs 15(12):388. https://doi.org/10.3390/md15120388

Notararigo S, Nácher-Vázquez M, Ibarburu I, Werning ML, De Palencia PF, Dueñas MT, et al (2013) Comparative analysis of production and purification of homo- and hetero-polysaccharides produced by lactic acid bacteria. Carbohydr Polym 93(1):57–64. https://doi.org/10.1016/j.carbpol.2012.05.016

Nagahawatta DP, Liyanage NM, Jayawardena TU, Yang F, Jayawardena HHACK, Kurera MJMS, et al. (2023) Functions and values of sulfated polysaccharides from seaweed. Algae 38(4): 217–40. https://doi.org/10.4490/algae.2023.38.12.1

Harding SE, Tombs MP, Adams GG, Paulsen BS, Inngjerdingen KT, Barsett H. (2017b) An Introduction to Polysaccharide Biotechnology [Internet]. 2nd ed. Second edition / Stephen E. Harding [and five others]. Boca: CRC Press; Available from: https://www.taylorfrancis.com/books/9781482248326

Jönsson M, Allahgholi L, Sardari RRR, Hreggviðsson GO, Nordberg Karlsson E. (2020) Extraction and Modification of Macroalgal Polysaccharides for Current and Next-Generation Applications. Molecules 25(4):930. https://doi.org/10.3390/molecules25040930

Sun Y, Hou S, Song S, Zhang B, Ai C, Chen X, et al. (2018) Impact of acidic, water and alkaline extraction on structural features, antioxidant activities of Laminaria japonica polysaccharides. Int J Biol Macromol 112:985–95. https://doi.org/10.1016/j.ijbiomac.2018.02.066

Dobrinčić A, Balbino S, Zorić Z, Pedisić S, Bursać Kovačević D, Elez Garofulić I, et al. (2020) Advanced Technologies for the Extraction of Marine Brown Algal Polysaccharides. Mar Drugs 18(3):168. https://doi.org/10.3390/md18030168

Fleurence J, Massiani L, Guyader O, Mabeau S. (1995) Use of enzymatic cell wall degradation for improvement of protein extraction from Chondrus crispus, Gracilaria verrucosa and Palmaria palmata. J Appl Phycol 7(4):393–7. https://doi.org/10.1007/BF00003796

Mirzadeh M, Arianejad MR, Khedmat L. (2020) Antioxidant, antiradical, and antimicrobial activities of polysaccharides obtained by microwave-assisted extraction method: A review. Carbohydr Polym 229:115421. https://doi.org/10.1016/j.carbpol.2019.115421

Shi L. (2016) Bioactivities, isolation and purification methods of polysaccharides from natural products: A review. Int J Biol Macromol 92:37–48. https://doi.org/10.1016/j.ijbiomac.2016.06.100

Stengel DB, Connan S, Popper ZA. (2011) Algal chemodiversity and bioactivity: Sources of natural variability and implications for commercial application. Biotechnol Adv 29(5):483–501. https://doi.org/10.1016/j.biotechadv.2011.05.016

Stevanović M, Filipović N. (2024) A Review of Recent Developments in Biopolymer Nano-Based Drug Delivery Systems with Antioxidative Properties: Insights into the Last Five Years. Pharmaceutics 16(5):670. https://doi.org/10.3390/pharmaceutics16050670

Silva TH, Alves A, Ferreira BM, Oliveira JM, Reys LL, Ferreira RJF, et al. (2012) Materials of marine origin: a review on polymers and ceramics of biomedical interest. Int Mater Rev 57(5): 276–306. https://doi.org/10.1179/1743280412Y.0000000002

Zayed A, El-Aasr M, Ibrahim ARS, Ulber R. (2020) Fucoidan Characterization: Determination of Purity and Physicochemical and Chemical Properties. Mar Drugs 18(11):571. https://doi.org/10.3390/md18110571

Silva MP, Fabi JP. (2022) Food biopolymers-derived nanogels for encapsulation and delivery of biologically active compounds: A perspective review. Food Hydrocoll Health 2:100079. https://doi.org/10.1016/j.fooh.2022.100079

Juneja A, Ceballos R, Murthy G. (2013) Effects of Environmental Factors and Nutrient Availability on the Biochemical Composition of Algae for Biofuels Production: A Review. Energies 6(9): 4607–38. https://doi.org/10.3390/en6094607

Feng M, Zhang M, Adhikari B, Chang L. (2024) Novel strategies for enhancing quality stability of edible flower during processing using efficient physical fields: A review. Food Chem 448: 139077. https://doi.org/10.1016/j.foodchem.2024.139077

Cardoso M, Costa R, Mano J. (2016) Marine Origin Polysaccharides in Drug Delivery Systems. Mar Drugs 14(2):34. https://doi.org/10.3390/md14020034

Barbosa AI, Coutinho AJ, Costa Lima SA, Reis S. (2019a) Marine Polysaccharides in Pharmaceutical Applications: Fucoidan and Chitosan as Key Players in the Drug Delivery Match Field. Mar Drugs 17(12):654. https://doi.org/10.3390/md17120654

Lin J, Jiao G, Kermanshahi-pour A. (2022) Algal Polysaccharides-Based Hydrogels: Extraction, Synthesis, Characterization, and Applications. Mar Drugs 20(5):306. https://doi.org/10.3390/md20050306

Colombo P, Bettini R, Santi P, De Ascentiis A, Peppas NA. (1996) Analysis of the swelling and release mechanisms from drug delivery systems with emphasis on drug solubility and water transport. J Controlled Release 39(2–3):231–7. https://doi.org/10.1016/0168-3659(95)00158-1

Lukova P, Katsarov P. (2023) Contemporary Aspects of Designing Marine Polysaccharide Microparticles as Drug Carriers for Biomedical Application. Pharmaceutics 15(8):2126. https://doi.org/10.3390/pharmaceutics15082126

Bayer IS. (2022) Recent Advances in Mucoadhesive Interface Materials, Mucoadhesion Characterization, and Technologies. Adv Mater Interfaces 9(18):2200211. https://doi.org/10.1002/admi.202200211

Makarova AO, Derkach SR, Khair T, Kazantseva MA, Zuev YF, Zueva OS. (2023) Ion-Induced Polysaccharide Gelation: Peculiarities of Alginate Egg-Box Association with Different Divalent Cations. Polymers 15(5):1243. https://doi.org/10.3390/polym15051243

Kraithong S, Bunyameen N, Theppawong A, Ke X, Lee S, Zhang X, et al. (2024) Potentials of Ulva spp.-derived sulfated polysaccharides as gelling agents with promising therapeutic effects. Int J Biol Macromol 273:132882. https://doi.org/10.1016/j.ijbiomac.2024.132882

Liu L, Yao W, Rao Y, Lu X, Gao J. (2017) pH-Responsive carriers for oral drug delivery: challenges and opportunities of current platforms. Drug Deliv 24(1):569–81. https://doi.org/10.1080/10717544.2017.1279238

Pacheco-Quito EM, Ruiz-Caro R, Veiga MD. (2020) Carrageenan: Drug Delivery Systems and Other Biomedical Applications. Mar Drugs 18(11):583. https://doi.org/10.3390/md18110583

Citkowska A, Szekalska M, Winnicka K. (2019) Possibilities of Fucoidan Utilization in the Development of Pharmaceutical Dosage Forms. Mar Drugs 17(8):458. https://doi.org/10.3390/md17080458

George M, Abraham TE. (2006) Polyionic hydrocolloids for the intestinal delivery of protein drugs: alginate and chitosan – a review. J Controlled Release 114(1):1–14. https://doi.org/10.1016/j.jconrel.2006.04.017

Sutapa BM, Dhruti A, Gopa RB. (2017) Pharmacological, pharmaceutical, cosmetic and diagnostic applications of sulfated polysaccharides from marine algae and bacteria. Afr J Pharm Pharmacol 11(5):68–77. https://doi.org/10.5897/AJPP2016.4695

Zhang C, Li M, Rauf A, Khalil AA, Shan Z, Chen C, et al. (2023) Process and applications of alginate oligosaccharides with emphasis on health beneficial perspectives. Crit Rev Food Sci Nutr 63(3):303–29. https://doi.org/10.1080/10408398.2021.1946008

Kumar Y, Tarafdar A, Badgujar PC. (2021) Seaweed as a Source of Natural Antioxidants: Therapeutic Activity and Food Applications. El-Sohaimy S, editor. J Food Qual 2021:1–17. https://doi.org/10.1155/2021/5753391

Lee, W.K., Lim, Y.Y., & Ho, C.L. (2022). Gracilaria as the Major Source of Agar for Food, Health and Biotechnology Applications. In A. Ranga Rao & G.A. Ravishankar (Eds.), Sustainable Global Resources of Seaweeds. Springer International Publishing. Volume 2 pp. 145–161.. https://doi.org/10.1007/978-3-030-92174-3_7.

Madany MA, Abdel-Kareem MS, Al-Oufy AK, Haroun M, Sheweita SA. (2021) The biopolymer ulvan from Ulva fasciata: Extraction towards nanofibers fabrication. Int J Biol Macromol 177: 401–12. https://doi.org/10.1016/j.ijbiomac.2021.02.047.

January GG, Naidoo RK, Kirby-McCullough B, Bauer R. Assessing methodologies for fucoidan extraction from South African brown algae. Algal Res. 2019 Jun;40:101517. https://doi.org/10.1016/j.algal.2019.101517.

Pomponi, S. A. (1999) The bioprocess-technological potential of the sea. Journal of Biotechnology 70(1–3), 5–13. https://doi.org/10.1016/S0168-1656(99)00053-9.

Sithranga Boopathy, N., & Kathiresan, K. (2010) Anticancer drugs from marine flora: An overview. Journal of Oncology, 2010, 1–18. https://doi.org/10.1155/2010/214186.

Skják-Bræk, G., & Draget, K. I. (2012) Alginates: Properties and applications. In K. Matyjaszewski & M. Möller (Eds.), Polymer science: A comprehensive reference (Vol. 10, pp. 213–219). Elsevier. https://doi.org/10.1016/B978-0-444-53349-4.00261-2.

Urbán-Morlán, Z., Serrano-Mora, L. E., Martínez-Acevedo, L., Leyva-Gómez, G., Mendoza-Muñoz, N., & Quintanar-Guerrero, D. (2020) New developments in intrauterine drug delivery systems and devices. In Elsevier eBooks (pp. 601–622). https://doi.org/10.1016/b978-0-12-819838-4.00018-3

Zhu, B., Ni, F., Xiong, Q., & Yao, Z. (2021) Marine oligosaccharides originated from seaweeds: Source, preparation, structure, physiological activity, and applications. Critical Reviews in Food Science and Nutrition, 61(1), 60–74. https://doi.org/10.1080/10408398.2020.1716207

I.P. Fernando, W. Lee, E.J. Han, G. Ahn (2020) Alginate-based nanomaterials: fabrication techniques, properties, and applications, Chem. Eng. J 21, 123823, https://doi.org/10.1016/j.cej.2019.123823

Shahiwala A. (2011) Formulation approaches in enhancement of patient compliance to oral drug therapy. Expert Opin Drug Deliv 8(11):1521–9. https://doi.org/10.1517/17425247.2011.628311

Atmaca H, Oguz F, Ilhan S. (2022) Drug Delivery Systems for Cancer Treatment: A Review of Marine-derived Polysaccharides. Curr Pharm Des 28(13):1031–45. https://doi.org/10.2174/1381612828666220211153931

Zhong H, Gao X, Cheng C, Liu C, Wang Q, Han X. (2020) The Structural Characteristics of Seaweed Polysaccharides and Their Application in Gel Drug Delivery Systems. Mar Drugs 18(12):658. https://doi.org/10.3390/md18120658

Negreanu-Pirjol BS, Negreanu-Pirjol T, Popoviciu DR, Anton RE, Prelipcean AM. (2022) Marine Bioactive Compounds Derived from Macroalgae as New Potential Players in Drug Delivery Systems: A Review. Pharmaceutics 4(9):1781. https://doi.org/10.3390/pharmaceutics14091781

Subramanian DA, Langer R, Traverso G. (2022) Mucus interaction to improve gastrointestinal retention and pharmacokinetics of orally administered nano-drug delivery systems. J Nanobiotechnology 20(1):362. https://doi.org/10.1186/s12951-022-01539-x

Azman M, Sabri AH, Anjani QK, Mustaffa MF, Hamid KA. (2022) Intestinal Absorption Study: Challenges and Absorption Enhancement Strategies in Improving Oral Drug Delivery. Pharmaceuticals 15(8):975. https://doi.org/10.3390/ph15080975

Yermak IM, Davydova VN, Volod'ko AV. (2022) Mucoadhesive Marine Polysaccharides. Mar Drugs 20(8):522. https://doi.org/10.3390/md20080522

Yuan H, Guo C, Liu L, Zhao L, Zhang Y, Yin T, et al. (2023) Progress and prospects of polysaccharide-based nanocarriers for oral delivery of proteins/peptides. Carbohydr Polym 312:120838. https://doi.org/10.1016/j.carbpol.2023.120838

S. Toumi, M.M. Yahoum, S. Lefnaoui, A. Hadjsadok, (2021)Synthesis, characterization and potential application of hydrophobically modified carrageenan derivatives as pharmaceutical excipients, Carbohydr. Polym. 2, 116997. https://doi.org/10.1016/j.carbpol.2020.116997

Ganesan, A. R., Saravana Guru, M., Balasubramanian, B., Mohan, K., Chao Liu, W., Valan Arasu, M., Abdullah Al-Dhabi, N., Duraipandiyan, V., Ignacimuthu, S., Sudhakar, M. P., &Seedevi, P. (2020) Biopolymer from edible marine invertebrates: A potential functional food. Fiji Journal of King Saud University—Science, 32(2), 17721777. https://doi.org/10.1016/j.jksus.2020.01.015

Grewal, A. K., Singh, T. G., Sharma, D., Sharma, V., Singh, M., Rahman, M. H., Najda, A., Walasek-Janusz, M., Kamel, M., Albadrani, G. M., Akhtar, M. F., Saleem, A., & Abdel-Daim, M. M. (2021) Mechanistic insights and perspectives involved in neuroprotective action of quercetin. Biomedicine and Pharmacotherapy, 140 https://doi.org/10.1016/j.biopha.2021.111729.

Iliou, K., Kikionis, S., Ioannou, E., & Roussis, V. (2022) Marine biopolymers as bioactive functional ingredients of electrospun nanofibrous scaffolds for biomedical applications. Marine Drugs, 20(5) https://doi.org/10.3390/md20050314.

Ahmed N, Prajapati V, Mishra P, Mishra NTP. (2024) Dosage form Design: From concept to Compliance—Navigating Regulatory Standards and Patient needs. Int J Drug Regul Aff 12(1): 24–35. https://doi.org/10.22270/ijdra.v12i1.647

Santhanes D, Teng LY, Sheng FS, Coombes AGA.(2018) Exploiting the versatility of oral capsule formulations based on high M-alginate for targeted delivery of poorly water soluble drugs to the upper and lower GI tract. J Drug Deliv Sci Technol 46:384–91. https://doi.org/10.1016/j.jddst.2018.04.004

Jacob, J., Haponiuk, J. T., Thomas, S., & Gopi, S. (2018b) Biopolymer based nanomaterials in drug delivery systems: A review. Materials Today Chemistry, 9, 4355 https://doi.org/10.1016/j.mtchem.2018.05.002.

Dhamecha, D.; Movsas, R.; Sano, U.; Menon, J.U. (2019) Applications of alginate microspheres in therapeutics delivery and cell culture: Past, present and future. Int. J. Pharm 569, 118627.

Abasalizadeh, F.; Moghaddam, S.V.; Alizadeh, E.; Akbari, E.; Kashani, E.; Fazljou, S.M.B.; Torbati, M.; Akbarzadeh, A. (2020) Alginate-based hydrogels as drug delivery vehicles in cancer treatment and their applications in wound dressing and 3D bioprinting. J. Biol. Eng 14, 8. https://doi.org/10.1016/j.ijpharm.2019.118627

Bulut, E. (2021) Development and optimization of Fe3+-crosslinked sodium alginate-methylcellulose semi-interpenetrating polymer network beads for controlled release of ibuprofen. Int. J. Biol. Macromol 168, 823–833. https://doi.org/10.1016/j.ijbiomac.2020.11.147

Tomić, S.L.; Babić Radić, M.M.; Vuković, J.S.; Filipović, V.V.; Nikodinovic-Runic, J.; Vukomanović, M. (2023) Alginate-Based Hydrogels and Scaffolds for Biomedical Applications. Mar. Drugs 2023, 21, 177. https://doi.org/10.3390/md21030177

Aderibigbe, B.A.; Buyana, B. (2018)Alginate in Wound Dressings. Pharmaceutics 10, 42. https://doi.org/10.3390/pharmaceutics10020042

Bui, V.T.N.T.; Nguyen, B.T.; Renou, F.; Nicolai, T. (2019) Rheology and microstructure of mixtures of iota and kappa-carrageenan. Food Hydrocoll 89, 180–187. https://doi.org/10.1016/j.foodhyd.2018.10.034

Stenner, R.; Matubayasi, N.; Shimizu, S. (2016) Gelation of carrageenan: Effects of sugars and polyols. Food Hydrocoll 54, 284–292. https://doi.org/10.1016/j.foodhyd.2015.10.007

Thakur, R.; Saberi, B.; Pristijono, P.; Golding, J.; Stathopoulos, C.; Scarlett, C.; Bowyer, M.; Vuong, Q. (2016) Characterization of rice starch-ι-carrageenan biodegradable edible film. Effect of stearic acid on the film properties. Int. J. Biol. Macromol 93, 952–960. https://doi.org/10.1016/j.ijbiomac.2016.09.053

Zhu, M.; Ge, L.; Lyu, Y.; Zi, Y.; Li, X.; Li, D.; Mu, C. (2017) Preparation, characterization and antibacterial activity of oxidized κ-carrageenan. Carbohydr. Polym 174, 1051–1058. https://doi.org/10.1016/j.carbpol.2017.07.029

Barbosa, A. I., Coutinho, A. J., Lima, S. a. C., & Reis, S. (2019b) Marine polysaccharides in pharmaceutical applications: Fucoidan and Chitosan as key players in the drug delivery match field. Marine Drugs, 17(12), 654. https://doi.org/10.3390/md17120654

Pelin, I. M., & Suflet, D. M. (2020) Mucoadhesive buccal drug delivery systems containing polysaccharides. Cellulose Chemistry and Technology 54(9–10) 889–902. https://doi.org/10.35812/cellulosechemtechnol.2020.54.86

Dubashynskaya, N. V., Petrova, V. A., & Skorik, Y. A. (2024) Biopolymer Drug Delivery Systems for Oromucosal Application: Recent Trends in Pharmaceutical R&D. International Journal of Molecular Sciences 25(10), 5359. https://doi.org/10.3390/ijms25105359

Sacramento, M. M. A., Borges, J., Correia, F. J. S., Calado, R., Rodrigues, J. M. M., Patrício, S. G., & Mano, J. F. (2022) Green approaches for extraction, chemical modification and processing of marine polysaccharides for biomedical applications. Frontiers in Bioengineering and Biotechnology, 10. https://doi.org/10.3389/fbioe.2022.1041102

Yuan, H.; Zhang, W.; Li, X.; Lü, X.; Li, N.; Gao, X.; Song, J. (2005) Preparation and in vitro antioxidant activity of kappa-carrageenan oligosaccharides and their oversulfated, acetylated, and phosphorylated derivatives. CarbohydrRes 340, 685–692. https://doi.org/10.1016/j.carres.2004.12.026

Aparna, V.; Melge, A.R.; Rajan, V.K.; Biswas, R.; Jayakumar, R.; Gopi Mohan, C. (2018) Carboxymethylated ι-carrageenan conjugated amphotericin B loaded gelatin nanoparticles for treating intracellular Candida glabrata infections. Int. J. Biol. Macromol 110, 140–149. https://doi.org/10.1016/j.ijbiomac.2017.11.126

Mihaila, S.M.; Gaharwar, A.K.; Reis, R.L.; Marques, A.P.; Gomes, M.E.; Khademhosseini, A. (2013) Photocrosslinkable kappa-carrageenan hydrogels for tissue engineering applications. Adv. Healthc. Mater 2, 895–907. https://doi.org/10.1002/adhm.201200317

Varghese, J.S.; Chellappa, N.; Fathima, N.N. (2014) Gelatin-carrageenan hydrogels: Role of pore size distribution on drug delivery process. Colloids Surf. B Biointerfaces 113, 346–351. https://doi.org/10.1016/j.colsurfb.2013.08.049

Liu, J.; Zhan, X.; Wan, J.; Wang, Y.; Wang, C. (2015) Review for carrageenan-based pharmaceutical biomaterials: Favourable physical features versus adverse biological effects. Carbohydr. Polym 121, 27–36. https://doi.org/10.1016/j.carbpol.2014.11.063

Keppeler, S.; Ellis, A.; Jacquier, J.C. (2009) Cross-linked carrageenan beads for controlled release delivery systems. Carbohydr. Polym 78, 973–977. https://doi.org/10.1016/j.carbpol.2009.07.029

Santo, V.E.; Frias, A.M.; Carida, M.; Cancedda, R.; Gomes, M.E.; Mano, J.F.; Reis, R.L. (2009) Carrageenan-based hydrogels for the controlled delivery of PDGF-BB in bone tissue engineering applications. Biomacromolecules 10, 1392–1401. https://doi.org/10.1021/bm8014973

Frederiksen K, Guy RH, Petersson K. (2015) Formulation considerations in the design of topical, polymeric film-forming systems for sustained drug delivery to the skin. Eur J Pharm Biopharm 91:9–15. https://doi.org/10.1016/j.ejpb.2015.01.002

Nickerson MT, Paulson AT. Rheological properties of gellan, κ-carrageenan and alginate polysaccharides: effect of potassium and calcium ions on macrostructure assemblages. CarbohydrPolym. 2004b Oct;58(1):15–24. https://doi.org/10.1016/j.carbpol.2004.06.006

Xie F, Gao C, Avérous L. (2024) Alginate-based materials: Enhancing properties through multiphase formulation design and processing innovation. Mater Sci Eng R Rep 159:100799. https://doi.org/10.1016/j.mser.2024.100799

Jiang, F.; Xu, X.-W.; Chen, F.-Q.; Weng, H.-F.; Chen, J.; Ru, Y.; Xiao, Q.; Xiao, A.-F. (2023) Extraction, Modification and Biomedical Application of Agarose Hydrogels: A Review. Drugs 21, 299. https://doi.org/10.3390/md21050299

Khodadadi Yazdi, M.; Taghizadeh, A.; Taghizadeh, M.; Stadler, F.J.; Farokhi, M.; Mottaghitalab, F.; Zarrintaj, P.; Ramsey, J.D.; Seidi, F.; Saeb, M.R.; et al. (2020)Agarose-based biomaterials for advanced drug delivery. J. Control 326, 523–543. https://doi.org/10.1016/j.jconrel.2020.07.028

Guastaferro, M.; Reverchon, E.; Baldino, L. (2021) Agarose, Alginate and Chitosan Nanostructured Aerogels for Pharmaceutical Applications: A Short Review. Front. Bioeng. Biotechnol 9, 688477. https://doi.org/10.3389/fbioe.2021.688477

Ninan, N.; Forget, A.; Shastri, V.P.; Voelcker, N.H.; Blencowe, A. (2016) Antibacterial and Anti-Inflammatory pH-Responsive Tannic Acid-Carboxylated Agarose Composite Hydrogels for Wound Healing. ACS Appl 8, 28511–28521. https://doi.org/10.1021/acsami.6b10491

Kolanthai, E.; Abinaya Sindu, P.; Thanigai Arul, K.; Sarath Chandra, V.; Manikandan, E.; Narayana Kalkura, S. (2017) Agarose encapsulated mesoporous carbonated hydroxyapatite nanocomposites powder for drug delivery. J. Photochem. Photobiol. B Biol 166, 220–231. https://doi.org/10.1016/j.jphotobiol.2016.12.005

Ajmal, G., Bonde, G. V., Mittal, P., Khan, G., Pandey, V. K., Bakade, B. V., & Mishra, B. (2019) Biomimetic PCL-gelatin based nanofibers loaded with ciprofloxacin hydrochloride and quercetin: A potential antibacterial and anti-oxidant dressing material for accelerated healing of a full thickness wound. International Journal of Pharmaceutics 567 https://doi.org/10.1016/j.ijpharm.2019.118480.

Bairagi, U., Mittal, P., Singh, J., & Mishra, B. (2018) Preparation, characterization, and in vivo evaluation of nano formulations of ferulic acid in diabetic wound healing. Drug Development and Industrial Pharmacy, 44(11), 17831796 https://doi.org/10.1080/03639045.2018.1496448.

Bansal, P., Katiyar, D., Prakash, S., Raghavendra Rao, N. G., Saxena, V., Kumar, V., & Kumar, A. (2022)Applications of some biopolymeric materials as medical implants: An overview. Materials Today: Proceedings, 65, 33773381 https://doi.org/10.1016/j.matpr.2022.05.480

Bonde, G. V., Yadav, S. K., Chauhan, S., Mittal, P., Ajmal, G., Thokala, S., & Mishra, B. (2018) Lapatinib nano-delivery systems: A promising future for breast cancer treatment. Expert Opinion on Drug Delivery, 15(5), 495507 https://doi.org/10.1080/17425247.2018.1449832

Lira, M. C., Santos-Magalhaes, N. S., Nicolas, V., Marsaud, V., Silva, M. P., Ponchel, G., & Vauthier, C. (2011) Cytotoxicity and cellular uptake of newly synthesized fucoidan-coated nanoparticles. European Journal of Pharmaceutics and Biopharmaceutics, 79(1), 162–170 . https://doi.org/10.1016/j.ejpb.2011.02.013

Etman, S. M., Elnaggar, Y. S. R., & Abdallah, O. Y. (2020) Fucoidan, a natural biopolymer in cancer combating: From edible algae to nanocarrier tailoring. International Journal of Biological Macromolecules, 147, 799–808. https://doi.org/10.1016/j.ijbiomac.2019.11.191

Chen, S., Li, Q., McClements, D. J., Han, Y., Dai, L., Mao, L., & Gao, Y. (2020) Co-delivery of curcumin and piperine in zein-carrageenan core-shell nanoparticles: Formation, structure, stability and in vitro gastrointestinal digestion. Food Hydrocolloids 99, 105334. https://doi.org/10.1016/j.foodhyd.2019.105334

Bonhome-Espinosa, A. B., Campos, F., Durand-Herrera, D., Sanchez-Lopez, J. D., Schaub, S., Duran, J. D. G., ... Carriel, V. (2020) In vitro characterization of a novel magnetic fibrin-agarose hydrogel for cartilage tissue engineering. Journal of the Mechanical Behavior of Biomedical Materials, 104, 103619. https://doi.org/10.1016/j.jmbbm.2020.103619

Cheba, B. A. (2011) Chitin and chitosan: Marine biopolymers with unique properties and versatile applications. Global Journal of Biotechnology & Biochemistry 6(3), 149153.

Fathiraja, P., Gopalrajan, S., Karunanithi, M., Obaiah, M. C., Rajasekaran, B., & Vedhi, C. (2022) Process optimization and characterization of composite biopolymer films obtained from fish scale gelatin, agar and chitosan using response surface methodology. Polymer Bulletin. https://doi.org/10.1007/s00289-022-04540-4

J. Pushpamalar, P. Meganathan, H.L. Tan, N.A. Dahlan, L.T. Ooi, B.N. Neerooa, R. Z. Essa, K. Shameli, S.Y. Teow, (2021) Development of a polysaccharide-based hydrogel drug delivery system (DDS): an update, Gels 4, 153. https://doi.org/10.3390/gels7040153.

E.A. Essa, T.T. Elebyary, M.M. Abdelquader, G.M. Maghraby, A.A. Elkordy (2021) Smart liquids for oral controlled drug release: an overview of alginate and non-alginate-based systems, J. Drug Delivery Sci. Technol. 12,102211 https://doi.org/10.1016/j.jddst.2020.102211.

Hariyadi D. M., Hendradi, E., & Sharon, N. (2019) Development of carrageenan polymer for encapsulation of ciprofloxacin HCL: in vitro characterization. Int. J. Drug Deliv. Technol. 9(01), 89–93 https://doi.org/10.25258/ijddt.9.1.14

Muhamad, I. I., Zulkifli, N., Selvakumaran, S. A., & Lazim, N. a. M. (2019) Bioactive Algal-Derived Polysaccharides: Multi-Functionalization, therapeutic potential and biomedical applications. Current Pharmaceutical Design 25(11), 1147–1162 https://doi.org/10.2174/1381612825666190618152133

Chiang, C., Huang, B., Chen, J., Chieng, W. W., Lim, S. H., Lee, W., Shyu, W., & Jeng, L. (2021) Fucoidan-Based Nanoparticles with Inherently Therapeutic Efficacy for Cancer Treatment. Pharmaceutics 13(12), 1986 https://doi.org/10.3390/pharmaceutics13121986

Du, B., Zhao, Q., Cheng, C., Wang, H., Liu, Y., Zhu, F., & Yang, Y. (2022) A critical review on extraction, characteristics, physicochemical activities, potential health benefits, and industrial applications of fucoidan. eFood 3(4) 10.1002/efd2.19

Kidgell, J. T., Magnusson, M., De Nys, R., & Glasson, C. R. (2019b) Ulvan: A systematic review of extraction, composition and function. Algal Research 39, 101422. https://doi.org/10.1016/j.algal.2019.101422

Wan, M., Qin, W., Lei, C., Li, Q., Meng, M., Fang, M., Song, W., Chen, J., Tay, F., & Niu, L. (2021) Biomaterials from the sea: Future building blocks for biomedical applications. Bioactive Materials 6(12), 4255–4285. https://doi.org/10.1016/j.bioactmat.2021.04.028

Bose, I., Nousheen, N., Roy, S., Yaduvanshi, P., Sharma, S., Chandel, V., & Biswas, D. (2023a) Unveiling the potential of marine biopolymers: sources, classification, and diverse food applications. Materials 16(13), 4840. https://doi.org/10.3390/ma16134840

Karthikeyan, A., Joseph, A., & Nair, B. G. (2022) Promising bioactive compounds from the marine environment and their potential effects on various diseases. Journal of Genetic Engineering and Biotechnology 20(1), 14. https://doi.org/10.1186/s43141-021-00290-4

Li, Y., & Li, Z. (2021) Cyclopeptide Derivatives from the Sponge-Derived Fungus Acremonium persicinum F10. Marine Drugs 19(10), 537 https://doi.org/10.3390/md19100537

Yang, Z., Liu, W., Liu, H., Li, R., Chang, L., Kan, S., Hao, M., & Wang, D. (2022). The applications of polysaccharides in dentistry. Frontiers in Bioengineering and Biotechnology, 10. https://doi.org/10.3389/fbioe.2022.970041

Miyazaki, S., Ishitani, M., Takahashi, A., Shimoyama, T., Itoh, K., & Attwood, D. (2011). Carrageenan gels for oral sustained delivery of acetaminophen to dysphagic patients. Biological and Pharmaceutical Bulletin, 34(1), 164–166. https://doi.org/10.1248/bpb.34.164

Venugopal, V. (2011) Marine polysaccharides. In CRC Press eBooks https://doi.org/10.1201/b10516

Syed, M. A., Aziz, G., Jehangir, M. B., Tabish, T. A., Zahoor, A. F., Khalid, S. H., Khan, I. U., Hosny, K. M., Rizg, W. Y., Hanif, S., Arshad, R., Qayyum, M. A., & Irfan, M. (2022). Evaluating novel Agarose-Based buccal gels Scaffold: Mucoadhesive and pharmacokinetic profiling in healthy volunteers. Pharmaceutics, 14(8), 1592. https://doi.org/10.3390/pharmaceutics14081592

D'Ayala, G. G., Malinconico, M., & Laurienzo, P. (2008). Marine derived polysaccharides for biomedical applications: Chemical modification approaches. Molecules, 13(9), 2069–2106. https://doi.org/10.3390/molecules13092069

Zhu, L., Ren, Y., Zhang, S., Guo, Y., Zong, J., & Liu, Y. (2024). Marine-derived polysaccharides: the potential agents against neurodegenerative diseases. Frontiers in Pharmacology 15 https://doi.org/10.3389/fphar.2024.1506789

De Anda-Flores Y, Carvajal-Millan E, Campa-Mada A, Lizardi-Mendoza J, Rascon-Chu A, Tanori-Cordova J, et al. (2021) Polysaccharide-Based Nanoparticles for Colon-Targeted Drug Delivery Systems. Polysaccharides 2(3):626–47. https://doi.org/10.3390/polysaccharides2030038

Lai SK, Wang YY, Hanes J. (2009) Mucus-penetrating nanoparticles for drug and gene delivery to mucosal tissues. Adv Drug Deliv Rev 61(2):158–71. https://doi.org/10.1016/j.addr.2008.11.002

Cui M, Zhang M, Liu K. (2021) Colon-targeted drug delivery of polysaccharide-based nanocarriers for synergistic treatment of inflammatory bowel disease: A review. Carbohydr Polym 272: 118530. https://doi.org/10.1016/j.carbpol.2021.118530

Kurl S, Kumar A, Reena, Mittal N, Singh D, Bassi P, et al. (2023) Challenges, opportunities, and future prospects of polysaccharide-based nanoparticles for colon targeting: A comprehensive review. CarbohydrPolym Technol Appl 6:100361. https://doi.org/10.1016/j.carpta.2023.100361

Wen H, Jung H, Li X. (2015) Drug Delivery Approaches in Addressing Clinical Pharmacology-Related Issues: Opportunities and Challenges. AAPS J 17(6):1327–40. https://doi.org/10.1208/s12248-015-9814-9

Cockburn DW, Koropatkin NM. (2016) Polysaccharide Degradation by the Intestinal Microbiota and Its Influence on Human Health and Disease. J Mol Biol 428(16):3230–52. https://doi.org/10.1016/j.jmb.2016.06.021

Anisha GS, Padmakumari S, Patel AK, Pandey A, Singhania RR. (2022) Fucoidan from Marine Macroalgae: Biological Actions and Applications in Regenerative Medicine, Drug Delivery Systems and Food Industry. Bioengineering 9(9):472. https://doi.org/10.3390/bioengineering9090472

Jiang Y, Yan C, Li M, Chen S, Chen Z, Yang L, et al. (2024) Delivery of natural products via polysaccharide-based nanocarriers for cancer therapy: A review on recent advances and future challenges. Int J Biol Macromol 278:135072. https://doi.org/10.1016/j.ijbiomac.2024.135072

Szymańska E, Winnicka K. (2015) Stability of Chitosan—A Challenge for Pharmaceutical and Biomedical Applications. Mar Drugs13(4):1819–46.https://doi.org/10.1016/j.ijbiomac.2024.135072

Bose I, Nousheen, Roy S, Yaduvanshi P, Sharma S, Chandel V, et al. (2023b) Unveiling the Potential of Marine Biopolymers: Sources, Classification, and Diverse Food Applications. Materials 16(13):4840. https://doi.org/10.3390/ma16134840

Quitério E, Soares C, Ferraz R, Delerue-Matos C, Grosso C. (2021) Marine Health-Promoting Compounds: Recent Trends for Their Characterization and Human Applications. Foods 10(12):3100. https://doi.org/10.3390/foods10123100

Long HL, Zhang JX, Guo JL, Sui GQ, Hou JJ, Yang WZ, et al. (2016) Development of specific and quantitative methods for the quality control of the polysaccharides from sea-tangle and sargassum. Chin J Nat Med 14(12):954–60. https://doi.org/10.1016/S1875-5364(17)30022-5

Choudhury PD, Ikbal AMA, Saha S, Debnath R, Debnath B, Singh LS, et al. (2025) Recent Advances in Multifaceted Drug Delivery Using Natural Polysaccharides and Polyacrylamide-based Nanomaterials in Nanoformulation. Curr Top Med Chem 25(4):395–408. https://doi.org/10.2174/0115680266316522241015143856

Wang H, Luan F, Shi Y, Yan S, Xin B, Zhang X, et al. (2024) Extraction, structural features, and pharmacological effects of the polysaccharides from Porphyra yezoensis: A review. Int J Biol Macromol 279:134745. https://doi.org/10.1016/j.ijbiomac.2023.134745

Lee, K. Y., & Mooney, D. J. (2011) Alginate: Properties and biomedical applications. Progress in Polymer Science 37(1), 106–126 https://doi.org/10.1016/j.progpolymsci.2011.06.003

Geng, H., Guo, C., Wang, W., & Chen, D. (2024) Marine Polysaccharides: Biological Activity and Drug Delivery. Marine Plant https://doi.org/10.2139/ssrn.4673644

Barbosa, A. I., Coutinho, A. J., Lima, S. a. C., & Reis, S. (2019c) Marine polysaccharides in pharmaceutical applications: Fucoidan and Chitosan as key players in the drug delivery match field. Marine Drugs 17(12), 654 https://doi.org/10.3390/md17120654

Da Silva, L. C. R. P., Todaro, V., Carmo, F. a. D., Frattani, F. S., De Sousa, V. P., Rodrigues, C. R., Sathler, P. C., & Cabral, L. M. (2018)A promising oral fucoidan-based antithrombotic nanosystem: development, activity and safety. Nanotechnology 29(16), 165102 10.1088/1361-6528/aaae5b

Hafiza, A. A., Khairunnisa-Atiqah, M. K., Mazlan, N. S. N., Salleh, K. M., & Zakaria, S. (2023) Biocompatible and biodegradable materials in medical applications. In Elsevier eBooks 331–358 https://doi.org/10.1016/b978-0-323-95169-2.00010-9

FDA floats regulating hyaluronic acid products as drugs, not devices. (2018). RAPS. https://www.raps.org/news-and-articles/news-articles/2018/12/fda-floats-regulating-hyaluronic-acid-products-as

Boychenko, Y., Budenkova, E., Kostyushina, N., Babich, O., & Kashinskikh, E. (2024) Porphyridium sp. Microalgae as a source of polysaccharides. Journal of Applied Biology &Biotechnology https://doi.org/10.7324/jabb.2024.165844

Hathcock, J. N., & Shao, A. (2006) Risk assessment for glucosamine and chondroitin sulfate. Regulatory Toxicology and Pharmacology 47(1), 78–83 https://doi.org/10.1016/j.yrtph.2006.07.004

Lahaye, M., Robic, A., & Biopolymères, I. A. (2007) Structure and Functional Properties of Ulvan, a Polysaccharide from Green Seaweeds. Biomacromolecules 8(6), 1765–1774. https://doi.org/10.1021/bm061185q

Pomin, V. H., & Mourao, P. a. S. (2008). Structure, biology, evolution, and medical importance of sulfated fucans and galactans. Glycobiology, 18(12), 1016–1027. https://doi.org/10.1093/glycob/cwn085

Cotas J, Lomartire S, Gonçalves AMM, Pereira L. From Ocean to Medicine: Harnessing Seaweed's Potential for Drug Development. Int J Mol Sci. 2024 Jan 8;25(2):797. https://doi.org/10.3390/ijms25020797

Alharbi H. (2024) Exploring the Frontier of Biopolymer-Assisted Drug Delivery: Advancements, Clinical Applications, and Future Perspectives in Cancer Nanomedicine. Drug Des Devel Ther 18:2063–87. https://doi.org/10.2147/DDDT.S441325

Alsaikhan F, Farhood B. (2024) Recent advances on chitosan/hyaluronic acid-based stimuli-responsive hydrogels and composites for cancer treatment: A comprehensive review. Int J Biol Macromol 280:135893. https://doi.org/10.1016/j.ijbiomac.2024.135893

Kidgell, J. T., Magnusson, M., De Nys, R., & Glasson, C. R. (2019c) Ulvan: A systematic review of extraction, composition and function. Algal Research 39, 101422 https://doi.org/10.1016/j.algal.2019.101422

Samalens, F., Thomas, M., Claverie, M., Castejon, N., Zhang, Y., Pigot, T., Blanc, S., & Fernandes, S. C. M. (2022) Progresses and future prospects in biodegradation of marine biopolymers and emerging biopolymer-based materials for sustainable marine ecosystems. Green Chemistry 24(5), 1762–1779 https://doi.org/10.1039/d1gc04327g

Jacob, J., Haponiuk, J. T., Thomas, S., & Gopi, S. (2018c) Biopolymer based nanomaterials in drug delivery systems: A review. Materials Today Chemistry 9, 43–55 https://doi.org/10.1016/j.mtchem.2018.05.002

Martins, A., Vieira, H., Gaspar, H., & Santos, S. (2014b) Marketed marine natural products in the pharmaceutical and cosmeceutical industries: Tips for success. Marine Drugs 12(2), 1066–1101. https://doi.org/10.3390/md12021066

https://www.fda.gov/science-research/fda-stem-outreach-education-and-engagement

Atanase, L., Desbrieres, J., & Riess, G. (2017) Micellization of synthetic and polysaccharides-based graft copolymers in aqueous media. Progress in Polymer Science 73, 32–60 https://doi.org/10.1016/j.progpolymsci.2017.06.001

Bai, L., Liu, L., Esquivel, M., Tardy, B. L., Huan, S., Niu, X., Liu, S., Yang, G., Fan, Y., & Rojas, O. J. (2022) Nanochitin: chemistry, structure, assembly, and applications. Chemical Reviews 122(13), 11604–11674. https://doi.org/10.1021/acs.chemrev.2c00125

Khrunyk, Y., Lach, S., Petrenko, I., & Ehrlich, H. (2020)Progress in modern marine biomaterials research. Marine Drugs, 18(12), 589. https://doi.org/10.3390/md18120589

Oyervides-Muñoz, E., Oyervides-Muñoz, M. A., & Garcia-Lobato, M. A. (2022)Chitin and Chitosan nanocomposites: From the synthesis to the application. In Engineering materials 101–118. https://doi.org/10.1007/978-3-031-18428-4_6

Singh, R., & Lillard, J. W. (2009) Nanoparticle-based targeted drug delivery. Exp. Mol. Pathol. 86(3), 215–223. https://doi.org/10.1016/j.yexmp.2008.12.004

Riess, G. (2003). Micellization of block copolymers. Progress in Polymer Science 28(7), 1107–1170. https://doi.org/10.1016/s0079-6700(03)00015-7

Domozych, D. S., &LoRicco, J. G. (2023). The extracellular matrix of green algae. Plant Physio. 194(1), 15–32. https://doi.org/10.1093/plphys/kiad384

Lindequist, U. (2016) Marine-Derived Pharmaceuticals—Challenges and opportunities. Biomol. Ther. 24(6), 561–571 https://doi.org/10.4062/biomolther.2016.181

Marine-Based Polysaccharides for Injectable Drug Delivery Approaches

Mohamed Ashraf, Hossam S. El-Sawy, and Mona M. A. Abdel-Mottaleb

Abstract Marine polysaccharides have emerged as versatile and biocompatible materials for the development of injectable drug delivery systems, offering a sustainable alternative to synthetic polymers. Derived from seaweed and marine organisms, polysaccharides such as alginate, chitosan, carrageenan, and fucoidan possess unique physicochemical properties, including biodegradability, gel-forming ability, and tunable viscosity, making them ideal candidates for parenteral applications. Their structural diversity allows for controlled drug release, targeted delivery, and enhanced therapeutic efficacy while minimizing systemic side effects. Recent advances have demonstrated their potential in encapsulating a wide range of therapeutics, including proteins, peptides, and small molecules, with promising results in cancer therapy, tissue engineering, and immunomodulation. Furthermore, marine polysaccharides are amenable to chemical modification and nanoparticle formulation, broadening their application in precision medicine. This review highlights the current progress, challenges, and future directions in utilizing marine-based polysaccharides for injectable drug delivery systems, underscoring their role in the advancement of biocompatible and effective pharmaceutical platforms.

Keywords Marine · Polysaccharides · Injectable · Drug delivery

M. Ashraf
Department of Pharmaceutics and Pharmaceutical Technology, Faculty of Pharmacy, Egyptian Russian University, Cairo, Egypt

H. S. El-Sawy
Department of Pharmaceutics and Pharmaceutical Technology, Faculty of Pharmacy, Egyptian Russian University, Cairo, Egypt

Department of Pharmaceutics, College of Pharmacy, University of Kut, Wasit, Iraq

M. M. A. Abdel-Mottaleb (✉)
Université de Franche-Comté, EFS, INSERM, UMR 1098 RIGHT, Besançon, France

Department of Pharmaceutics and industrial Pharmacy, Faculty of Pharmacy, Ain Shams University, Cairo, Egypt
e-mail: mona.abdelmottaleb@pharma.asu.edu.eg

S. Jana et al. (eds.), *Multifunctional Marine Polysaccharides*,
https://doi.org/10.1007/978-981-95-4126-3_3

1 Introduction

Polysaccharides originating from marine organisms are considered one of the most plentiful materials in the ocean, including alginate, carrageenan, kombucha polysaccharide, rockweed polysaccharide, chitin, chitin derivatives, rockweed glycan extracted from algae, hyaluronic acid, and chitosan obtained from animal sources, such as crustacean bones and cartilaginous fish tissue, while some polysaccharides like prokaryotes come from marine microorganisms. Polysaccharides of marine origin can in general be designated as a large complicated group of different macromolecules, which could have various biological characteristics (Dongre 2022). Marine polysaccharides possess significant biological appealing properties such as biocompatibility, biodegradability, anti-inflammatory activity, adhesion, and antimicrobial effects. Algal polysaccharides have long been revealed to have anti-inflammatory activity both in vitro and in vivo, attributed to their unique structural and physicochemical properties. Since sulfate is partially involved in the interaction between polysaccharides and cell surface receptors, sulfate content is important in manipulating macrophages. Several studies have shown that polysaccharides inhibit the migration of leukocytes to sites of inflammation (Carrasqueira et al. 2025).

Conventional drug delivery methods have many drawbacks ranging from a lack of selectivity, limited solubility, short duration of action due to rapid elimination, and extensive side effects on the healthy tissues. As a result, drug delivery systems (DDS) that can selectively target drugs to the specific site of interest are widely needed to enhance bioavailability and minimize drug side effects (Mousa et al. 2025; Sedky et al. 2024; Kotb et al. 2021). Target-specific nanocarriers can be directed to the target site tissue. Further, they can enter the cell via the endocytic pathway for drug release in response to a specific environment. Microparticle and nanoparticle formulations are of great interest as materials for drug delivery. Microparticles enhance the preparation of long-term stability and can be administered by intramuscular and/or subcutaneous injection. Stimulus-responsive nano-/microcarriers are drug delivery vehicles that are capable of altering their structure (e.g., degradation or disintegration), conformation, or composition in response to stimuli either internal or external physicochemical environmental variations, facilitating the controlled release of the encapsulated drug into the diseased tissue (Adepu and Ramakrishna 2021).

In recent years, DDS based on marine polysaccharides have gained increasing attention because of the advantages offered by the incorporated marine polysaccharides such as biocompatibility, biodegradability, non-toxicity, low cost, and high utility (Ramadan et al. 2025). This leads to various applications in biomedical materials and applications, such as targeted delivery of drugs, tissue engineering, wound healing dressings, etc. (Fig. 1). Marine polysaccharide-based DDS allow the controlled distribution of drugs in time, space, and dose (Sun et al. 2021). Drug loading efficiency, reduction of toxic side effects, and improvement of target drug delivery can also be achieved. Natural marine polysaccharides such as hyaluronic acid and rockweed polysaccharides have been shown to target the CD44 receptor

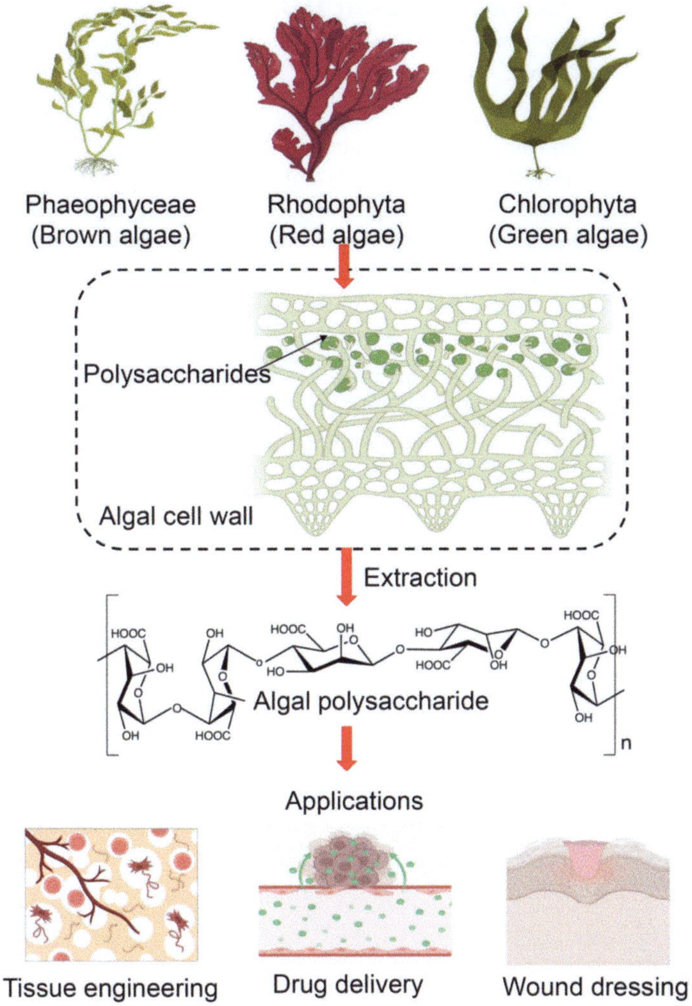

Fig. 1 Source and different biomedical applications of polysaccharides. (Reproduced with permission from Ramadan et al. (2025), Elsevier)

and the inflammatory site P-selectin specifically. Therefore, they can be easily modified by chemical reactions and functional modifications to synthesize nanoparticles with heterogeneous structures. For example, introducing disulfide or imine bonds between the active molecule and the polysaccharide backbone allows for the reactive release of the tumor microenvironment. DDS that depend on marine-derived polysaccharides possess the pharmacological activity of polysaccharides and the advantage of specific or selective targeted drug delivery. Furthermore, the DDS based on different marine polysaccharides have a wide range of applications (Joshi et al. 2019), which are displayed in the following sections.

2 Marine Polysaccharide-Based DDS

2.1 Alginate-Based DDS

Alginate is considered one of the most abundant and commonly used polysaccharides of marine origin. It is anionic in nature and composed mainly of interconnected units of β-D-mannuronic acid (M) and α-L-glucuronic acid (G). The mechanical characteristics of alginate depend mainly on the length of the G unit; on the other side, the number of the M units is more connected to immunogenicity. The presence of many active sites on the M units of alginate provides a high potential for various targeting modifications as well as tailored biological properties (Abka Khajouei et al. 2022). Wang et al. fabricated nanosized DDS incorporating an iRGD tumor-penetrating peptide-modified propylene glycol sodium alginate in addition to combination with a disulfide-containing hydrophobic kernel that is sensitive to both pH and redox reactions. iRGD surface modification revealed an enhanced tumor penetration/cellular internalization, which lead to enhanced activity against breast cancer (Chen et al. 2022).

Alginate hydrogels loaded with nitric oxide were proposed as an excellent tool to provide sustained release leading to outstanding antibacterial properties (Fig. 2) in addition to the water absorption and swelling capacity of the produced hydrogels (Zheng et al. 2023).

Huang et al. reported and constructed multifunctional platforms for realizing synergistic treatment against hepatocellular carcinoma (HCC). They achieved that *via* utilization of the ability of the G units in alginate to interact specifically with mannose receptors, and also by utilization of the G unit as a binding site that can be used as a highly reactive response to biotin, together they have constructed a

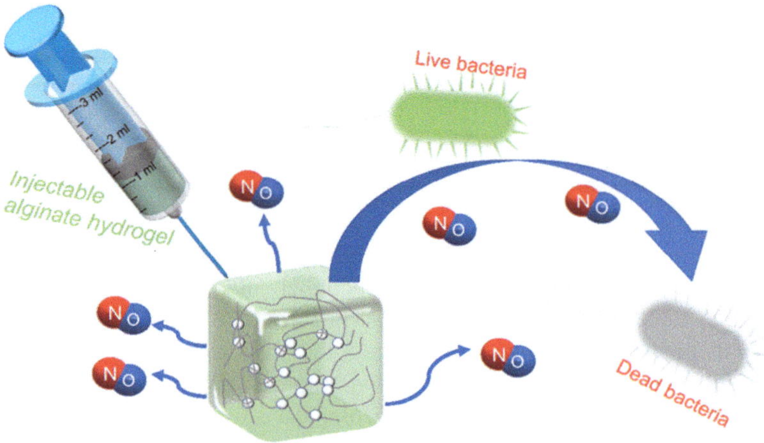

Fig. 2 Controllable release of nitric oxide from an injectable alginate hydrogel. (Reproduced with permission from Zheng et al. (2023). Elsevier)

dual-targeted carrier-loaded doxorubicin nanomicelles. Overall, findings revealed that alginate has a significant therapeutic ability to improve liver fibrosis triggering chemotherapeutic efficacy and enhance therapeutic outcome (Huang et al. 2023).

Another example on the use of alginate is their utilization as a basic polymer to produce nanocarriers by utilizing the electrostatic attraction between alginate, especially when dissolved in media of neutral or slightly alkaline pH values, to oppositely charged natural materials, such as the positively charged aminated chitosan, for construction of advanced drug delivery systems used for various applications such as gene delivery. The early developed systems used for gene delivery were usually based on the encapsulation of genetic material into viral vectors (Hariyadi and Islam 2020). It was also used for the delivery of hormones such as testosterone, which was used in treatment of osteoporosis and coronary heart diseases, and testosterone-loaded alginate nanocapsules were fabricated. In situ polymeric nanoemulsification cross-linking method was used. The pharmacokinetic data showed that alginate nanocapsules loaded with testosterone have shown better bioavailability in comparison with commercial testosterone injection and pure testosterone (Jana et al. 2015).

Vaccine delivery is necessary to enhance immunity for prophylaxis of a wide range of infectious diseases. Attenuated *Androctonus australis hector* (Aah) venom and its toxic fraction "FtoxG50" were loaded into calcium alginate nanoparticles to be used against scorpion envenomation. Ionic gelation technique was used. Venom is entrapped inside nanoparticles to induce protective immunity. Its results revealed the influence of different parameters on the suitable nanoparticle formation and no toxicity or inflammation due to free nanoparticles, but only by Aah venom. Encapsulation efficiency of the nanoparticles was 94.99%. The specific IgG titer and IgG1/IgG2a isotype balance evaluation showed a protective effect and have cellular phagocytosis in comparison to free proteins to more enhancement of immune processing. Thus, calcium alginate nanoparticles proved to provide a promising vaccine delivery system against scorpion envenomation (Laraba-djebari 2016).

2.2 Carrageenan-Based DDS

Carrageenan is a linear sulfated polysaccharide composed of D-galactose with alternating α-1,3 and β-1,4 bonds. It is considered also an anionic polysaccharide due to its high content of sulfate groups. It can be classified as k, I, and λ based on the number of sulfate groups in its structure, for one, two, and three sulfate groups, respectively. It was reported that carrageenan possesses various interesting therapeutic activities such as anticancer, anti-inflammatory, and antioxidant actions. They also have protective effects against bacteria and fungi, in addition to 370 viruses. It was also reported that carrageenan gum exerts an anticoagulant activity via the enhancement of the activity of antithrombin III (Yermak et al. 2017).

Usually the high molecular weight carrageenan suffers from very poor aqueous solubility, which necessitates its degradation to oligosaccharides first to produce different drug delivery systems. It has been used to produce a novel multi-stimulus-responsive nanoparticle with triple responses to pH, temperature, and magnetic forces loaded with the cytotoxic drug fluorouracil. The production of these k-carrageenan-based nanoparticles and their multiple responses led to enhanced antitumor and immune-enhancing activities in addition to the optimum drug loading and delivery making them easily categorized as a smart responsive antitumor delivery system (Küçükbalcı Geyik and Işıklan 2021).

2.3 Fucoidan-Based DDS

This is a highly hydrophilic polysaccharide with sulfate groups and consisting mainly of L-fucose, uronic acid, galactose, xylose, mannose, rhamnose, glucose, arabinose, and xylose, extracted from the cell walls of algae and some marine invertebrates (Yu et al. 2014), as it possesses biological activity. Studies have shown that rockweed polysaccharides have unique biological activities in terms of antioxidant (Jia et al. 2016), anti-inflammatory, immunomodulatory, antiviral, and antitumor activities (Thinh et al. 2013)

Self-assembly curcumin-loaded nanocellular micelles of fucoidan were fabricated for kidney targeting. By utilization of the ability of fucoidan to target P-selectin, which is highly expressed in the inflamed renal endothelial cells, the uptake of loaded drug was enhanced, and the treatment outcome on the renal activity was improved (Shu et al. 2021).

Fucoidan nanoparticles loaded with doxorubicin targeting the breast cancer abundant P-selectin receptors were also fabricated. It was found that the P-selectin-targeted nanodelivery system showed a greater efficacy and lower side effects. It could effectively adhere to living platelets via P-selectin resulting in increasing deposition of the drug in the cancerous tissues and specifically that P-selectin expression is strongly connected with the higher risk of vascular metastatic dissemination (Shu et al. 2021).

On the same line of work, fucoidan-based P-selectin-targeted microwave stimulation-responsive nanoparticles were fabricated, in which a dual encapsulation of both the cytotoxic agent doxorubicin and a photosensitizer was achieved. Adjuvant microwave exposure permits the magnificent accumulation and localized release of doxorubicin *in the liver cancerous tissue*. This can lead to efficient targeting and controlled drug release via using fucoidan-based DDS (Xu et al. 2019).

2.4 Chitosan-Based DDS

Chitosan is a naturally derived polysaccharide obtained through the deacetylation of chitin, a major structural component found in the exoskeletons of marine crustaceans such as shrimp, crabs, and lobsters. It is widely recognized for its exceptional biocompatibility, biodegradability, and nontoxic nature, making it highly suitable for biomedical applications, particularly in injectable drug delivery systems (Abuelella et al. 2022a, b). One of chitosan's most valuable properties is its cationic nature, which allows it to interact readily with negatively charged biological membranes and drugs. This facilitates efficient drug encapsulation and enhances cellular uptake. Its mucoadhesive properties also prolong the residence time of drugs at the site of administration, which can improve therapeutic efficacy (Piekarska et al. 2023). Additionally, chitosan is amenable to chemical modification, allowing for the introduction of functional groups that can enhance its solubility, responsiveness to physiological stimuli (e.g., pH or temperature), and targeting capabilities. For example, grafting polyethylene glycol (PEG) or adding targeting ligands can improve its pharmacokinetics and tissue specificity. Biological properties of chitosan differ according to different molecular weights as solubility of high molecular weight chitosan in water is low, with high viscosity in dilute acidic solution. This solubility drawback may hinder the use of chitosan in many biological applications. However, low molecular weight chitosan (LMWC) has higher solubility and lower viscosity so it can be used for a variable kind of pharmaceutical applications. It also has polycationic properties enabling interaction with the negative wall lipopolysaccharide and protein components of bacteria (Román-Doval et al. 2023).

Dual pH-responsive nanomicelles loaded with genistein based on chitosan were fabricated by Wang et al. The amino group is protonated at pH of the tumor microenvironment allowing the interaction to the negatively charged surface of cancer cells, and thus higher rate of internalization, while the imine group is hydrolyzed by pH change sensitivity to release genistein at the tumor site achieving potential formulation as drug delivery system for targeting solid tumor micromilieu (Wang et al. 2019).

Nanoparticles can be coated with chitosan either by chemical bond formation or simply via physical attachment using electrostatic interaction (Salama et al. 2025), which provides a positive charge on the surface of these nanoparticles rendering their interaction and attachment to the negatively charged cell membranes much easier and prolonged. On the same line of work, remote folic acid-grafted chitosan-coated magnetic nanoparticles loaded with doxorubicin were constructed, and the results showed an enhanced localization of drug release at tumor cells, providing more safe profile and lower side effects (Yang et al. 2017). Liposomes containing ursolic acid coated with chitosan by electrostatic adsorption were also constructed. Induction of positive charge enables targeting to the negative charged tumor cells. Also, the low pH environment in the tumor allowed the targeted drug release and its uptake by the tumor cells (Wang et al. 2017).

Another study investigated the fabrication of silymarin incorporation into galactosylated chitosan nanoparticles successfully aiming to make use of asialoglycoprotein receptors, which are present in liver cells. Results based on pharmacokinetic profile, plasma drug concentration level, and levels of liver enzymes indicated the suitability of nanoparticles to target liver cells for the aim of treating liver cirrhosis (Venugopal et al. 2015).

It is without question that the intravenous injections can overcome various shortages of the oral route such as degradation problems and poor absorption. However, in case of gene delivery, genes are expected to be susceptible to nuclease degradation before even reaching the target site. Therefore, novel systems with higher stability in the bloodstream and other biological fluids should be established to assure the efficacy of the loaded gene. Developed chitosan-coated poly(isohexyl cyanoacrylate) nanoparticles were developed through anionic emulsion polymerization to increase stability of antisense phosphodiester oligonucleotide in a mouse Ewing sarcoma model. Results showed tumor suppression by a significant degree after injection of nanoparticles. Also, the expression level of target gene silence exceeds 40%, which participate in further inhibition of the tumor growth, suggesting an efficient gene delivery system to overcome certain diseases (Li et al. 2012).

2.5 *Ulvan-Based DDS*

Ulvan is a sulfated polysaccharide composed mainly of glucose, rhamnose, xylose, and glucuronic and iduronic acid linked with each other by (1N4) linkage and extracted mainly from the *Ulva* green algae (Jalal et al. 2019). Because of ulvan ability to form complexes with different metal ions, ulvan could be used as a chelating agent that proved to be useful in the treatment of different poisoning conditions as well as various food and cosmetic industries (Sulastri et al. 2021). Ulvan enjoys various interesting biological properties that made it suitable for applications in tissue engineering and regenerative medicine, in addition to its antiviral, antioxidant, antitumor, anticoagulant, and immune system-enhancing activities. Ulvan has been also used in the construction of nanocarriers for biomolecules. Additionally, it is also possible to obtain three-dimensional ulvan-based structures. In this work line, three-dimensional scaffold of ulvan/chitosan combined with D,L-lactic acid loaded with dexamethasone was produced for bone tissue regeneration application. Assays of in vitro release demonstrated a burst release, followed by a sustained cumulative release in the next 3 weeks (Alves et al. 2012). Ulvan-tyramine solution optimization was carried out using horseradish peroxide as a catalyst and adjustment of the amount of H_2O_2 amount. This tyramine modification was performed in order that polymer can be easily identified by enzymes. New formulation showed excellent biocompatibility enzymatic catalysis susceptibility in addition to appropriate gelation time suitable with in situ gelling systems and enhancement of cell (Morelli et al. 2015)

2.6 *Hyaluronan-Based DDS*

Hyaluronan, is the main family member of glycosaminoglycans composed mainly of units of N-acetyl-D-glucosamine and D-glucuronic linked by glycosidic bonds, which can be broken by the action of hydrolases such as hyaluronidase giving the character of biodegradability to hyaluronan (Burdick and Prestwich 2011). Hyaluronan is a chief component of extracellular matrix, synovial fluid, and cartilage tissue. Hyaluronan has also a vital role in several biological functions such as tissue regeneration and wound healing (Abuelella et al. 2023, 2025) and cell proliferation and migration (Kogan et al. 2007). We can make use of the presence of hyaluronan in the synovial fluid in joint as a biological marker for rheumatoid arthritis diagnosis (Lee et al. 2008).

Hyaluronan is extracted directly from marine animal sources, such as cartilage and vitreous humor of many fish species. Hyaluronan-based hydrogels were developed with dual stimuli responsiveness to both pH and temperature. Gentamicin was incorporated as a model drug. Assays of in vitro release showed a burst release of around 25% in the first hour, followed by a controlled release of up to 30% over the following 20 h. Increasing hyaluronan incorporation led to increasing release rate and more complete release afterward. The designed hydrogel showed response to variations in temperature, making it a potential vehicle for biomolecules to achieve smart controlled release system (Santos et al. 2010).

Another study investigated hyaluronan-tyramine (HA-Tyr) conjugates formed by enzymatic cross-linking, which are characterized by their biodegradability and encapsulation efficiency and continuous release of entrapped protein by the action of hyaluronidase on the network of the polymer. Hyaluronan-tyramine hydrogel was fabricated to incorporate trastuzumab anti-breast cancer drug. In vitro release studies showed release controlled of trastuzumab and depends mainly on concentration of hyaluronidase by the hydrogel degradation controlled by the concentration of hyaluronidase. Single subcutaneous of HA-Tyr conjugate inhibited tumor growth significantly with improved pharmacokinetic profile compared to trastuzumab alone (Xu et al. 2015).

Liposomes are well-known DDS candidate as templates for hyaluronan coatings. Jiang et al. presented a new liposome coated with hyaluronan in order to improve drug targeting and increase cellular uptake by cancer cells in addition to its shielding effect against plasma protein attack in blood circulation. Controlled drug release was achieved by degradation action of hyaluronidase present in extracellular matrix, and once the outer layer is degraded, pH environment variation allows the release of active drug achieving dual responsive action function of drug delivery system. Results showed significant antitumor activity, remarkable cytotoxicity, and efficient cellular uptake during in vivo tests. Hyaluronan hydrogels can be used as reservoirs of bioactive agents obtained via various methods of constructions (Jiang et al. 2012).

Hyaluronic acid can be also utilized to enhance the delivery of celastrol into tumor cells and improve its selectivity and efficacy. Celastrol-loaded cationic liposomes were then formulated via conjugation to hyaluronic acid (HA) by electrostatic binding interaction. Results showed enhanced delivery of active constituent into mitochondria achieving apoptosis of cells and higher antitumor efficacy in addition to improved safety profile due to lower associated side effects and higher cellular uptake by recognizing CD44-rich receptors on surfaces (Xiao et al. 2023).

Mentioning another example of utilization of the overexpression of CD44 receptors on activated macrophages during rheumatoid arthritis (RA), hyaluronic acid (HA)-coated acid-sensitive polymer nanoparticles loaded with dexamethasone were fabricated. In this example, the pH-responsive characteristic and targeting privilege of the abovementioned formulation were utilized to target CD44 receptors. Results showed improved cellular uptake and suppression of rheumatoid arthritis (RA) (Yu et al. 2019). HA-coated liposome loaded with Adriamycin was developed to achieve higher concentration of anticancer drug at tumor cells, utilizing the interaction of hyaluronic acid and CD44 on the surfaces of tumor cells. It was concluded that hyaluronic acid succeeded to yield a smart nano-DDS (Tian et al. 2018).

Another example displayed glutathione-responsive hyaluronic acid conjugate micelles, which were fabricated for the targeted delivery of DOX. Hyaluronic acid was chosen as the hydrophilic end of the polymeric micelles. The formulation achieved significant tumor suppression and higher cellular uptake offering potential delivery system to overcome side effects of antitumor drugs and safety profile (Yan et al. 2022).

2.7 *Chondroitin Sulfate-Based DDS*

Chondroitin sulfate is another sulfated glycosaminoglycan consisting mainly of a single chain of repeating disaccharide units of glucuronic acid (GlcA) and N-acetylgalactosamine (GalNAc). It can be extracted from some different marine animals, like whales and sharks, in addition to other non-mammalian marine animal sources, such as rays, salmon fishes, and sea cucumbers (Silva et al. 2012). Chondroitin sulfate has anticoagulant properties in addition to anti-inflammatory effect. This made it suitable to be used as anticoagulant agent and as a supplement to alleviate arthritis, and its hydrogels are widely used in tissue regeneration applications. Therefore, chondroitin sulfate is considered an interesting material to build DDS with different applications. It was reported that chondroitin sulfate/PEG hydrogels were proposed for many applications in biomedicine, such as in wound healing and regenerative medicine (Cardoso et al. 2016). Construction from hydroxyapatite and chondroitin sulfate porous tubular structure was performed for the delivery of chemotherapeutics. Results showed doxorubicin hydrochloride release in controlled manner, along with high encapsulation capacity of around 91% of efficacy attributed to the designed scaffold geometry, in addition to the in vitro dependent controlled release at different pH values (5, 6, and 7.4) (Guo et al. 2014).

There are several types of glycosaminoglycans; although they have low bioavailability, they are widely used due to their unique biological properties. Intra-articular injection of 40 mg of chondroitin and 40 mg of hyaluronic acid for treatment of knee arthritis was assessed. Pain relief and consumption of analgesic drugs were decreased, and improved mobility was also observed indicating safety and efficacy of the injection (Rivera et al. 2016). Another study investigated the protective effect of intramuscular injection of pure chondroitin sulfate after injection of chymopapain. Results showed positive outcomes and suggested that daily treatment with chondroitin sulfate participates in protecting and enhancing the damaged cartilage (Uebelhart et al. 1998). Another study demonstrated the healing effect of the submucosal injection of solution containing chondroitin sulfate combined with hyaluronic acid and poloxamer 407 on endoscopic mucosal resection. It showed early healing effect and proliferation of collagen and elastic fibers (Córdova et al. 2019). Fabrication of bovine serum albumin-loaded chitosan microspheres has been also performed, which are incorporated into hydrogel of carboxymethyl chitosan and oxidized chondroitin sulfate hydrogel. The scaffold properties showed improvement and lower swelling ratio, decreased gelation time, and controlled release pattern. In addition, the chondrocyte embedded in gel scaffold showed higher viability, which makes the scaffold a potential drug delivery system in tissue engineering (Fan et al. 2017). Chondroitin sulfate-chitosan nanoparticles incorporating doxorubicin were fabricated *via* ionotropic gelation and electrostatic interaction technique, which allow high drug loading. Formulation achieved a sustained release profile and appropriate cellular uptake by tumor cells and suppression of tumor in higher proportion than pure doxorubicin solution, which indicated potential of scaffold to effectively deliver antitumor drugs into cancer cells (Hu et al. 2014). For bone repair, recombinant human bone morphogenetic protein-2 was loaded into scaffold of chondroitin sulfate to be a vehicle for its gene delivery in mesenchymal stem cells. Results showed enhanced controlled release and comparable volume of bone formation and repairing of critical bone defect segments (Andrews et al. 2019).

2.8 Heparan Sulfate-Based DDS

Another glycosaminoglycan is heparan sulfate, which has a structure of high similarity to the structure of heparin. Biological activity depends mainly on different interactions with different biological biomolecules such as heparin and antithrombin. It consists in a linear chain of alternating D-glucuronic acid or iduronic acid and sulfated or deacylated D-glucosamine residues (Gandhi and Mancera 2008). Its affinity to interact with other proteins can be influenced by the number of sulfate groups, which in turn can influence their biological properties and processes such as coagulation. The heparan sulfate polysaccharide is highly biodegradable, principally by enzymatic action of heparanase (Meneghetti et al. 2015).

Cartilage repair is the main concern in drug development field as cartilage lacks basic repair mechanism. So, injected biomaterials to support chondrogenesis were developed in order to enhance cartilage tissue engineering. Scaffold composed of transforming growth factor (which is necessary for cartilage formation and hemostasis) and heparan (known to bind with growth factor and conjugated with hyaluronan hydrogel) was engineered. Results showed sustained release of transforming growth observed through the absence of matrix deposition and excellent chondrogenesis and improved safety profile due to localization of transforming growth factor injection (Levinson et al. 2019).

Loading of heparan into suitable drug delivery system can be occurred by specific interaction between heparan and cargo molecules. Polyelectrolyte complex hydrogels were developed by chemical interaction between chitosan and heparan sulfate and conjugated to surface of magnetic or metallic nanoparticles. These nanoparticles can be coupled with hemoglobin, other functional proteins, and DNA for different potential applications (Chauvierre et al. 2004). Nanoparticles containing low molecular weight heparan (fragmin)/protamine were produced and injected locally to lesions of Cushing syndrome. Results showed enhanced repairing damaged muscle tissue and improved motor function and blood flow (Takikawa et al. 2015).

2.9 Agarose-Based DDS

Another commonly used marine-derived polysaccharide is the agarose. Its structure resembles to a great extent the carrageenan, and it is commonly found in the cell wall of the red algae. Its structure comprises two main monosaccharide units connected in an alternate conformation (AB). The main difference between carrageenan and agar is that the carrageenan unit A is always in the D-conformation, while the agar unit A can only be in the L-conformation. Another difference compared to carrageenan is that agarose is not classified according to the sulfation degree, since the best known type of agarose is a neutral type without any sulfated group.

Agarose is utilized mainly in food industry and used widely in as a rich culture medium. It is also involved in different biomedical applications especially as hydrogels for the release of bioactive agents, taking advantage of its ability to jellify, biocompatibility, and native biodegradability. One of the most significant challenges that present in clinical practice is overcoming bacterial infection. A good example is the injectable hydrogels, which were developed based on agarose, carboxymethylcellulose, and silk fibroin to load vancomycin hydrochloride. The finding revealed a sustained release, perfect gelation time, and desirable antibacterial activity and wound healing (Babaluei et al. 2023).

Another utilization of beneficial combination between methylcellulose and agarose holding nerve guidance channel in place loaded with therapeutic agents. This combination maintained elastic modulus, and the ganglion with dissociated dorsal roots wasn't altered indicating the effective therapeutic delivery to the nervous system (Martin et al. 2008). Design of injectable hydrogels for tissue engineering participating in cell adhesion and proliferation promoting tissue engineering and nerve regeneration in addition fibroblast and olfactory bulb which are in contact with hydrogel have normal cell morphology and normal cells migration through porous hydrogel (Tonda-Turo et al. 2017). Minimally invasive approach (injectable hydrogels) can be utilized for tissue engineering, and scaffold from agarose, gelatin, and methacrylate is designed. The hydrogel showed appropriate injectability and porosity, offering a good delivery system for all osteochondral tissue engineering applications (Mokhtarzade et al. 2023). Agarose-based biomaterials can also be a suitable solution for restoration of injured cartilages and maintaining its hemostasis as they have unique mechanical properties facility upon static and dynamic loading. Agarose with low concentration of around 1% resulted in collagen deposition and enhanced matrix deposition in addition to enhancing cellular activity and regeneration of cartilage (Salati et al. 2020).

3 Conclusion: Future Perspective

Marine polysaccharides have demonstrated significant promise as materials for injectable drug delivery systems due to their inherent biocompatibility, biodegradability, and versatile physicochemical properties. Their ability to form hydrogels, nanoparticles, and in situ gelling systems enables the controlled and targeted release of therapeutic agents, making them particularly attractive for applications in oncology, regenerative medicine, and chronic disease management. Polysaccharides such as alginate, chitosan, carrageenan, and fucoidan have shown potential not only as drug carriers but also as bioactive components that can enhance therapeutic outcomes.

Looking forward, future research should focus on the structural modification of marine polysaccharides to improve their stability, drug-loading capacity, and responsiveness to physiological stimuli. The integration of advanced technologies, such as 3D bioprinting, injectable nanogels, and stimuli-responsive systems, holds promise for the development of next-generation injectable platforms. Furthermore, deeper insights into their interactions with biological systems, supported by in vivo studies and clinical trials, will be essential to translate laboratory findings into real-world therapies. With growing interest in sustainable and marine-based biomaterials, marine polysaccharides are poised to play a pivotal role in the evolution of safe, effective, and eco-friendly injectable drug delivery systems.

References

Abka Khajouei R, Tounsi L, Shahabi N, Patel A, Abdelkafi S, Michaud P (2022) Structures, Properties and Applications of Alginates. Marine Drugs 20:364. https://doi.org/10.3390/md20060364

Abuelella, K.E., Abd-Allah, H., Soliman, S.M., Abdel-Mottaleb, M.M.A., 2023. Skin targeting by chitosan/hyaluronate hybrid nanoparticles for the management of irritant contact dermatitis: In vivo therapeutic efficiency in mouse-ear dermatitis model. International Journal of Biological Macromolecules 232, 123458. https://doi.org/10.1016/j.ijbiomac.2023.123458

Abuelella, K.E., Abd-Allah, H., Soliman, S.M., Abdel-Mottaleb, M.M.A., 2022a. Polysaccharide Based Biomaterials for Dermal Applications, in: Jana, Sougata, Jana, Subrata (Eds.), Functional Biomaterials: Drug Delivery and Biomedical Applications. Springer Singapore, Singapore, pp. 105–127. https://doi.org/10.1007/978-981-16-7152-4_4

Abuelella, K.E., Abd-Allah, H., Soliman, S.M., Abdel-Mottaleb, M.M.A., 2022b. Chitosan based polyelectrolyte complex nanoparticles: preparation and characterization. Bulletin of Pharmaceutical Sciences. Assiut 45, 53–62. https://doi.org/10.21608/bfsa.2022.239176

Abuelella, K.E., Abd-Allah, Hend, Soliman, Sara M., and Abdel-Mottaleb, M.M.A., 2025. Intra-articular treatment of osteoarthritis using novel biocompatible etoricoxib chitosan-hyaluronate hybrid microparticles. Journal of Microencapsulation 1–15. https://doi.org/10.1080/02652048.2025.2490033

Adepu S, Ramakrishna S (2021) Controlled Drug Delivery Systems: Current Status and Future Directions. Molecules 26:5905. https://doi.org/10.3390/molecules26195905

Alves A, Duarte ARC, Mano JF, Sousa RA, Reis RL (2012) PDLLA enriched with ulvan particles as a novel 3D porous scaffold targeted for bone engineering. The Journal of Supercritical Fluids 65:32–38. https://doi.org/10.1016/j.supflu.2012.02.023

Andrews S, Cheng A, Stevens H, Logun MT, Webb R, Jordan E, Xia B, Karumbaiah L, Guldberg RE, Stice S (2019) Chondroitin Sulfate Glycosaminoglycan Scaffolds for Cell and Recombinant Protein-Based Bone Regeneration. Stem Cells Transl Med 8:575–585. https://doi.org/10.1002/sctm.18-0141

Babaluei M, Mojarab Y, Mottaghitalab F, Farokhi M (2023) Injectable hydrogel based on silk fibroin/carboxymethyl cellulose/agarose containing polydopamine functionalized graphene oxide with conductivity, hemostasis, antibacterial, and anti-oxidant properties for full-thickness burn healing. International Journal of Biological Macromolecules 249:126051. https://doi.org/10.1016/j.ijbiomac.2023.126051

Burdick JA, Prestwich GD (2011) Hyaluronic acid hydrogels for biomedical applications. Adv Mater 23:H41-56. https://doi.org/10.1002/adma.201003963

Cardoso MJ, Costa RR, Mano JF (2016) Marine Origin Polysaccharides in Drug Delivery Systems. Marine Drugs 14:34. https://doi.org/10.3390/md14020034

Carrasqueira J, Bernardino S, Bernardino R, Afonso C (2025) Marine-Derived Polysaccharides and Their Potential Health Benefits in Nutraceutical Applications. Marine Drugs 23:60. https://doi.org/10.3390/md23020060

Chauvierre C, Marden MC, Vauthier C, Labarre D, Couvreur P, Leclerc L (2004) Heparin coated poly(alkylcyanoacrylate) nanoparticles coupled to hemoglobin: a new oxygen carrier. Biomaterials 25:3081–3086. https://doi.org/10.1016/j.biomaterials.2003.09.097

Chen B, Liu X, Li Y, Shan T, Bai L, Li C, Wang Y (2022) iRGD Tumor-Penetrating Peptide-Modified Nano-Delivery System Based on a Marine Sulfated Polysaccharide for Enhanced Anti-Tumor Efficiency Against Breast Cancer. Int J Nanomedicine 17:617–633. https://doi.org/10.2147/IJN.S343902

Córdova H, Cuatrecasas M, García-Rodríguez A, Montenegro A, Melo J, Miguel CR, Martínez-Pallí G, Garcés-Durán R, Llach J, Fernández-Esparrach G (2019) Successful outcomes of a new combined solution of hyaluronic acid, chondroitin sulfate and poloxamer 407 for submucosal injection: animal survival study. Endoscopy International Open 07:E576–E582. https://doi.org/10.1055/a-0869-7757

Dongre R (2022) Marine Polysaccharides in Pharmaceutical Uses: Chitin, Chitosan, Alginate, and Carrageenan. p 33 (745–779l)

Fan M, Ma Y, Tan H, Jia Y, Zou S, Guo S, Zhao M, Huang H, Ling Z, Chen Y, Hu X (2017) Covalent and injectable chitosan-chondroitin sulfate hydrogels embedded with chitosan microspheres for drug delivery and tissue engineering. Materials Science and Engineering: C 71:67–74. https://doi.org/10.1016/j.msec.2016.09.068

Gandhi NS, Mancera RL (2008) The structure of glycosaminoglycans and their interactions with proteins. Chem Biol Drug Des 72:455–482. https://doi.org/10.1111/j.1747-0285.2008.00741.x

Guo Y, Shi X, Fang Q, Zhang J, Fang H, Jia W, Yang G, Yang L (2014) Facile preparation of hydroxyapatite–chondroitin sulfate hybrid mesoporous microrods for controlled and sustained release of antitumor drugs. Materials Letters 125:111–115. https://doi.org/10.1016/j.matlet.2014.03.084

Hariyadi DM, Islam N (2020) Current Status of Alginate in Drug Delivery. Advances in Pharmacological and Pharmaceutical Sciences 2020:8886095. https://doi.org/10.1155/2020/8886095

Hu C-S, Tang S-L, Chiang C-H, Hosseinkhani H, Hong P-D, Yeh M-K (2014) Characterization and anti-tumor effects of chondroitin sulfate–chitosan nanoparticles delivery system. J Nanopart Res 16:2672. https://doi.org/10.1007/s11051-014-2672-z

Huang C, Xie T, Liu Y, Yan S, OuYang F, Zhang H, Lei L, He D, Wei H, Yu C-Y (2023) A Sodium Alginate-Based Multifunctional Nanoplatform for Synergistic Chemo-Immunotherapy of Hepatocellular Carcinoma. Advanced Materials 35:2301352. https://doi.org/10.1002/adma.202301352

Jalal S, Hama Amin HB, Aziz S, Sha A, Hassan S, Abdul Aziz J, Rahman H (2019) Structural Characterization, Antimicrobial Activity, and In Vitro Cytotoxicity Effect of Black Seed Oil. Evidence-Based Complementary and Alternative Medicine 2019:1–9. https://doi.org/10.1155/2019/6515671

Jana S, Gangopadhaya A, Bhowmik B, Nayak A, Mukhrjee A (2015) Pharmacokinetic evaluation of testosterone-loaded nanocapsules in rats. International Journal of Biological Macromolecules 72:28–30. https://doi.org/10.1016/j.ijbiomac.2014.08.001

Jia Y, Sun Y, Weng L, Li Y, Zhang Q, Zhou H, Yang B (2016) Low molecular weight fucoidan protects renal tubular cells from injury induced by albumin overload. Sci Rep 6:31759. https://doi.org/10.1038/srep31759

Jiang T, Zhang Z, Zhang Y, Lv H, Zhou J, Li C, Hou L, Zhang Q (2012) Dual-functional liposomes based on pH-responsive cell-penetrating peptide and hyaluronic acid for tumor-targeted anticancer drug delivery. Biomaterials 33:9246–9258. https://doi.org/10.1016/j.biomaterials.2012.09.027

Joshi S, Eshwar S, Jain V (2019) Marine Polysaccharides: Biomedical and Tissue Engineering Applications. pp 443–487

Kogan G, Šoltés L, Stern R, Gemeiner P (2007) Hyaluronic acid: a natural biopolymer with a broad range of biomedical and industrial applications. Biotechnol Lett 29:17–25. https://doi.org/10.1007/s10529-006-9219-z

Y. Kotb, M. Hegazy, K. Abdelrahman, Z. Nour, M. Al-Jebzi, O. Ibrahim, A. Gouda, M. Abdel-Mottaleb, M. Serry, 2021. IoT-Based Reconfigurable Micropump for Drug Delivery Applications, in: 2021 IEEE Sensors. Presented at the 2021 IEEE Sensors, pp. 1–4. https://doi.org/10.1109/SENSORS47087.2021.9639776

Küçükbalcı Geyik G, Işıklan N (2021) Multi-stimuli-sensitive superparamagnetic κ-carrageenan based nanoparticles for controlled 5-fluorouracil delivery. Colloids and Surfaces A: Physicochemical and Engineering Aspects 634:127960. https://doi.org/10.1016/j.colsurfa.2021.127960

Laraba-djebari F (2016) Development and characterization of a new carrier for vaccine delivery based on calcium-alginate nanoparticles: Safe immunoprotective approach against scorpion envenoming. Vaccine

Lee H, Lee K, Kim IK, Park TG (2008) Synthesis, characterization, and in vivo diagnostic applications of hyaluronic acid immobilized gold nanoprobes. Biomaterials 29:4709–4718. https://doi.org/10.1016/j.biomaterials.2008.08.038

Levinson C, Lee M, Applegate LA, Zenobi-Wong M (2019) An injectable heparin-conjugated hyaluronan scaffold for local delivery of transforming growth factor β1 promotes successful chondrogenesis. Acta Biomaterialia 99:168–180. https://doi.org/10.1016/j.actbio.2019.09.017

Li P, Liu D, Miao L, Liu C, Sun X, Liu Y, Zhang N (2012) A pH-sensitive multifunctional gene carrier assembled via layer-by-layer technique for efficient gene delivery. Int J Nanomedicine 7: 925–939. https://doi.org/10.2147/IJN.S26955

Martin BC, Minner EJ, Wiseman SL, Klank RL, Gilbert RJ (2008) Agarose and methylcellulose hydrogel blends for nerve regeneration applications. J Neural Eng 5:221. https://doi.org/10.1088/1741-2560/5/2/013

Meneghetti MCZ, Hughes AJ, Rudd TR, Nader HB, Powell AK, Yates EA, Lima MA (2015) Heparan sulfate and heparin interactions with proteins. J R Soc Interface 12:0589. https://doi.org/10.1098/rsif.2015.0589

Mokhtarzade A, Imani R, Shokrollahi P (2023) A gradient four-layered gelatin methacrylate/agarose construct as an injectable scaffold for mimicking osteochondral tissue. J Mater Sci 58:5735–5755. https://doi.org/10.1007/s10853-023-08374-x

Morelli A, Betti M, Puppi D, Bartoli C, Gazzarri M, Federica C (2015) Enzymatically Crosslinked Ulvan Hydrogels as Injectable Systems for Cell Delivery. Macromolecular Chemistry and Physics 217:n/a-n/a. https://doi.org/10.1002/macp.201500353

Mousa, A.M., Abdelraof, M., Hassabo, A.A., Darwish, D.A., Abdel-Mottaleb, M.M.A., Allam, R. M., 2025. Marine L-arginase encapsulated in poly (lactic-co-glycolic acid) nanoparticles: A novel anti-cancer strategy for effective hepatocellular carcinoma treatment in vitro and in vivo. Journal of Drug Delivery Science and Technology 109, 106980. https://doi.org/10.1016/j.jddst.2025.106980

Piekarska K, Sikora M, Owczarek M, Jóźwik-Pruska J, Wiśniewska-Wrona M (2023) Chitin and Chitosan as Polymers of the Future—Obtaining, Modification, Life Cycle Assessment and Main Directions of Application. Polymers 15:793. https://doi.org/10.3390/polym15040793

Ramadan, N.E., Youssef, F.R., Alshishtawy, A.A.K., Elshikh, F.M., Newir, O., Abdelazeem, S.H., Ma'ruf, N.K., Shouman, H., Ali, S.S., El-Sheekh, M.M., 2025. Marine algal polysaccharides for drug delivery applications: A review. International Journal of Biological Macromolecules 295, 139551. https://doi.org/10.1016/j.ijbiomac.2025.139551

Rivera F, Bertignone L, Grandi G, Camisassa R, Comaschi G, Trentini D, Zanone M, Teppex G, Vasario G, Fortina G (2016) Effectiveness of intra-articular injections of sodium hyaluronate-chondroitin sulfate in knee osteoarthritis: a multicenter prospective study. J Orthopaed Traumatol 17:27–33. https://doi.org/10.1007/s10195-015-0388-1

Román-Doval R, Torres-Arellanes SP, Tenorio-Barajas AY, Gómez-Sánchez A, Valencia-Lazcano AA (2023) Chitosan: Properties and Its Application in Agriculture in Context of Molecular Weight. Polymers 15:2867. https://doi.org/10.3390/polym15132867

Salati MA, Khazai J, Tahmuri AM, Samadi A, Taghizadeh A, Taghizadeh M, Zarrintaj P, Ramsey JD, Habibzadeh S, Seidi F, Saeb MR, Mozafari M (2020) Agarose-Based Biomaterials: Opportunities and Challenges in Cartilage Tissue Engineering. Polymers 12:1150. https://doi.org/10.3390/polym12051150

Santos JR, Alves NM, Mano JF (2010) New Thermo-responsive Hydrogels Based on Poly (N-isopropylacrylamide)/ Hyaluronic Acid Semi-interpenetrated Polymer Networks: Swelling Properties and Drug Release Studies. Journal of Bioactive and Compatible Polymers 25:169–184. https://doi.org/10.1177/0883911509357863

Salama, R.M., Yehia, R., Elmongy, N.F., Sallam, A.A., Abd-Elgalil, M.M., Schaalan, M.F., Abdel-Mottaleb, M.M.A., Bazan, L.S., 2025. Evaluation of betanin-loaded liposomal nanocarriers in AlCl3-induced Alzheimer's disease in rats: Impact on cognitive function, neurodegeneration, and TREM2/ADAM10 pathways. Archiv der Pharmazie 358, e2400641. https://doi.org/10.1002/ardp.202400641

Sedky, M., Ali, A., Abdel-Mottaleb, M., Serry, M., 2024. A new rapid-release SMA-activated micropump with incorporated microneedle arrays and polymeric nanoparticles for optimized transdermal drug delivery. Sensors and Actuators B: Chemical 408, 135549. https://doi.org/10.1016/j.snb.2024.135549

Shu G, Lu C, Wang Z, Du Y, Xu X, Xu M, Zhao Z, Chen M, Dai Y, Weng Q, Fang S, Fan K, Liu D, Du Y, Ji J (2021) Fucoidan-based micelles as P-selectin targeted carriers for synergistic treatment of acute kidney injury. Nanomedicine 32:102342. https://doi.org/10.1016/j.nano.2020.102342

Silva TH, Alves A, Popa EG, Reys LL, Gomes ME, Sousa RA, Silva SS, Mano JF, Reis RL (2012) Marine algae sulfated polysaccharides for tissue engineering and drug delivery approaches. Biomatter 2:278–289. https://doi.org/10.4161/biom.22947

Sulastri E, Lesmana R, Zubair M, Elamin K, Wathoni N (2021) A Comprehensive Review on Ulvan Based Hydrogel and Its Biomedical Applications. Chemical & pharmaceutical bulletin 69:432–443. https://doi.org/10.1248/cpb.c20-00763

Sun Y, Ma X, Hu H (2021) Marine Polysaccharides as a Versatile Biomass for the Construction of Nano Drug Delivery Systems. Mar Drugs 19:345. https://doi.org/10.3390/md19060345

Takikawa M, Nakamura S, Ishihara M, Takabayashi Y, Fujita M, Hattori H, Kushibiki T, Ishihara M (2015) Improved angiogenesis and healing in crush syndrome by fibroblast growth factor-2-containing low-molecular-weight heparin (Fragmin)/protamine nanoparticles. J Surg Res 196: 247–257. https://doi.org/10.1016/j.jss.2015.03.022

Thinh PD, Menshova RV, Ermakova SP, Anastyuk SD, Ly BM, Zvyagintseva TN (2013) Structural characteristics and anticancer activity of fucoidan from the brown alga Sargassum mcclurei. Mar Drugs 11:1456–1476. https://doi.org/10.3390/md11051456

Tian Z, Liu J, Li N, Garamus VM, Zou A (2018) Hyaluronic acid-coated liposome for active targeting on CD44 expressing tumors. J Nanopart Res 20:235. https://doi.org/10.1007/s11051-018-4324-1

Tonda-Turo C, Gnavi S, Ruini F, Gambarotta G, Gioffredi E, Chiono V, Perroteau I, Ciardelli G (2017) Development and characterization of novel agar and gelatin injectable hydrogel as filler for peripheral nerve guidance channels. Journal of Tissue Engineering and Regenerative Medicine 11:197–208. https://doi.org/10.1002/term.1902

Uebelhart D, Thonar EJ, Zhang J, Williams JM (1998) Protective effect of exogenous chondroitin 4,6-sulfate in the acute degradation of articular cartilage in the rabbit. Osteoarthritis Cartilage 6 Suppl A:6–13. https://doi.org/10.1016/s1063-4584(98)80005-8

Venugopal V, RAJA KUMAR J, Muralidharan S (2015) TARGETED DELIVERY OF SILYMARIN TO LIVER CELLS BY GALACTOSYLATED NA-NOPARTICLES: IN-VITRO & IN-VIVO EVALUATION STUDIES. Albanian Journal of Pharmaceutical Sciences 2

Wang M, Zhao T, Liu Y, Wang Q, Xing S, Li L, Wang L, Liu L, Gao D (2017) Ursolic acid liposomes with chitosan modification: Promising antitumor drug delivery and efficacy. Materials Science and Engineering: C 71:1231–1240. https://doi.org/10.1016/j.msec.2016.11.014

Wang Y, Khan A, Liu Y, Feng J, Dai L, Wang G, Alam N, Tong L, Ni Y (2019) Chitosan oligosaccharide-based dual pH responsive nano-micelles for targeted delivery of hydrophobic drugs. Carbohydrate Polymers 223:115061. https://doi.org/10.1016/j.carbpol.2019.115061

Xiao S, Huang S, Yang X, Lei Y, Chang M, Hu J, Meng Y, Zheng G, Chen X (2023) The development and evaluation of hyaluronic acid coated mitochondrial targeting liposomes for celastrol delivery. Drug Deliv 30:2162156. https://doi.org/10.1080/10717544.2022.2162156

Xu J, Cheng X, Tan L, Fu C, Ahmed M, Tian J, Dou J, Zhou Q, Ren X, Wu Q, Tang S, Zhou H, Meng X, Yu J, Liang P (2019) Microwave Responsive Nanoplatform via P-Selectin Mediated Drug Delivery for Treatment of Hepatocellular Carcinoma with Distant Metastasis. Nano Lett 19:2914–2927. https://doi.org/10.1021/acs.nanolett.8b05202

Xu K, Lee F, Gao S, Tan M-H, Kurisawa M (2015) Hyaluronidase-incorporated hyaluronic acid–tyramine hydrogels for the sustained release of trastuzumab. Journal of Controlled Release 216: 47–55. https://doi.org/10.1016/j.jconrel.2015.08.015

Yan K, Feng Y, Gao K, Shi X, Zhao X (2022) Fabrication of hyaluronic acid-based micelles with glutathione-responsiveness for targeted anticancer drug delivery. J Colloid Interface Sci 606: 1586–1596. https://doi.org/10.1016/j.jcis.2021.08.129

Yang C-L, Chen J-P, Wei K-C, Chen J-Y, Huang C-W, Liao Z-X (2017) Release of Doxorubicin by a Folate-Grafted, Chitosan-Coated Magnetic Nanoparticle. Nanomaterials (Basel) 7:85. https://doi.org/10.3390/nano7040085

Yermak IM, Mischchenko NP, Davydova VN, Glazunov VP, Tarbeeva DV, Kravchenko AO, Pimenova EA, Sorokina IV (2017) Carrageenans-Sulfated Polysaccharides from Red Seaweeds as Matrices for the Inclusion of Echinochrome. Mar Drugs 15:337. https://doi.org/10.3390/md15110337

Yu C, Li X, Hou Y, Meng X, Wang D, Liu J, Sun F, Li Y (2019) Hyaluronic Acid Coated Acid-Sensitive Nanoparticles for Targeted Therapy of Adjuvant-Induced Arthritis in Rats. Molecules 24:146. https://doi.org/10.3390/molecules24010146

Yu L, Xue C, Chang Y, Xu X, Ge L, Liu G, Wang Y (2014) Structure elucidation of fucoidan composed of a novel tetrafucose repeating unit from sea cucumber Thelenota ananas. Food Chemistry 146:113–119. https://doi.org/10.1016/j.foodchem.2013.09.033

Zheng, G., Li, R., Wu, P., Zhang, L., Qin, Y., Wan, S., Pei, J., Yu, P., Fu, K., Meyerhoff, M.E., Liu, Y., Zhou, Y., 2023. Controllable release of nitric oxide from an injectable alginate hydrogel. International Journal of Biological Macromolecules 252, 126371. https://doi.org/10.1016/j.ijbiomac.2023.126371

Marine Seaweed Polysaccharide in Antiviral Activities

Fatma Sa'eed El-Tokhy and Mona M. A. Abdel-Mottaleb

Abstract Marine biotechnology is an evolving field that employs marine organisms to generate, alter, or enhance biological resources for nutritional, industrial, medicinal, or environmental purposes. Given the pharmacological importance of marine bioactive compounds, numerous metabolic products derived from marine biomass were examined for their medicinal efficacy. The identification of algal polysaccharides exhibiting antiviral properties has notably risen over the last few decades. Additionally, distinct polysaccharides derived from seaweeds, including carrageenan, alginates, fucoidans, galactans, laminarins, and ulvans, have demonstrated efficacy in combating viral infection. New antiviral therapies could be developed using seaweed polysaccharides because of their various characteristics that are similar to effective antiviral drugs. In this chapter, we describe the most important marine seaweed polysaccharides with potential antiviral activities and the mechanism of their action as well as examples of their successful use in the treatment of various viral infections.

Keywords Seaweed · Polysaccharides · Antiviral · Marine

1 Introduction

Marine biotechnology is an evolving field that employs marine living organisms to generate, alter, or enhance biologic resources for nutritional, industrial, medicinal, or environmental purposes. Given the pharmacological importance of marine bioactive

F. S. El-Tokhy
Department of Pharmaceutics and Industrial Pharmacy, Faculty of Pharmacy, Badr University in Cairo (BUC), Cairo, Egypt

M. M. A. Abdel-Mottaleb (✉)
Université de Franche-Comté, EFS, INSERM, UMR 1098 RIGHT, Besançon, France

Department of Pharmaceutics and industrial Pharmacy, Faculty of Pharmacy, Ain Shams University, Cairo, Egypt
e-mail: mona.abdelmottaleb@pharma.asu.edu.eg

S. Jana et al. (eds.), *Multifunctional Marine Polysaccharides*,
https://doi.org/10.1007/978-981-95-4126-3_4

compounds, numerous metabolic products derived from marine biomass were examined for their medicinal efficacy (Bai and Tuvikene 2021; Mousa et al. 2025). Seaweed informally denotes macroscopic, multi-cellular marine algae. Such algae are devoid of root systems, leaves, flowers, fruits, stems, and seeds. Typically, they flourish and are anchored to rocks or sturdy substrates situated below the maximum water level, or they may freely float in the oceans (Akter et al. 2024).

Marine algae encounter environmental stresses such as low temperatures, elevated salinity, high pressure, and nutrient deficiency, leading to the evolution of various polysaccharides with multifaceted functions (Wei et al. 2022). Therefore, polysaccharides represent the main composition of seaweeds, accounting for up to 70% of their dry weight (Xu et al. 2017). Polysaccharides like cellulose and agar confer both rigidity and flexibility to the cell walls of seaweed, enabling them to endure water currents while preserving their structural integrity. Other polysaccharides act as energy reserves such as laminarin and floridean starch, which store glucose for metabolic activities during periods when photosynthesis is restricted, such as at night or in deep aquatic environments. Hydrocolloids such as alginate and carrageenan facilitate water retention in seaweed, thereby mitigating dehydration in low tide zones.

Recently, polysaccharides derived from seaweed are receiving considerable focus in biomedical research due to their varied biological activities, particularly in regenerative medicine, tissue engineering, and prospective uses in pharmaceutical drug delivery (Bai and Tuvikene 2021). Few examples would include their use in bone regeneration, where seaweed polysaccharides can serve as scaffolding framework for the extracellular matrix of osseous tissue (Jin et al. 2023). Carrageenan and fucoidan showed remarkable osteogenic inducing potential that could be utilized in clinical applications (Cao et al. 2021; Citkowska et al. 2019). Increasing evidence suggests that sulfated polysaccharides can disrupt the leukocytes' migration to inflammatory sites. The heterofucan mitigates inflammation through direct interaction with the cell surface of leukocytes, particularly polymorphonuclear cells (PMNs). It entirely prevents the migration of leukocytes into the injured tissue (De Jesus Raposo et al. 2015). The significant antitumor properties of seaweed polysaccharides have been highlighted by many researches. Fucoidan, alginate, and carrageenan have been recognized for apoptosis induction and inhibition of cancer cell proliferation and interference with tumor growth by modulation of various signaling pathways (Guo et al. 2022; Jin et al. 2022a, b). Other interesting characteristics such as biocompatibility, biodegradability, and structure-forming ability make seaweed polysaccharides promising candidates for drug delivery applications whether as formulation ingredients, such as alginate and carrageenan that are used as gel-forming and thickening agents, or as intrinsically active substances in cancer, infections, or inflammation therapy (Abuelella et al. 2022).

The identification of algal polysaccharides exhibiting antiviral properties has notably risen over the last few decades. Additionally, distinct polysaccharides derived from seaweeds, including carrageenan, alginates, galactans, fucoidans, ulvans, and laminarins, have demonstrated efficacy in combating viral infections (Damonte et al. 2004). New antiviral therapies could be developed using seaweed polysaccharides because of their various characteristics that are similar to effective antiviral drugs (Hans et al. 2021). The complex polysaccharides are able to hinder the viral adherence and entrance as well as crucial replication processes, demonstrating an outstanding ability to disrupt many phases of the viral life cycle (Ahmadi et al. 2015). With their broad range of viral targets, capacity to modulate the immune response, and low toxicity to human cells, they hold great promise as a means of combating viral infections while preserving the well-being of hosts. A primary criterion for an antiviral medication is its minimal cytotoxic effects on human cells. Furthermore, their natural origin and capacity to mitigate viral resistance offer an innovative perspective on the field of antiviral pharmaceutical development, which may one day overcome the limitations and difficulties associated with current treatments (Liyanage et al. 2023) especially that viral infections continue to pose a significant and pressing challenge to the well-being of populations worldwide. At present, more than 500 viruses have been identified as infecting agents in humans.

2 Viral Life Cycle and Antiviral Targets

Despite the variation in life cycles among different viral species, there are three fundamental stages common to all. First is a viral cell entry stage that encompasses the viral attachment, entry, and uncoating. The replication phase comes next followed by post-replication where the assembly and release of mature virions from the host cell occur (Rampersad and Tennant 2018).

These stages represent potential targets for inhibitory agents. Antiviral medications may exert an inhibitory influence on the complete replication cycle. Classification can be based on the specific stage to which they are directed.

2.1 Viral Cell Entry Stage

The viral cell entrance phase represents a pivotal moment in the viral life cycle, involving the virus's binding to the host cell followed by its internalization into the cellular environment. This process is crucial for the onset of viral infection and subsequent replication and its interruption can reduce the viral load and limit the spread of infection within the host.

This phase commences with viral attachment, during which viruses utilize glycoproteins on their surfaces to adhere to specific receptors located on the host cell membrane. This interaction is precise and defines the virus's tropism. A stable complex is established between viral glycoproteins and host cell receptors, enabling subsequent interactions essential for entry. Certain viruses penetrate host cells via endocytosis, a process in which the cell encapsulates the virus within a vesicle. Enveloped viruses possess the ability to merge their lipid envelope with the host cell membrane, thereby facilitating the release of the viral genome into the cytoplasm.

Upon cell penetration, the viral capsid undergoes disassembly (uncoating), facilitating the release of the viral genome into the cytoplasm. Diverse approaches are available to block viral adsorption and entry, each targeting different aspects of this phase. Targeting the surface glycoproteins, hemagglutinin-neuraminidase (HN) proteins in Newcastle disease virus (NDV) via 1-formyl-β-carboline derivatives could block the viral attachment to sialic acid receptors on host cells (Wang et al. 2021). Similarly, fucoidan, a sulfated polysaccharide, can block influenza A virus (IAV) infection by targeting the same proteins (Wang et al. 2017). Enfuvirtide serves as a peptidic mimic of the HR2 domain of HIV-1 gp41, playing a crucial role in the fusion process, thereby blocking viral entry. Anionic molecules interact with the positively charged amino acids found in viral surface glycoproteins, thereby preventing binding with host cell receptors. This mechanism prevents the fusion of the virion envelope with the cell membrane, thereby inhibiting viral entry (Meyer et al. 2020).

2.2 Viral Replication Stage

Similar to how our DNA encodes the information necessary for protein synthesis, a viral genome serves as the blueprint for the production of viral proteins. The viral replication objective is to facilitate the production and perpetuation of its species. Through the prolific replication of its genome and subsequent encapsulation into virions, the virus effectively perpetuates its ability to infect new hosts. Consequently, all viruses must express their genes as functional mRNAs at the onset of infection to guide the cellular translational machinery in synthesizing viral proteins. The replication strategy of a virus typically hinges on the nature of its nucleic acid genome (Louten 2016). RNA viruses reproduce their genetic material via two unique processes: RNA-dependent RNA synthesis and, in the context of retroviruses, RNA-dependent DNA synthesis (reverse transcription) that is then followed by further DNA replication and transcription. Both pathways necessitate enzymatic activities typically absent in uninfected host cells. Subsequently, these viruses encode the necessary enzymes, which are either expressed early in the infection process or co-packaged with the viral genome during virion assembly, preparing for subsequent infection cycles. DNA viruses primarily focus on mRNA generation, employing well-established strategies in normal cell biology: the transcription of mRNA from double-stranded DNA and the replication of double-stranded DNA within the cell nucleus. Numerous organisms utilize host enzymes for these processes, whereas certain larger viruses encode their own enzymes. The process comprises three primary phases: initiation, elongation, and termination. This stage includes the organization of the viral genome in readiness for replication. Viral polymerases commence nucleic acid synthesis through diverse mechanisms that are tailored to the host cell environment. In DNA viruses, the initiation process typically takes place within the nucleus, where host enzymes are readily accessible. In RNA viruses, the initiation process generally takes place within the cytoplasm.

Nucleotides are appended to the extending strand of the viral genetic material during elongation. This process entails the activity of viral or host polymerases that generate new strands utilizing the viral template. DNA viruses utilize host DNA polymerases for elongation, whereas RNA viruses employ viral RNA-dependent RNA polymerase. Termination signifies the end of replication phase, culminating in the end of the replication process and the production of new viral genome copies. This stage guarantees the complete replication of the viral genome, preparing it for assembly into new virions (Hangyu et al. 2024).

Antiviral agents that target this phase of viral infections aim to obstruct the mechanisms that enable viruses to replicate their genetic material. Their targets encompass enzymes and processes critical for viral genome replication such as viral polymerases. Viral polymerases are formally classified as DNA-dependent DNA polymerases, RNA-dependent DNA polymerases, and RNA-dependent RNA polymerases (RdRp), based on the type of viral nucleic acid and replication method (Hangyu et al. 2024). Numerous polymerase inhibitors have been designed to target these specific subunits: polymerase base 1 (PB1), polymerase base 2 (PB2), and polymerase acidic (PA). As influenza virus RdRp inhibitors, baloxavir, a PA-specific inhibitor, is effective against both influenza A and B virus strains, whereas ribavirin and favipiravir are nucleoside analogues and function as PB1 antagonists (Massari et al. 2021). Remdesivir and favipiravir serve as SARS-CoV-2 RdRp inhibitors. These nucleoside analogues selectively inhibit the RdRp of SARS-CoV-2. The reverse transcriptase of HIV possesses RNA/DNA-dependent DNA polymerase activity. The inaugural anti-HIV medication, suramin, targets the viral reverse transcriptase to obstruct the virus's replication cycle (De Clercq 2021). Currently, non-nucleoside agents exemplified by etravirine and its derivatives are the primary HIV polymerase inhibitors utilized in clinical practice (Havens et al. 2020). Recent investigations have unveiled compelling evidence suggesting that liquid-liquid phase separation (LLPS) during the process of viral replication presents a promising target for antiviral therapeutic strategies. Research indicates that various viral proteins and nucleic acids participate in liquid-liquid phase separation, leading to the formation of condensates that facilitate viral replication. Cyclopamine, a steroidal alkaloid, along with its chemical analogue A3E, impedes the replication of respiratory syncytial virus (RSV) by disrupting and solidifying the viral inclusion body condensates, which are crucial sites for viral RNA synthesis (York 2021).

2.3 Post-replication Stage

The stages that follow replication in the viral life cycle encompass assembly, maturation, and release. Following the replication of the viral genome, these stages play a vital role in the generation of infectious viruses (Bird and Kirkegaard 2015). Assembly begins to take place in diverse regions of the host cell, including the cytoplasm, nucleus, or endoplasmic reticulum. Recently synthesized viral elements, encompassing genomes and proteins, are meticulously organized into nascent

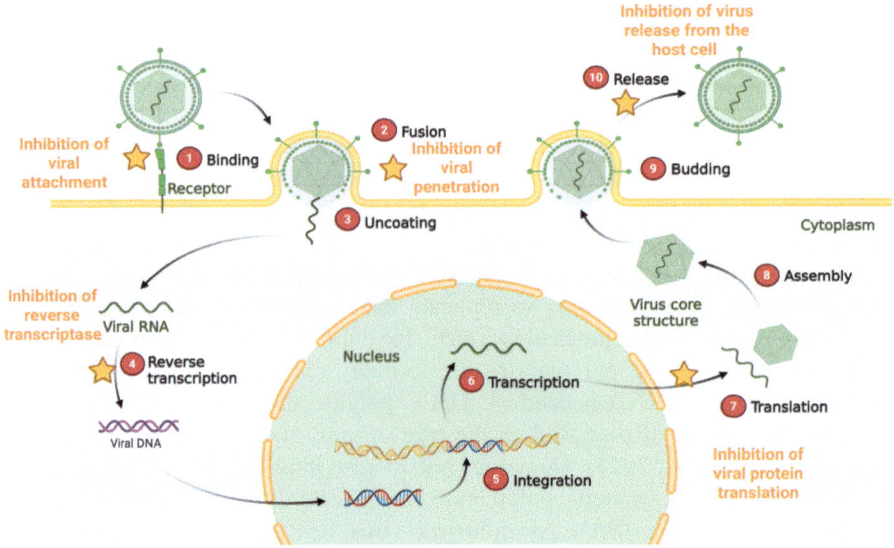

Fig. 1 The viral replication stages with the potential mechanisms of different antiviral agents

virions. In certain viruses, the capsid assembles around the genome during its replication, whereas in others, the genome is incorporated into an already constructed capsid. Afterward, the assembled virions experience structural transformations—maturation step—which render them infectious. This process frequently entails alterations to the viral capsid or envelope, which may be facilitated by enzymes from either the host or the virus itself. Viruses possess various mechanisms to exit the host cell. Budding is where the virus envelops itself in a portion of the host cell membrane, subsequently emerging without inducing cell lysis (Bird and Kirkegaard 2015). Lysis occurs when the host cell ruptures, resulting in the release of newly formed viral particles (Koca and Çetinkaya 2024). This phenomenon is characteristic of cytolytic viruses such as influenza, smallpox, and herpes viruses (Koca and Çetinkaya 2024). Exocytosis involves the release of viruses, which are encapsulated within vesicles before being expelled from the cell (Gerges et al. 2024). The antiviral mechanisms that target this stage could be achieved via inhibition of critical key elements and key players. For instance, disrupting the interaction between viral proteins and host factors can inhibit the formation of new virions. Another strategy is the inhibition of viral proteases, which are responsible for maturation of viral particles. This inhibition could occur via blocking the cleavage of precursor proteins into functional proteins like HIV protease inhibitors (Kausar et al. 2021). On the other hand, the release of new virions from infected cells can be disrupted using neuraminidase inhibitors (e.g., oseltamivir), which are the first choice in the prevention and treatment of influenza (Bassetti et al. 2024). Figure 1 summarizes the viral replication stages with the potential mechanisms of different antiviral agents.

3 Superior Antiviral Activity of Sulfated Polysaccharides

Seaweed-derived sulfated polysaccharides demonstrate a remarkable antiviral efficacy when compared with their non-sulfated variants. This enhanced activity can be attributed to the presence of sulfate groups, which significantly bolster their capacity to engage with viral entities and the components of host cells (Jiao et al. 2011). The presence of negatively charged sulfate groups allows sulfated polysaccharides to form robust interactions with positively charged areas on viral surface proteins, including glycoproteins and capsid proteins, thereby effectively hindering viral attachment and subsequent entry into host cells (Wang et al. 2012). For instance, carrageenans and fucoidans, two thoroughly explored sulfated polysaccharides, have shown significant inhibitory effects against a diverse array of viruses, such as herpes simplex virus (HSV), human immunodeficiency virus (HIV), influenza virus, and hepatitis C virus (HCV) (Panggabean et al. 2022; Song et al. 2020). The sulfate groups are crucial in compromising viral envelopes, resulting in the direct inactivation of enveloped viruses. Furthermore, sulfated polysaccharides possess the ability to disrupt viral replication through the inhibition of essential viral enzymes, including reverse transcriptase and proteases. Sulfated polysaccharides can also emulate heparan sulfate, which present promising antiviral properties. Since they can obscure the positive charge of viral surface receptors, thereby hindering their ability to attach to heparan sulfate proteoglycans located on the surface of host cells. Hence, they are capable of disrupting the initial phases of viral replication. They also engage with viral nucleic acids, thereby obstructing their replication process (Kang et al. 2022). In addition to their direct antiviral properties, sulfated polysaccharides play a pivotal role in augmenting the host immune response. They stimulate the production of antiviral cytokines, activate immune cells, and enhance phagocytosis, collectively offering a comprehensive defense against viral infections (Shen et al. 2024). The distinctive structural characteristics, especially the extent and arrangement of sulfation, play a crucial role in determining their antiviral effectiveness, rendering them more effective than non-sulfated polysaccharides in the fight against viral infections (Bandyopadhyay et al. 2011). The interplay of direct virucidal activity, immune modulation, and extensive antiviral effects highlights the promising therapeutic efficiency of the sulfated polysaccharides as natural antiviral agents.

4 Antiviral Activity of Prominent Algal Polysaccharides

4.1 Carrageenan

Carrageenan is a water-soluble sulfated galactan extracted from red seaweed, predominantly from the genera *Chondrus*, *Eucheuma*, and *Gigartina*. Carrageenan consists of linear sulfated galactans, characterized by extensive chains of galactose units interconnected through alternating α-(1 $\rightarrow$ 3) and β-(1 $\rightarrow$ 4) glycosidic bonds.

The extent and configuration of sulfation differ among the three principal varieties of carrageenan—kappa (κ), iota (ι), and lambda (λ)—thereby affecting their physical characteristics and biological functions. Lambda-carrageenans consist of galactose units, while iota- and kappa-carrageenans are composed of equal proportions of galactose and 3,6-anhydrogalactose. The relationship between the structure and activity of carrageenan is intricately linked to its pattern of sulfation, with the negatively charged sulfate groups being pivotal in their interactions with viral particles and host cells (Álvarez-Viñas et al. 2021). Notably, an increased level of sulfation in carrageenan does not inherently equate to enhanced antiviral activity. The biological activity of these polymers is influenced by their chemical structure, which encompasses factors such as the degree of sulfation, molecular weight, constituent sugars, and stereochemistry (Álvarez-Viñas et al. 2021). The capacity of sulfated polysaccharides to penetrate tissues might be limited by their large molecular weight, which significantly constrains their potential for antiviral use in humans. Consequently, depolymerized derivatives of carrageenan, oligosaccharides, are regarded as promising alternatives for the prevention of various diseases, particularly those induced by enveloped viruses (Guo et al. 2019). Low-molecular-weight λ-carrageenan demonstrates superior performance in these areas. Carrageenan effectively inactivates viruses by destabilizing their envelopes, highlighting its broad-spectrum antiviral prowess. This is especially potent against enveloped viruses that depend on their lipid bilayer for infection. Carrageenan's sulfated polysaccharide structure engages with the viral envelope, compromising its integrity and making the virus non-infectious (Girond et al. 1991). Sulfate groups in carrageenan, carrying a negative charge, attach to positively charged areas on viral envelope proteins, causing conformational shifts that weaken the envelope. This destabilization may lead to viral content leakage and even total disintegration of the viral particle (Carlucci et al. 1999; Girond et al. 1991). The studies carried out both in vitro and in vivo on the effects of carrageenans on the herpes simplex virus (HSV) demonstrated a virucidal effect, the inactivation of virions, a protective role against viral replication, and an improvement in mortality outcomes (Carlucci et al. 1999, 2004).

The antiviral activity of carrageenan is primarily attributed to its ability to interfere with viral attachment and entry into host cells. The sulfated polysaccharides in carrageenan mimic the heparan sulfate proteoglycans on cell surfaces, which many viruses use as receptors for attachment. By binding to viral surface proteins, carrageenan prevents the virus from interacting with host cells, thereby inhibiting infection (Álvarez-Viñas et al. 2021).

Some carrageenans may disrupt viral internalization and uncoating, in addition to blocking viral attachment. Carrageenans can also prevent papilloma virus infection through heparin sulfate-independent mechanism following attachment. The inhibitory effect arises from the blockage of binding between virion surfaces and cellular proteins during infection, along with the disruption of necessary conformational changes in virion proteins (Buck et al. 2006; Campo et al. 2009). Dengue virus retains the ability to infiltrate host cells even when carrageenans are present. The direct engagement of carrageenans with the viral membrane glycoprotein E may obstruct the subsequent uncoating and liberation of DENV from endosomes. During viral transcription and replication stages, reports indicated that low-molecular-weight k-carrageenan oligosaccharides and their sulfated derivatives have the potential to inhibit the replication of influenza A virus in both in vitro and in vivo investigations. The antiviral activities of k-carrageenan oligosaccharides largely hinge on their molecular weight and the extent of sulfation, which encompasses both the sulfate content and the specific positions of sulfation. Oligosaccharides with molecular weights ranging from 1 to 3 kDa and varying sulfate contents (0.8–1.0 mol/disaccharide mole) exhibit the most potent antiviral activity. Wang et al. concluded that carrageenan oligosaccharides have the capability to penetrate host cells, subsequently inhibiting influenza A virus mRNA and protein expression with increasing doses. Furthermore, ί-carrageenans have the potential to hinder the dengue virus replication inside mosquito cells by affecting specific targets within the host cells. Additionally, carrageenan has been shown to induce an immune response by stimulating the production of interferons and other cytokines, which further enhances its antiviral effects. Its mechanism is broad-spectrum, making it effective against a variety of enveloped and non-enveloped viruses, including influenza, herpes simplex virus (HSV), human papillomavirus (HPV), and respiratory syncytial virus (RSV) (Wei et al. 2022).

Carrageenans have demonstrated efficacy primarily in combating enveloped viruses. The family Herpesviridae has been the subject of extensive research, particularly focusing on herpes simplex virus types I and II (Boulho et al. 2017; Harden et al. 2009), cytomegalovirus (Baba et al. 1988; Hamasuna et al. 1994), bovine herpes virus (Diogo et al. 2015), and varicella zoster virus (Abu-Galiyun et al. 2019). Carrageenans were also found to exert antiviral activity against human immunodeficiency virus (Baba et al. 1988; Shulgin et al. 2024), rabies virus (Luo et al. 2015), respiratory syndrome virus (Guo et al. 2019), influenza viruses, and severe acute respiratory syndrome (Bansal et al. 2020; Jang et al. 2021). The activity of carrageenans has been claimed against many non-enveloped viruses including human papillomavirus (Alli et al. 2023; Buck et al. 2006) and human rhinovirus (Grassauer et al. 2008).

4.2 Galactans

Red algae primarily exhibit sulfated galactans as their principal polysaccharides. Carrageenans and agarans display a linear configuration of galactose molecules, characterized by only minor deviations from this recognized structure. The chains are composed of alternating moieties of G units (3-β-d-galactopyranose) and either 4-3,6-anhydrogalactopyranose or 4-α-d-galactopyranose residues, which collectively form the central backbone. Carrageenans are distinguished by their d-series units, whereas agarans are composed of l-series units. DL-hybrids represent a unique category of galactans, defined by the presence of a G unit that is connected to D and L units together. The varied structural arrangements of galactans have shown considerable antiviral effectiveness against a range of enveloped viruses such as

HSV-1 and HSV-2, HIV-1, DENV, HIV-2, as well as the hepatitis A virus (Akter et al. 2024). The investigation focused on the antiviral characteristics of a D, L-galactan hybrid, C2S-3, derived from *Cryptonemia crenulata*, Brazilian marine alga, assessing its effectiveness against the replication of DENV-2 in the Vero cell line. The lack of negative effects on the cell line emphasizes the activity of this molecule against different DENV-2 strains, demonstrating an IC50 range of 0.8–16 μg/mL (Ahmadi et al. 2015).

4.3 Fucoidan

Fucoidans, also known as fucan or fucosan, are polysaccharides primarily composed of L-fucose and sulfate ester groups, extracted from brown seaweed and certain marine invertebrates, including sea cucumbers and sea urchins. Fucoidans are high-molecular-weight sulfated polysaccharides consisting of a core backbone of either 2-sulfate-O-fucose or 4-sulfate-O-fucose. Several sugars, including glucose, mannose, xylose, and glucuronic acid, have been identified in fucoidans derived from diverse species of brown seaweeds (Li et al. 2008). Fucoidans are water-soluble branched matrix sulfated polysaccharides with sulfate moieties that are commonly located in C2 or C4 positions. Fucans can be categorized into three primary groups: fucoidans, xylofucoglycuronans, and glycuronogalactofucans. This classification relies on a multitude of factors, such as the basic backbone, branch structure, linkage mode, sulfate content, and positioning characteristics (Claus-Desbonnet et al. 2022). Fucans don't possess direct virucidal effect (Lomartire and Gonçalves 2022). Fucoidans primarily obstruct the attachment of viruses to host cells by disrupting the external viral glycoproteins that play a crucial role in the binding to target cells (Harden et al. 2009; Lee et al. 2004). Fucoidan inhibits viral adsorption onto cells, thereby preventing viral entrance, and so prevents HIV, HSV, influenza, and human CMV (Dinesh et al. 2016; Mandal et al. 2007). The most prominent antiviral activity of fucans against RNA and DNA viruses is mediated through inhibition of reverse transcriptase. At concentrations ranging from 0.5 to 1.0 mg/mL, fucans derived from *Fucus vesiculosus* clearly inhibit HIV reverse transcriptase (RT) (Queiroz et al. 2008). In order to suppress the transcription of viral DNA, fucans use unique sugar rings that spatially orient and alter configuration to recognize the enzyme and determine the binding (Dinesh et al. 2016). *Undaria pinnatifida*-derived fucoidan inhibits HSV-1 replication and stimulates innate and adaptive immune responses, making it an effective weapon against the virus (Hayashi et al. 2008). Fucoidan from *Kjellmaniella crassifolia* successfully inhibited IAV infection in vitro while maintaining low toxicity. It demonstrated a wide anti-IAV spectrum and a minimal induction of viral resistance, outperforming the anti-IAV drug amantadine. The studied fucoidan effectively inactivated virus particles prior to infection and hindered certain stages post-adsorption. It may attach to viral neuraminidase, hindering its function and preventing the release of IAV. On the other side, it disrupted the activation of EGFR, PKCα, NF-κB, and Akt while also hindering IAV endocytosis and EGFR internalization in infected cells, indicating the inhibition of the cellular EGFR pathway (Wang et al. 2017).

4.4 Ulvan

Ulvan is the predominant water-soluble polysaccharide present in green seaweed belonging to the order Ulvales (specifically *Ulva* and *Enteromorpha* species), accounting for 8–29% of the dry weight of the algae (Andrieux et al. 1998; Kumar et al. 2024). Ulvan is a sulfated polysaccharide predominantly extracted from the cell walls of green algae, particularly species belonging to the genera *Ulva* and *Enteromorpha*. Its primary constituents include rhamnose, glucuronic acid, iduronic acid, xylose, and sulfate groups, forming a heterogeneous anionic polysaccharide. The structural backbone is characterized by repeating disaccharide units, such as ulvanobiuronic acid (A3S: → 4)-β-D-GlcA-(1 → 4)-α-L-Rha 3S-(1→) and ulvanobioses (B3S:→4)-α-L-IdoA-(1 → 4)-α-L-Rha 3S-(1→), with variable sulfation patterns influencing its physicochemical properties (Kidgell et al. 2019). The degree of sulfation and monosaccharide composition can vary depending on algal species, environmental conditions, and extraction techniques. Due to its gel-forming ability and bioactive potential, ulvan has gained interest for applications in biomedicine, nutraceuticals, and biodegradable materials (Barakat et al. 2022).

Ulvan exhibits significant antiviral activity through multiple mechanisms, primarily attributed to its high sulfate content and anionic properties (Kidgell et al. 2019). Studies suggest that ulvan interferes with viral attachment and entry by competitively binding to viral envelope proteins or host cell receptors, thereby blocking viral adhesion (Binsuwaidan et al. 2024). The process by which NDV enters host cells is predominantly dependent on the attachment protein HN and the fusion protein F, both of which play crucial roles in the formation of syncytia associated with NDV. Ulvans impede viral fusion by obstructing the cleavage of the intact protein F0 into its mature form. Ulvans demonstrated superior anti-cell-cell fusion effects compared to fucoidans, and their efficacy can be further enhanced through combined application (Chi et al. 2020). The extract of ulvan derived from *Ulva lactuca* exhibits antiviral properties in relation to the Japanese encephalitis virus (JEV) (Chiu et al. 2012). This flavivirus, transmitted by mosquitoes, results in the onset of acute encephalitis in humans. Ulvan has the capacity to impede JEV infection in Vero cells by blocking the adsorption of the virus and thwarting its entry into the cells (Chiu et al. 2012). Ulvan from *Ulva clathrata* and fucoidan from *Cladosiphon okamuranus* were successfully isolated by Aguilar-Briseño et al. (2015). The antiviral properties and mechanisms of action of isolated ulvan, fucoidan, and their combination against Newcastle disease virus (NDV) were evaluated. Their antiviral efficacy was assessed through a syncytia reduction assay. Their statement indicates that the inhibition of syncytia formation is contingent upon the prior addition of ulvan and its combination before the process of protein cleavage takes place. Following the cleavage of the protein via trypsin digestion, ulvan will lose its capacity to inhibit the formation of syncytia. The results reveal that ulvan achieved a 67% reduction in syncytia formation, whereas fucoidan showed a 47% reduction. The interplay between the two substances led to a notable 59% reduction in syncytia formation (Aguilar-Briseño et al. 2015). Ulvan produced from *Ulva pertusa* was tested for vesicular stomatitis virus (VSV) antiviral activity. Ulvan-F1, ulvan-F2, and ulvan-F3 were generated via enzymatic (lyase) degradation and ultrafiltration at 38.5, 17.8, and 5.2 kDa, respectively. Ulvans have no cytotoxic effects on Vero cells when tested for antiviral activity. Ulvan-F0 and ulvan-F1 at 100 μg/mL showed antiviral efficacy, suppressing VSV infection and replication. Antiviral activity interrelated with percentage molecular weight. The molecular weight of ulvan may affect its bioactivities (Chi et al. 2020). The polysaccharide derived from Ulvaceae, specifically from *Enteromorpha compressa*, was evaluated for its efficacy against HSV. A fraction of sulfated ulvan designated as SU1F1 was employed to evaluate its antiviral efficacy against HSV in HEp-2 cells. The results indicated significant antiviral activity of SU1F1, evidenced by a low IC50 value of 28.25 μg/mL. The antiviral activity is intricately connected to the content of sulfate groups and the molecular weight. Consequently, the antiviral efficacy of SU1F1 observed up to 8 h post-infection at elevated concentrations indicates a suppression of DNA replication and transcription, accompanied by a reduction in HSV protein synthesis (Lopes et al. 2017). Ulvans have been identified as antagonists to fucoidans in the context of viral attachment or entry, as they operate through the same mechanism during the infection process (Liyanage et al. 2023).

5 Modulation of Host Antiviral Immune Responses with Seaweed Polysaccharides

The viral infection has the capacity to provoke antiviral immune responses within the host cell. The type I interferon system (IFN), alongside host natural killer (NK) cells and phagocytic cells, plays a crucial role in the defense against viral infections. Interferon engages with receptors located on the cell membrane, leading to the production of antiviral proteins and the amplification of natural killer cells, T lymphocytes, and macrophages (Akter et al. 2024). Different polysaccharides derived from seaweed contribute to the indirect suppression of viral infections and enhance the efficiency of virus elimination by activating natural killer cells and stimulating antiviral immune responses.

λ-Carrageenan polysaccharide has demonstrated the ability to stimulate the synthesis of interferon, thereby exerting a significant influence on the biological effects of the immune response. Research indicates that the microwave degradation of λ-carrageenan derived from *Chondrus ocellatus* can impede tumor growth by boosting interferon activity and promoting lymphocyte proliferation (Liu et al. 2019). Fucoidan exhibits a range of immune-modulating effects, including the stimulation of NK cell production, the promotion of dendritic cell development, and the enhancement of cytotoxic lymphocyte function. Furthermore, it amplifies the Th1-type immune response through the generation of antibodies that specifically target antigen determinants while also fostering the maturation of memory T cells that are tailored to the virus (Zhang et al. 2015). Carrageenan derived from *Kappaphycus striatum* influences the immune response by boosting the activity of macrophages and NK cells, in addition to elevating the expression levels of interleukin-2 (IL-2) and tumor necrosis factor-alpha (TNF-α) (Yuan et al. 2006). The sulfated polysaccharides derived from *Enteromorpha prolifera* have the capacity to stimulate macrophage cells. Moreover, it has the capacity to promote the production of several cytokines, including interferon-gamma (IFN-γ) and interleukin-2 (IL-2), thereby augmenting the Th1 response (Kim et al. 2011).

The impact of polysaccharides on immune function is fundamentally shaped by their distinctive structural features, including branching regions, molecular weight, the presence of acetyl or sulfate groups, conformation, monosaccharide composition, and glycosidic linkages (Sasaki et al. 2020). The molecular weight of polysaccharides holds considerable significance. Polysaccharides with lower molecular weight demonstrate improved immunomodulatory properties. Compounds characterized by varying molecular weights demonstrate a range of effects on the regulation of the immune system. Research indicates that the influence of *Schisandra chinensis* polysaccharides on the immune system shows an inverse correlation with their molecular weight (Zhao et al. 2014). Polysaccharides demonstrate a remarkable capacity to navigate cellular barriers with relative ease, a characteristic linked to their lower molecular weight and simpler structural arrangements (Chen et al. 2020). The impact of polysaccharide molecular weights on immune responses is both complex and significant. Typically, polysaccharides characterized by low molecular weight demonstrate improved immune activation capabilities. Their capacity to stimulate immune cells, such as natural killer cells, dendritic cells, and macrophages, leads to an increased production of cytokines and signaling molecules throughout immune responses (Jiang et al. 2018). Low-molecular-weight polysaccharides, distinguished by their simple structures, can be readily recognized by the pattern recognition receptors (PRRs) found on immune cells. This identification activates intrinsic immune responses, consequently enhancing adaptive immunological resistance to infection (Cai et al. 2023). Lowered concentrations of polysaccharides could enhance the phagocytic function of immune cells, thereby aiding in the absorption and eradication of infections (Bi et al. 2018). This enhances the immune response and eliminates pathogens. A variety of low-molecular-weight polysaccharides demonstrate significant antiviral and anticancer activities (Kasai et al. 2015). They concurrently hinder the advancement of tumors and viruses while also bolstering the immune response, thereby enabling targeted strategies against diseases or malignant cells. The molecular weights of polysaccharides can affect immune reactivity via various mechanisms.

6 Sulfated Polysaccharides and COVID-19

The coronavirus pandemic disease (COVID-19) has emerged in China, in late December 2019. COVID-19 is a recently identified enveloped betacoronavirus that primarily targets the respiratory and gastrointestinal systems (Zhu et al. 2020). The virus's outer membrane comprises spike proteins that extend from the cell surface. The internal virus encompasses capsid protein along with its genome and a single-stranded RNA. It is reported that the surface glycoproteins of coronavirus interact with the host cell receptors. This interaction leads to the viral entry inside the host cell. Nevertheless, spike proteins on the virus surface bind with blood vessel cells of the heart and kidney and with epithelial cells of the lungs and intestine via angiotensin-converting enzyme (Xu et al. 2020).

Marine sulfated polysaccharides have gained attention lately due to their antiviral properties, as well as evidence has demonstrated their antiviral effects and promising inhibition against various viruses. Carrageenan was found to effectively disrupt the binding of the virus to receptors on the host cell, thereby preventing the entry of viral particles. A clinical trial was conducted to evaluate a nasal spray formulated with carrageenan, demonstrating its efficacy in treating a patient afflicted with a common cold induced by OC43 (beta) and 229E (alpha)coronaviruses. The findings from clinical trials demonstrated that this treatment resulted in a 2.5-fold decrease in the probability of symptom relapses and enhanced viral elimination when contrasted with individuals who were administered a placebo (Koenighofer et al. 2014). Scientists have developed lozenges containing 10 mg of ί-carrageenan to counteract throat infections caused by OC43 human coronavirus. The results indicated the denaturation of glycoproteins located on the coronavirus surface during the presence of the lozenge in the oral cavity. The acidic environment of the oral cavity induced alterations in the glycoproteins as a result of the carrageenan present in the lozenges. The denaturation of glycoproteins hinders the virucidal effects of coronaviruses (Morokutti-Kurz et al. 2017). A recent study conducted amidst the SARS-CoV-2 outbreak revealed that marine sulfated polysaccharides, particularly iota-CG, possess the ability to inhibit viral attachment and entry into host cells. Iota-CG has the potential to restrict infection when given at concentrations of 125 μg/mL or above. Consequently, it is evident that marine polysaccharides demonstrate notable antiviral properties against a range of viruses by obstructing viral attachment. This strategically places them in a favorable position for both the prevention and treatment of coronavirus disease 2019 (COVID-19) (Song et al. 2020).

7 Applications of Marine Polysaccharides in Nanotechnology

Seaweed polysaccharides have emerged as pivotal biomaterials in the development of nanodelivery systems due to their biocompatibility, biodegradability, low immunogenicity, and tunable physicochemical properties. Key polysaccharides such as alginate, carrageenan, and fucoidan have been extensively explored for their ability to form nanoparticles (NPs) via methods like ionic gelation, polyelectrolyte complexation (PEC), and emulsion techniques. These NPs exhibit controlled drug release, high encapsulation efficiency, and targeted delivery, making them ideal for therapeutic applications. In Table 1, we summarize the most important applications of marine polysaccharides in nanotechnology for different drug delivery applications.

8 Conclusion

Marine seaweed polysaccharides with antiviral activities represent a potential class of natural antiviral agents with diverse structures and mechanisms of action. Their ability to inhibit a broad spectrum of viruses underscores their potential in both therapeutic and preventive antiviral applications. Sulfated polysaccharides such as carrageenans, fucoidans, and ulvans have shown particularly strong antiviral properties by blocking viral entry, replication, or assembly. Continued research into their structure-activity relationships, bioavailability, and synergistic effects with existing antiviral drugs will allow full use of their biomedical potential. Looking ahead, future research should also focus on the development of standardized extraction and purification methods to ensure the consistency of quality and efficacy of the marine-derived polysaccharides. As antiviral resistance continues to challenge conventional treatments, marine seaweed polysaccharides can offer a valuable alternative.

Table 1 Applications of marine polysaccharides in nanotechnology-based drug delivery

Polysaccharide	Nanosystem	Preparation technique	Encapsulated active material	Therapeutic activity	References
Alginate	Calcium alginate microspheres containing niosomes and chitosomes	Thin-layer evaporation Ionotropic gelation	Metformin hydrochloride	Type II diabetes mellitus	Maestrelli et al. (2017)
	Polymeric nanoparticles	Ionotropic gelation	Curcumin	Wound healing	Shahnia (2017)
	pH-sensitive sodium alginate, hydroxyapatite bilayer-coated iron oxide nanoparticle composite	Co-precipitation	Curcumin 6-Gingerol	Anticancer	Manatunga et al. (2017)
	Alginate/chitosan microspheres	Cross-linking	Nanoselenium	Antioxidant	Cavalu et al. (2017)
	Calcium alginate nanoparticles	Emulsification and cross-linking	Curcumin and resveratrol	Prostate cancer cell line	Saralkar and Dash (2017)
	Sodium alginate-modified graphene oxide	Cross-linking	5-Fluorouracil	Colorectal liver metastasis	Zhang et al. (2017)
	Self-assembled nanomicelles	Cross-linking	Curcumin	Anticancer	Lachowicz et al. (2019)
	Porous silica nanospheres encapsulated in sodium alginate (SA) microgel spheres wrapped by pH-sensitive $CaCO_3$	Cross-linking and freeze-drying	Green tea polyphenol	Bone infection	
	Alginate-gelatin microfibers	Ionotropic gelation and needle extrusion	Curcumin	Wound healing	Sharma et al. (2020)
	Chitosan-alginate polyelectrolyte microparticles	Ionotropic gelation	Vancomycin chloride	Antibacterial	Unagolla and Jayasuriya (2018)
Carrageenan	Chitosan-carrageenan nanoparticles	Ionotropic gelation	Recombinant human erythropoietin	Renal anemia and chemotherapy-induced anemia	Bulmer et al. (2012)
	Polymeric nanoparticles	Ionic complexation	Ovalbumin	–	Grenha et al. (2010)

	Lectin-functionalized carboxymethylated kappa-carrageenan microparticles	Ionic gelation	Insulin	Type I diabetes	Leong et al. (2011)
Fucoidan	Fucoidan-coated mesoporous silica nanoparticles	Cross-linking	Curcumin	Antitumor	Zhang et al. (2022)
	Zein-fucoidan composite nanoparticles	Antisolvent precipitation	Resveratrol	–	Liu et al. (2022)
	Zein/γ-polyglutamic acid/low-molecular-weight chitosan/fucoidan nanosystem	Layer-by-layer ionotropic gelation	Quercetin	Endothelial blood vessel inflammation	Lu et al. (2024)
	O-Carboxymethyl chitosan/FU NPs	Ionic cross-linking	Curcumin	Anticancer	Venkatesan et al. (2016)
	Fucoidan polymeric nanoparticles	Covalent conjugation	Doxorubicin	Anticancer	Jafari et al. (2020)
	Fucoidan/PLGA nanoparticles	Emulsification—solvent evaporation	–	Anticancer	Chiang et al. (2021)
	Fucoidan-adsorbed nano-hydroxyapatite/hydroxypropyl chitosan composite scaffolds	Cross-linking	–	Bone regeneration	Lu et al. (2019)

References

Abuelella, K.E., Abd-Allah, H., Soliman, S.M., Abdel-Mottaleb, M.M.A., 2022. Polysaccharide Based Biomaterials for Dermal Applications, in: Jana, Sougata, Jana, Subrata (Eds.), Functional Biomaterials: Drug Delivery and Biomedical Applications. Springer Singapore, Singapore, pp. 105–127. https://doi.org/10.1007/978-981-16-7152-4_4

Abu-Galiyun, E., Huleihel, M., & Levy-Ontman, O. (2019). Antiviral bioactivity of renewable polysaccharides against Varicella Zoster. *Cell Cycle, 18*, 3540–3549. https://doi.org/10.1080/15384101.2019.1691363

Aguilar-Briseño, J. A., Cruz-Suarez, L. E., Sassi, J. F., Ricque-Marie, D., Zapata-Benavides, P., Mendoza-Gamboa, E., Rodríguez-Padilla, C., & Trejo-Avila, L. M. (2015). Sulphated polysaccharides from Ulva clathrata and Cladosiphon okamuranus seaweeds both inhibit viral attachment/entry and cell-cell fusion, in NDV infection. *Marine Drugs, 13*, 697–712. https://doi.org/10.3390/md13020697

Ahmadi, A., Zorofchian Moghadamtousi, S., Abubakar, S., & Zandi, K. (2015). Antiviral potential of algae polysaccharides isolated from marine sources: A review. *BioMed Research International, 2015*. https://doi.org/10.1155/2015/825203

Akter, A., Sobuj, M. K. A., Islam, Md. S., Chakroborty, K., Tasnim, N., Ayon, M. H., Hossain, Md. F., & Rafiquzzaman, S. M. (2024). Seaweed polysaccharides: Sources, structure and biomedical applications with special emphasis on antiviral potentials. *Future Foods, 10*, 100440. https://doi.org/10.1016/j.fufo.2024.100440

Alli, B. Y., Madathil, S., Tran, S. D., & Nicolau, B. (2023). Protocol: carrageenan for the prevention of oral HPV infection—a feasibility randomised clinical trial. *BMJ Open, 13*. https://doi.org/10.1136/bmjopen-2023-074498

Álvarez-Viñas, M., Souto, S., Flórez-Fernández, N., Torres, M. D., Bandín, I., & Domínguez, H. (2021). Antiviral activity of carrageenans and processing implications. *Marine Drugs, 19*. https://doi.org/10.3390/md19080437

Andrieux, C., Hibert, A., Houari, A. M., Bensaada, M., Popot, F., & Szylit, O. (1998). Ulva lactuca is poorly fermented but alters bacterial metabolism in rats inoculated with human faecal flora from methane and non-methane producers. *Journal of the Science of Food and Agriculture, 77*, 25–30. https://doi.org/10.1002/(sici)1097-0010(199805)77:1<25::aid-jsfa989>3.3.co;2-3

Baba, M., Snoeck, R., Pauwels, R., & De Clercq, E. (1988). Sulfated polysaccharides are potent and selective inhibitors of various enveloped viruses, including herpes simplex virus, cytomegalovirus, vesicular stomatitis virus, and human immunodeficiency virus. *Antimicrobial Agents and Chemotherapy, 32*, 1742–1745. https://doi.org/10.1128/AAC.32.11.1742

Bai, R. G., &Tuvikene, R. (2021). Potential antiviral properties of industrially important marine algal polysaccharides and their significance in fighting a future viral pandemic. In *Viruses* (Vol. 13, Issue 9). MDPI. https://doi.org/10.3390/v13091817

Bandyopadhyay, S. S., Navid, M. H., Ghosh, T., Schnitzler, P., & Ray, B. (2011). Structural features and in vitro antiviral activities of sulfated polysaccharides from Sphacelaria indica. *Phytochemistry, 72*, 276–283. https://doi.org/10.1016/j.phytochem.2010.11.006

Bansal, S., Jonsson, C. B., Taylor, S. L., Figueroa, J. M., Dugour, A. V., Palacios, C., & César Vega, J. (2020). *Iota-carrageenan and Xylitol inhibit SARS-CoV-2 in cell culture*. https://doi.org/10.1101/2020.08.19.225854

Barakat, K. M., Ismail, M. M., Abou El Hassayeb, H. E., El Sersy, N. A., & Elshobary, M. E. (2022). Chemical characterization and biological activities of ulvan extracted from Ulva fasciata (Chlorophyta). *Rendiconti Lincei, 33*, 829–841. https://doi.org/10.1007/s12210-022-01103-7

Bassetti, M., Sepulcri, C., Giacobbe, D. R., & Fusco, L. (2024). Treating influenza with neuraminidase inhibitors: an update of the literature. In *Expert Opinion on Pharmacotherapy* (Vol. 25, pp. 1163–1174). Taylor and Francis Ltd. https://doi.org/10.1080/14656566.2024.2370895

Bi, D., Yu, B., Han, Q., Lu, J., White, W. L., Lai, Q., Cai, N., Luo, W., Gu, L., Li, S., Xu, H., Hu, Z., Nie, S., & Xu, X. (2018). Immune Activation of RAW264.7 Macrophages by Low Molecular

Weight Fucoidan Extracted from New Zealand *Undaria pinnatifida*. *Journal of Agricultural and Food Chemistry*, *66*(41), 10721–10728. https://doi.org/10.1021/acs.jafc.8b03698

Binsuwaidan, R., El-Masry, T. A., El-Sheekh, M., Seadawy, M. G., Makhlof, M. E. M., Aboukhatwa, S. M., El-Shitany, N. A., Elmorshedy, K. E., El-Nagar, M. M. F., & El-Bouseary, M. M. (2024). Prospective Antiviral Effect of Ulva lactuca Aqueous Extract against COVID-19 Infection. *Marine Drugs*, *22*. https://doi.org/10.3390/md22010030

Bird, S. W., & Kirkegaard, K. (2015). Escape of non-enveloped virus from intact cells. In *Virology* (Vols. 479–480, pp. 444–449). Academic Press Inc. https://doi.org/10.1016/j.virol.2015.03.044

Boulho, R., Marty, C., Freile-Pelegrín, Y., Robledo, D., Bourgougnon, N., &Bedoux, G. (2017). Antiherpetic (HSV-1) activity of carrageenans from the red seaweed Solieria chordalis (Rhodophyta, Gigartinales) extracted by microwave-assisted extraction (MAE). *Journal of Applied Phycology*, *29*, 2219–2228. https://doi.org/10.1007/s10811-017-1192-5

Buck, C. B., Thompson, C. D., Roberts, J. N., Müller, M., Lowy, D. R., & Schiller, J. T. (2006). Carrageenan is a potent inhibitor of papillomavirus infection. *PLoS Pathogens*, *2*, 0671–0680. https://doi.org/10.1371/journal.ppat.0020069

Bulmer, C., Margaritis, A., & Xenocostas, A. (2012). Encapsulation and Controlled Release of Recombinant Human Erythropoietin from Chitosan-Carrageenan Nanoparticles. *Current Drug Delivery*, *9*, 527–537. https://doi.org/10.2174/156720112802650680

Cai, Y., Si, Z., Jiang, Y., Ye, M., Wang, F., Yang, X., Yu, J., Gao, X., & Liu, W. (2023). Structure-activity relationship of low molecular weight Astragalus membranaceus polysaccharides produced by Bacteroides. *Carbohydrate Polymers*, *316*. https://doi.org/10.1016/j.carbpol.2023.121036

Campo, V. L., Kawano, D. F., Silva, D. B. da, & Carvalho, I. (2009). Carrageenans: Biological properties, chemical modifications and structural analysis—A review. In *Carbohydrate Polymers* (Vol. 77, pp. 167–180). https://doi.org/10.1016/j.carbpol.2009.01.020

Cao, W., Jin, J., Wu, G., Bravenboer, N., Helder, M. N., Pathak, J. L., Zandieh-Doulabi, B., Hogervorst, J. M. A., Matsukawa, S., Geonzon, L. C., Bacabac, R. G., Schulten, E. A. J. M., & Klein-Nulend, J. (2021). K-carrageenan stimulates pre-osteoblast proliferation and osteogenic differentiation: A potential factor for the promotion of bone regeneration? *Molecules*, *26*. https://doi.org/10.3390/molecules26206131

Carlucci, M. J., Ciancia, M., Matulewicz, M. C., Cerezo, A. S., & Damonte, E. B. (1999). Antiherpetic activity and mode of action of natural carrageenans of diverse structural types. *Antiviral Research*, *43*, 93–102. https://doi.org/10.1016/S0166-3542(99)00038-8

Carlucci, M. J., Scolaro, L. A., Noseda, M. D., Cerezo, A. S., & Damonte, E. B. (2004). Protective effect of a natural carrageenan on genital herpes simplex virus infection in mice. *Antiviral Research*, *64*, 137–141. https://doi.org/10.1016/j.antiviral.2004.07.001

Cavalu, S., Prokisch, J., Laslo, V., & Vicas, S. (2017). Preparation, structural characterisation and release study of novel hybrid microspheres entrapping nanoselenium, produced by green synthesis. *IET Nanobiotechnology*, *11*, 426–432. https://doi.org/10.1049/iet-nbt.2016.0107

Chen, J. Y., Sun, X. Y., & Ouyang, J. M. (2020). Modulation of calcium oxalate crystal growth and protection from oxidatively damaged renal epithelial cells of corn silk polysaccharides with different molecular weights. *Oxidative Medicine and Cellular Longevity*, *2020*. https://doi.org/10.1155/2020/6982948

Chi, Y., Zhang, M., Wang, X., Fu, X., Guan, H., & Wang, P. (2020). Ulvan lyase assisted structural characterization of ulvan from Ulva pertusa and its antiviral activity against vesicular stomatitis virus. *International Journal of Biological Macromolecules*, *157*, 75–82. https://doi.org/10.1016/j.ijbiomac.2020.04.187

Chiang, C. S., Huang, B. J., Chen, J. Y., Chieng, W. W., Lim, S. H., Lee, W., Shyu, W. C., & Jeng, L. Bin. (2021). Fucoidan-based nanoparticles with inherently therapeutic efficacy for cancer treatment. *Pharmaceutics*, *13*. https://doi.org/10.3390/pharmaceutics13121986

Chiu, Y. H., Chan, Y. L., Li, T. L., & Wu, C. J. (2012). Inhibition of Japanese Encephalitis Virus Infection by the Sulfated Polysaccharide Extracts from Ulva lactuca. *Marine Biotechnology*, *14*, 468–478. https://doi.org/10.1007/s10126-011-9428-x

Citkowska, A., Szekalska, M., & Winnicka, K. (2019). Possibilities of fucoidan utilization in the development of pharmaceutical dosage forms. In *Marine Drugs* (Vol. 17). MDPI AG. https://doi.org/10.3390/md17080458

Claus-Desbonnet, H., Nikly, E., Nalbantova, V., Karcheva-Bahchevanska, D., Ivanova, S., Pierre, G., Benbassat, N., Katsarov, P., Michaud, P., Lukova, P., & Delattre, C. (2022). Polysaccharides and Their Derivatives as Potential Antiviral Molecules. In *Viruses* (Vol. 14, Issue 2). MDPI. https://doi.org/10.3390/v14020426

Damonte, E., Matulewicz, M., & Cerezo, A. (2004). Sulfated Seaweed Polysaccharides as Antiviral Agents. *Current Medicinal Chemistry, 11*(18), 2399–2419. https://doi.org/10.2174/0929867043364504

De Clercq, E. (2021). 1984-Discovery of the first anti-HIV drug, suramin. *Viruses, 13*. https://doi.org/10.3390/v13081646

De Jesus Raposo, M. F., De Morais, A. M. B., & De Morais, R. M. S. C. (2015). Marine polysaccharides from algae with potential biomedical applications. In *Marine Drugs* (Vol. 13, pp. 2967–3028). MDPI AG. https://doi.org/10.3390/md13052967

Dinesh, S., Menon, T., Hanna, L. E., Suresh, V., Sathuvan, M., & Manikannan, M. (2016). In vitro anti-HIV-1 activity of fucoidan from Sargassum swartzii. *International Journal of Biological Macromolecules, 82*, 83–88. https://doi.org/10.1016/j.ijbiomac.2015.09.078

Diogo, J. V., Novo, S. G., González, M. J., Ciancia, M., & Bratanich, A. C. (2015). Antiviral activity of lambda-carrageenan prepared from red seaweed (Gigartina skottsbergii) against BoHV-1 and SuHV-1. *Research in Veterinary Science, 98*, 142–144. https://doi.org/10.1016/j.rvsc.2014.11.010

Gerges, D., Abd El-Ghany, K., Hevesi, Z., Aiad, M., Omic, H., Baumgartner, C., Winnicki, W., Eder, M., Schmidt, A., Eskandary, F., & Wagner, L. (2024). Shedding Light on Viral Shedding: Novel Insights into Nuclear Assembly, Cytoplasmic Transformation and Extracellular Vesicle Release of the BK Virus. *International Journal of Molecular Sciences, 25*. https://doi.org/10.3390/ijms25169130

Girond, S., Crance, J. M., Van Cuyck-Gandre, H., Renaudet, J., & Deloince, R. (1991). Antiviral activity of carrageenan on hepatitis A virus replication in cell culture. *Research in Virology, 142*, 261–270. https://doi.org/10.1016/0923-2516(91)90011-Q

Grassauer, A., Weinmuellner, R., Meier, C., Pretsch, A., Prieschl-Grassauer, E., & Unger, H. (2008). Iota-Carrageenan is a potent inhibitor of rhinovirus infection. *Virology Journal, 5*. https://doi.org/10.1186/1743-422X-5-107

Grenha, A., Gomes, M. E., Rodrigues, M., Santo, V. E., Mano, J. F., Neves, N. M., & Reis, R. L. (2010). Development of new chitosan/carrageenan nanoparticles for drug delivery applications. *Journal of Biomedical Materials Research—Part A, 92*, 1265–1272. https://doi.org/10.1002/jbm.a.32466

Guo, C., Zhu, Z., Yu, P., Zhang, X., Dong, W., Wang, X., Chen, Y., & Liu, X. (2019). Inhibitory effect of iota-carrageenan on porcine reproductive and respiratory syndrome virus in vitro. *Antiviral Therapy, 24*, 261–270. https://doi.org/10.3851/IMP3295

Guo, R., Chen, M., Ding, Y., Yang, P., Wang, M., Zhang, H., He, Y., & Ma, H. (2022). Polysaccharides as Potential Anti-tumor Biomacromolecules—A Review. In *Frontiers in Nutrition* (Vol. 9). Frontiers Media S.A. https://doi.org/10.3389/fnut.2022.838179

Hamasuna, R., Eizuru, Y., & Minamishima, Y. (1994). Inhibition by iota-carrageenan of the spread of murine cytomegalovirus from the peritoneal cavity to the blood plasma. *Journal of General Virology, 75*, 111–116. https://doi.org/10.1099/0022-1317-75-1-111

Hangyu, W., Panpan, L., Jie, S., Hongyan, W., Linmiao, W., Kangning, H., Yichen, S., Shuai, W., & Cheng, W. (2024). Advancements in Antiviral Drug Development: Comprehensive Insights into Design Strategies and Mechanisms Targeting Key Viral Proteins. In *Journal of Microbiology and Biotechnology* (Vol. 34, pp. 1376–1384). Korean Society for Microbiolog and Biotechnology. https://doi.org/10.4014/jmb.2403.03008

Hans, N., Malik, A., & Naik, S. (2021). Antiviral activity of sulfated polysaccharides from marine algae and its application in combating COVID-19: Mini review. In *Bioresource Technology Reports* (Vol. 13). Elsevier Ltd. https://doi.org/10.1016/j.biteb.2020.100623

Harden, E. A., Falshaw, R., Carnachan, S. M., Kern, E. R., & Prichard, M. N. (2009). Virucidal activity of polysaccharide extracts from four algal species against herpes simplex virus. *Antiviral Research, 83*, 282–289. https://doi.org/10.1016/j.antiviral.2009.06.007

Havens, J. P., Podany, A. T., Scarsi, K. K., & Fletcher, C. V. (2020). Clinical Pharmacokinetics and Pharmacodynamics of Etravirine: An Updated Review. In *Clinical Pharmacokinetics* (Vol. 59, pp. 137–154). Adis. https://doi.org/10.1007/s40262-019-00830-9

Hayashi, K., Nakano, T., Hashimoto, M., Kanekiyo, K., & Hayashi, T. (2008). Defensive effects of a fucoidan from brown alga Undaria pinnatifida against herpes simplex virus infection. *International Immunopharmacology, 8*(1), 109–116. https://doi.org/10.1016/j.intimp.2007.10.017

Jafari, M., Sriram, V., Xu, Z., Harris, G. M., & Lee, J. Y. (2020). Fucoidan-Doxorubicin Nanoparticles Targeting P-Selectin for Effective Breast Cancer Therapy. *Carbohydrate Polymers, 249*. https://doi.org/10.1016/j.carbpol.2020.116837

Jang, Y., Shin, H., Lee, M. K., Kwon, O. S., Shin, J. S., Kim, Y. il, Kim, C. W., Lee, H. R., & Kim, M. (2021). Antiviral activity of lambda-carrageenan against influenza viruses and severe acute respiratory syndrome coronavirus 2. *Scientific Reports, 11*. https://doi.org/10.1038/s41598-020-80896-9

Jiang, L., Yu, Z., Lin, Y., Cui, L., Yao, S., Lv, L., & Liu, J. (2018). Low-molecular-weight polysaccharides from agaricus blazei Murrill modulate the Th1 response in cancer immunity. *Oncology Letters, 15*, 3429–3436. https://doi.org/10.3892/ol.2018.7794

Jiao, G., Yu, G., Zhang, J., & Ewart, H. S. (2011). Chemical structures and bioactivities of sulfated polysaccharides from marine algae. *Marine Drugs, 9*, 196–233. https://doi.org/10.3390/md9020196

Jin, H., Li, M., Tian, F., Yu, F., & Zhao, W. (2022a). An Overview of Antitumour Activity of Polysaccharides. In *Molecules* (Vol. 27). MDPI. https://doi.org/10.3390/molecules27228083

Jin, J. O., Yadav, D., Madhwani, K., Puranik, N., Chavda, V., & Song, M. (2022b). Seaweeds in the Oncology Arena: Anti-Cancer Potential of Fucoidan as a Drug—A Review. In *Molecules* (Vol. 27). MDPI. https://doi.org/10.3390/molecules27186032

Jin, Y., Yu, Q., Li, S., Chen, T., & Liu, D. (2023). Application of seaweed polysaccharide in bone tissue regeneration. In *Frontiers in Marine Science* (Vol. 10). Frontiers Media SA. https://doi.org/10.3389/fmars.2023.1202422

Kang, J., Jia, X., Wang, N., Xiao, M., Song, S., Wu, S., Li, Z., Wang, S., Cui, S. W., & Guo, Q. (2022). Insights into the structure-bioactivity relationships of marine sulfated polysaccharides: A review. In *Food Hydrocolloids* (Vol. 123). Elsevier B.V. https://doi.org/10.1016/j.foodhyd.2021.107049

Kasai, A., Arafuka, S., Koshiba, N., Takahashi, D., & Toshima, K. (2015). Systematic synthesis of low-molecular weight fucoidan derivatives and their effect on cancer cells. *Organic and Biomolecular Chemistry, 13*, 10556–10568. https://doi.org/10.1039/c5ob01634g

Kausar, S., Said Khan, F., Ishaq Mujeeb Ur Rehman, M., Akram, M., Riaz, M., Rasool, G., Hamid Khan, A., Saleem, I., Shamim, S., & Malik, A. (2021). A review: Mechanism of action of antiviral drugs. In *International Journal of Immunopathology and Pharmacology* (Vol. 35). SAGE Publications Inc. https://doi.org/10.1177/20587384211002621

Kidgell, J. T., Magnusson, M., de Nys, R., & Glasson, C. R. K. (2019). Ulvan: A systematic review of extraction, composition and function. In *Algal Research* (Vol. 39). Elsevier B.V. https://doi.org/10.1016/j.algal.2019.101422

Kim, J. K., Cho, M. L., Karnjanapratum, S., Shin, I. S., & You, S. G. (2011). In vitro and in vivo immunomodulatory activity of sulfated polysaccharides from Enteromorpha prolifera. *International Journal of Biological Macromolecules, 49*, 1051–1058. https://doi.org/10.1016/j.ijbiomac.2011.08.032

Koca, R., & Çetinkaya, E. A. (2024). *Herpes Simplex Viruses in Children* (pp. 859–879). https://doi.org/10.1007/978-3-031-74853-0_71

Koenighofer, M., Lion, T., Bodenteich, A., Prieschl-Grassauer, E., Grassauer, A., Unger, H., Mueller, C. A., & Fazekas, T. (2014). Carrageenan nasal spray in virus confirmed common cold: individual patient data analysis of two randomized controlled trials. *Multidisciplinary Respiratory Medicine, 9*. https://doi.org/10.4081/mrm.2014.392

Kumar, A., Hart, P., & Thakur, V. K. (2024). Seaweed Based Hydrogels: Extraction, Gelling Characteristics, and Applications in the Agriculture Sector. *ACS Sustainable Resource Management*. https://doi.org/10.1021/acssusresmgt.4c00043

Lachowicz, D., Karabasz, A., Bzowska, M., Szuwarzyński, M., Karewicz, A., & Nowakowska, M. (2019). Blood-compatible, stable micelles of sodium alginate—Curcumin bioconjugate for anti-cancer applications. *European Polymer Journal, 113*, 208–219. https://doi.org/10.1016/j.eurpolymj.2019.01.058

Lee, J. B., Hayashi, K., Hashimoto, M., Nakano, T., & Hayashi, T. (2004). Novel antiviral fucoidan from sporophyll of Undaria pinnatifida (Mekabu). *Chemical and Pharmaceutical Bulletin, 52*, 1091–1094. https://doi.org/10.1248/cpb.52.1091

Leong, K. H., Chung, L. Y., Noordin, M. I., Onuki, Y., Morishita, M., & Takayama, K. (2011). Lectin-functionalized carboxymethylated kappa-carrageenan microparticles for oral insulin delivery. *Carbohydrate Polymers, 86*, 555–565. https://doi.org/10.1016/j.carbpol.2011.04.070

Li, B., Lu, F., Wei, X., & Zhao, R. (2008). Fucoidan: Structure and bioactivity. In *Molecules* (Vol. 13, pp. 1671–1695). https://doi.org/10.3390/molecules13081671

Liu, Q., Qin, Y., Jiang, B., Chen, J., & Zhang, T. (2022). Development of self-assembled zein-fucoidan complex nanoparticles as a delivery system for resveratrol. *Colloids and Surfaces B: Biointerfaces, 216*. https://doi.org/10.1016/j.colsurfb.2022.112529

Liu, Z., Gao, T., Yang, Y., Meng, F., Zhan, F., Jiang, Q., & Sun, X. (2019). Anti-Cancer Activity of Porphyran and Carrageenan from Red Seaweeds. *Molecules, 24*(23), 4286. https://doi.org/10.3390/molecules24234286

Liyanage, N. M., Nagahawatta, D. P., Jayawardena, T. U., Sanjeewa, K. K. A., Jayawrdhana, H. H. A. C. K., Kim, J. Il, & Jeon, Y. J. (2023). Sulfated Polysaccharides from Seaweeds: A Promising Strategy for Combatting Viral Diseases—A Review. In *Marine Drugs* (Vol. 21, Issue 9). Multidisciplinary Digital Publishing Institute (MDPI). https://doi.org/10.3390/md21090461

Lomartire, S., & Gonçalves, A. M. M. (2022). Antiviral Activity and Mechanisms of Seaweeds Bioactive Compounds on Enveloped Viruses—A Review. *Marine Drugs, 20*. https://doi.org/10.3390/md20060385

Lopes, N., Ray, S., Espada, S. F., Bomfim, W. A., Ray, B., Faccin-Galhardi, L. C., Linhares, R. E. C., & Nozawa, C. (2017). Green seaweed Enteromorpha compressa (Chlorophyta, Ulvaceae) derived sulphated polysaccharides inhibit herpes simplex virus. *International Journal of Biological Macromolecules, 102*, 605–612. https://doi.org/10.1016/j.ijbiomac.2017.04.043

Louten, J. (2016). Virus Replication. In *Essential Human Virology* (pp. 49–70). Elsevier. https://doi.org/10.1016/b978-0-12-800947-5.00004-1

Lu, H. T., Lu, T. W., Chen, C. H., & Mi, F. L. (2019). Development of genipin-crosslinked and fucoidan-adsorbed nano-hydroxyapatite/hydroxypropyl chitosan composite scaffolds for bone tissue engineering. *International Journal of Biological Macromolecules, 128*, 973–984. https://doi.org/10.1016/j.ijbiomac.2019.02.010

Lu, H. Y., Mi, F. L., Chou, C. M., Lin, C., Chen, Y. Y., Chu, C. Y., Liu, C. Y., Lee, Y. L. A., Shih, C. C., & Cheng, C. H. (2024). Layer-by-layer assembly of quercetin-loaded zein/γPGA/low-molecular-weight chitosan/fucoidan nanosystem for targeting inflamed blood vessels. *International Journal of Biological Macromolecules, 267*. https://doi.org/10.1016/j.ijbiomac.2024.131369

Luo, Z., Tian, D., Zhou, M., Xiao, W., Zhang, Y., Li, M., Sui, B., Wang, W., Guan, H., Chen, H., Fu, Z. F., & Zhao, L. (2015). λ-carrageenan P32 is a potent inhibitor of rabies virus infection. *PLoS ONE, 10*. https://doi.org/10.1371/journal.pone.0140586

Maestrelli, F., Mura, P., González-Rodríguez, M. L., Cózar-Bernal, M. J., Rabasco, A. M., Di Cesare Mannelli, L., & Ghelardini, C. (2017). Calcium alginate microspheres containing metformin hydrochloride niosomes and chitosomes aimed for oral therapy of type 2 diabetes mellitus. *International Journal of Pharmaceutics, 530*, 430–439. https://doi.org/10.1016/j.ijpharm.2017.07.083

Manatunga, D. C., de Silva, R. M., de Silva, K. M. N., de Silva, N., Bhandari, S., Yap, Y. K., & Costha, N. P. (2017). pH responsive controlled release of anti-cancer hydrophobic drugs from sodium alginate and hydroxyapatite bi-coated iron oxide nanoparticles. *European Journal of Pharmaceutics and Biopharmaceutics, 117*, 29–38. https://doi.org/10.1016/j.ejpb.2017.03.014

Mandal, P., Mateu, C. G., Chattopadhyay, K., Pujol, C. A., Damonte, E. B., & Ray, B. (2007). Structural features and antiviral activity of sulphated fucans from the brown seaweed Cystoseira indica. *Antiviral Chemistry and Chemotherapy, 18*, 153–162. https://doi.org/10.1177/095632020701800305

Massari, S., Desantis, J., Nizi, M. G., Cecchetti, V., & Tabarrini, O. (2021). Inhibition of Influenza Virus Polymerase by Interfering with Its Protein-Protein Interactions. In *ACS Infectious Diseases* (Vol. 7). American Chemical Society. https://doi.org/10.1021/acsinfecdis.0c00552

Meyer, H., Ehmann, R., & Smith, G. L. (2020). Smallpox in the post-eradication Era. *Viruses, 12*. https://doi.org/10.3390/v12020138

Morokutti-Kurz, M., Graf, C., &Prieschl-Grassauer, E. (2017). Amylmetacresol/2,4-dichlorobenzyl alcohol, hexylresorcinol, or carrageenan lozenges as active treatments for sore throat. *International Journal of General Medicine, 10*, 53–60. https://doi.org/10.2147/IJGM.S120665

Mousa, A.M., Abdelraof, M., Hassabo, A.A., Darwish, D.A., Abdel-Mottaleb, M.M.A., Allam, R. M., 2025. Marine L-arginase encapsulated in poly (lactic-co-glycolic acid) nanoparticles: A novel anti-cancer strategy for effective hepatocellular carcinoma treatment in vitro and in vivo. Journal of Drug Delivery Science and Technology 109, 106980. https://doi.org/10.1016/j.jddst.2025.106980

Panggabean, J. A., Adiguna, S. P., Rahmawati, S. I., Ahmadi, P., Zainuddin, E. N., Bayu, A., & Putra, M. Y. (2022). Antiviral Activities of Algal-Based Sulfated Polysaccharides. In *Molecules* (Vol. 27). MDPI. https://doi.org/10.3390/molecules27041178

Queiroz, K. C. S., Medeiros, V. P., Queiroz, L. S., Abreu, L. R. D., Rocha, H. A. O., Ferreira, C. V., Jucá, M. B., Aoyama, H., & Leite, E. L. (2008). Inhibition of reverse transcriptase activity of HIV by polysaccharides of brown algae. *Biomedicine and Pharmacotherapy, 62*, 303–307. https://doi.org/10.1016/j.biopha.2008.03.006

Rampersad, S., & Tennant, P. (2018). Replication and Expression Strategies of Viruses. In *Viruses: Molecular Biology, Host Interactions, and Applications to Biotechnology* (pp. 55–82). Elsevier. https://doi.org/10.1016/B978-0-12-811257-1.00003-6

Saralkar, P., & Dash, A. K. (2017). Alginate Nanoparticles Containing Curcumin and Resveratrol: Preparation, Characterization, and In Vitro Evaluation Against DU145 Prostate Cancer Cell Line. *AAPS PharmSciTech, 18*, 2814–2823. https://doi.org/10.1208/s12249-017-0772-7

Sasaki, D., Sasaki, K., & Kondo, A. (2020). Glycosidic Linkage Structures Influence Dietary Fiber Fermentability and Propionate Production by Human Colonic Microbiota In Vitro. *Biotechnology Journal, 15*. https://doi.org/10.1002/biot.201900523

Shahnia, M. (2017). *Formulating curcumin in a biodegradable polymeric composite material: A step towards wound healing applications*. http://orcid.org/0000-0001-5565-881X

Sharma, A., Mittal, A., Puri, V., Kumar, P., & Singh, I. (2020). Curcumin-loaded, alginate–gelatin composite fibers for wound healing applications. *3 Biotech, 10*. https://doi.org/10.1007/s13205-020-02453-5

Shen, Y., Zhao, H., Wang, X., Wu, S., Wang, Y., Wang, C., Zhang, Y., & Zhao, H. (2024). Unraveling the web of defense: the crucial role of polysaccharides in immunity. In *Frontiers in Immunology* (Vol. 15). Frontiers Media SA. https://doi.org/10.3389/fimmu.2024.1406213

Shulgin, A., Spirin, P., Lebedev, T., Kravchenko, A., Glasunov, V., Yermak, I., & Prassolov, V. (2024). Comparative study of HIV-1 inhibition efficiency by carrageenans from red seaweeds family gigartinaceae, Tichocarpaceae and Phyllophoraceae, *Heliyon, 10*, e33407. https://doi.org/10.1016/j.heliyon.2024.e33407

Song, S., Peng, H., Wang, Q., Liu, Z., Dong, X., Wen, C., Ai, C., Zhang, Y., Wang, Z., & Zhu, B. (2020). Inhibitory activities of marine sulfated polysaccharides against SARS-CoV-2. *Food and Function, 11*, 7415–7420. https://doi.org/10.1039/d0fo02017f

Unagolla, J. M., & Jayasuriya, A. C. (2018). Drug transport mechanisms and in vitro release kinetics of vancomycin encapsulated chitosan-alginate polyelectrolyte microparticles as a controlled drug delivery system. *European Journal of Pharmaceutical Sciences, 114*, 199–209. https://doi.org/10.1016/j.ejps.2017.12.012

Venkatesan, J., Anil, S., Kim, S.-K., & Shim, M. (2016). Seaweed Polysaccharide-Based Nanoparticles: Preparation and Applications for Drug Delivery. *Polymers, 8*(2), 30. https://doi.org/10.3390/polym8020030

Wang, C., Wang, T., Dai, J., An, Z., Hu, R., Duan, L., Chen, H., Wang, X., Chu, Z., Liu, H., Wang, J., Li, N., Yang, Z., & Wang, J. (2021). 1-formyl-β-carboline derivatives block Newcastle disease virus proliferation through suppressing viral adsorption and entry processes. *Biomolecules, 11*. https://doi.org/10.3390/biom11111687

Wang, W., Wang, S. X., & Guan, H. S. (2012). The antiviral activities and mechanisms of marine polysaccharides: An overview. In *Marine Drugs* (Vol. 10, pp. 2795–2816). MDPI AG. https://doi.org/10.3390/md10122795

Wang, W., Wu, J., Zhang, X., Hao, C., Zhao, X., Jiao, G., Shan, X., Tai, W., & Yu, G. (2017). Inhibition of influenza A virus infection by fucoidan targeting viral neuraminidase and cellular EGFR pathway. *Scientific Reports, 7*. https://doi.org/10.1038/srep40760

Wei, Q., Fu, G., Wang, K., Yang, Q., Zhao, J., Wang, Y., Ji, K., & Song, S. (2022). Advances in Research on Antiviral Activities of Sulfated Polysaccharides from Seaweeds. In *Pharmaceuticals* (Vol. 15, Issue 5). MDPI. https://doi.org/10.3390/ph15050581

Xu, S. Y., Huang, X., & Cheong, K. L. (2017). Recent advances in marine algae polysaccharides: Isolation, structure, and activities. In *Marine Drugs* (Vol. 15). MDPI AG. https://doi.org/10.3390/md15120388

Xu, X., Chen, P., Wang, J., Feng, J., Zhou, H., Li, X., Zhong, W., & Hao, P. (2020). Evolution of the novel coronavirus from the ongoing Wuhan outbreak and modeling of its spike protein for risk of human transmission. In *Science China Life Sciences* (Vol. 63, pp. 457–460). Science in China Press. https://doi.org/10.1007/s11427-020-1637-5

York, A. (2021). Targeting viral liquid–liquid phase separation. *Nature Reviews Microbiology, 19*, 550. https://doi.org/10.1038/s41579-021-00608-6

Yuan, H., Song, J., Li, X., Li, N., & Dai, J. (2006). Immunomodulation and antitumor activity of κ-carrageenan oligosaccharides. *Cancer Letters, 243*, 228–234. https://doi.org/10.1016/j.canlet.2005.11.032

Zhang, B., Yan, Y., Shen, Q., Ma, D., Huang, L., Cai, X., & Tan, S. (2017). A colon targeted drug delivery system based on alginate modificated graphene oxide for colorectal liver metastasis. *Materials Science and Engineering C, 79*, 185–190. https://doi.org/10.1016/j.msec.2017.05.054

Zhang, W., Oda, T., Yu, Q., & Jin, J. O. (2015). Fucoidan from Macrocystis pyrifera has powerful immune-modulatory effects compared to three other fucoidans. *Marine Drugs, 13*, 1084–1104. https://doi.org/10.3390/md13031084

Zhang, X., Zhu, Y., Fan, L., Ling, J., Yang, L. Y., Wang, N., & Ouyang, X. kun. (2022). Delivery of curcumin by fucoidan-coated mesoporous silica nanoparticles: Fabrication, characterization, and in vitro release performance. *International Journal of Biological Macromolecules, 211*, 368–379. https://doi.org/10.1016/j.ijbiomac.2022.05.086

Zhao, T., Feng, Y., Li, J., Mao, R., Zou, Y., Feng, W., Zheng, D., Wang, W., Chen, Y., Yang, L., & Wu, X. (2014). Schisandra polysaccharide evokes immunomodulatory activity through TLR 4-mediated activation of macrophages. *International Journal of Biological Macromolecules, 65*, 33–40. https://doi.org/10.1016/j.ijbiomac.2014.01.018

Zhu, N., Zhang, D., Wang, W., Li, X., Yang, B., Song, J., Zhao, X., Huang, B., Shi, W., Lu, R., Niu, P., Zhan, F., Ma, X., Wang, D., Xu, W., Wu, G., Gao, G. F., & Tan, W. (2020). A Novel Coronavirus from Patients with Pneumonia in China, 2019. *New England Journal of Medicine, 382*, 727–733. https://doi.org/10.1056/nejmoa2001017

Marine Animal Polysaccharide in Targeted Drug Delivery

Sarra Akermi, Moufida Chaari, Khaoula Elhadef, Bouthaina Hadj Hmida, Gulzar Rather, Fakhreddine Ben Amara, Ashwani Sharma, and Slim Smaoui

Abstract Polysaccharides sourced from marine animal have gained an extensive interest as bioactive carriers used in targeted drug delivery systems, providing a variety of therapeutic options with the respect of ecological sustainability. In this sense, numerous compounds including chitosan, alginate, fucoidan, and carrageenan, derived from organisms such as crustaceans, mollusks, and algae-associated species, were found to exhibit remarkable properties including biocompatibility, enzymatic degradability, mucoadhesiveness, and reactive functional groups. These valuable characteristics facilitate their incorporation into a large range of delivery systems such as hydrogels, nanoparticles, microspheres, and nanofibrous scaffolds, ensuring an effective and proper control of drug release.

The present chapter emphasizes the importance of marine polysaccharides and studies their potential properties for responsive delivery. It also discusses the recent innovations related to drug delivery systems including smart release systems and composite formulations that synergize marine polysaccharides with other materials. Furthermore, challenges and limitations are discussed as well as emerging strategies to improve delivery performance. Finally, the chapter highlights future directions and perspectives in marine-based drug delivery technologies, outlining their role in the era of next generation of precision therapeutics and regenerative remedies.

S. Akermi · M. Chaari · K. Elhadef · F. B. Amara · S. Smaoui (✉)
Laboratory of Microbial Biotechnology, Enzymatic and Biomolecules, Centre of Biotechnology of Sfax, Sfax, Tunisia

B. H. Hmida
Laboratory of Biochemistry and Enzymatic Engineering of Lipases, National Engineering School of Sfax (ENIS), Sfax, Tunisia

G. Rather
AMR and Nanotherapeutics Lab, Department of Pharmacology, Saveetha Dental College and Hospital, Saveetha Institute of Medical and Technical Sciences, Chennai, India

A. Sharma
Insight Biosolutions, Biopole Rennes, Rennes, France

S. Jana et al. (eds.), *Multifunctional Marine Polysaccharides*,
https://doi.org/10.1007/978-981-95-4126-3_5

Keywords Marine animal · Polysaccharides · Drug delivery · Recent innovations · Sustainability · Challenges and limitations

1 Introduction

The continuous development and design of drugs have considerably expanded with the innovations related to targeted drug delivery systems. These latter are largely used to enhance therapeutic functions by rapidly and properly delivering bioactive molecules to their precise site of action (Ezike et al. 2023). This strategy could improve drug efficacy, reduce possible side effects, and minimize the required dosage especially in the treatment of diseases such as cancer, autoimmune disorders, and chronic infections (Zhao et al. 2020). Targeted delivery systems are tightly linked to smart carriers that can cross biological barriers, recognize their specific targets, and control the release of drugs (Singh 2024).

Among the various systems dedicated for drug delivery, biopolymers came to light as a keystone owing to their unique combination of various properties including bioavailability, adaptability, and physiological compatibility (Trucillo 2024). These macromolecules can be chemically modified to enhance different parameters, such as solubility, surface charge, or degradation rate, required in drug transport (Joye and McClements 2016). Their natural source also makes them safe for human use and less immunogenic compared to synthetic alternatives. However, a vast number of biopolymers originated from marine organisms are still underexplored resources (Thomas et al. 2020). Marine ecosystems offer a multitude of polysaccharides sourced from animals such as crustaceans (shrimp and crab), echinoderms (sea cucumbers), mollusks (squid and shellfish), as well as algae-associated organisms (Bose et al. 2023). These marine polysaccharides are diverse in terms of structures and functions, making them ideal alternatives to conventional synthetic delivery platforms (Fig. 1). Among the most well-known marine-derived biopolymers, we cite chitosan, alginate, fucoidan, and carrageenan characterized by particular properties that make them valuable in targeted drug delivery systems (Ege et al. 2024). In this sense, the chitosan, extracted from the exoskeletons of crustaceans, exhibits mucoadhesive and antimicrobial characteristics (Abere et al. 2022); the alginate, extracted from brown algae, showed great gel-forming capability and excellent biocompatibility (Tiwari et al. 2022). In addition, the fucoidan, a sulfated polysaccharide found in brown seaweed, possesses anti-inflammatory and anticancer potential, and the carrageenan, derived from red algae, is largely exploited owing to its precious properties such as viscosity and utility in controlled-release formulations (Alfinaikh et al. 2025).

These biopolymers can be converted into various delivery carriers such as nanoparticles, hydrogels, liposomes, and microspheres, in order to facilitate the transport of therapeutic agents to their specific destination (Gopi et al. 2018). Beyond their biochemical versatility, marine polysaccharides were suggested to be sustainable and eco-conscious alternative to synthetic polymers, aligning with the growing demands related to green healthcare techniques (Shokrak et al. 2024). Their

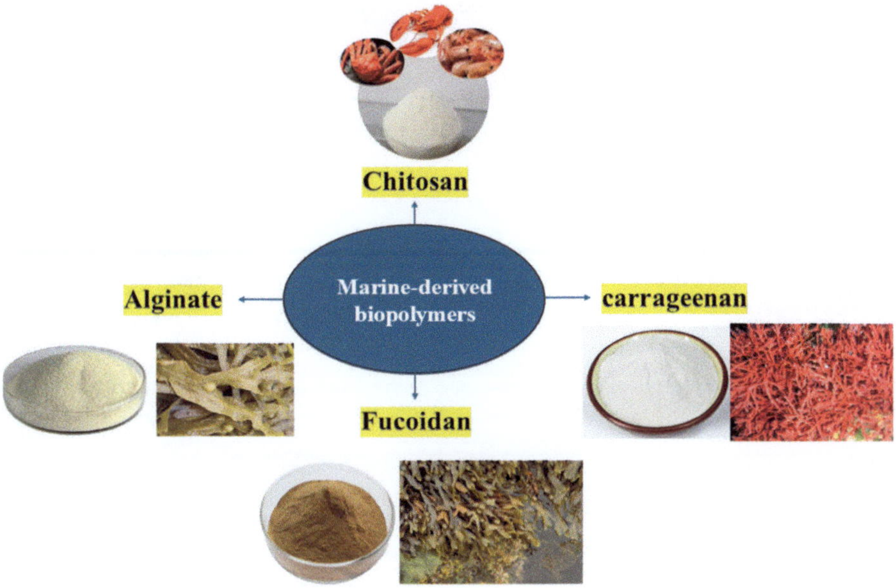

Fig. 1 Examples of marine-derived biopolymers

fast interaction with physiological stimuli (pH, temperature, and enzymatic activity) improves their ability to form smart drug delivery systems that release therapeutics precisely at the desired site (Raza et al. 2019). As a result, marine animal polysaccharides are redefining the future of targeted drug delivery by offering biologically inspired scaffolds that are not only effective and safe but also environmentally responsible (Chellapandian et al. 2025).

2 Sources of Marine Polysaccharides

Marine polysaccharides can be derived from a variety of oceanic sources, with marine animals offering several unique types that differ from those found in seaweeds or microorganisms (Fig. 2).

2.1 Biopolymers Derived from Seaweed

Seaweed-derived biopolymers have emerged as a compelling class of natural materials in the field of drug delivery, offering a sustainable and biocompatible alternative to synthetic polymers (Krishnan et al. 2024). Extracted from marine macroalgae such as brown (*Laminaria*), red (*Gracilaria*, *Gelidium*), and green (*Ulva*) seaweeds,

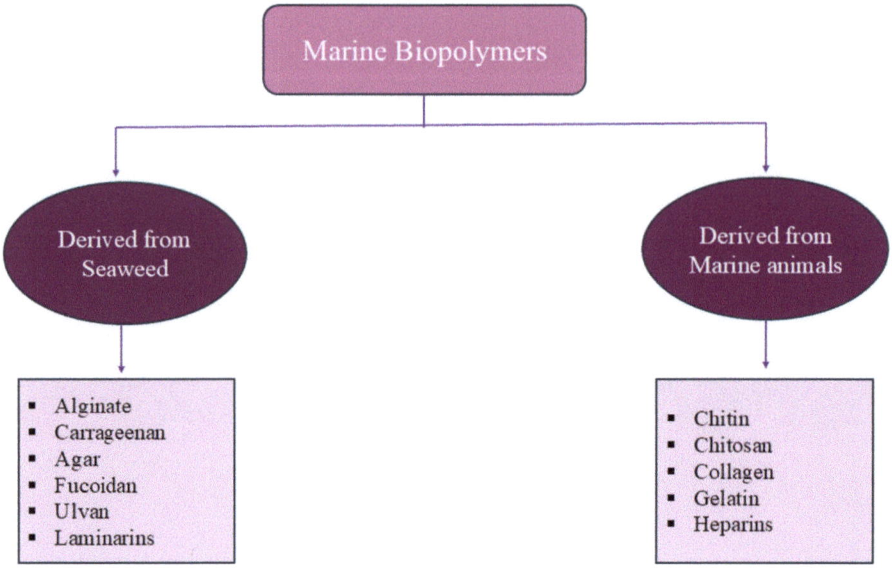

Fig. 2 Different sources of marine polysaccharides

these polysaccharides include alginate, carrageenan, agar, fucoidan, and ulvan (Table 1), each possessing unique physicochemical properties that make them ideal for biomedical applications (Jönsson et al. 2020). Their inherent characteristics such as gel-forming ability, mucoadhesiveness, and responsiveness to physiological stimuli enable the development of advanced drug delivery systems including hydrogels, nanoparticles, and transdermal patches (Zamboulis et al. 2020).

These biopolymers are not only biodegradable and non-toxic but also exhibit excellent encapsulation efficiency and controlled-release profiles, making them suitable carriers for a wide range of therapeutic agents, from small molecules to proteins and peptides (Kučuk et al. 2023). Moreover, their anionic nature and surface functional groups (sulfate, carboxyl, hydroxyl) facilitate targeted delivery and interaction with biological tissues (Miao et al. 2018). As the demand for eco-friendly and patient-specific therapies grows, seaweed-based biopolymers are gaining traction in regenerative medicine, cancer treatment, and wound healing ushering in a new era of marine-inspired pharmaceutical innovation (Jeong et al. 2022).

2.1.1 Alginate

Alginate is a naturally occurring anionic polysaccharide predominantly extracted from brown seaweeds such as *Laminaria*, *Ascophyllum*, and *Macrocystis* (Rahman et al. 2024). It consists of linear chains of two uronic acid monomers including β-D-mannuronic acid (M) and α-L-guluronic acid (G) arranged in homopolymeric (MM or GG) and heteropolymeric (MG or GM) blocks (Abka-khajouei et al.

Table 1 Seaweed-derived biopolymers and their properties and applications

Biopolymer	Source	Functional properties	Applications	References
Alginate	Brown algae (*Laminaria, Ascophyllum*, and *Macrocystis*)	Gel-forming Biocompatible Absorbent	Wound dressings and drug delivery	Abourehab et al. (2022)
Agar	Red algae (*Gracilaria, Gelidium*)	Thermo-reversible gel Clarity	Hydrogels Microparticles Nanoparticles Beads and capsules	Salave et al. (2022)
Carrageenan	Red algae (*Kappaphycus, Gigartina*)	Thickening Stabilizing Antiviral	Oral delivery of poorly soluble drugs Wound healing, tissue engineering Extended release of oral formulations	Omidian and Wilson (2024)
Ulvan	Green algae (*Ulva*)	Antioxidant Immunomodulatory	Biomedical coatings	Pari et al. (2025)
Fucoidans	Brown algae (*Fucus, Undaria*)	Anticoagulant Anti-inflammatory	Nutraceuticals and cancer therapy	Iqbal et al. (2024)
Laminarins	Brown algae	Antitumor Prebiotic	Functional foods and pharmaceuticals	Berezhnaya et al. (2024)

2022). The ratio and sequence of these blocks significantly influence alginate physicochemical properties, including gel strength, porosity, and degradation rate (Ramdhan et al. 2020). One of the alginate most valuable features is its ability to undergo ionic gelation in the presence of divalent cations such as Ca^{2+}, Ba^{2+}, or Sr^{2+}, forming hydrogels through the well-known "egg-box" model (Malektaj 2024). This mild gelation process occurs under physiological conditions, making alginate highly suitable for encapsulating sensitive bioactives like proteins, peptides, and live cells (Li et al. 2021a, b). The resulting gel matrix is biocompatible, non-toxic, and thermally stable, offering protection against environmental stressors such as heat, moisture, and pH fluctuations, key factors in enhancing drug stability and shelf-life (Kothale et al. 2020).

The alginate possesses mucoadhesive properties, pH responsiveness, and controlled-release behavior, which have made it a cornerstone material in the development of oral, transdermal, and injectable drug delivery systems (Sarkar et al. 2025). Its affordability, ease of processing, and neutral taste and odor further contribute to its widespread use in both pharmaceutical and nutraceutical formulations (Gheorghita Puscaselu et al. 2020). Moreover, alginate can be chemically modified or blended with other polymers to tailor its mechanical strength, degradation rate, and bioactivity, expanding its utility in tissue engineering, wound healing, and targeted therapy (Abourehab et al. 2022).

2.1.2 Agar

Agar is a natural polysaccharide extracted primarily from red seaweeds such as *Gracilaria*, *Gelidium*, and *Ahnfeltia* and is composed of two main fractions: agarose and agaropectin (Padmesh and Singh 2021). Agarose is a neutral, linear polymer made up of repeating units of D-galactose and 3,6-anhydro-L-galactopyranose, while agaropectin is a branched, sulfated polysaccharide containing acidic side groups like sulfate, pyruvate, and uronic acids (Zia et al. 2017). These structural features contribute to agar unique thermo-reversible gelation behavior forming a firm gel at temperatures below 40–45 °C and melting above 80–90 °C (Rhein-Knudsen et al. 2017). Additionally, the double-helix molecular structure of agar aggregates into a three-dimensional network capable of entrapping water and bioactive compounds, making it an excellent candidate for controlled drug release (Biscari 2023). Its biocompatibility, non-toxicity, and mechanical stability allow it to be used in various pharmaceutical formulations, including hydrogels, microparticles, nanocomposites, and film-based delivery systems (Salave et al. 2022). Agar-based carriers can encapsulate drugs, protect them from degradation, and release them in response to physiological conditions, such as temperature or pH (Gupta et al. 2023).

In drug delivery, agar has been explored for oral, pulmonary, and topical applications, with promising results in antibiotic, antiviral, and anticancer therapies (Shahruzzaman et al. 2019). Its ability to form stable matrices and interact with other polymers or nanoparticles further enhances its versatility. Moreover, agar's low cost, ease of processing, and renewable marine origin make it a sustainable alternative to synthetic excipients in modern pharmaceutical design (Lazim and Muhamad 2025).

2.1.3 Carrageenan

Carrageenan is a family of high-molecular-weight sulfated galactans predominantly found in the cell walls of red seaweeds belonging to the Rhodophyceae class, such as *Chondrus crispus*, *Gigartina*, and *Eucheuma* (Tuvikene 2021). Structurally, carrageenan is composed of alternating units of D-galactose and 3,6-anhydro-D-galactose, linked via α-1,3 and β-1,4 glycosidic bonds (Ali and Ahmed 2018). The degree and position of sulfate ester groups on these sugar units give rise to various types of carrageenan, primarily kappa (κ), iota (ι), and lambda (λ), each with distinct gelling, viscosity, and solubility profiles (Pereira et al. 2017).

In drug delivery, the hydrophilic nature of carrageenan, its biocompatibility, and non-toxic profile make it an attractive candidate for developing hydrogels, films, nanoparticles, and microspheres (Mirzaei et al. 2023). Its ability to form thermo-reversible gels and viscoelastic matrices enables the encapsulation and controlled release of a wide range of therapeutic agents, including small molecules, proteins, and vaccines (Omidian and Wilson 2024). *Kappa* and *iota* carrageenan exhibit strong gelation in the presence of potassium and calcium ions, respectively, forming three-dimensional networks that mimic extracellular matrices ideal for tissue engineering and cell delivery (Qamar et al. 2024). Moreover, carrageenan sulfated functional groups contribute to its bioactivity, including antiviral, anticoagulant, and immunomodulatory effects, which can enhance therapeutic outcomes (Nagahawatta et al. 2023). Recent innovations involve chemical modifications and hybrid formulations with other polymers or nanoparticles to improve mechanical strength, responsiveness to stimuli (such as pH and temperature), and targeting capabilities (Mokhtari et al. 2021).

2.1.4 Ulvan

Ulvans are water-soluble sulfated heteropolysaccharides predominantly found in the cell walls of green macroalgae from the genus *Ulva*, commonly known as "sea lettuce" (Yu-Qing et al. 2016). Widely distributed across coastal regions worldwide, *Ulva* species are among the most abundant members of the *Chlorophyta* phylum and have long been utilized in food, agriculture, and traditional medicine (Bajaj et al. 2023). Ulvan comprises approximately 9–36% of the dry weight of *Ulva* biomass and is structurally rich in rhamnose 3-sulfate, xylose, xylose 2-sulfate, glucuronic acid, and iduronic acid, contributing to its highly sulfated and bioactive nature (Tran et al. 2023). The unique chemical architecture of ulvan including its resemblance to mammalian glycosaminoglycans, including heparan sulfate and chondroitin sulfate, makes it a promising candidate for biomedical applications (Sulastri et al. 2021). Its anionic charge, hydrophilicity, and biocompatibility allow it to form hydrogels, nanoparticles, and films capable of encapsulating and releasing therapeutic agents in a controlled manner. Ulvan-based hydrogels have shown potential in wound healing, tissue engineering, and oral drug delivery, with studies highlighting their antioxidant, anti-inflammatory, antiviral, and anticancer properties (Pari et al. 2025). Structurally, *Ulva* cell walls contain two major polysaccharide groups. The primary group is composed of soluble ulvan and insoluble cellulose. However, the secondary group is composed of alkali-soluble xyloglucan and glucuronan (Li et al. 2023).

These components contribute to ulvan gel-forming ability, mechanical stability, and bioactivity, making it suitable for stimuli-responsive drug delivery systems (Kumar et al. 2022). Additionally, ulvan fiber-rich composition supports gut health and has been linked to reduced risk of chronic diseases, further enhancing its value in nutraceutical formulations (Harsha Mohan et al. 2025).

2.1.5 Fucoidans

Fucoidan is a water-soluble, sulfated heteropolysaccharide predominantly synthesized by brown macroalgae such as *Fucus vesiculosus*, *Undaria pinnatifida*, and *Ascophyllum nodosum* (Saeed et al. 2021). It is primarily composed of L-fucose, a deoxyhexose sugar ($C_6H_{12}O_5$), along with varying amounts of galactose, mannose, xylose, and uronic acids, depending on the algal species and extraction conditions (Kurera et al. 2024). The presence of sulfate ester groups imparts a negative charge to the molecule, contributing to its mucoadhesive behavior, pH responsiveness, and bioactivity (Haggag et al. 2023). Furthermore, fucoidan has garnered significant attention in pharmaceutical research due to its multifunctional therapeutic properties, including anticoagulant, antithrombotic, anti-obesity, immunomodulatory, and anticancer effects (Iqbal et al. 2024). These biological activities are largely attributed to its sulfation pattern, molecular weight, and glycosidic linkages, which influence its interaction with cellular receptors and biological membranes (Wang et al. 2019).

In drug delivery, fucoidan serves as a biocompatible carrier capable of forming nanoparticles, hydrogels, and film-based systems for the controlled release of active pharmaceutical ingredients (Negreanu-Pirjol et al. 2022). Its ability to respond to physiological stimuli such as pH changes in the gastrointestinal tract makes it particularly useful for oral and mucosal delivery routes. Moreover, the non-toxic nature of fucoidan, biodegradability, and ability to bind bioactive compounds position it as a promising material for targeted therapy, especially in oncology, wound healing, and regenerative medicine (Anisha et al. 2022).

2.1.6 Laminarins

Laminarin is a low-molecular-weight β-glucan predominantly stored in the vacuoles of brown macroalgae, especially in species such as *Laminaria digitata*, *Saccharina japonica*, *Ecklonia kurome*, and *Eisenia bicyclis* (Chen et al. 2021). Structurally, it consists of β-(1 → 3)-linked glucose units with occasional β-(1 → 6) branches, forming a compact and water-soluble polysaccharide (Olatunji 2020). Its molecular weight typically ranges between 5 and 10 kDa, depending on species, harvest season, and extraction method (Kadam et al. 2015). In addition, laminarin is primarily composed of neutral carbohydrates, with minor contributions from uronic acids and mannitol residues, which influence its solubility and biological activity (Li et al. 2021b). It can be chemically modified through sulfation using chlorosulfonic acid in pyridine and sulfur dioxide at sub-zero temperatures to enhance its anticoagulant and antitumor properties (Berezhnaya et al. 2024). These modifications improve its interaction with biological targets and expand its utility in targeted drug delivery systems. Recent studies have shown that laminarin-based microparticles can achieve sustained release, stimuli-responsive behavior, and non-cytotoxicity in human cell lines (Zhang et al. 2022). Additionally, its fermentable nature allows hydrolysis into glucose, which can be utilized in bioethanol production, supporting circular bioeconomy models (Immanuel Suresh and Divyeswari 2024).

2.2 *Biopolymers Derived from Marine Animals*

Biopolymers sourced from marine animals represent a unique class of naturally occurring macromolecules with remarkable structural diversity and functional versatility (Biplajit et al. 2021). Extracted from organisms such as crustaceans, mollusks, echinoderms, and fish, these compounds primarily proteins and polysaccharides have gained increasing attention for their roles in biomedical, pharmaceutical, and environmental applications (Romano et al. 2022). Notable examples include chitin and chitosan from shrimp and crab shells, collagen and gelatin from fish skin and scales, and glycosaminoglycans like hyaluronic acid and chondroitin sulfate from marine invertebrates and cartilaginous fish (Kim 2018).

These biopolymers exhibit key properties such as biodegradability, biocompatibility, and low immunogenicity, making them ideal candidates for developing drug delivery systems, wound dressings, tissue scaffolds, and bioactive coatings (Biswas et al. 2022). Their ability to form hydrogels, nanoparticles, and films enables controlled release of therapeutic agents and targeted delivery to specific tissues. Moreover, the valorization of marine by-products such as shells, cartilage, and skin aligns with sustainable development goals by reducing waste and promoting circular bioeconomy practices (Ore Areche et al. 2024). As research continues to uncover the molecular intricacies and bioactivities of these marine-derived materials, their integration into advanced medical technologies and green industrial processes is expected to expand, offering innovative solutions rooted in oceanic biodiversity (Lagopati et al. 2023).

2.2.1 Chitin and Chitosan

Chitin is a naturally occurring structural polysaccharide found abundantly in the exoskeletons of marine crustaceans, particularly crabs, shrimp, and lobsters (Bastiaens et al. 2019). It serves as a protective and supportive component, forming a rigid matrix that contributes to the mechanical strength of these organisms (Moussian 2019). Among marine sources, crab shells are considered one of the most commercially viable and concentrated reservoirs of chitin and its derivative, chitosan (Suryawanshi et al. 2019). Chemically, chitin is composed of β-(1 $\rightarrow$ 4)-linked N-acetyl-D-glucosamine units, structurally similar to cellulose but distinguished by the presence of acetamide groups (Ahmed et al. 2025). This configuration allows chitin to form crystalline microfibrils, which are insoluble in water but highly stable (Xu 2017). The term "chitin" was first introduced in the early nineteenth century, derived from the Greek word chiton, meaning "mail coat," reflecting its protective role in nature (Terkula Iber et al. 2022).

In biomedical contexts, chitin has gained recognition for its biocompatibility, biodegradability, and low immunogenicity, making it suitable for applications such as wound dressings, tissue scaffolds, and drug delivery systems (Baharlouei and Rahman 2022). Its antibacterial activity, moisture retention, and ability to promote cell proliferation further enhance its utility in regenerative medicine. Additionally, chitin is bioabsorbable, meaning it can be broken down and assimilated by biological systems without adverse effects (Wijesekara and Xu 2024).

Through a process known as N-deacetylation, chitin is chemically converted into chitosan, a more soluble and reactive derivative (Table 2). The degree of deacetylation (DDA), which varies based on species, extraction method, and processing conditions, directly influences chitosan solubility, charge density, and biological activity (Pellis et al. 2022). Chitosan, with its free amino groups, is widely used in drug encapsulation, gene delivery, and antimicrobial coatings (Mikušová and Mikuš 2021). Due to its renewable nature, low cost, and abundant availability from seafood industry by-products, chitin represents a sustainable and versatile material for both biomedical and food industry innovations (Iroegbu and Ray 2023). Its transformation into chitosan further expands its functional range, making it a cornerstone of marine biopolymer research.

Table 2 Differences and applications of chitin and chitosan in drug delivery

Properties	Chitin	Chitosan
Chemical structure	β-(1 → 4)-linked N-acetylglucosamine units	Partially deacetylated chitin with glucosamine and N-acetylglucosamine units
Solubility	Insoluble in water and most solvents	Soluble in acidic aqueous solutions
Biodegradability	Slow biodegradability	Biodegradable with faster degradation rate
Biocompatibility	Good	Excellent
Antimicrobial properties	Mild	Strong antimicrobial activity
Mechanical strength	High (rigid structure)	Moderate (more flexible)
Drug delivery uses	Limited due to poor solubility and processability	Widely used due to solubility, bioadhesion, and modifiability
Forms used in delivery	Films, scaffolds (mainly structural)	Nanoparticles, hydrogels, microspheres, coatings
Targeted delivery	Less effective	Effective for oral, nasal, ocular, and transdermal delivery routes

2.2.2 Marine Collagen

Growing attention has been directed toward the utilization of by-products from the fishing industry, such as fish skin, scales, and bones, as an eco-conscious and cost-effective source for extracting collagen (Baksi et al. 2025). This marine-derived collagen is increasingly favored due to its excellent biocompatibility, biodegradability, and minimal immunogenicity, making it suitable for diverse biomedical and industrial applications, including tissue engineering, wound healing, and cosmetic formulations (Wosicka-Frąckowiak et al. 2024). In this sense, marine collagen exhibits both fibrillar and non-fibrillar structures, yet it differs significantly from its terrestrial counterparts (Coppola et al. 2021). Notably, it possesses higher viscosity than bovine collagen, which can influence its behavior in solution and its performance in formulations (Farooq et al. 2024). However, it also has lower gelling and melting temperatures, a consequence of its unique amino acid composition and reduced hydroxyproline content (Shaik et al. 2024). These thermal properties stem from the less stable intermolecular cross-links found in fish collagen, which render it more sensitive to heat and enzymatic degradation compared to mammalian sources.

Structurally, most fish collagens are composed of two polypeptide chains commonly designated as $\alpha 1$ and $\alpha 2$, which form the characteristic triple helix of type I collagen (Jafari et al. 2020). This configuration supports its role in maintaining structural integrity in connective tissues while also offering flexibility for modification and incorporation into advanced biomaterials. Furthermore, its unique molecular structure characterized by reduced hydroxyproline content and lower thermal stability enables faster enzymatic degradation, which is ideal for controlled drug release (Lim et al. 2019). In this context, marine collagen has been successfully integrated into various delivery platforms including hydrogels, nanoparticles, microspheres, and bioactive films. These systems enhance drug stability and absorption, particularly for oral, topical, and wound-related applications (Debele and Su 2022). Its positive impact on cell adhesion and tissue regeneration also supports advanced applications like gene therapy and regenerative implants (Geahchan et al. 2022). By leveraging its functional versatility, marine collagen continues to drive innovation in targeted and sustained-release therapies.

2.2.3 Marine Gelatin

Gelatin, a hydrolyzed form of collagen, is rich in amino acids such as glycine, proline, and hydroxyproline, which contribute to its structural integrity and biological activity (Dille et al. 2021). When derived from marine sources particularly fish skin, scales, and bones, it offers a sustainable and culturally inclusive alternative to mammalian gelatin, which dominates the global market (Abd Aziz et al. 2025). Marine gelatin has gained traction not only in food packaging but also in biomedical applications, especially drug delivery, due to its biodegradability, biocompatibility, and low immunogenicity (Al-Nimry et al. 2021).

On the other side, marine gelatin serves as a versatile matrix for encapsulating and releasing therapeutic agents (Jia et al. 2024). Its hydrophilic nature and ability to form gels at low temperatures make it suitable for injectable formulations and temperature-sensitive drugs. Marine gelatin-based hydrogels, nanogels, and microspheres have been engineered to deliver small-molecule drugs, proteins, and even genetic material with controlled-release profiles (Delgado-Pujol et al. 2025). For instance, gelatin methacryloyl (GelMA) derived from fish has been used to fabricate nanogels that exhibit high drug-loading efficiency and pH-responsive release behavior, ideal for targeting tumor microenvironments (Du et al. 2025). Despite its promise, fish gelatin presents challenges such as variable amino acid composition, lower mechanical strength, and distinct sensory properties (such as odor and color), which can affect formulation consistency (Joy et al. 2024). However, these limitations are being addressed through chemical modifications, blending with other polymers like chitosan or alginate, and cross-linking techniques that enhance its functional properties (Shi et al. 2022). As demand for marine-derived biomaterials grows alongside concerns over mammalian sources, fish gelatin continues to evolve as a key component in eco-friendly and effective drug delivery platforms (Chegu Krishnamurthi et al. 2023).

2.2.4 Heparins

Heparin, a highly sulfated glycosaminoglycan (GAG), is naturally present in the tissues of both terrestrial and marine organisms, including vertebrates and invertebrates (Volpi and Maccari 2016). It was first identified in 1916 by Jay McLean during research aimed at discovering thromboplastic agents, and it later became the first clinically used anticoagulant (Green 2020). Structurally, heparin consists of repeating disaccharide units composed of uronic acid and glucosamine, extensively modified by sulfation, which imparts its strong negative charge and biological activity (Sultana and Kamihira 2024).

In drug delivery, heparin has evolved far beyond its traditional anticoagulant role. Its unique physicochemical properties such as high charge density, biocompatibility, and ability to bind various proteins make it a promising candidate for advanced therapeutic systems (Banik et al. 2021). Heparin-based carriers have been developed for targeted delivery of chemotherapeutics, anti-inflammatory agents, and even nucleic acids (Kundu et al. 2018). These systems often exploit heparin affinity for growth factors and its ability to inhibit angiogenesis and metastasis, particularly in cancer therapy (Atallah et al. 2020). Recent innovations include the integration of heparin into nanomaterials, such as nanoparticles, hydrogels, and micelles, to enhance bioavailability and control drug release kinetics (Delgado-Pujol et al. 2025). For instance, ionically complexed nanoparticles using chitosan as a cationic matrix have been shown to improve oral delivery of heparin by protecting it from degradation in the gastrointestinal tract (Maretti et al. 2021). Additionally, heparin coatings on medical devices like stents and catheters have been employed to improve blood compatibility and reduce thrombogenicity (Biran and Pond 2017).

Despite its widespread use, there remains a gap in the literature regarding the recovery and application of heparins or heparan sulfates from marine species, particularly in the form of electrospun nanofibers (Alfinaikh et al. 2025). Such marine-derived variants could offer novel structural and functional properties, potentially expanding the scope of heparin-based drug delivery systems.

3 Mechanisms and Strategies of Drug Delivery

The delivery of pharmaceutical agents within the human body is a multidimensional process shaped by biological barriers, chemical properties of the drug, and the design of the delivery platform itself (Ezike et al. 2023). At its foundation, drug delivery systems aim to optimize therapeutic efficacy while minimizing side effects by controlling when, where, and how a drug is released (Adepu and Ramakrishna 2021). Fundamentally, mechanisms of drug delivery include passive diffusion, where molecules traverse cellular membranes based on concentration gradients; facilitated transport via protein carriers, useful for transporting polar or charged compounds; and endocytic pathways that allow cellular uptake of complex macromolecules or particulate formulations (Kokate et al. 2023). These mechanisms are often fine-tuned to align with the physicochemical characteristics of the drug and its target site.

Strategically, modern drug delivery designs embrace technologies that go beyond simple administration. Controlled-release systems incorporate biodegradable carriers such as polymers, lipids, or gels that disassemble at predictable rates, offering prolonged therapeutic action (Pillai et al. 2023). Moreover, targeted delivery methods utilize biological markers or receptors specific to diseased tissues, enabling precise deposition and reducing systemic exposure (Zhao et al. 2020). For example, nanocarriers functionalized with ligands can home in on tumor cells while evading healthy tissue (Mi et al. 2020). Responsive or "smart" delivery systems represent another frontier, engineered to react to endogenous triggers like pH fluctuations, enzymatic activity, or oxidative stress (Raza et al. 2019). This enables spatial and temporal precision in drug release, particularly useful in inflammatory conditions, cancer, and microbial infections. Additionally, advances in transdermal patches, pulmonary aerosols, and implantable microdevices are expanding the horizons of drug administration routes, accommodating patients' lifestyles and clinical needs (Cojocaru et al. 2024).

Finally, the integration of emerging tools like 3D bioprinting, biosensors, and computational modeling continues to shape the evolution of drug delivery systems (Alzoubi et al. 2023). With growing interest in personalization and precision medicine, future strategies will likely combine biological insights with engineering ingenuity offering smarter, safer, and more adaptive therapeutics to meet individual health profiles (Nawaz 2024).

4 Recent Advances and Innovations

Marine animal polysaccharides have emerged as powerful tools in the development of targeted drug delivery systems, offering a sustainable and biologically active alternative to synthetic polymers. Recent innovations have focused on engineering stimuli-responsive delivery platforms using marine polysaccharides (Srivastava et al. 2021). For instance, one of the most transformative innovations involves chitosan-based nanoparticles, which have been modified to enhance mucosal adhesion and facilitate transcellular transport (Iacob et al. 2021). These carriers are particularly effective for oral and nasal delivery, where they protect sensitive drugs from enzymatic degradation and promote absorption across epithelial barriers (Mura et al. 2022). For example, chitosan nanoparticles loaded with insulin have demonstrated improved glycemic control in diabetic models by bypassing gastrointestinal breakdown (Seyam et al. 2020).

Additionally, fucoidan, a sulfated polysaccharide derived from brown algae, has gained attention for its tumor-targeting capabilities (Wang et al. 2024). Its affinity for P-selectin receptors overexpressed in certain cancer cells enables selective delivery of chemotherapeutics, reducing off-target toxicity (Haggag et al. 2023). Fucoidan has also been incorporated into dual-drug nanocomposites, allowing simultaneous delivery of anticancer agents and immunomodulators for synergistic therapy (Guo et al. 2025).

Alginate, known for its gel-forming properties, has been used to develop pH-sensitive hydrogels that release drugs in the alkaline environment of the intestine (Singh and Nayak 2023). This is particularly useful for drugs that degrade in the stomach but require absorption in the lower GI tract. Recent studies have also explored alginate-chitosan hybrid systems for sustained release of antibiotics and anti-inflammatory agents in wound healing applications (Saberian et al. 2024). Another breakthrough is the fabrication of electrospun nanofibers using marine polysaccharides. These fibers can be loaded with growth factors, antimicrobial peptides, or small-molecule drugs and applied directly to wounds or surgical sites (Riaz et al. 2025). Their high surface area and porosity enhance drug diffusion and tissue integration, making them ideal for localized therapy and regenerative medicine (Ding et al. 2019). Moreover, marine-derived exopolysaccharides from cyanobacteria and marine bacteria are being explored for their unique structural motifs and bioactivities (Zayed et al. 2022). These novel polysaccharides offer customizable backbones for gene delivery, vaccine carriers, and biosensing platforms, expanding the therapeutic landscape beyond conventional small molecules (Nguyen et al. 2024).

In summary, the convergence of marine biotechnology, nanotechnology, and polymer chemistry has propelled marine animal polysaccharides into the spotlight of targeted drug delivery research (Jain et al. 2025). Their ability to be chemically tailored, combined with their natural abundance and low toxicity, positions them as key players in the development of personalized, responsive, and sustainable therapeutic systems.

5 Challenges and Future Perspectives

Marine animal polysaccharides have gained significant attention in targeted drug delivery due to their ability to be chemically modified for therapeutic applications. However, their integration into advanced pharmaceutical systems is not without challenges (Table 3). One of the primary limitations lies in the structural variability of these biopolymers, which can differ based on species, habitat, and extraction methods (Sacramento et al. 2022). This inconsistency affects reproducibility in drug formulations and complicates regulatory approval. Additionally, some marine polysaccharides exhibit low mechanical strength and limited stability under physiological conditions, which may hinder their performance in sustained-release systems (Dattilo et al. 2023).

Another concern is the batch-to-batch variability in molecular weight and sulfation patterns, particularly in compounds like fucoidan and carrageenan (Inácio et al. 2022). These variations can influence bioactivity and drug-binding efficiency, making standardization difficult. Moreover, the sensory properties of marine-derived materials such as odor and color can pose formulation challenges, especially for oral or topical applications (Harinisri Ram and Thamarai Selvi 2024). From a scalability perspective, sustainable harvesting and purification of marine polysaccharides require careful ecological management to avoid overexploitation of marine resources (Sacramento et al. 2022).

Despite these hurdles, the future of marine polysaccharides in drug delivery is promising. Advances in biotechnological synthesis and genetic engineering are paving the way for controlled production of uniform polysaccharide structures. Emerging techniques like microfluidics, 3D bioprinting, and stimuli-responsive systems are expanding the versatility of these materials in personalized medicine (Sadraei and Naghib 2025). For instance, chitosan-based nanocarriers are being explored for gene therapy, while alginate hydrogels are showing potential in

Table 3 Summary of the main limitations of marine polysaccharide uses

Challenges and limitations		References
Structural variability	Differences due to species, habitat, and extraction methods affect reproducibility and regulatory approval	Sacramento et al. (2022)
Mechanical and physiological stability	Some polysaccharides lack sufficient mechanical strength and degrade too quickly in physiological environments	Sepe et al. (2025)
Batch-to-batch inconsistency	Variations in molecular weight and sulfation as well as the complicated standardization	Chi and Wang (2023)
Sensory attributes	Odor, color, and taste of marine materials may limit their use in oral or topical formulations	Harinisri Ram and Thamarai Selvi (2024) and Guillerme et al. (2017)
Scalability and sustainability	Harvesting and purification methods must be eco-conscious to prevent resource depletion	Sacramento et al. (2022)

localized cancer treatment (Patra et al. 2024). Furthermore, the development of marine-inspired hybrid systems, combining polysaccharides with synthetic polymers or inorganic nanoparticles, offers new avenues for enhancing drug stability, targeting precision, and therapeutic efficacy (Fernandes et al. 2022). As research continues to bridge the gap between marine biology and pharmaceutical engineering, marine animal polysaccharides are poised to become integral components of next-generation drug delivery platforms.

6 Conclusion

Marine animal polysaccharides have showed an interesting potential in the field of targeted drug delivery, providing an effective and eco-friendly alternative to synthetic carriers. Their valuable properties (including biocompatibility, biodegradability, and structural diversity) facilitate the design of delivery systems that could manage physiological needs and ameliorate therapeutic precision. For that reason, marine-derived biopolymers have been successfully involved into different carriers such as nanoparticles, hydrogels, and electrospun fibers for proper drug administration.

Despite challenges and limitations related to their uses, recent advancements in marine biotechnology and polymer engineering continue to highlight their potent functionality and their safe applicability. Innovations including stimuli-responsive systems and bioactive composites are predominating the future perspectives for assisted medicine and regenerative remedies. As research permanently continues, marine animal polysaccharides are suggested to play a pivotal role in the development of next-generation drug delivery systems in order to fill the gap between nature-inspired materials and clinical innovation.

References

Abd Aziz, Mohd Aizudin, Khairunnisa Abdul Aziz, Syed Radzi Rahamaddulla, et al. 2025. 'Unlocking Halal Gelatin: Exploring Sustainable Sourcing and Applications'. In *Proceedings of the 4th International Conference on Biomass Utilization and Sustainable Energy; ICoBiomasSE 2024; 2–3 September; Penang, Malaysia*, edited by Hui Lin Ong, Siti Jamilah Hanim Mohd Yusof, Noor Hasyierah Mohd Salleh, Khairul Farihan Kasim, and Noor Shazliana Aizee Abidin. Springer Nature. https://doi.org/10.1007/978-981-96-3785-0_43.

Abere, Dare Victor, Sammy A. Ojo, Maria Belen Paredes-Epinosa, and Ali Hakami. 2022. 'Derivation of Composites of Chitosan-Nanoparticles from Crustaceans Source for Nanomedicine: A Mini Review'. *Biomedical Engineering Advances* 4 (December): 100058. https://doi.org/10.1016/j.bea.2022.100058.

Abka-khajouei, Roya, Latifa Tounsi, Nasim Shahabi, Anil Kumar Patel, Slim Abdelkafi, and Philippe Michaud. 2022. 'Structures, Properties and Applications of Alginates'. *Marine Drugs* 20 (6): 6. https://doi.org/10.3390/md20060364.

Abourehab, Mohammad A. S., Rahul R. Rajendran, Anshul Singh, et al. 2022. 'Alginate as a Promising Biopolymer in Drug Delivery and Wound Healing: A Review of the State-of-the-Art'. *International Journal of Molecular Sciences* 23 (16): 16. https://doi.org/10.3390/ijms23169035.

Adepu, Shivakalyani, and Seeram Ramakrishna. 2021. 'Controlled Drug Delivery Systems: Current Status and Future Directions'. *Molecules* 26 (19): 19. https://doi.org/10.3390/molecules26195905.

Ahmed, Shakeel, Soumeia Zeghoud, Hadia Hemmami, and Ilham Ben Amor. 2025. *Chitin and Chitosan: Physical and Chemical Properties*. CRC Press.

Ali, Akbar, and Shakeel Ahmed. 2018. 'Carrageenans: Structure, Properties and Applications'. In *Marine Polysaccharides*. Jenny Stanford Publishing.

Al-Nimry, Suhair, Alaa Abu Dayah, Inas Hasan, and Rawand Daghmash. 2021. 'Cosmetic, Biomedical and Pharmaceutical Applications of Fish Gelatin/Hydrolysates'. *Marine Drugs* 19 (3): 3. https://doi.org/10.3390/md19030145.

Alzoubi, Lorca, Alaa A. A. Aljabali, and Murtaza M. Tambuwala. 2023. 'Empowering Precision Medicine: The Impact of 3D Printing on Personalized Therapeutic'. *AAPS PharmSciTech* 24 (8): 228. https://doi.org/10.1208/s12249-023-02682-w.

Anisha, Grace Sathyanesan, Savitha Padmakumari, Anil Kumar Patel, Ashok Pandey, and Reeta Rani Singhania. 2022. 'Fucoidan from Marine Macroalgae: Biological Actions and Applications in Regenerative Medicine, Drug Delivery Systems and Food Industry'. *Bioengineering* 9 (9): 9. https://doi.org/10.3390/bioengineering9090472.

Atallah, Johnny, Hussein H. Khachfe, Juliett Berro, and Hazem I. Assi. 2020. 'The Use of Heparin and Heparin-like Molecules in Cancer Treatment: A Review'. *Cancer Treatment and Research Communications* 24 (January): 100192. https://doi.org/10.1016/j.ctarc.2020.100192.

Baharlouei, Parnian, and Azizur Rahman. 2022. 'Chitin and Chitosan: Prospective Biomedical Applications in Drug Delivery, Cancer Treatment, and Wound Healing'. *Marine Drugs* 20 (7): 7. https://doi.org/10.3390/md20070460.

Bajaj, Taruni, Hina Alim, Ahmad Ali, and Nimisha Patel. 2023. 'Phytochemical and Bioactive Compounds of Green Algae (Chlorophyta) and Their Applications'. In *Aquatic Medicinal Plants*. CRC Press.

Baksi, Sibojyoti, Pritha Pal, and Sibashish Baksi. 2025. 'Green Valorization Protocols for Marine Food Waste: Collagen and Chitin Recovery'. In *Food Waste Valorization : Green Techniques in Sustainable Management*, edited by Tanmay Sarkar. Springer US. https://doi.org/10.1007/978-1-0716-4646-5_15.

Banik, Nipa, Seong-Bin Yang, Tae-Bong Kang, Ji-Hong Lim, and Jooho Park. 2021. 'Heparin and Its Derivatives: Challenges and Advances in Therapeutic Biomolecules'. *International Journal of Molecular Sciences* 22 (19): 19. https://doi.org/10.3390/ijms221910524.

Bastiaens, Leen, Lise Soetemans, Els D'Hondt, and Kathy Elst. 2019. 'Sources of Chitin and Chitosan and Their Isolation'. In *Chitin and Chitosan*. John Wiley & Sons, Ltd. https://doi.org/10.1002/9781119450467.ch1.

Berezhnaya, Yaroslava D., Aleksandr S. Kazachenko, Anna S. Kazachenko, Yuriy N. Malyar, and Valentina S. Borovkova. 2024. 'Sulfation of Various Polysaccharide Structures: Different Methods and Perspectives'. *Chemistry* 6 (4): 4. https://doi.org/10.3390/chemistry6040038.

Biplajit, Das, Paul Sujata, and Sharma Hemanta Kumar. 2021. 'A Review on Bio-Polymers Derived from Animal Sources with Special Reference to Their Potential Applications. | EBSCOhost'. March 1. https://doi.org/10.22270/jddt.v11i2.4763.

Biran, Roy, and Daniel Pond. 2017. 'Heparin Coatings for Improving Blood Compatibility of Medical Devices'. *Advanced Drug Delivery Reviews*, Drug Device Combinations, vol. 112 (March): 12–23. https://doi.org/10.1016/j.addr.2016.12.002.

Biscari, G. 2023. *MULTIFUNCTIONAL POLYSACCHARIDES-DERIVED HYDROGELS WITH ANTIMICROBIAL PROPERTIES FOR INFECTED SKIN WOUND HEALING*. December 12. https://iris.unipa.it/handle/10447/619058.

Biswas, Manik Chandra, Bodiuzzaman Jony, Pranab Kumar Nandy, et al. 2022. 'Recent Advancement of Biopolymers and Their Potential Biomedical Applications'. *Journal of Polymers and the Environment* 30 (1): 51–74. https://doi.org/10.1007/s10924-021-02199-y.

Bose, Ipsheta, Nousheen, Swarup Roy, et al. 2023. 'Unveiling the Potential of Marine Biopolymers: Sources, Classification, and Diverse Food Applications'. *Materials* 16 (13): 13. https://doi.org/10.3390/ma16134840.

Chegu Krishnamurthi, Madhubalaji, Sonal Tiwari, Pallaval Veera Bramhachari, and G. V. Swarnalatha. 2023. 'Exploitation of Marine-Derived Multifunctional Biomaterials in Biomedical Engineering and Drug Delivery'. In *Marine Bioactive Molecules for Biomedical and Pharmacotherapeutic Applications*, edited by Pallaval Veera Bramhachari and Chanda Vikrant Berde. Springer Nature. https://doi.org/10.1007/978-981-99-6770-4_12.

Chellapandian, Hethesh, Sivakamavalli Jeyachandran, Kiyun Park, and Ihn-sil Kwak. 2025. 'Marine-Derived Functional Biomaterials: Advancements in Biomedicine and Drug Delivery Applications'. *Natural Product Communications* 20 (6): 1934578X241302009. https://doi.org/10.1177/1934578X241302009.

Chen, Jichen, Jianchao Yang, Hong Du, et al. 2021. 'Laminarin, a Major Polysaccharide in Stramenopiles'. *Marine Drugs* 19 (10): 10. https://doi.org/10.3390/md19100576.

Chi, Yongzhou, and Peng Wang. 2023. 'Structure, Preparation, and Biological Activity of Sulfated Polysaccharides from the Genus Caulerpa (Chlorophyta): A Review'. *Journal of Applied Phycology* 35 (6): 3069–85. https://doi.org/10.1007/s10811-023-03090-0.

Cojocaru, Elena, Ovidiu Rusalim Petriş, and Cristian Cojocaru. 2024. 'Nanoparticle-Based Drug Delivery Systems in Inhaled Therapy: Improving Respiratory Medicine'. *Pharmaceuticals* 17 (8): 8. https://doi.org/10.3390/ph17081059.

Coppola, Daniela, Chiara Lauritano, Fortunato Palma Esposito, Gennaro Riccio, Carmen Rizzo, and Donatella de Pascale. 2021. 'Fish Waste: From Problem to Valuable Resource'. *Marine Drugs* 19 (2): 2. https://doi.org/10.3390/md19020116.

Dattilo, Marco, Francesco Patitucci, Sabrina Prete, Ortensia Ilaria Parisi, and Francesco Puoci. 2023. 'Polysaccharide-Based Hydrogels and Their Application as Drug Delivery Systems in Cancer Treatment: A Review'. *Journal of Functional Biomaterials* 14 (2): 2. https://doi.org/10.3390/jfb14020055.

Debele, Tilahun Ayane, and Wen-Pin Su. 2022. 'Polysaccharide and Protein-Based Functional Wound Dressing Materials and Applications'. *International Journal of Polymeric Materials and Polymeric Biomaterials* 71 (2): 87–108. https://doi.org/10.1080/00914037.2020.1809403.

Delgado-Pujol, Ernesto J., Guillermo Martínez, David Casado-Jurado, et al. 2025. 'Hydrogels and Nanogels: Pioneering the Future of Advanced Drug Delivery Systems'. *Pharmaceutics* 17 (2): 2. https://doi.org/10.3390/pharmaceutics17020215.

Dille, M. J., I. J. Haug, and K. I. Draget. 2021. 'Chapter 34—Gelatin and Collagen'. In *Handbook of Hydrocolloids (Third Edition)*, edited by Glyn O. Phillips and Peter A. Williams. Woodhead Publishing Series in Food Science, Technology and Nutrition. Woodhead Publishing. https://doi.org/10.1016/B978-0-12-820104-6.00028-0.

Ding, Yaping, Wei Li, Feng Zhang, et al. 2019. 'Electrospun Fibrous Architectures for Drug Delivery, Tissue Engineering and Cancer Therapy'. *Advanced Functional Materials* 29 (2): 1802852. https://doi.org/10.1002/adfm.201802852.

Du, Bowei, Shuhan Feng, Jiajun Wang, et al. 2025. 'Collagen-Based Micro/Nanogel Delivery Systems: Manufacturing, Release Mechanisms, and Biomedical Applications'. *Chinese Medical Journal* 138 (10): 1135–52. https://doi.org/10.1097/CM9.0000000000003611.

Ege, Hasan, Zeynep Ruya Ege, and Oguzhan Gunduz. 2024. 'Marine-Derived Materials for the Development of Advanced Drug Delivery Systems'. In *Handbook of the Extracellular Matrix*. Springer, Cham. https://doi.org/10.1007/978-3-031-56363-8_55.

Ezike, Tobechukwu Christian, Ugochukwu Solomon Okpala, Ufedo Lovet Onoja, et al. 2023. 'Advances in Drug Delivery Systems, Challenges and Future Directions'. *Heliyon* 9 (6). https://doi.org/10.1016/j.heliyon.2023.e17488.

Farooq, Shahzad, Muhammad Ijaz Ahmad, Shijie Zheng, et al. 2024. 'A Review on Marine Collagen: Sources, Extraction Methods, Colloids Properties, and Food Applications'. *Collagen and Leather* 6 (1): 11. https://doi.org/10.1186/s42825-024-00152-y.

Fernandes, Andreia S., Catarina Oliveira, Rui L. Reis, Albino Martins, and Tiago H. Silva. 2022. 'Marine-Inspired Drugs and Biomaterials in the Perspective of Pancreatic Cancer Therapies'. *Marine Drugs* 20 (11): 11. https://doi.org/10.3390/md20110689.

Geahchan, Sarah, Parnian Baharlouei, and Azizur Rahman. 2022. 'Marine Collagen: A Promising Biomaterial for Wound Healing, Skin Anti-Aging, and Bone Regeneration'. *Marine Drugs* 20 (1): 1. https://doi.org/10.3390/md20010061.

Gheorghita Puscaselu, Roxana, Andrei Lobiuc, Mihai Dimian, and Mihai Covasa. 2020. 'Alginate: From Food Industry to Biomedical Applications and Management of Metabolic Disorders'. *Polymers* 12 (10): 10. https://doi.org/10.3390/polym12102417.

Gopi, Sreeraj, Augustine Amalraj, Nimisha P. Sukumaran, Józef T. Haponiuk, and Sabu Thomas. 2018. 'Biopolymers and Their Composites for Drug Delivery: A Brief Review'. *Macromolecular Symposia* 380 (1): 1800114. https://doi.org/10.1002/masy.201800114.

Green, David. 2020. *The Heparins: Basic and Clinical Aspects*. Academic Press.

Guillerme, Jean-Baptiste, Céline Couteau, and Laurence Coiffard. 2017. 'Applications for Marine Resources in Cosmetics'. *Cosmetics* 4 (3): 3. https://doi.org/10.3390/cosmetics4030035.

Guo, Yu, Min Wang, Yuzhong Zhang, Zeyun Zhao, and Jiannan Li. 2025. 'Advanced Hydrogel Material for Colorectal Cancer Treatment'. *Drug Delivery* 32 (1): 2446552. https://doi.org/10.1080/10717544.2024.2446552.

Gupta, N. Vishal, Souvik Chakraborty, K. Trideva Sastri, M. Sharadha, Balamuralidhara Veeranna, and A. Ramkishan. 2023. 'Agar-Based Drug Delivery Systems for Respiratory Disease'. In *Natural Polymeric Materials Based Drug Delivery Systems in Lung Diseases*, edited by Harish Dureja, Jon Adams, Raimar Löbenberg, Terezinha de Jesus Andreoli Pinto, and Kamal Dua. Springer Nature. https://doi.org/10.1007/978-981-19-7656-8_21.

Haggag, Yusuf A., Abeer A. Abd Elrahman, Roland Ulber, and Ahmed Zayed. 2023. 'Fucoidan in Pharmaceutical Formulations: A Comprehensive Review for Smart Drug Delivery Systems'. *Marine Drugs* 21 (2): 2. https://doi.org/10.3390/md21020112.

Harinisri Ram, K., and B. Thamarai Selvi. 2024. 'Inventive Applications of Marine Resources in Cosmetic Production: A Review'. In *Multidisciplinary Applications of Marine Resources: A Step towards Green and Sustainable Future*, edited by Mohd Rafatullah, Masoom Raza Siddiqui, Moonis Ali Khan, and Riti Thapar Kapoor. Springer Nature. https://doi.org/10.1007/978-981-97-5057-3_19.

Harsha Mohan, E., S. Madhusudan, B. S. Roopa, Nandini P. Shetty, Asha Martin, and Revathy Baskaran. 2025. 'Characterisation of Seaweed (Ulva lactuca) Powder and Its Incorporation for the Development of Vegetable Patty Enriched with Dietary Fibre, Protein and Antioxidants'. *Journal of Food Science and Technology* 62 (8): 1449–59. https://doi.org/10.1007/s13197-024-06115-9.

Iacob, Andreea Teodora, Florentina Geanina Lupascu, Maria Apotrosoaei, et al. 2021. 'Recent Biomedical Approaches for Chitosan Based Materials as Drug Delivery Nanocarriers'. *Pharmaceutics* 13 (4): 4. https://doi.org/10.3390/pharmaceutics13040587.

Immanuel Suresh, J., and S. Divyeswari. 2024. 'Seaweeds Are Potential Source for Production of Sustainable Bioethanol for the Imminent Future'. In *Multidisciplinary Applications of Marine Resources: A Step towards Green and Sustainable Future*, edited by Mohd Rafatullah, Masoom Raza Siddiqui, Moonis Ali Khan, and Riti Thapar Kapoor. Springer Nature. https://doi.org/10.1007/978-981-97-5057-3_7.

Inácio, Ana Rita, Ana C. Carvalho, Catarina Oliveira, et al. 2022. 'Sulfated Seaweed Polysaccharides'. In *Polysaccharides of Microbial Origin*. Springer, Cham. https://doi.org/10.1007/978-3-030-42215-8_17.

Iqbal, Muhammad Waheed, Tahreem Riaz, Shahid Mahmood, et al. 2024. 'Fucoidan-Based Nanomaterial and Its Multifunctional Role for Pharmaceutical and Biomedical Applications'. *Critical Reviews in Food Science and Nutrition* 64 (2): 354–80. https://doi.org/10.1080/10408398.2022.2106182.

Iroegbu, Austine Ofondu Chinomso, and Suprakas Sinha Ray. 2023. 'Chitin Nanomaterials as Multifunctional Systems in Advanced Applications—Progress and Challenges toward Sustainability'. *Macromolecular Materials and Engineering* 308 (9): 2300053. https://doi.org/10.1002/mame.202300053.

Jafari, Hafez, Alberto Lista, Manuela Mafosso Siekapen, et al. 2020. 'Fish Collagen: Extraction, Characterization, and Applications for Biomaterials Engineering'. *Polymers* 12 (10): 10. https://doi.org/10.3390/polym12102230.

Jain, Pooja, Rahmuddin Khan, Bushra Ahmed, et al. 2025. 'Marine-Polysaccharides as Nano-Drug Delivery Vehicles'. In *Handbook of Research in Marine Pharmaceutics*. Apple Academic Press.

Jeong, Geum-Jae, Sohail Khan, Nazia Tabassum, Fazlurrahman Khan, and Young-Mog Kim. 2022. 'Marine-Bioinspired Nanoparticles as Potential Drugs for Multiple Biological Roles'. *Marine Drugs* 20 (8): 8. https://doi.org/10.3390/md20080527.

Jia, Xiaoyu, Xin Fan, Cheng Chen, et al. 2024. 'Chemical and Structural Engineering of Gelatin-Based Delivery Systems for Therapeutic Applications: A Review'. *Biomacromolecules* 25 (2): 564–89. https://doi.org/10.1021/acs.biomac.3c01021.

Jönsson, Madeleine, Leila Allahgholi, Roya R. R. Sardari, Guðmundur O. Hreggviðsson, and Eva Nordberg Karlsson. 2020. 'Extraction and Modification of Macroalgal Polysaccharides for Current and Next-Generation Applications'. *Molecules* 25 (4): 4. https://doi.org/10.3390/molecules25040930.

Joy, Jean Mary, Amruth Padmaprakashan, Akshay Pradeep, Preethy Treesa Paul, Rosemol Jacob Mannuthy, and Suseela Mathew. 2024. 'A Review on Fish Skin-Derived Gelatin: Elucidating the Gelatin Peptides—Preparation, Bioactivity, Mechanistic Insights, and Strategies for Stability Improvement'. *Foods* 13 (17): 17. https://doi.org/10.3390/foods13172793.

Joye, Iris J., and D. Julian McClements. 2016. 'Biopolymer-Based Delivery Systems: Challenges and Opportunities'. *Current Topics in Medicinal Chemistry* 16 (9): 1026–39. https://doi.org/10.2174/1568026615666150825143130.

Kadam, Shekhar U, Brijesh K Tiwari, and Colm P O'Donnell. 2015. 'Extraction, Structure and Biofunctional Activities of Laminarin from Brown Algae'. *International Journal of Food Science and Technology* 50 (1): 24–31. https://doi.org/10.1111/ijfs.12692.

Kim, Se-Kwon. 2018. *Healthcare Using Marine Organisms*. CRC Press.

Kokate, Amit, Jae H. Chang, and Miki S. Park. 2023. 'Absorption of Drugs Via Passive Diffusion and Carrier-Mediated Pathways'. In *Oral Bioavailability and Drug Delivery*. John Wiley & Sons, Ltd. https://doi.org/10.1002/9781119660699.ch5.

Kothale, Dhalendra, Utsav Verma, Nagesh Dewangan, Partha Jana, Ankit Jain, and Dharmendra Jain. 2020. 'Alginate as Promising Natural Polymer for Pharmaceutical, Food, and Biomedical Applications'. *Current Drug Delivery* 17 (9): 755–75. https://doi.org/10.2174/1567201817666200810110226.

Krishnan, Lakshmi, Nandhini Ravi, Anjon Kumar Mondal, et al. 2024. 'Seaweed-Based Polysaccharides—Review of Extraction, Characterization, and Bioplastic Application'. *Green Chemistry* 26 (10): 5790–823. https://doi.org/10.1039/D3GC04009G.

Kučuk, Nika, Mateja Primožič, Željko Knez, and Maja Leitgeb. 2023. 'Sustainable Biodegradable Biopolymer-Based Nanoparticles for Healthcare Applications'. *International Journal of Molecular Sciences* 24 (4): 4. https://doi.org/10.3390/ijms24043188.

Kumar, Manish, Abhishek Jha, and Brahmeshwar Mishra. 2022. 'Marine Biopolymers for Transdermal Drug Delivery'. In *Marine Biomaterials : Drug Delivery and Therapeutic Applications*, edited by Sougata Jana and Subrata Jana. Springer Nature. https://doi.org/10.1007/978-981-16-4787-1_6.

Kundu, Amit, Prasanta Dey, Subham Banerjee, et al. 2018. 'Heparin and Its Derivatives-Based Nanoparticles for Cancer Therapy'. In *Polysaccharide Based Nano-Biocarrier in Drug Delivery*. CRC Press.

Kurera, Mihidukulasuriya Jude Michael Shehan, Dineth Pramuditha Nagahawatta, and You Jin Jeon. 2024. 'Structure of Fucoidan and Isolation Techniques'. In *The Role of Seaweeds in Blue Bioeconomy*. Bentham Science Publishers. https://www.benthamdirect.com/content/books/9789815223644.chapter-5.

Lagopati, Nefeli, Natassa Pippa, Maria-Anna Gatou, et al. 2023. 'Marine-Originated Materials and Their Potential Use in Biomedicine'. *Applied Sciences* 13 (16): 16. https://doi.org/10.3390/app13169172.

Lazim, Nurul Asmak Md, and Ida Idayu Muhamad. 2025. '13—Agar Agar in Drug Delivery'. In *Natural Biopolymers for Drug Delivery*, edited by Amit Kumar Nayak, Md Saquib Hasnain, and Tejraj M. Aminabhavi. Woodhead Publishing Series in Biomaterials. Woodhead Publishing. https://doi.org/10.1016/B978-0-323-95367-2.00012-0.

Li, Chen, Tiancheng Tang, Yuguang Du, et al. 2023. 'Ulvan and Ulva Oligosaccharides: A Systematic Review of Structure, Preparation, Biological Activities and Applications'. *Bioresources and Bioprocessing* 10 (1): 66. https://doi.org/10.1186/s40643-023-00690-z.

Li, Duoduo, Zihao Wei, and Changhu Xue. 2021a. 'Alginate-Based Delivery Systems for Food Bioactive Ingredients: An Overview of Recent Advances and Future Trends'. *Comprehensive Reviews in Food Science and Food Safety* 20 (6): 5345–69. https://doi.org/10.1111/1541-4337.12840.

Li, Yanping, Yuting Zheng, Ye Zhang, et al. 2021b. 'Brown Algae Carbohydrates: Structures, Pharmaceutical Properties, and Research Challenges'. *Marine Drugs* 19 (11): 11. https://doi.org/10.3390/md19110620.

Lim, Ye-Seon, Ye-Jin Ok, Seon-Yeong Hwang, Jong-Young Kwak, and Sik Yoon. 2019. 'Marine Collagen as A Promising Biomaterial for Biomedical Applications'. *Marine Drugs* 17 (8): 8. https://doi.org/10.3390/md17080467.

Malektaj, Haniyeh. 2024. 'Mechanical properties, swelling and structural characterization of biocompatible hydrogels for biomedical applications'. Aalborg University. https://doi.org/10.54337/aau755548293.

Maretti, Eleonora, Barbara Pavan, Cecilia Rustichelli, et al. 2021. 'Chitosan/Heparin Polyelectrolyte Complexes as Ion-Paring Approach to Encapsulate Heparin in Orally Administrable SLN: In Vitro Evaluation'. *Colloids and Surfaces A: Physicochemical and Engineering Aspects* 608 (January): 125606. https://doi.org/10.1016/j.colsurfa.2020.125606.

Mi, Peng, Horacio Cabral, and Kazunori Kataoka. 2020. 'Ligand-Installed Nanocarriers toward Precision Therapy'. *Advanced Materials* 32 (13): 1902604. https://doi.org/10.1002/adma.201902604.

Miao, Tianxin, Junqing Wang, Yun Zeng, Gang Liu, and Xiaoyuan Chen. 2018. 'Polysaccharide-Based Controlled Release Systems for Therapeutics Delivery and Tissue Engineering: From Bench to Bedside'. *Advanced Science* 5 (4): 1700513. https://doi.org/10.1002/advs.201700513.

Mikušová, Veronika, and Peter Mikuš. 2021. 'Advances in Chitosan-Based Nanoparticles for Drug Delivery'. *International Journal of Molecular Sciences* 22 (17): 17. https://doi.org/10.3390/ijms22179652.

Mirzaei, Akbar, Maryam Esmkhani, Mahsa Zallaghi, Zahra Nezafat, and Shahrzad Javanshir. 2023. 'Biomedical and Environmental Applications of Carrageenan-Based Hydrogels: A Review'. *Journal of Polymers and the Environment* 31 (5): 1679–705. https://doi.org/10.1007/s10924-022-02726-5.

Mokhtari, Hamidreza, Shima Tavakoli, Fereshteh Safarpour, et al. 2021. 'Recent Advances in Chemically-Modified and Hybrid Carrageenan-Based Platforms for Drug Delivery, Wound Healing, and Tissue Engineering'. *Polymers* 13 (11): 11. https://doi.org/10.3390/polym13111744.

Moussian, Bernard. 2019. 'Chitin: Structure, Chemistry and Biology'. In *Targeting Chitin-Containing Organisms*, edited by Qing Yang and Tamo Fukamizo. Springer. https://doi.org/10.1007/978-981-13-7318-3_2.

Mura, Paola, Francesca Maestrelli, Marzia Cirri, and Natascia Mennini. 2022. 'Multiple Roles of Chitosan in Mucosal Drug Delivery: An Updated Review'. *Marine Drugs* 20 (5): 5. https://doi.org/10.3390/md20050335.

Nagahawatta, D. P., N. M. Liyanage, Thilina U. Jayawardena, et al. 2023. 'Functions and Values of Sulfated Polysaccharides from Seaweed'. *ALGAE* 38 (4): 217–40. https://doi.org/10.4490/algae.2023.38.12.1.

Nawaz, Dr Ali. 2024. 'The Role of Biotechnology in Personalized Medicine: Tailoring Treatments through Genomic Insights'. *Life Sciences Perspectives* 1 (02): 02.

Negreanu-Pirjol, Bogdan-Stefan, Ticuta Negreanu-Pirjol, Dan Razvan Popoviciu, Ruxandra-Elena Anton, and Ana-Maria Prelipcean. 2022. 'Marine Bioactive Compounds Derived from Macroalgae as New Potential Players in Drug Delivery Systems: A Review'. *Pharmaceutics* 14 (9): 9. https://doi.org/10.3390/pharmaceutics14091781.

Nguyen, Huu-Thanh, Thuy-Trang Pham, Phu-Tho Nguyen, Hélène Le-Buanec, Holy N. Rabetafika, and Hary L. Razafindralambo. 2024. 'Advances in Microbial Exopolysaccharides: Present and Future Applications'. *Biomolecules* 14 (9): 9. https://doi.org/10.3390/biom14091162.

Olatunji, Ololade. 2020. 'Laminarins'. In *Aquatic Biopolymers: Understanding Their Industrial Significance and Environmental Implications*, edited by Ololade Olatunji. Springer International Publishing. https://doi.org/10.1007/978-3-030-34709-3_9.

Omidian, Hossein, and Renae L. Wilson. 2024. 'Long-Acting Gel Formulations: Advancing Drug Delivery across Diverse Therapeutic Areas'. *Pharmaceuticals* 17 (4): 4. https://doi.org/10.3390/ph17040493.

Ore Areche, Franklin, Juan Alberto Julcahuanga Dominguez, Jovencio Ticsihua Huaman, et al. 2024. 'Maximizing the Potential of Marine Resources: A Sustainable Approach to High-Value Product Development from Seafood by-Products and Waste. | EBSCOhost'. December 1. https://doi.org/10.12944/CRNFSJ.12.3.7.

Padmesh, Sudhakar, and Aditi Singh. 2021. 'Agars: Properties and Applications'. In *Polysaccharides*. John Wiley & Sons, Ltd. https://doi.org/10.1002/9781119711414.ch5.

Pari, Rizfi Fariz, Uju Uju, Safrina Dyah Hardiningtyas, et al. 2025. 'Ulva Seaweed-Derived Ulvan: A Promising Marine Polysaccharide as a Sustainable Resource for Biomaterial Design'. *Marine Drugs* 23 (2): 2. https://doi.org/10.3390/md23020056.

Patra, Pratikshya, Tarun Kumar Upadhyay, Nawaf Alshammari, Mohd Saeed, and Kavindra Kumar Kesari. 2024. 'Alginate-Chitosan Biodegradable and Biocompatible Based Hydrogel for Breast Cancer Immunotherapy and Diagnosis: A Comprehensive Review'. *ACS Applied Bio Materials* 7 (6): 3515–34. https://doi.org/10.1021/acsabm.3c00984.

Pellis, Alessandro, Georg M. Guebitz, and Gibson Stephen Nyanhongo. 2022. 'Chitosan: Sources, Processing and Modification Techniques'. *Gels* 8 (7): 7. https://doi.org/10.3390/gels8070393.

Pereira, Leonel, Fabiana Soares, Ana Cristina Freitas, Armando C. Duarte, and Paulo Ribeiro-Claro. 2017. 'Extraction, Characterization, and Use of Carrageenans'. In *Industrial Applications of Marine Biopolymers*. CRC Press.

Pillai, Akhilraj, Dhanashree Bhande, and Vinal Pardhi. 2023. 'Controlled Drug Delivery System'. In *Advanced Drug Delivery: Methods and Applications*, edited by Tuhin Subhra Santra and Ashwini Uma Surendra Shinde. Springer Nature. https://doi.org/10.1007/978-981-99-6564-9_11.

Qamar, Sarmad Ahmad, Muhammad Junaid, Areej Riasat, Muhammad Jahangeer, Muhammad Bilal, and Bo-Zhong Mu. 2024. 'Carrageenan-Based Hybrids with Biopolymers and Nano-Structured Materials for Biomimetic Applications'. *Starch—Stärke* 76 (1–2): 2200018. https://doi.org/10.1002/star.202200018.

Rahman, Md. Mostafizur, Md. Abdus Shahid, Md. Tanvir Hossain, et al. 2024. 'Sources, Extractions, and Applications of Alginate: A Review'. *Discover Applied Sciences* 6 (8): 443. https://doi.org/10.1007/s42452-024-06151-2.

Ramdhan, Tezar, Su Hung Ching, Sangeeta Prakash, and Bhesh Bhandari. 2020. 'Physical and Mechanical Properties of Alginate Based Composite Gels'. *Trends in Food Science & Technology* 106 (December): 150–59. https://doi.org/10.1016/j.tifs.2020.10.002.

Raza, Ali, Tahir Rasheed, Faran Nabeel, Uzma Hayat, Muhammad Bilal, and Hafiz M. N. Iqbal. 2019. 'Endogenous and Exogenous Stimuli-Responsive Drug Delivery Systems for Programmed Site-Specific Release'. *Molecules* 24 (6): 6. https://doi.org/10.3390/molecules24061117.

Rhein-Knudsen, Nanna, Marcel Tutor Ale, Fatemeh Ajalloueian, Liyun Yu, and Anne S. Meyer. 2017. 'Rheological Properties of Agar and Carrageenan from Ghanaian Red Seaweeds'. *Food Hydrocolloids* 63 (February): 50–58. https://doi.org/10.1016/j.foodhyd.2016.08.023.

Riaz, Zakia, Yu Xuan Fong, Yunn Yee Chan, Vincent Chan, Neethu Ninan, and Vi Khanh Truong. 2025. 'Therapeutics-Loaded Electrospun Nanofibers: Rational Design and Mechanistic Insights on Managing Chronic Wound Infection'. *Regenerative Medicine and Dentistry*, June 24, 9. https://doi.org/10.53941/rmd.2025.100009.

Romano, Giovanna, Mariana Almeida, Ana Varela Coelho, et al. 2022. 'Biomaterials and Bioactive Natural Products from Marine Invertebrates: From Basic Research to Innovative Applications'. *Marine Drugs* 20 (4): 4. https://doi.org/10.3390/md20040219.

Saberian, Mostafa, Raha Safari Roudsari, Neda Haghshenas, Ali Rousta, and Shaban Alizadeh. 2024. 'How the Combination of Alginate and Chitosan Can Fabricate a Hydrogel with Favorable Properties for Wound Healing'. *Heliyon* 10 (11). https://doi.org/10.1016/j.heliyon.2024.e32040.

Sacramento, Margarida M. A., João Borges, Fernando J. S. Correia, et al. 2022. 'Green Approaches for Extraction, Chemical Modification and Processing of Marine Polysaccharides for Biomedical Applications'. *Frontiers in Bioengineering and Biotechnology* 10 (December). https://doi.org/10.3389/fbioe.2022.1041102.

Sadraei, Alireza, and Seyed Morteza Naghib. 2025. '4D Printing of Physical Stimuli-Responsive Hydrogels for Localized Drug Delivery and Tissue Engineering'. *Polymer Reviews* 65 (1): 104–68. https://doi.org/10.1080/15583724.2024.2427184.

Saeed, Muhammad, Muhammad A. Arain, Sarfraz Ali Fazlani, et al. 2021. 'A Comprehensive Review on the Health Benefits and Nutritional Significance of Fucoidan Polysaccharide Derived from Brown Seaweeds in Human, Animals and Aquatic Organisms'. *Aquaculture Nutrition* 27 (3): 633–54. https://doi.org/10.1111/anu.13233.

Salave, Sagar, Dhwani Rana, Amit Sharma, et al. 2022. 'Polysaccharide Based Implantable Drug Delivery: Development Strategies, Regulatory Requirements, and Future Perspectives'. *Polysaccharides* 3 (3): 3. https://doi.org/10.3390/polysaccharides3030037.

S. Alfinaikh, Reem, Khalid A. Alamry, and Mahmoud A. Hussein. 2025. 'Sustainable and Biocompatible Hybrid Materials-Based Sulfated Polysaccharides for Biomedical Applications: A Review'. *RSC Advances* 15 (6): 4708–67. https://doi.org/10.1039/D4RA07277D.

Sarkar, Arindam, Shila Barman, and Sanchita Mandal. 2025. 'Sodium Alginate in Mucoadhesive Drug Delivery Systems: A Comprehensive Review of Properties, Dosage Forms, And Characterization Methods 906-928 |'. *International Journal of Pharmaceutical Sciences* 3 (January): 906–28. https://doi.org/10.5281/zenodo.14636331.

Sepe, Fabrizia, Anna Valentino, Loredana Marcolongo, et al. 2025. 'Marine-Derived Polysaccharide Hydrogels as Delivery Platforms for Natural Bioactive Compounds'. *International Journal of Molecular Sciences* 26 (2): 2. https://doi.org/10.3390/ijms26020764.

Seyam, Salma, Norsyafikah Asyilla Nordin, and Mulham Alfatama. 2020. 'Recent Progress of Chitosan and Chitosan Derivatives-Based Nanoparticles: Pharmaceutical Perspectives of Oral Insulin Delivery'. *Pharmaceuticals* 13 (10): 10. https://doi.org/10.3390/ph13100307.

Shahruzzaman, Md, Shanta Biswas, Md Nurus Sakib, Papia Haque, Mohammed Mizanur Rahman, and Abul K. Mallik. 2019. 'Pharmaceutical Applications of Agar-Agar'. In *Natural Polymers for Pharmaceutical Applications*. Apple Academic Press.

Shaik, Mannur Ismail, Siti Hajar Abdul Rahman, Anis Syafiqah Yusri, Mohammad Rashedi Ismail-Fitry, Nune Satya Sampath Kumar, and Norizah Mhd Sarbon. 2024. 'A Review on the Processing Technique, Physicochemical, and Bioactive Properties of Marine Collagen'. *Journal of Food Science* 89 (9): 5205–29. https://doi.org/10.1111/1750-3841.17273.

Shi, Xiao-Dan, Jing-Jing Huang, Jiu-Lin Wu, et al. 2022. 'Fabrication, Interaction Mechanism, Functional Properties, and Applications of Fish Gelatin-Polysaccharide Composites: A Review'. *Food Hydrocolloids* 122 (January): 107106. https://doi.org/10.1016/j.foodhyd.2021.107106.

Shokrak, Nermeen M., Hadeer A. Elkhouly, Nourhan A. Abozahra, et al. 2024. 'Application of Marine Green Algae for Development of Bioplastics: Current Status and Future Challenges'. In *Biomass Valorization: A Sustainable Approach towards Carbon Neutrality and Circular Economy*, edited by Riti Thapar Kapoor, Mika Sillanpää, Jakub Zdarta, and Mohd Rafatullah. Springer Nature. https://doi.org/10.1007/978-981-97-8557-5_5.

Singh, Dilpreet. 2024. 'Beyond the Maze: Recent Advancements in Molecular and Cellular Tethered Drug Delivery Systems'. *ASSAY and Drug Development Technologies* 22 (4): 203–15. https://doi.org/10.1089/adt.2024.025.

Singh, Jagtar, and Pallavi Nayak. 2023. 'pH-Responsive Polymers for Drug Delivery: Trends and Opportunities'. *Journal of Polymer Science* 61 (22): 2828–50. https://doi.org/10.1002/pol.20230403.

Srivastava, Nishi, Arti Singh, Puja Kumari, et al. 2021. 'Chapter 21—Advances in Extraction Technologies: Isolation and Purification of Bioactive Compounds from Biological Materials'. In *Natural Bioactive Compounds*, edited by Rajeshwar p. Sinha and Donat-P Häder. Academic Press. https://doi.org/10.1016/B978-0-12-820655-3.00021-5.

Sulastri, Evi, Ronny Lesmana, Muhammad Sulaiman Zubair, Khaled M. Elamin, and Nasrul Wathoni. 2021. 'A Comprehensive Review on Ulvan Based Hydrogel and Its Biomedical Applications'. *Chemical and Pharmaceutical Bulletin* 69 (5): 432–43. https://doi.org/10.1248/cpb.c20-00763.

Sultana, Razia, and Masamichi Kamihira. 2024. 'Multifaceted Heparin: Diverse Applications beyond Anticoagulant Therapy'. *Pharmaceuticals* 17 (10): 10. https://doi.org/10.3390/ph17101362.

Suryawanshi, N., S. E. Jujjavarapu, and S. Ayothiraman. 2019. 'Marine Shell Industrial Wastes–an Abundant Source of Chitin and Its Derivatives: Constituents, Pretreatment, Fermentation, and Pleiotropic Applications-a Revisit'. *International Journal of Environmental Science and Technology* 16 (7): 3877–98. https://doi.org/10.1007/s13762-018-02204-3.

Terkula Iber, Benedict, Nor Azman Kasan, Donald Torsabo, and Jenifer Wese Omuwa. 2022. 'A Review of Various Sources of Chitin and Chitosan in Nature'. *Journal of Renewable Materials* 10 (4): 1097–123. https://doi.org/10.32604/jrm.2022.018142.

Thomas, Sabu, Sreeraj Gopi, and Augustine Amalraj. 2020. *Biopolymers and Their Industrial Applications: From Plant, Animal, and Marine Sources, to Functional Products*. Elsevier.

Tiwari, Sonal, E. Amala Claret, and Vikas S. Chauhan. 2022. 'Algae as a Source of Polysaccharides and Potential Applications'. In *Algal Biorefineries and the Circular Bioeconomy*. CRC Press.

Tran, Vy Ha Nguyen, Maria Dalgaard Mikkelsen, Hai Bang Truong, et al. 2023. 'Structural Characterization and Cytotoxic Activity Evaluation of Ulvan Polysaccharides Extracted from the Green Algae Ulva Papenfussii'. *Marine Drugs* 21 (11): 11. https://doi.org/10.3390/md21110556.

Trucillo, Paolo. 2024. 'Biomaterials for Drug Delivery and Human Applications'. *Materials* 17 (2): 2. https://doi.org/10.3390/ma17020456.

Tuvikene, R. 2021. 'Chapter 25—Carrageenans'. In *Handbook of Hydrocolloids (Third Edition)*, edited by Glyn O. Phillips and Peter A. Williams. Woodhead Publishing Series in Food Science, Technology and Nutrition. Woodhead Publishing. https://doi.org/10.1016/B978-0-12-820104-6.00006-1.

Volpi, Nicola, and Francesca Maccari. 2016. 'Heparin from Marine Mollusks: Occurrence, Structure, and Biological Role'. In *Marine Glycobiology*. CRC Press.

Wang, Hui, Roger Hunter, Quanbin Zhang, et al. 2024. 'The Application of Marine Polysaccharides to Antitumor Nanocarriers'. *Carbohydrate Polymers* 342 (October): 122407. https://doi.org/10.1016/j.carbpol.2024.122407.

Wang, Yu, Maochen Xing, Qi Cao, Aiguo Ji, Hao Liang, and Shuliang Song. 2019. 'Biological Activities of Fucoidan and the Factors Mediating Its Therapeutic Effects: A Review of Recent Studies'. *Marine Drugs* 17 (3): 3. https://doi.org/10.3390/md17030183.

Wijesekara, Tharuka, and Baojun Xu. 2024. 'New Insights into Sources, Bioavailability, Health-Promoting Effects, and Applications of Chitin and Chitosan'. *Journal of Agricultural and Food Chemistry* 72 (31): 17138–52. https://doi.org/10.1021/acs.jafc.4c02162.

Wosicka-Frąckowiak, Hanna, Kornelia Poniedziałek, Stanisław Woźny, et al. 2024. 'Collagen and Its Derivatives Serving Biomedical Purposes: A Review'. *Polymers* 16 (18): 18. https://doi.org/10.3390/polym16182668.

Xu, Zhenbo. 2017. *Solubility of Polysaccharides*. BoD – Books on Demand.

Yu-Qing, Tang, Kaiser Mahmood, Ruqyia Shehzadi, and Muhammad Furqan Ashraf. 2016. 'Ulva Lactuca and Its Polysaccharides: Food and Biomedical Aspects'. *Journal of Biology*.

Zamboulis, Alexandra, Stavroula Nanaki, Georgia Michailidou, et al. 2020. 'Chitosan and Its Derivatives for Ocular Delivery Formulations: Recent Advances and Developments'. *Polymers* 12 (7): 7. https://doi.org/10.3390/polym12071519.

Zayed, Ahmed, Mai K. Mansour, Mohamed S. Sedeek, Mohamed H. Habib, Roland Ulber, and Mohamed A. Farag. 2022. 'Rediscovering Bacterial Exopolysaccharides of Terrestrial and Marine Origins: Novel Insights on Their Distribution, Biosynthesis, Biotechnological Production, and Future Perspectives'. *Critical Reviews in Biotechnology* 42 (4): 597–617. https://doi.org/10.1080/07388551.2021.1942779.

Zhang, Hengtong, Xixi Wu, Liang Quan, and Qiang Ao. 2022. 'Characteristics of Marine Biomaterials and Their Applications in Biomedicine'. *Marine Drugs* 20 (6): 6. https://doi.org/10.3390/md20060372.

Zhao, Zongmin, Anvay Ukidve, Jayoung Kim, and Samir Mitragotri. 2020. 'Targeting Strategies for Tissue-Specific Drug Delivery'. *Cell* 181 (1): 151–67. https://doi.org/10.1016/j.cell.2020.02.001.

Zia, Khalid Mahmood, Mohammad Zuber, and Muhammad Ali. 2017. *Algae Based Polymers, Blends, and Composites: Chemistry, Biotechnology and Materials Science*. Elsevier.

Marine-Based Polysaccharides in Nose-to-Brain Drug Delivery

Shubhrat Maheshwari, Aditya Singh, Amita Verma, Vaseem A. Ansari, Juber Akhtar, and Bhupendra G. Prajapati

Abstract This chapter explores the potential of marine-based polysaccharides in nose-to-brain drug delivery systems, focusing on their applications for treating central nervous system (CNS) disorders. Marine polysaccharides, including alginates, chitosan, and carrageenans, offer unique advantages due to their natural biocompatibility, biodegradability, and ability to form gels with desirable mechanical properties for drug delivery. These polysaccharides exhibit excellent mucoadhesive properties, enhancing the sustained release and absorption of therapeutic agents through the nasal mucosa. They can effectively bypass the blood-brain barrier (BBB) via olfactory and trigeminal nerve pathways, providing a noninvasive alternative to traditional drug delivery methods. The chapter highlights various synthesis strategies for marine polysaccharide-based hydrogels, including chemical crosslinking and physical stimuli-responsive gelation, and discusses their combination with nanoparticles for enhanced drug release and targeting. In vitro and in vivo studies demonstrate the successful application of these systems in nose-to-brain (N2B) drug delivery, with improved drug retention, reduced side effects, and enhanced therapeutic effects. While challenges remain in improving mechanical strength and optimizing drug release profiles, marine polysaccharides offer great promise as drug carriers for CNS treatments. Further research and development are essential to realize their full potential for treating neurological diseases.

S. Maheshwari · A. Verma
Bioorganic and Medicinal Chemistry Research Laboratory, Department of Pharmaceutical Sciences, Sam Higginbottom University of Agriculture, Technology and Sciences, Prayagraj, Uttar Pradesh, India

A. Singh · V. A. Ansari · J. Akhtar
Department of Pharmacy, Faculty of Pharmacy, Integral University, Lucknow, Uttar Pradesh, India

B. G. Prajapati (✉)
Department of Pharmaceutics, Parul Institute of Pharmacy, Faculty of Pharmacy, Parul University, Vadodara, Gujarat, India
e-mail: bhupendra.prajapati40731@paruluniversity.ac.in

S. Jana et al. (eds.), *Multifunctional Marine Polysaccharides*,
https://doi.org/10.1007/978-981-95-4126-3_6

Keywords Marine polysaccharides · Nose-to-brain drug delivery · Alginates · Chitosan · Carrageenans · Central nervous system · Blood-brain barrier · Drug delivery systems · Mucoadhesion · Nasal drug delivery · Drug release · Nanoparticles

1 Introduction

Marine ecosystems harbor an extraordinary diversity of organisms that produce a wide array of bioactive compounds with unique biological properties (Bhatnagar and Kim 2010). Among these, marine polysaccharides have emerged as a focal point of interest in the biomedical and pharmaceutical sciences. Their biocompatibility, biodegradability, and nontoxic nature, coupled with their ability to form complex structures and exhibit diverse biological activities, make them ideal candidates for advanced drug delivery systems (DDSs). In particular, their application in nose-to-brain drug delivery has attracted considerable attention as a novel approach to overcome the challenges of treating central nervous system (CNS) disorders (Karthikeyan et al. 2022). Nose-to-brain (N2B) drug delivery presents an innovative and noninvasive route to bypass the blood-brain barrier (BBB) (Fig. 1), a physiological obstacle that limits the effective delivery of therapeutic agents to the brain (El-Regal and Satheesh 2023). This approach exploits the unique anatomical and physiological features of the nasal cavity, including its close proximity to the brain and its connection to the olfactory and trigeminal neural pathways. This direct route not only ensures rapid drug delivery to the brain but also minimizes systemic side effects and enhances drug bioavailability (Paul et al. 2021). Marine-based

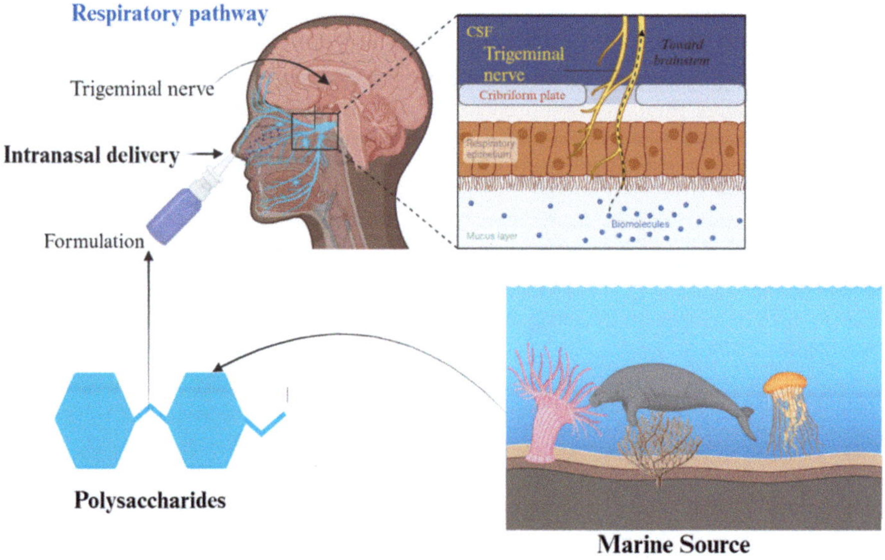

Fig. 1 Schematic representation of the nose-to-brain pathway

polysaccharides, with their inherent mucoadhesive properties, capacity to form hydrogels, and ability to undergo chemical modifications, hold immense potential as carriers for facilitating this delivery route. Marine polysaccharides are predominantly derived from algae, crustaceans, fish, and marine microorganisms (Kim 2013). Algae, in particular, serve as a rich source of polysaccharides such as agar, carrageenan, and alginate, while crustacean exoskeletons yield chitosan, a polysaccharide widely recognized for its remarkable biomedical applications. Sulfated polysaccharides, a unique subclass of these biomaterials, are of special interest due to their diverse biological activities, including antioxidant, anticoagulant, anti-inflammatory, and anticancer properties (Debbab et al. 2010). These characteristics further enhance their applicability in developing therapeutic systems for complex CNS disorders such as Alzheimer's disease (AD), Parkinson's disease (PD), depression, and epilepsy. One of the most compelling attributes of marine polysaccharides is their ability to form stable, biocompatible, and biodegradable drug delivery systems. These systems can encapsulate therapeutic agents, protect them from enzymatic degradation, and provide controlled and sustained drug release (Ahmed et al. 2024). For nose-to-brain delivery, these properties are critical for ensuring effective transport of drugs across the nasal mucosa and into the brain. Furthermore, advancements in nanotechnology have enabled the development of innovative polysaccharide-based nanoparticles, hydrogels, and hybrid systems that significantly improve drug targeting and delivery efficiency (Table 1). Marine polysaccharides have demonstrated potential as carriers for genetic material, peptides, and other macromolecules. These applications are particularly relevant for emerging therapeutic modalities such as gene therapy, which faces challenges related to the safety and efficiency of viral vectors. Polysaccharide-based systems provide a safer and more versatile alternative, offering stabilization, improved solubility, and enhanced delivery to specific brain regions. The integration of marine polysaccharides into N2B drug delivery systems also aligns with the growing emphasis on personalized medicine (Banday et al. 2024). By enabling lower drug dosages and reducing systemic toxicity, these systems offer a more patient-centric approach to treating CNS disorders. Moreover, the ability to chemically modify these polysaccharides allows for the development of tailored drug delivery platforms that meet the specific needs of individual patients or disease states (Snelgrove 2016). This book chapter aims to provide a comprehensive overview of the role of marine-based polysaccharides in nose-to-brain drug delivery. It explores their sources, structural properties, and biological functions, highlighting recent advancements in their application to CNS drug delivery. By delving into the intersection of marine biotechnology and advanced drug delivery, this chapter seeks to illuminate the transformative potential of marine polysaccharides in addressing some of the most pressing challenges in modern medicine (Sugumaran et al. 2022).

Table 1 Polysaccharide-based drug delivery products, marketed formulations, dosages, and active pharmaceutical ingredients (APIs)

Product on the market	Dosage	API	Polysaccharide	Form
Nasonex	50 μg/actuation	Mometasone furoate	Cellulose	Suspension (Giddings et al. 2015)
Aerodiol	150 μg/actuation	Estradiol	Methylbetadex	Aqueous solution (Subramani and Aalbersberg 2013)
Tosymra	Single dose 10 mg	Sumatriptan	n-Dodecyl β-D-maltoside	Aqueous solution (Egan et al. 2008)
Baqsimi	Single dose 3 mg	Glucagon	Betadex (E459, β-cyclodextrin)	Nasal powder (Conte et al. 2020)
PecFent	100 μg/actuation and 400 μg/actuation	Fentanyl	Pectin	Aqueous solution (Sable et al. 2017)
Valtoco	Available in 5 mg, 7.5 mg, and 10 mg/ 0.1 mL solution	Diazepam	n-Dodecyl β-D-maltoside	Nonaqueous solution (Poli et al. 2017)

2 Alginate in N2B Drug Delivery

Alginate, a linear anionic polysaccharide derived from brown algae, is one of the most widely studied marine polysaccharides for drug delivery applications. Its ability to form hydrogels under mild conditions, such as in the presence of divalent cations like calcium, makes it an attractive material for encapsulating and delivering therapeutic agents (Xu et al. 2023). Alginate gels can encapsulate drugs, protect them from enzymatic degradation, and provide controlled and sustained release, which is critical for effective nose-to-brain delivery. The gelation process, based on the "egg-box" model, occurs when calcium ions interact with the guluronic acid blocks in alginate, forming a stable three-dimensional network (Nawaz et al. 2023). This property ensures that alginate-based formulations remain stable during nasal administration while releasing the drug over time. Furthermore, alginate's ability to encapsulate both hydrophilic and hydrophobic drugs broadens its applicability for various CNS disorders, including AD, PD, and depression. In N2B systems, alginate can be used to create nanoparticles, microparticles, or in situ gelling formulations that adhere to the nasal mucosa, enhancing drug residence time and absorption (Trapani et al. 2021). Chemical modifications of alginate, such as oxidation or conjugation with other polymers, can improve its mucoadhesive properties and drug-loading efficiency. For instance, oxidized alginate has been shown to enhance drug permeation across the nasal epithelium, making it a valuable tool for delivering macromolecules like peptides and proteins, which are otherwise challenging to transport through conventional methods. These advancements highlight alginate's versatility in developing N2B systems that meet the specific needs of CNS therapies (Nafee et al. 2020).

3 Chitosan in N2B Drug Delivery

Chitosan, derived from the deacetylation of chitin found in crustacean shells, is another marine-based polysaccharide with immense potential for N2B drug delivery. Its unique properties, including bioadhesion, permeability enhancement, and antimicrobial activity, make it a powerful candidate for formulating nasal drug delivery systems (Clementino et al. 2025a). Chitosan's bioadhesive nature allows it to adhere to the nasal mucosa, prolonging drug residence time and increasing the likelihood of drug absorption. Chitosan opens tight junctions between epithelial cells, facilitating the paracellular transport of large or hydrophilic molecules, such as peptides, proteins, and genetic materials (Hao et al. 2016). N2B delivery, chitosan-based nanoparticles, and in situ gels have demonstrated significant potential. These systems not only enhance drug stability and bioavailability but also enable targeted and sustained delivery to the brain. For example, chitosan nanoparticles loaded with neuroprotective peptides have been shown to achieve efficient brain delivery, improving therapeutic outcomes for neurodegenerative disorders. Moreover, chitosan's chemical structure can be easily modified to improve its drug-binding capacity, solubility, and biocompatibility (Kaur et al. 2016). Derivatives such as trimethyl chitosan and carboxymethyl chitosan have been extensively studied for their enhanced mucoadhesive and permeability properties, making them ideal for N2B applications. By incorporating chitosan into N2B systems, researchers can overcome key challenges associated with nasal drug delivery, such as enzymatic degradation and rapid mucociliary clearance (Majgainya et al. 2015).

3.1 Sulfated Polysaccharides and Their Role in N2B Delivery

Sulfated polysaccharides, including fucoidan and carrageenan, are unique marine-based biomaterials known for their diverse biological activities, such as antioxidant, anti-inflammatory, and neuroprotective properties. These characteristics make them particularly attractive for developing N2B drug delivery systems targeting CNS disorders (Sonvico et al. 2018). Fucoidan, a sulfated polysaccharide derived from brown algae, has shown promise in protecting neurons from oxidative stress and inflammation, both of which are hallmarks of neurodegenerative diseases like AD and PD. Its ability to form hydrogels and nanoparticles enhances its potential as a carrier for delivering therapeutic agents to the brain. Carrageenan, extracted from red algae, is another sulfated polysaccharide with unique gelling properties that can be exploited for nasal drug delivery (Bonaccorso et al. 2017). Its ability to form strong hydrogels at low concentrations makes it suitable for encapsulating and releasing drugs in a controlled manner. Carrageenan-based systems have been shown to enhance drug stability and bioavailability, making them ideal for N2B applications. Furthermore, the sulfate groups in these polysaccharides contribute to their mucoadhesive properties, allowing them to adhere to the nasal epithelium and improve drug absorption (Lombardo et al. 2021). Recent advancements in nanotechnology have further expanded the potential of marine polysaccharides in N2B drug delivery. The development of polysaccharide-based nanoparticles, nanogels, and hybrid systems has provided new avenues for delivering drugs directly to the brain with high precision and efficiency. These nanoscale systems offer several advantages, including enhanced drug stability, controlled release, and targeted delivery. For example, alginate and chitosan nanoparticles have been successfully used to deliver neuroprotective agents and genetic materials, achieving significant therapeutic effects in preclinical models of neurodegenerative diseases (Yagi et al. 2024). Hybrid systems that combine different polysaccharides or incorporate other biopolymers, such as hyaluronic acid or polyethylene glycol, have also shown promise in improving drug delivery efficiency. These systems leverage the unique properties of each component to create multifunctional carriers that can overcome the limitations of individual materials (Cote et al. 2019). For instance, combining alginate with chitosan can enhance the mucoadhesive and permeability properties of the delivery system, while incorporating sulfated polysaccharides can provide additional biological benefits, such as antioxidant and anti-inflammatory effects (Spindler et al. 2021).

3.2 Chitin and Chitosan in N2B

Chitin and its derivative chitosan, obtained from the exoskeletons of crustaceans and certain fungi, have garnered significant attention in biomedical applications due to their remarkable biocompatibility, biodegradability, mucoadhesive properties, and ease of chemical modification. While chitin serves primarily as a precursor, its derivative, chitosan, has emerged as a versatile biomaterial with a wide range of applications in N2B drug delivery (Yui et al. 2021). Chitosan's unique properties, including its ability to enhance mucosal permeability and its inherent bioadhesion, make it an excellent candidate for formulating effective drug delivery systems targeting the CNS. The positively charged amino groups in chitosan interact with the negatively charged mucin layer of the nasal epithelium, enhancing its retention time in the nasal cavity. This mucoadhesive property is particularly important for N2B delivery, as it helps to overcome rapid mucociliary clearance and increases the time available for drug absorption (Su et al. 2020). Chitosan facilitates the opening of tight junctions between epithelial cells, enabling paracellular transport of hydrophilic and large-molecular-weight drugs, such as peptides, proteins, and nucleic acids. Chitosan has been extensively utilized to develop nanoparticles and in situ gelling systems for N2B drug delivery. Nanoparticles formulated using chitosan can encapsulate drugs, protect them from enzymatic degradation, and provide controlled and sustained release profiles. These nanoparticles also enhance the bioavailability of therapeutic agents by ensuring efficient drug delivery to the brain via the olfactory and trigeminal pathways (Li et al. 2012). For example, chitosan-based nanoparticles loaded with neuroprotective drugs have demonstrated significant success in preclinical studies targeting AD and PD, showcasing improved therapeutic outcomes compared to conventional delivery methods (Clementino et al. 2025b). In situ gelling systems based on chitosan have also shown promise in N2B applications. These formulations remain in a liquid state during administration and undergo gelation upon contact with the nasal mucosa, forming a localized drug reservoir. This enhances drug retention and absorption, making such systems highly effective for sustained brain delivery. The gelation properties of chitosan can be further optimized by chemical modifications or by combining it with other polymers, such as hyaluronic acid or alginate, to enhance its functional properties (Finetti et al. 2023). Chemical modifications of chitosan have been widely explored to improve its solubility, stability, and functional properties for N2B delivery. Derivatives such as N-trimethyl chitosan (TMC) and carboxymethyl chitosan (CMC) have shown enhanced mucoadhesion and permeability, making them ideal for delivering challenging therapeutics like peptides and genetic materials. TMC, for instance, has been reported to increase drug absorption across the nasal epithelium due to its ability to open tight junctions more effectively than unmodified chitosan. Similarly, carboxymethyl chitosan offers improved water solubility and drug-loading capacity, broadening its applicability for diverse N2B systems (Patharapankal et al. 2023). Enhancing drug delivery efficiency, chitosan derivatives have demonstrated potential as carriers for advanced therapeutics, including RNA-based drugs and CRISPR-Cas9 gene-editing systems. By stabilizing these sensitive molecules and facilitating their targeted delivery to the brain, chitosan-based carriers open new avenues for treating complex CNS disorders. Chitosan-based N2B systems hold immense promise for the treatment of various CNS disorders, including neurodegenerative diseases, brain tumors, epilepsy, and depression (Adscheid et al. 2024). These systems can deliver neuroprotective agents, anti-inflammatory drugs, and even genetic therapies directly to the brain, bypassing the limitations of conventional delivery routes. For instance, chitosan nanoparticles have been used to deliver curcumin, a neuroprotective compound, to the brain, demonstrating enhanced therapeutic efficacy in models of AD (Du et al. 2023).

3.3 Mechanisms of N2B Drug Delivery

This mechanism leverages the unique anatomical and physiological properties of the nasal cavity, particularly its close proximity to the brain and the presence of direct neural pathways such as the olfactory and trigeminal routes (Fig. 2). The nasal cavity, divided into two non-connected symmetrical chambers, is lined by distinct regions, each with specific anatomical and functional characteristics (Saha et al. 2023). The anterior region, or nasal vestibule, consists of stratified, squamous, and keratinized epithelium, which provides resistance to environmental pollutants but offers minimal drug permeability. The respiratory region, characterized by pseudostratified columnar epithelium with ciliated and goblet cells, serves as the primary site for drug absorption and warming, filtering, and humidifying inhaled air

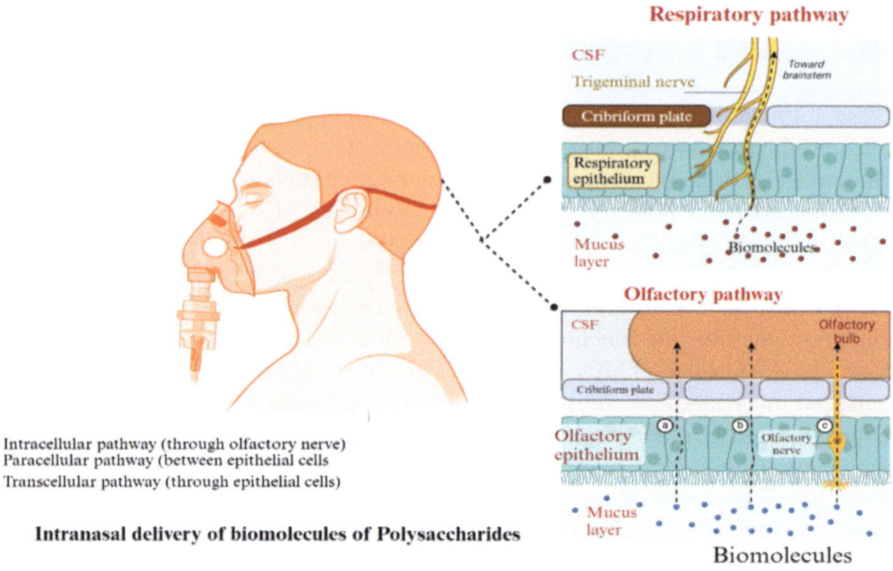

Fig. 2 The nasal cavity, with its close proximity to the brain and the presence of direct neural pathways, including the respiratory and olfactory routes, facilitates efficient drug delivery to the central nervous system

(Ogawa et al. 2020). The vascularization and lymphatic drainage of this region enhance systemic drug absorption, while the mucociliary clearance mechanism removes inhaled particulates and nasally administered drugs, limiting their residence time (Okmen Altas et al. 2024). The cutting-edge approach in pharmaceutical sciences aimed at overcoming the limitations of conventional drug delivery systems for CNS disorders. The effectiveness of this route lies in the unique anatomical and physiological features of the nasal cavity, as well as the intricate neural connections that bypass the restrictive BBB (Mwema et al. 2023). By leveraging these pathways, N2B drug delivery facilitates the direct transport of therapeutic agents to the brain, enabling rapid onset of action, improved bioavailability, and minimized systemic side effects. This method has proven particularly advantageous for treating neurodegenerative diseases, brain tumors, psychiatric disorders, and acute conditions such as stroke and epilepsy, where traditional routes often fail to deliver adequate drug concentrations to the brain. The nasal cavity is divided into distinct regions, each contributing uniquely to drug absorption (Haasbroek-Pheiffer et al. 2024). The anterior vestibule, composed of keratinized epithelial cells, acts as a protective barrier, offering limited permeability. Beyond this lies the respiratory region, which constitutes the primary site for systemic drug absorption due to its highly vascularized pseudostratified columnar epithelium. This region includes goblet cells that secrete mucus, ciliated columnar cells that facilitate mucociliary clearance, and basal cells that maintain epithelial integrity (Bennion et al. 2018). The total surface area of the respiratory region, approximately 150 cm^2, and its rich blood supply make it highly suitable for drug absorption into the systemic circulation. The olfactory region, though smaller (around 10 cm^2), holds the key to direct brain delivery. Located at the roof of the nasal cavity, it is characterized by specialized olfactory neurons that extend from the nasal epithelium to the olfactory bulb, providing a direct anatomical link to the CNS (Katare et al. 2024). These neurons are supported by basal and sustentacular cells, forming an intricate network capable of transporting molecules directly to the brain. This pathway is unique in its ability to bypass the BBB, which ordinarily restricts the entry of large or hydrophilic molecules into the CNS (Ladel et al. 2019). The extracellular pathway involves the diffusion of drugs through paracellular clefts or the perineural space surrounding neuronal axons, providing a relatively rapid transport mechanism to the brain. The intracellular pathway relies on endocytosis and axonal transport, wherein drugs are internalized by olfactory or trigeminal neurons and carried to the brain along the neuronal axons. While slower than the extracellular route, the intracellular pathway ensures targeted delivery to specific brain regions (Agnihotri et al. 2025). The trigeminal nerve pathway, which innervates the respiratory and olfactory regions, also plays a significant role in delivering drugs to deeper brain areas, further enhancing the scope of N2B delivery systems. N2B drug delivery offers several advantages over traditional routes such as oral, intravenous, or intrathecal administration. The most significant benefit is the ability to bypass the BBB, a formidable obstacle that limits the penetration of most drugs into the brain. This barrier, composed of tightly joined endothelial cells, restricts the entry of large molecules, hydrophilic substances, and therapeutic agents, often requiring invasive techniques or high systemic doses to achieve therapeutic concentrations in the CNS (Laurienzo 2010). N2B delivery circumvents these limitations by providing a direct route for drugs to reach the brain, enabling the administration of a wide range of molecules, including peptides, proteins, nucleic acids, and hydrophilic compounds. Another key advantage is the rapid onset of action associated with N2B delivery. The proximity of the nasal cavity to the brain and the absence of first-pass metabolism allow drugs to achieve therapeutic levels in the CNS within minutes of administration. This is particularly beneficial for acute conditions such as seizures, migraines, or stroke, where immediate intervention is crucial (Borgogna et al. 2011). N2B delivery minimizes systemic side effects by localizing drug action to the CNS, reducing off-target interactions and improving the therapeutic index of the administered agents. The noninvasive nature of intranasal drug delivery enhances patient compliance, especially for chronic conditions requiring long-term treatment. Compared to intravenous injections or intrathecal infusions, nasal sprays and gels are more user-friendly, eliminating the need for trained medical personnel and specialized equipment (Tudu and Samanta 2023). Moreover, the potential for self-administration makes this route particularly appealing for outpatient care and home-based therapies. N2B drug delivery faces several challenges that limit its widespread application. One of the primary obstacles is the rapid clearance of drugs from the nasal cavity due to mucociliary clearance. This natural defense mechanism, which involves the movement of mucus along the ciliated epithelium, efficiently removes foreign particles and pathogens but also reduces the residence time of nasally administered drugs, thereby limiting their absorption. Strategies to overcome this include the use of mucoadhesive formulations, such as chitosan-based nanoparticles (Lee et al. 2017), which enhance drug retention by adhering to the nasal mucosa. Enzymatic degradation is another significant challenge. The nasal epithelium is rich in enzymes such as cytochrome P450 isoforms, esterases, and proteases, which can metabolize drugs before they reach the brain. This "nasal pseudo first-pass effect" reduces the bioavailability of sensitive molecules, particularly peptides and proteins. Formulation approaches such as encapsulating drugs in protective carriers, co-administering enzyme inhibitors, or modifying the drug structure to resist enzymatic degradation have been explored to address this issue (Manivasagan and Oh 2016). The limited absorption surface area of the nasal cavity and the small volume of administrable formulations (25–200 μL) pose additional challenges, particularly for drugs with low solubility or requiring high doses. Nanoparticles, liposomes, and in situ gelling systems have been developed to enhance the solubility, stability, and bioavailability of such drugs, enabling efficient use of the available nasal surface area. Physicochemical properties of the drug, such as molecular weight, lipophilicity, and ionization, also play a crucial role in determining its suitability for N2B delivery (Venkatesan et al. 2016). Low-molecular-weight, lipophilic, and non-ionized drugs are typically absorbed more efficiently through the nasal epithelium. For hydrophilic or macromolecular drugs, permeation enhancers, surfactants, and advanced carrier systems are often required to facilitate transport across the nasal barrier. The anatomical and physiological variability of the nasal cavity among individuals adds another layer of complexity to N2B delivery. Factors such as age, gender, nasal pathologies (e.g., rhinitis, sinusitis, nasal polyps), and environmental conditions (e.g., temperature, humidity) can influence drug absorption and efficacy. Personalized approaches and adaptable formulations are being developed to address these variations and ensure consistent therapeutic outcomes (Beaumont et al. 2021). Regulatory and safety concerns also need to be addressed for the successful translation of N2B delivery systems from research to clinical practice. The long-term effects of repeated nasal administration, potential irritation or toxicity to the nasal mucosa, and the risk of contamination or infection are critical considerations. Rigorous preclinical and clinical testing is required to evaluate the safety, efficacy, and biocompatibility of N2B formulations. Nanotechnology plays a pivotal role in advancing N2B drug delivery, with nanoparticles, nanogels, and nanostructured lipid carriers offering enhanced drug stability, controlled release, and targeted delivery to specific brain regions (Barbosa et al. 2019). Mucoadhesive polymers, such as chitosan and alginate, are being utilized to improve drug retention and absorption, while in situ gelling systems provide prolonged release and better patient compliance. Functionalization of delivery carriers with targeting ligands, such as antibodies or peptides, enables precise delivery to specific brain receptors or regions, enhancing therapeutic efficacy. The development of dry powder formulations and advanced nasal spray devices has improved the stability, usability, and patient acceptance of N2B delivery systems (Rajasekaran and Viswanathan 2023). The integration of personalized medicine with N2B delivery holds immense promise for tailoring therapies to individual patients based on their genetic, physiological, and pathological profiles. Moreover, the combination of N2B delivery with advanced therapeutic modalities, such as gene editing, RNA-based therapies, and immunotherapy, opens new avenues for treating CNS disorders that were previously considered untreatable (Popa et al. 2015).

4 Application of Marine Polysaccharides in Formulation Development

Hydrogels, nanoparticles, and microparticles have emerged as leading platforms for delivering small molecules (Fig. 3), peptides, proteins, nucleic acids, and other therapeutic agents. These formulations address challenges such as low bioavailability, poor solubility, and systemic side effects, providing a pathway to enhance drug stability, targeted delivery, and controlled release (Khanna et al. 2019). Hydrogels (Table 2), three-dimensional polymeric networks capable of retaining significant amounts of water while maintaining structural integrity, are a cornerstone of polysaccharide-based drug delivery. Marine-derived polysaccharides like alginate, carrageenan, and chitosan are widely used for hydrogel formation due to their unique gelling properties. Alginate hydrogels, formed through ionic crosslinking with divalent cations like calcium, exhibit excellent biocompatibility and a gentle gelation process suitable for encapsulating sensitive therapeutic agents (Besednova et al.

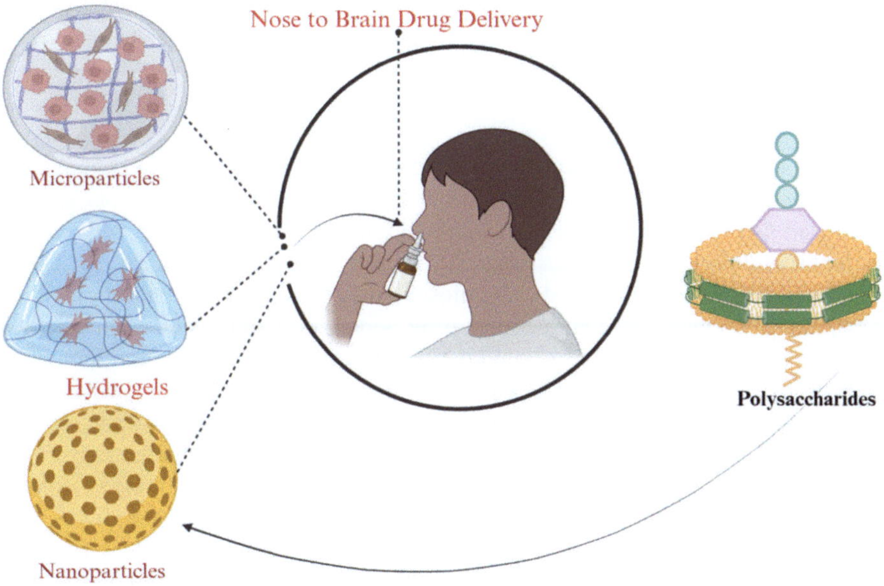

Fig. 3 Hydrogels, nanoparticles, and microparticles have emerged as leading platforms for the delivery of small molecules

Table 2 Overview of polysaccharide-based matrices, their synthesis/loading procedures, and types of carriers for drug delivery systems

Polysaccharide matrix	Synthesis/loading procedure	Type of carrier	References
Cellulose + alginate	Polymerization + spray-drying	Microspheres	Wang et al. (2017)
Cellulose	Coprecipitation + dispersion	Hydrogel beads	Ahmed and Aljaeid (2016)
Cellulose + pectin	Extrusion-spheronization	Pellet (0.8–1.0 mm)	Bodnar et al. (2005)
Cellulose + chitosan	Wrapping method	Beads (4–5 mm)	Pistone et al. (2017)
Chitosan	Gelation and crosslinking method	MPs (130–160 μm)	Cheng et al. (2020)
Chitosan + pectin	Emulsification	NPs	Delair (2011)
Pectin	Dissolution, emulsification, self-assembly, and lyophilization	NPs	Holtekjølen et al. (2006)
Alginate	Emulsification	Microsphere	Mudgil et al. (2014)
Dextran	Microfluidized crosslinking reaction	NPs (110 nm)	Wang et al. (2023)
Starch	High-speed shearing emulsification	NPs (300 nm)	Luo and Wang (2014)
Guar gum	Wet granulation	Tablet (0.588 g/cm^3)	Halder et al. (2024)
Cyclodextrin	Encapsulation	NPs (110 nm)	Kumari et al. (2022)
Pectin + chitosan	Dispersion + superhydrophobic surface-based encapsulation	Microgel (280 and 557 μm)	Ruocco et al. (2016)

2020). These hydrogels are extensively used in wound healing, tissue engineering, and controlled drug release, where their ability to form localized depots ensures prolonged therapeutic effects. For example, alginate hydrogels loaded with growth factors or antibiotics provide sustained delivery at wound sites, enhancing healing and minimizing infection risks. Chitosan hydrogels, formed through ionic crosslinking or chemical modifications, offer additional functionalities due to their cationic nature, enabling electrostatic interactions with anionic drugs and biological membranes. These hydrogels are widely employed in cancer therapy, where they facilitate localized delivery of chemotherapeutic agents, reducing systemic toxicity (Ghosh et al. 2017). Chitosan's mucoadhesive properties make it particularly effective for intranasal and gastrointestinal drug delivery, ensuring prolonged contact time with mucosal surfaces and enhanced absorption. Carrageenan hydrogels, derived from red algae, are another example of marine-based hydrogels with excellent gelation properties. These hydrogels are commonly used in oral and transdermal drug delivery systems, where their ability to form strong, thermally reversible gels enhances drug stability and controlled release. Functionalization of marine polysaccharides has further expanded the scope of hydrogels in drug delivery (Lukova and Katsarov 2023). For instance, thiolated chitosan hydrogels demonstrate enhanced mucoadhesion and swelling properties, making them ideal for delivering drugs to the nasal cavity or gastrointestinal tract. Similarly, chemically modified alginates with grafted functional groups, such as polyethylene glycol (PEG) or cyclodextrins, enhance the hydrophilic or hydrophobic balance of hydrogels, improving their drug-loading capacity and release kinetics. In tissue engineering, hybrid hydrogels combining alginate and chitosan have been developed to provide a balanced combination of mechanical strength and bioactivity, supporting cell adhesion, proliferation, and differentiation. These hybrid systems are particularly useful for the localized delivery of growth factors and stem cells, facilitating regenerative processes in damaged tissues (Oliveira and Mano 2011).

Nanoparticles, typically ranging in size from 1 to 100 nanometers, represent a transformative approach in drug delivery, providing enhanced solubility, stability, and bioavailability for poorly soluble drugs. Marine polysaccharides have proven to be exceptional materials for nanoparticle fabrication, offering tunable properties and functional groups for drug encapsulation and release (Hussein et al. 2022). Chitosan nanoparticles, prepared through ionic gelation, emulsion, or coacervation techniques, are among the most extensively studied systems. Their positive charge at physiological pH enables strong interactions with negatively charged mucosal surfaces, enhancing mucoadhesion and drug absorption. These nanoparticles are widely used for delivering anticancer drugs, insulin, vaccines, and siRNA, where their ability to protect therapeutic agents from enzymatic degradation and provide sustained release is critical (Miao et al. 2018). Surface modification of chitosan nanoparticles has enabled the development of targeted delivery systems. For example, chitosan nanoparticles conjugated with folic acid or transferrin target specific receptors on cancer cells, enhancing drug accumulation in tumor tissues while minimizing off-target effects. Similarly, lactoferrin-conjugated chitosan nanoparticles have been developed for nose-to-brain delivery, targeting the transferrin receptor to enhance drug transport across the BBB. Functionalized nanoparticles with PEG or polyethyleneimine improve stability and circulation time, making them suitable for intravenous administration (Severino et al. 2019). Alginate nanoparticles, often prepared through ionic gelation with calcium ions, are another example of marine polysaccharide-based nanoparticles with excellent biocompatibility and drug-loading capabilities. These nanoparticles are commonly used for the oral delivery of proteins and peptides, where their ability to form protective barriers against acidic gastric environments ensures the stability and bioavailability of encapsulated drugs. Alginate nanoparticles have also been used for gene delivery, where their gentle encapsulation process preserves the integrity of DNA or RNA molecules, enhancing their therapeutic potential. Carrageenan and fucoidan nanoparticles, derived from red and brown algae, respectively, have also shown promise as drug carriers (Mondal et al. 2018). Carrageenan nanoparticles, with their anionic nature, are particularly useful for encapsulating cationic drugs and proteins, while fucoidan nanoparticles exhibit unique biological activities such as anticoagulant, antioxidant, and anti-inflammatory properties. These nanoparticles are being explored for their potential in cancer therapy, where they provide both therapeutic and synergistic effects. Recent advancements in nanotechnology have enabled the development of hybrid nanoparticles combining marine polysaccharides with synthetic polymers or inorganic materials. For instance, chitosan-coated gold or silver nanoparticles exhibit enhanced antibacterial and anticancer properties, while alginate-based hybrid nanoparticles with lipids or surfactants improve drug solubility and targeting. These hybrid systems represent a new frontier in nanomedicine, offering customizable platforms for a wide range of therapeutic applications (Rescignano et al. 2015).

Microparticles, typically ranging in size from 1 to 1000 micrometers, offer unique advantages for drug delivery, particularly for controlled and localized release. Marine polysaccharides, with their ability to form stable matrices, are widely used for microparticle fabrication. Alginate microparticles, prepared through emulsification or spray-drying techniques, are commonly employed for oral and injectable drug delivery (Wang et al. 2022). These microparticles provide a protective matrix for encapsulated drugs, ensuring stability and controlled release. For example, alginate microparticles loaded with probiotics or peptides protect these sensitive agents from harsh gastric conditions, enabling their delivery to the intestinal tract. Chitosan microparticles, formed through ionic gelation or coacervation methods, are particularly effective for mucoadhesive drug delivery. Their ability to adhere to mucosal surfaces prolongs the residence time of drugs, enhancing their absorption and bioavailability. Chitosan microparticles are widely used for intranasal and pulmonary drug delivery, where they provide localized effects with minimal systemic exposure (Saravanakumar et al. 2020). For instance, chitosan microparticles loaded with antiasthmatic drugs deliver therapeutic agents directly to the lungs, reducing inflammation and improving respiratory function. Carrageenan microparticles, with their gel-forming properties, are commonly used for encapsulating hydrophilic drugs and proteins. These microparticles provide sustained release profiles, making them suitable for long-acting injectable formulations. Fucoidan microparticles, on the other hand, offer additional biological activities such as anti-inflammatory and antioxidant effects, making them attractive for wound healing and tissue regeneration applications. Hybrid and composite microparticles have been developed to enhance the functionality of marine polysaccharide-based carriers. For example, alginate-chitosan composite microparticles combine the strengths of both polymers, providing improved mechanical stability, mucoadhesion, and drug-loading capacity. These systems are particularly useful for the oral delivery of poorly soluble drugs, where they enhance solubility and bioavailability. Similarly, microparticles combining carrageenan with synthetic polymers or lipids provide tailored release profiles, making them suitable for a wide range of therapeutic applications (Carrion et al. 2021).

5 Future Perspectives and Challenges

The development of nanotechnology-based delivery systems, such as nanoparticles, nanogels, and nanofibers, holds immense promise for enhancing the efficiency of marine polysaccharide-based N2B drug delivery. By leveraging nanotechnology, researchers can optimize the size, surface charge, and functionalization of polysaccharide carriers to improve their mucoadhesive properties, stability, and drug-loading capacities. For instance, chitosan nanoparticles have demonstrated significant potential for delivering drugs across the nasal mucosa and into the brain, owing to their mucoadhesive and permeation-enhancing properties. Future advancements in hybrid and composite nanoparticles, incorporating other polymers or inorganic materials, could further enhance targeting specificity and therapeutic efficacy. In this chapter, we provide an overview of marine-based polysaccharides and their promising potential in nose-to-brain drug delivery applications. Marine polysaccharides, including alginates, chitosan, and carrageenans, offer a unique advantage for drug delivery systems, especially for CNS. These polysaccharides, derived from marine organisms, have gained attention due to their natural biocompatibility, biodegradability, and their ability to form gels with desirable mechanical properties for drug delivery. Marine polysaccharides exhibit excellent mucoadhesive properties, which make them ideal candidates for nasal drug delivery, facilitating sustained release and enhanced absorption of therapeutic agents through the nasal mucosa. Marine-based polysaccharides have been classified based on their chemical structure, solubility, and crosslinking potential. Alginates, derived from brown seaweeds, are widely used in drug delivery systems because of their ability to form hydrogels through ionic crosslinking, which helps in encapsulating drugs and releasing them in a controlled manner. Chitosan, a biopolymer derived from the shells of crustaceans, has shown great potential in nasal delivery due to its ability to enhance drug absorption and promote mucoadhesion. Carrageenans, extracted from red seaweeds, also possess excellent gelling properties and have been explored for their potential in nasal drug delivery. Marine polysaccharides, in combination with nanoparticles or other active agents, offer a dual-functional approach to drug delivery, providing therapeutic benefits while enhancing the stability, bioavailability, and targeting of drugs. In vitro and in vivo studies have demonstrated the successful application of marine polysaccharide-based systems for nose-to-brain delivery, with improved drug retention, reduced systemic side effects, and enhanced therapeutic effects compared to traditional drug delivery methods (Bharathi and Lee 2024).

6 Conclusion

In summary, marine-based polysaccharides hold immense potential as carriers for nose-to-brain drug delivery, offering biocompatibility, biodegradability, and low toxicity. The combination of marine polysaccharides with nanoparticles or other therapeutic agents further enhances the drug delivery capabilities, making these systems highly promising for the treatment of CNS disorders. However, challenges such as improving the mechanical strength of these hydrogels and optimizing drug release profiles still remain. Continued research is needed to fully realize the potential of marine polysaccharides for nose-to-brain drug delivery systems, with the goal of developing safe, effective, and commercially viable products for treating a range of neurological diseases. The future of this field is bright, and further advancements in formulation strategies, as well as understanding the underlying mechanisms, will pave the way for innovative therapeutic solutions targeting the brain.

References

Bhatnagar I, Kim SK. Immense essence of excellence: marine microbial bioactive compounds. Marine drugs. 2010 Oct 15;8(10):2673–701.

Karthikeyan A, Joseph A, Nair BG. Promising bioactive compounds from the marine environment and their potential effects on various diseases. Journal of Genetic Engineering and Biotechnology. 2022 Dec 1;20(1):14.

El-Regal MA, Satheesh S. Biodiversity of Marine Ecosystems. Marine Ecosystems: A Unique Source of Valuable Bioactive Compounds. 2023 Nov 6;3:1–42.

Paul SI, Majumdar BC, Ehsan R, Hasan M, Baidya A, Bakky MA. Bioprospecting potential of marine microbial natural bioactive compounds. Journal of Applied Biotechnology Reports. 2021 Jun 1;8(2):96–108.

Kim SK, editor. Marine microbiology: bioactive compounds and biotechnological applications. John Wiley & Sons; 2013 Jun 21.

Debbab A, Aly AH, Lin WH, Proksch P. Bioactive compounds from marine bacteria and fungi. Microbial biotechnology. 2010 Sep;3(5):544–63.

Ahmed N, Sheikh MA, Ubaid M, Chauhan P, Kumar K, Choudhary S. Comprehensive exploration of marine algae diversity, bioactive compounds, health benefits, regulatory issues, and food and drug applications. Measurement: Food. 2024 Mar 30:100163.

Banday AH, ul Azha N, Farooq R, Sheikh SA, Ganie MA, Parray MN, Mushtaq H, Hameed I, Lone MA. Exploring the potential of marine natural products in drug development: A comprehensive review. Phytochemistry Letters. 2024 Feb 1;59:124–35.

Snelgrove PV. An ocean of discovery: Biodiversity beyond the census of marine life. Planta medica. 2016 Jun;82(09/10):790–9.

Sugumaran A, Pandiyan R, Kandasamy P, Antoniraj MG, Navabshan I, Sakthivel B, Dharmaraj S, Chinnaiyan SK, Ashokkumar V, Ngamcharussrivichai C. Marine biome-derived secondary metabolites, a class of promising antineoplastic agents: A systematic review on their classification, mechanism of action and future perspectives. Science of the Total Environment. 2022 Aug 25;836:155445.

Giddings LA, Newman DJ, Giddings LA, Newman DJ. Bioactive compounds from marine extremophiles. Springer International Publishing; 2015.

Subramani R, Aalbersberg W. Culturable rare Actinomycetes: diversity, isolation and marine natural product discovery. Applied microbiology and biotechnology. 2013 Nov;97:9291-321.

Egan S, Thomas T, Kjelleberg S. Unlocking the diversity and biotechnological potential of marine surface associated microbial communities. Current opinion in microbiology. 2008 Jun 1;11(3): 219–25.

Conte M, Fontana E, Nebbioso A, Altucci L. Marine-derived secondary metabolites as promising epigenetic bio-compounds for anticancer therapy. Marine drugs. 2020 Dec 31;19(1):15.

Sable R, Parajuli P, Jois S. Peptides, peptidomimetics, and polypeptides from marine sources: a wealth of natural sources for pharmaceutical applications. Marine drugs. 2017 Apr 22;15(4): 124.

Poli A, Finore I, Romano I, Gioiello A, Lama L, Nicolaus B. Microbial diversity in extreme marine habitats and their biomolecules. Microorganisms. 2017 May 16;5(2):25.

Xu BL, Wang YY, Dong CM. Study on Marine actinomycetes and analysis of their secondary metabolites. Life Res. 2023;6(4):18.

Nawaz T, Gu L, Fahad S, Saud S, Jiang Z, Hassan S, Harrison MT, Liu K, Khan MA, Liu H, El-Kahtany K. A comprehensive review of the therapeutic potential of cyanobacterial marine bioactives: Unveiling the hidden treasures of the sea. Food and Energy Security. 2023 Sep;12 (5):e495.

Trapani A, Corbo F, Agrimi G, Ditaranto N, Cioffi N, Perna F, Quivelli A, Stefàno E, Lunetti P, Muscella A, Marsigliante S. Oxidized alginate dopamine conjugate: in vitro characterization for nose-to-brain delivery application. Materials. 2021 Jun 23;14(13):3495.

Nafee N, Ameen AE, Abdallah OY. Patient-friendly, olfactory-targeted, stimuli-responsive hydrogels for cerebral degenerative disorders ensured> 400% brain targeting efficiency in rats. AAPS PharmSciTech. 2020 Nov 22;22(1):6.

Clementino A, Climani G, Bianchera A, Buttini F, Sonvico F. Polysaccharides: New Frontiers for Nasal Administration of Medicines. Polysaccharides. 2025a Jan 15;6(1):6.

Hao J, Zhao J, Zhang S, Tong T, Zhuang Q, Jin K, Chen W, Tang H. Fabrication of an ionic-sensitive in situ gel loaded with resveratrol nanosuspensions intended for direct nose-to-brain delivery. Colloids and Surfaces B: Biointerfaces. 2016 Nov 1;147:376–86.

Kaur P, Garg T, Rath G, Goyal AK. In situ nasal gel drug delivery: A novel approach for brain targeting through the mucosal membrane. Artificial cells, nanomedicine, and biotechnology. 2016 May 18;44(4):1167–76.

Majgainya S, Soni S, Bhat P. Novel approach for nose-to-brain drug delivery bypassing blood brain barrier by pressurized olfactory delivery device. J App Pharm. 2015 Jul;7(3):148–63.

Sonvico F, Clementino A, Buttini F, Colombo G, Pescina S, Stanisçuaski Guterres S, Raffin Pohlmann A, Nicoli S. Surface-modified nanocarriers for nose-to-brain delivery: from bioadhesion to targeting. Pharmaceutics. 2018 Mar 15;10(1):34.

Bonaccorso A, Musumeci T, Serapide MF, Pellitteri R, Uchegbu IF, Puglisi G. Nose to brain delivery in rats: Effect of surface charge of rhodamine B labeled nanocarriers on brain subregion localization. Colloids and Surfaces B: Biointerfaces. 2017 Jun 1;154:297–306.

Lombardo R, Musumeci T, Carbone C, Pignatello R. Nanotechnologies for intranasal drug delivery: an update of literature. Pharmaceutical development and technology. 2021 Sep 14;26(8): 824–45.

Yagi H, Tomono T, Abe K, Tsutsumi Y, Makabe M, Mitsuhashi H, Kimura T, Kobayashi H, Miyata K, Shigeno K, Sakuma S. Validation of the Absorption-Enhancing Ability of Oligoarginines Grafted onto a Backbone of Hyaluronic Acid through Animal Studies from Rodents to Primates. Molecular Pharmaceutics. 2024 May 28.

Cote B, Rao D, Alany RG, Kwon GS, Alani AW. Lymphatic changes in cancer and drug delivery to the lymphatics in solid tumors. Advanced Drug Delivery Reviews. 2019 Apr 1;144:16–34.

Spindler LM, Feuerhake A, Ladel S, Günday C, Flamm J, Günday-Türeli N, Türeli E, Tovar GE, Schindowski K, Gruber-Traub C. Nano-in-micro-particles consisting of PLGA nanoparticles embedded in chitosan microparticles via spray-drying enhances their uptake in the olfactory mucosa. Frontiers in Pharmacology. 2021 Sep 1;12:732954.

Yui T, Uto T, Ogawa K. Molecular and Crystal Structure of a Chitosan– Zinc Chloride Complex. Nanomaterials. 2021 May 26;11(6):1407.

Su Y, Sun B, Gao X, Liu S, Hao R, Han B. Chitosan hydrogel doped with PEG-PLA nanoparticles for the local delivery of miRNA-146a to treat allergic rhinitis. Pharmaceutics. 2020 Sep 23;12 (10):907.

Li P, Zhou C, Rayatpisheh S, Ye K, Poon YF, Hammond PT, Duan H, Chan-Park MB. Cationic peptidopolysaccharides show excellent broad-spectrum antimicrobial activities and high selectivity. Advanced Materials. 2012 Aug 8;24(30):4130.

Clementino A, Climani G, Bianchera A, Buttini F, Sonvico F. Polysaccharides: New Frontiers for Nasal Administration of Medicines. Polysaccharides. 2025b Jan 15;6(1):6.

Finetti L, Benetti L, Leyria J, Civolani S, Bernacchia G. Topical delivery of dsRNA in two hemipteran species: Evaluation of RNAi specificity and non-target effects. Pesticide Biochemistry and Physiology. 2023 Jan 1;189:105295.

Patharapankal EJ, Ajiboye AL, Mattern C, Trivedi V. Nose-to-Brain (N2B) Delivery: An Alternative Route for the Delivery of Biologics in the Management and Treatment of Central Nervous System Disorders. Pharmaceutics. 2023 Dec 31;16(1):66.

Adscheid SA, Türeli AE, Günday-Türeli N, Schneider M. Nanotechnological approaches for efficient N2B delivery: from small-molecule drugs to biopharmaceuticals. Beilstein Journal of Nanotechnology. 2024 Nov 12;15(1):1400–14.

Du L, Chen L, Liu F, Wang W, Huang H. Nose-to-brain drug delivery for the treatment of CNS disease: New development and strategies. International Review of Neurobiology. 2023 Jan 1;171:255–97.

Saha P, Kathuria H, Pandey MM. Intranasal nanotherapeutics for brain targeting and clinical studies in Parkinson's disease. Journal of Controlled Release. 2023 Jun 1;358:293–318.

Ogawa K, Kato N, Kawakami S. Recent strategies for targeted brain drug delivery. Chemical and Pharmaceutical Bulletin. 2020 Jul 1;68(7):567–82.

Okmen Altas B, Kalaycioglu GD, Lifshiz-Simon S, Talmon Y, Aydogan N. Tadpole-Like Anisotropic Polymer/Lipid Janus Nanoparticles for Nose-to-Brain Drug Delivery: Importance of Geometry, Elasticity on Mucus-Penetration Ability. Molecular pharmaceutics. 2024 Jan 2;21 (2):633–50.

Mwema A, Muccioli GG, Des Rieux A. Innovative drug delivery strategies to the CNS for the treatment of multiple sclerosis. Journal of Controlled Release. 2023 Dec 1;364:435–57.

Haasbroek-Pheiffer A, Viljoen A, Steenekamp J, Chen W, Hamman J. An ex vivo investigation on drug permeability of sheep nasal epithelial tissue membranes from the respiratory and olfactory regions. Current Drug Delivery. 2024 Jan 1;21(1):115–25.

Bennion DM, Jones CH, Dang AN, Isenberg J, Graham JT, Lindblad L, Domenig O, Waters MF, Poglitsch M, Sumners C, Steckelings UM. Protective effects of the angiotensin II AT2 receptor agonist compound 21 in ischemic stroke: a nose-to-brain delivery approach. Clinical Science. 2018 Mar 15;132(5):581–93.

Katare P, Pawar Medhe T, Nadkarni A, Deshpande M, Tekade RK, Benival D, Jain A. Nasal drug delivery system and devices: an overview on health effects. ACS Chemical Health & Safety. 2024 Feb 9;31(2):127–43.

Ladel S, Schlossbauer P, Flamm J, Luksch H, Mizaikoff B, Schindowski K. Improved in vitro model for intranasal mucosal drug delivery: Primary olfactory and respiratory epithelial cells compared with the permanent nasal cell line RPMI 2650. Pharmaceutics. 2019 Aug 1;11(8):367.

Agnihotri TG, Dahifale A, Gomte SS, Rout B, Peddinti V, Jain A. Nanosystems at Nexus: Navigating Nose-to-Brain Delivery for Glioblastoma Treatment. Molecular Pharmaceutics. 2025 Jan 8.

Laurienzo P. Marine polysaccharides in pharmaceutical applications: an overview. Marine drugs. 2010 Sep 2;8(9):2435–65.

Borgogna M, Bellich B, Cesàro A. Marine polysaccharides in microencapsulation and application to aquaculture:"from sea to sea". Marine drugs. 2011 Dec 8;9(12):2572–604.

Tudu M, Samanta A. Natural polysaccharides: Chemical properties and application in pharmaceutical formulations. European Polymer Journal. 2023 Feb 7;184:111801.

Lee YE, Kim H, Seo C, Park T, Lee KB, Yoo SY, Hong SC, Kim JT, Lee J. Marine polysaccharides: therapeutic efficacy and biomedical applications. Archives of Pharmacal Research. 2017 Sep;40:1006–20.

Manivasagan P, Oh J. Marine polysaccharide-based nanomaterials as a novel source of nanobiotechnological applications. International journal of biological macromolecules. 2016 Jan 1;82:315–27.

Venkatesan J, Anil S, Kim SK, Shim MS. Seaweed polysaccharide-based nanoparticles: Preparation and applications for drug delivery. Polymers. 2016 Jan 26;8(2):30.

Beaumont M, Tran R, Vera G, Niedrist D, Rousset A, Pierre R, Shastri VP, Forget A. Hydrogel-forming algae polysaccharides: From seaweed to biomedical applications. Biomacromolecules. 2021 Feb 12;22(3):1027–52.

Barbosa AI, Coutinho AJ, Costa Lima SA, Reis S. Marine polysaccharides in pharmaceutical applications: Fucoidan and chitosan as key players in the drug delivery match field. Marine Drugs. 2019 Nov 21;17(12):654.

Rajasekaran J, Viswanathan P. Anti-bacterial and antibiofilm properties of seaweed polysaccharide-based nanoparticles. Aquaculture International. 2023 Oct;31(5):2799–823.

Popa EG, Reis RL, Gomes ME. Seaweed polysaccharide-based hydrogels used for the regeneration of articular cartilage. Critical Reviews in Biotechnology. 2015 Jul 3;35(3):410–24.

Khanna P, Kaur A, Goyal D. Algae-based metallic nanoparticles: Synthesis, characterization and applications. Journal of microbiological methods. 2019 Aug 1;163:105656.

Besednova NN, Zaporozhets TS, Kuznetsova TA, Makarenkova ID, Kryzhanovsky SP, Fedyanina LN, Ermakova SP. Extracts and marine algae polysaccharides in therapy and prevention of inflammatory diseases of the intestine. Marine drugs. 2020 May 31;18(6):289.

Ghosh PR, Fawcett D, Sharma SB, Poinern GE. Production of high-value nanoparticles via biogenic processes using aquacultural and horticultural food waste. Materials. 2017 Jul 25;10 (8):852.

Lukova P, Katsarov P. Contemporary Aspects of Designing Marine Polysaccharide Microparticles as Drug Carriers for Biomedical Application. Pharmaceutics. 2023 Aug 11;15(8):2126.

Oliveira MB, Mano JF. Polymer-based microparticles in tissue engineering and regenerative medicine. Biotechnology progress. 2011 Jul;27(4):897–912.

Hussein HA, Nazir MS, Azra N, Qamar Z, Seeni A, Tengku Din TA, Abdullah MA. Novel drug and gene delivery system and imaging agent based on marine diatom biosilica nanoparticles. Marine Drugs. 2022 Jul 27;20(8):480.

Miao T, Wang J, Zeng Y, Liu G, Chen X. Polysaccharide-based controlled release systems for therapeutics delivery and tissue engineering: from bench to bedside. Advanced science. 2018 Apr;5(4):1700513.

Severino P, da Silva CF, Andrade LN, de Lima Oliveira D, Campos J, Souto EB. Alginate nanoparticles for drug delivery and targeting. Current pharmaceutical design. 2019 Mar 1;25 (11):1312–34.

Mondal S, Dorozhkin SV, Pal U. Recent progress on fabrication and drug delivery applications of nanostructured hydroxyapatite. Wiley Interdisciplinary Reviews: Nanomedicine and Nanobiotechnology. 2018 Jul;10(4):e1504.

Rescignano N, Fortunati E, Armentano I, Hernandez R, Mijangos C, Pasquino R, Kenny JM. Use of alginate, chitosan and cellulose nanocrystals as emulsion stabilizers in the synthesis of biodegradable polymeric nanoparticles. Journal of colloid and interface science. 2015 May 1;445:31–9.

Wang L, Hao F, Tian S, Dong H, Nie J, Ma G. Targeting polysaccharides such as chitosan, cellulose, alginate and starch for designing hemostatic dressings. Carbohydrate Polymers. 2022 Sep 1;291:119574.

Saravanakumar K, Sathiyaseelan A, Mariadoss AV, Xiaowen H, Wang MH. Physical and bioactivities of biopolymeric films incorporated with cellulose, sodium alginate and copper oxide nanoparticles for food packaging application. International Journal of Biological Macromolecules. 2020 Jun 15;153:207–14.

Carrion CC, Nasrollahzadeh M, Sajjadi M, Jaleh B, Soufi GJ, Iravani S. Lignin, lipid, protein, hyaluronic acid, starch, cellulose, gum, pectin, alginate and chitosan-based nanomaterials for

cancer nanotherapy: Challenges and opportunities. International Journal of Biological Macromolecules. 2021 May 1;178:193–228.
Wang C, Gao X, Chen Z, Chen Y, Chen H. Preparation, characterization and application of polysaccharide-based metallic nanoparticles: a review. Polymers. 2017 Dec 8;9(12):689.
Ahmed TA, Aljaeid BM. Preparation, characterization, and potential application of chitosan, chitosan derivatives, and chitosan metal nanoparticles in pharmaceutical drug delivery. Drug design, development and therapy. 2016 Jan 28:483–507.
Bodnar M, Hartmann JF, Borbely J. Preparation and characterization of chitosan-based nanoparticles. Biomacromolecules. 2005 Sep 12;6(5):2521–7.
Pistone S, Goycoolea FM, Young A, Smistad G, Hiorth M. Formulation of polysaccharide-based nanoparticles for local administration into the oral cavity. European Journal of Pharmaceutical Sciences. 2017 Jan 1;96:381–9.
Cheng D, Jiang C, Xu J, Liu Z, Mao X. Characteristics and applications of alginate lyases: A review. International Journal of Biological Macromolecules. 2020 Dec 1;164:1304–20.
Delair T. Colloidal polyelectrolyte complexes of chitosan and dextran sulfate towards versatile nanocarriers of bioactive molecules. European Journal of Pharmaceutics and Biopharmaceutics. 2011 May 1;78(1):10–8.
Holtekjølen AK, Uhlen AK, Bråthen E, Sahlstrøm S, Knutsen SH. Contents of starch and non-starch polysaccharides in barley varieties of different origin. Food Chemistry. 2006 Feb 1;94(3):348–58.
Mudgil D, Barak S, Khatkar BS. Guar gum: processing, properties and food applications—a review. Journal of food science and technology. 2014 Mar;51:409–18.
Wang S, Wei Y, Wang Y, Cheng Y. Cyclodextrin regulated natural polysaccharide hydrogels for biomedical applications-a review. Carbohydrate Polymers. 2023 Aug 1;313:120760.
Luo Y, Wang Q. Recent development of chitosan-based polyelectrolyte complexes with natural polysaccharides for drug delivery. International journal of biological macromolecules. 2014 Mar 1;64:353–67.
Halder D, Das S, Joseph A. An insight into structure-activity relationship of naturally derived biological macromolecules for the treatment of Alzheimer's disease: a review. Journal of Biomolecular Structure and Dynamics. 2024 Aug 12;42(12):6455–71.
Kumari R, Vivekanand V, Pareek N. Marine-Based Carbohydrates as a Valuable Resource for Nutraceuticals and Biotechnological Application. InMarine Biochemistry 2022 Oct 12 (pp. 1-29). CRC Press.
Ruocco N, Costantini S, Guariniello S, Costantini M. Polysaccharides from the marine environment with pharmacological, cosmeceutical and nutraceutical potential. Molecules. 2016 Apr 27;21 (5):551.
Bharathi D, Lee J. Recent Advances in Marine-Derived Compounds as Potent Antibacterial and Antifungal Agents: A Comprehensive Review. Marine Drugs. 2024 Jul 29;22(8):348.

Marine Algae Polysaccharides in Anticancer Drug Delivery

Souad A. Elfeky, Gamal El-ghannam, Mostafa Zedan, and Nayer Qenawi

Abstract Marine algae polysaccharides are gaining attention in anticancer drug delivery because they are biocompatible, demonstrate unique biological activities, and are multifunctional. These are naturally derived polysaccharides that come from various sea algae species and include alginates, fucoidans, carrageenans, ulvans, and agars. The polysaccharides have their own inherent anticancer, anti-inflammatory, and immunomodulatory properties. Given that they can form hydrogels, nanoparticles, and capsules, marine algae polysaccharides can lead to controlled and sustained drug release, which is advantageous for treatment efficacy while reducing potential toxicity. Marine algae also respond dynamically to environmental stimuli (pH and enzymes), which enhances targeted delivery to the tumor site while avoiding off-target effects. Although there are potential challenges related to scalability and structural complexity, improvements and advancements in extraction and biotechnological development continue to diminish these challenges. Overall, marine algae polysaccharides represent a novel and more organic strategy to enhance the safety and efficacy of anticancer drug therapy, with development avenues toward further integration into personalized medicine and the creation of combination therapies.

Keywords Marine algae polysaccharides · Anticancer drug delivery · Nanoparticles · Biocompatibility · Hydrogels · Controlled drug release

1 Introduction

1.1 Overview of Marine Algae and Their Polysaccharides

Marine algae, a broad category of aquatic photosynthetic organisms, are essential to the complex dynamics of the world's oceans. This broad group includes anything

S. A. Elfeky (✉) · G. El-ghannam · M. Zedan · N. Qenawi
Department of Laser Applications in Metrology, Photochemistry, and Agriculture (LAMPA), National Institute of Laser Enhanced Science (NILES), Cairo University, Giza, Egypt
e-mail: dr_souad_elfeky@niles.cu.edu.eg

S. Jana et al. (eds.), *Multifunctional Marine Polysaccharides*,
https://doi.org/10.1007/978-981-95-4126-3_7

from microscopic phytoplankton to massive seaweeds, and it plays a vital role in essential functions such as oxygen synthesis, carbon dioxide absorption, and the general preservation of ecological equilibrium (Veluchamy and Palaniswamy 2020). These organisms vary in size from tiny phytoplankton to large seaweeds, and they can generally be categorized into three basic groups (relying on their color and chemical structure), which include green algae (Chlorophyta), brown algae (Phaeophyceae), and red algae (Rhodophyta) (Manzelat et al. 2018). Numerous research conducted in recent years has demonstrated the significance of marine algae as sources of bioactive natural compounds that have a direct bear on the modulation of chronic disease. To date, a number of algal chemical bioactivities have been reported, including anti-inflammatory, anticancer, antimicrobial, antifungal, and antiviral properties; anti-obesity and antidiabetic properties; and antiparasitic properties. As a result, a novel approach of separating and characterizing bioactive substances and components from marine algae has surfaced (Stengel and Connan 2015). Seaweeds produce a variety of polysaccharides, such as laminaran, carrageenan, fucoidan, and alginate. Over the past 20 years, a great deal of research has been done on the potential biomedical uses of seaweed-derived polysaccharides. The polysaccharides are very appropriate for a variety of applications in biomedicine, especially in tissue engineering and pharmaceutical administration, due to their capacity to form hydrogels in response to particular pH levels, their biocompatibility, and their nontoxic properties. The field of polysaccharide biotechnology is now seeing rapid and substantial growth. All seaweed provides a wide variety of biofunctional compounds with real-world applications in the fields of medicine and functional foods, such as tissue engineering and pharmaceutical research (Venkatesan et al. 2015).

1.2 Importance of Marine Algae Polysaccharides in Biomedical Applications

Marine algae have an extensive range of polysaccharides, which are of interest for a number of biomedical applications. Polysaccharides such as alginates, agar, carrageenan, and fucoidans have good biocompatibility, biodegradability, and versatility, allowing them to be incorporated as functional components in healthcare and pharmaceutical formulations (Bilal and Iqbal 2020). Given their capacity to engage with biological systems in a nontoxic and often beneficial manner, marine algae polysaccharides have garnered much interest in drug delivery systems, wound healing, tissue engineering, and immunotherapy. Perhaps the most interesting feature of marine algae polysaccharides is their ability to form gels and films, which have important ramifications for controlled drug delivery systems. Polysaccharides can be tailored to entrap therapeutics, allowing for sustained drug release profiles and enhancing the bioavailability or effectiveness of drugs, in part by protecting the drug from degradation (Cardoso et al. 2016). Researchers have the capability to develop a patient-specific delivery system for different types of therapy, such as pain management and anticancer therapies, due to their ability to alter the physical and chemical properties. This versatility is what identifies algal polysaccharides from marine sources as a renewable source in the development of next-generation biomedical products. Furthermore, algal polysaccharides exhibit a wide range of bioactivities, such as anti-inflammatory, antioxidant, and antimicrobial properties, which contribute to their ability to enhance tissue repair and modulate inflammation (Matin et al. 2024). Furthermore, the natural anti-inflammatory, antimicrobial, and immunomodulatory characteristics of marine algae polysaccharides may promote wound healing and minimize risk of infection, which is beneficial in chronic wound healing and burns. The exploration of polysaccharides derived from marine algae for use in biomedicine is not just an exciting opportunity for innovative solutions but also explores a sustainable approach to global health issues. By leveraging abundant and naturally occurring resources, researchers are creating possibilities for a very promising realm of developing new therapies that are effective and environmentally friendly, where new developments can take advantage of the vast and valuable oceanic resources to advance human health.

1.3 Relevance to Anticancer Drug Delivery

Marine algae and their polysaccharides have emerged as promising agents in anticancer drug delivery. The polysaccharides produced by marine algae are recognized for their bioactivity and diversity and include alginates, agar, carrageenans, and fucoidans. Researchers are studying the possibility of using marine algae polysaccharides as antifolates to enhance the poor solubility and bioavailability of many anticancer drugs, as well as to ameliorate the adverse side effects associated with traditional therapies (Hsu et al. 2024). These polymers from nature are biodegradable, biocompatible, and nontoxic; hence, they are ideal for drug delivery systems, helping to alleviate chemotherapy toxicity and/or enhance efficacy. The primary advantage of marine algae polysaccharides for anticancer delivery systems is that they can be easily modified for targeted drug delivery. These polysaccharides can be chemically tailored to enable the direct delivery of anticancer agents to tumor sites, thereby decreasing systemic toxicity and increasing therapeutic response rates. In addition to this possibility, certain polysaccharides (e.g., alginates and carrageenans) also exhibit specific properties, such as gel-forming properties and the ability to control drug release rate from an encapsulated structure, which are important specifically for sustained and controlled drug release in cancer therapy (Yadav et al. 2022). It is feasible to improve drug release efficacy at the tumor site by encapsulating chemotherapy agents within polysaccharide carriers, allowing for more effective and selective treatment. Furthermore, polysaccharides derived from marine algae display innate bioactive properties, including anti-inflammatory, antioxidant, and immunomodulatory properties, which can enhance their function in anticancer therapy. Fucoidan, for instance, is a sulfated polysaccharide derived from brown algae that has exhibited anticancer activity through the induction of apoptosis and inhibition of tumor cell proliferation (Bhuyan et al. 2023; Elfeky and Qenawi 2024). Not only do these bioactive properties facilitate the direct delivery of cancer therapeutics, but they also influence the immune system to boost, potentially, the body's natural defenses against tumor growth. Hence, the incorporation of polysaccharides derived from marine algae within anticancer drug delivery systems holds great promise as an opportunity for the development of safer and more effective cancer treatment options.

2 Marine Algae Polysaccharides: Types and Properties

2.1 Classification of Polysaccharides

Polysaccharides derived from seaweeds are a prominent form of natural polymer. These natural polymers can be classified into two specific types of polysaccharides based on their function and location in the seaweed: the cell-wall polysaccharides and the storage polysaccharides. This type of classification suggests the functional and structural aspects of polysaccharides that enable the survival, growth, and reproduction of the algal organism. Algal polysaccharides are predominantly cell-wall polysaccharides, wherein the cell wall provides structural support and protection properties. Contrasting with cell-wall polymers, storage carbohydrates are mainly found in plastids for energy storage (Şahin 2021). Cell-wall polysaccharides are the main class of chemicals found in seaweed and are key for preserving the structural integrity of the algae. As cell-wall polysaccharides, they serve a vital purpose as a form of support and protection from mechanical stress or loss of water. Classifications of cell-wall polysaccharides in seaweed are typically defined as alginate, carrageenan, agar, and ulvan. These polysaccharides are critical in allowing physical properties of seaweeds such as gel formation, thickening ability, and water retention (Synytsya et al. 2015). Alginate, which is found in brown algae, is widely used for its gelling properties and its ability to form a matrix for controlled drug release systems (Łabowska et al. 2019). Carrageenans are a class of biopolymers that are commonly present in red seaweed. In food products, commercial carrageenans have long been utilized as thickening, gelling, stabilizing, and emulsifying agents. It is believed that carrageenans are bioactive polysaccharides with disease-modifying and microbiota-modulating activities (Liu et al. 2023). Likewise, agar is a red algae-derived gelling agent that is widely utilized in microbiological media, food products, and as a stabilizer in the cosmetic industry (Ganjoo et al. 2023). Ulvan, a sulfated polysaccharide from green algae, has demonstrated a range of biological properties, including antiviral, antibacterial, anticancer, anti-inflammatory, and antioxidant properties (Mo'o et al. 2020). On the other hand, storage polysaccharides are located primarily in the plastids and serve as energy and carbon reserves. These polysaccharides will be stored within the cell for times when the algae need energy, such as during times of low light or when conditions limit photosynthesis. The storage

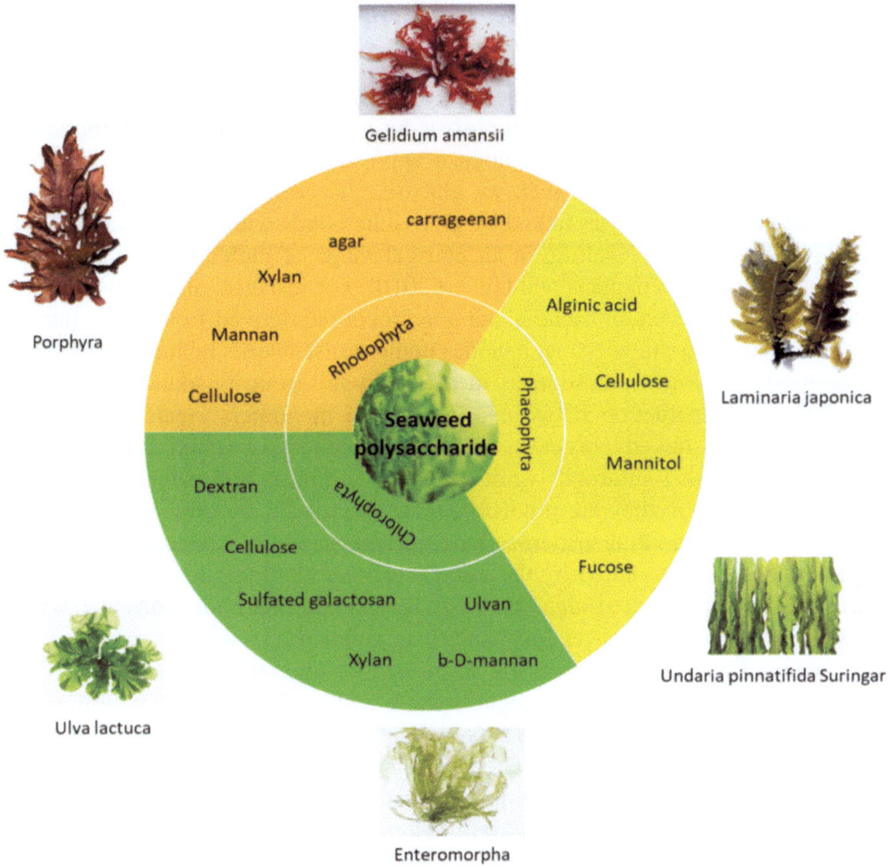

Fig. 1 The major kinds of algae and their products (seaweed polysaccharides). (Reproduced from Zhong et al. (2020) under the terms and conditions of the Creative Commons Attribution (CC BY) license http://creativecommons.org/licenses/by/4.0/)

polysaccharide that is best recognized in seaweeds is laminarin and floridean starch. Laminarin, a β-glucan in brown algae, is the main energy reserve and can be hydrolyzed back to glucose when needed by the algae (Kadam et al. 2015). Floridean starch (found in red algae) is similar in structure to starch in land plants and is utilized for energy storage. The seaweed's ability to store carbohydrates in the form of polysaccharide allows it to survive and grow in variable environments (Yu et al. 2021). Seaweed polysaccharides come in a variety of forms from various sources and are categorized as Rhodophyta, Fucophyta, Chlorophyta, and others. Figure 1 shows the major kinds of algae and their products (Zhong et al. 2020).

2.2 Structural and Chemical Properties

The structural and chemical characteristics of the polysaccharides derived from marine sources are important for the diversity of their functional and application potential in both industrial and biological applications. Polysaccharides are made from monosaccharide units, such as glucose, galactose, mannose, fucose, and xylose. Monosaccharides are linked by glycosidic bonds with different orientations and types of linkages, resulting in an unusual range of molecular structures with different properties (Vilaplana and Gilbert 2010). For instance, alginate is an extracellular polymer of certain bacteria and a hydrocolloid derived from algae, particularly brown algae, a category that includes numerous seaweeds including kelps. One of the most well-known substances in the hydrogel group is sodium alginate. A straightforward interaction between one or more monomers creates hydrogel, a network of cross-linked polymers which is expanded by water. It is based on d-mannuronic and l-guluronic acids and has a linear (unbranched) structure. Depending on where they are produced, these monomers are arranged in random, sequential, and alternating patterns. This polysaccharide's chemical and physical characteristics can be altered by the same monomer configuration (Abka-khajouei et al. 2022). Similarly, red algae-derived carrageenan is a high molecular weight linear polymer made up of repeated galactose units and 3,6-anhydrogalactose (3,6 AG), both sulfated and non-sulfated, connected by alternating α-(1,3) and β-(1,4) glycosidic bonds. The most straightforward and well-known alteration is the so-called alkaline treatment, which is only feasible in carrageenans with ß-D-galactose 6-sulfate units, as they increase the gelling characteristics of the polysaccharide by converting these units into 3,6-anhydrogalactose. The change in the negative charge such as oxidation at C-6, desulfation, or oversulfation can significantly influence its biological activity and physicochemical properties Cosenza et al. 2016; McArdle and Hamill 2011). Agar, also a polysaccharide derived from red algae, consists of agarose and agaropectin, with agarose being the principal active agent credited with its gelling properties (Pandya et al. 2022). Besides their fundamental structure, polysaccharides identified in marine algae can have several chemical modifications (sulfation, acetylation, and esterification), which alter their solubility, viscosity, and functionality. These modifications can not only improve gel-forming capacity but also influence water-holding ability and bioactivity. For instance, sulfation of polysaccharides such as fucans and carrageenans has been related to their biological activities, such as antioxidant, antimicrobial, and antiviral properties. Further, the characteristics of these polysaccharides, which also describe the size distribution of their respective polymer chains, specifically, molecular weight and polydispersity, will affect their physical properties as well. In general, polysaccharides with a higher average molecular weight have been associated with higher solution viscosity and stronger gel formation, both of which are important in food products, drug delivery systems, and industrial processes (Pomin and Mourão 2008; Sharma et al. 2024). Together, the unique structural and chemical features of polysaccharides from marine algae represent an important resource and can be utilized in multiple sectors, including food, pharmaceuticals, biotechnology, and cosmetics. Their unique capacity to interact with water, create gels, and display biological activities has resulted in their wide use in various industries, ranging from thickening and stabilizing agents in food, developing biocompatible materials, and using topical applications in cosmetic and medicinal formulations. Understanding these characteristics will be instrumental in future applications and will enhance our ability to use marine algae polysaccharides (Flórez-Fernández et al. 2017).

2.3 Biological Activities Relevant to Cancer Therapy

Polysaccharides from marine algae have attracted a great deal of interest for cancer treatment due to their biological activities, including the potential to inhibit cancer growth, promote apoptosis, modulate the immune response, and enhance the efficacy of other therapies. These polysaccharides such as fucoidans, alginate, carrageenan, and agar possess unique chemical structures and bioactivities that contribute to their effectiveness. The therapeutic potential of polysaccharides is likely a result of the interactions of polysaccharides with cellular pathways, including immune cells and components of the extracellular matrix, which make them good candidates for alternative or adjunct cancer therapies. Algal-derived polysaccharides have demonstrated anticancer properties in both in vitro and in vivo conditions. The anticancer properties of algal polysaccharides are attributed to the following mechanisms: (1) cell cycle arrest, (2) mitochondrial membrane depolarization, (3) nitric oxide generation, (4) immune system activation against cancer cells, and (5) tumor apoptosis (Vaikundamoorthy et al. 2018). In the area of immune modulation and antitumor activity, a number of polysaccharides produced from marine algae, including fucoidans (i.e., sulfated polysaccharides derived from brown algae), have been shown to enhance immune system function, an integral component of the body's defense against cancer. In particular, fucoidans are capable of promoting the immune response by stimulating the production of immune-related molecules (e.g., cytokines) and activating macrophages, natural killer (NK) cells, and dendritic cells. Overall, immune modulation allows the body to more effectively combat cancer cells and disrupt tumor growth and metastasis. However, fucoidans have also been shown to increase the phagocytic activity of immune cells, increase tumor identification, and enhance the cytotoxic activity of immune cells—all of which contribute to reducing tumor growth and spread (Li et al. 2023).

Induction of apoptosis. Apoptosis, also known as programmed cell death, is an essential target in cancer treatment, as it enables the removal of abnormal or cancerous cells with minimal harm to surrounding healthy tissue. Polysaccharides from marine algae, specifically carrageenans and fucoidans, have shown the ability to induce cancer cell death in cancer cell lines through apoptosis. Carrageenans have been shown to induce cancer cell death through the activation of the apoptotic program in the mitochondria leading to DNA fragmentation and, consequently, the activation of caspases. Fucoidans have also been shown to modulate key regulatory proteins that control the mitochondrial pathway-regulated apoptotic program, such as Bcl-2 and Bax. In addition, the ability of these polysaccharides to sensitize cancer cells to drug-induced apoptosis may enhance the efficacy of conventional agents of chemotherapeutic cancer treatments (Duan et al. 2020; Jazzara et al. 2016).

Inhibition of tumor angiogenesis. Angiogenesis (the generation of new blood vessels) is a critical aspect of tumor growth and metastasis. Angiogenesis allows tumors to grow and metastasize by providing oxygen and nutrients to proliferating cancer cells. Marine algae polysaccharides (particularly alginate and fucoidans) have shown antiangiogenic properties because they can interfere with the signaling pathways of angiogenesis. For example, fucoidans can inhibit the vascular endothelial growth factor (VEGF) pathway, which is necessary for generating new blood vessels in tumors. By inhibiting angiogenesis, these polysaccharides limit the size of tumors and their potential to metastasize, making them an interesting opportunity for cancer therapy (Ferreira et al. 2017; Matou-Nasri et al. 2002). Metastasis, or the spreading of cancer cells from the primary tumor to distant sites in the body, is one of the main contributors to cancer-related deaths. Marine algal polysaccharides (especially fucoidans and carrageenans) have been shown to disrupt cancer cell adhesion, migration, and invasion, which are all important steps in the metastatic process. Fucoidans have also been shown to induce changes in the expression of adhesion molecules and matrix metalloproteinases (MMPs) that are involved in the breakdown of the extracellular matrix and promote directional movement of cancer cells. These polysaccharides, then, may be beneficial not only to slow the advancement of cancer but also to hinder recurrences post-treatment (Calvo et al. 2019; Lee and Seyedian 2012). Oxidative stress is strongly associated with cancer initiation and progression in part due to chronic inflammation. Marine algae polysaccharides possess antioxidant and anti-inflammatory properties that may inhibit cancer; for example, alginate has been shown to scavenge free radicals and reduce oxidative injury to macromolecules, including DNA, proteins, and lipids, which can lead to carcinogenesis (Tusi et al. 2011). In addition, the anti-inflammatory properties of marine algae polysaccharides, such as fucoidans and carrageenans, are attributed to their ability to regulate the expression of inflammatory cytokines and inflammatory mediators, including cycloxygenase-2 (COX-2) and nitrous oxide synthase (iNOS), both of which are associated with tumorigenesis. With regard to cancer prevention, the polysaccharides mentioned have the potential to mitigate inflammation and oxidative stress, reduce cancer risk, and improve the therapeutic effects of conventional treatments (Komisarska et al. 2024; Mensah et al. 2023).

Synergistic effects with standard therapies. Marine algae polysaccharides have been shown to work synergistically with standard cancer drugs such as chemotherapy and radiation. Polysaccharides such as fucoidans and carrageenans can sensitize cancer cells to chemotherapy agents, thereby enhancing drug effectiveness and leading to a greater therapeutic impact. This may allow for reduced dosing, thereby minimizing side effects. In addition, the polysaccharides' immune modulatory and apoptotic pathway regulatory effects can act in concert with other therapeutic agents. Polysaccharides derived from marine algae exhibit synergistic effects and represent a promising addition to standard treatment regimens by aiding in the management of chemoresistant tumors and enhancing overall therapeutic efficacy of standard treatment (Atashrazm et al. 2015; Elfeky et al. 2024; Ping-Hsiu et al. 2019).

3 Mechanisms of Action in Cancer Treatment

3.1 Anticancer Properties of Marine Polysaccharides

Marine algae polysaccharides have been recognized as a plentiful source of bioactive compounds with potent anticancer activities, which has attracted a lot of attention to their potential in cancer chemoprevention and treatment. Primarily derived from brown, red, and green macroalgae, these polysaccharides—fucoidan, carrageenan, alginate, laminarin, and ulvan exert anticancer properties based on their impact on various biological mechanisms that target multiple cancer hallmarks (Ouyang et al. 2021). Not surprisingly, one of the highlighted mechanisms relates to their induction of programmed cell death, known as apoptosis. This process can occur via the intrinsic (mitochondria-mediated) or extrinsic (death receptor-mediated) apoptotic pathways, both of which are characterized by caspase activation, cytochrome c release, and alterations in apoptosis-related proteins (e.g., Bcl-2 and Bax). One example is fucoidan induction of caspase-3 and caspase-9; loss of mitochondrial membrane potential; and increased DNA fragmentation in tumor cells, processes that lead to apoptosis while sparing normal cells from significant harm (Kokoulin et al. 2025). Besides inducing apoptosis, marine polysaccharides also perform a significant role in inducing cell cycle arrest, which is important in anticancer activity. The polysaccharides can regulate cyclin-dependent kinases (CDKs) and their cyclin regulators, which regulate the checkpoint for cell cycle arrest, primarily the G0/G1 or G2/M phases, to momentarily inhibit cancer cell proliferation and prevent the replication of damaged DNA and hyperproliferation (Dalisay et al. 2024). In addition, certain polysaccharides exhibit an antiangiogenic effect by inhibiting the formation of new blood vessels that tumors need to obtain oxygen and nutrients. They achieve this by downregulating pro-angiogenic factors, which include vascular endothelial growth factor (VEGF) and its receptors, thereby disrupting the vascular network that supports tumor growth and metastasis (Banerjee et al. 2023). Polysaccharides derived from marine macroalgae also exhibit effective anti-metastatic functions by inhibiting matrix metalloproteinases (MMPs), particularly MMP-2 and MMP-9, enzymes responsible for degrading the extracellular matrix and aiding in cancer cell invasion and migration. By maintaining tissue integrity and reducing cancer cell dissemination, these polysaccharides may assist in managing metastasis, which is one of the leading causes of cancer-related deaths (Zheng et al. 2022). The polysaccharides enhance both innate and adaptive immune responses by activating macrophages, dendritic cells, T-lymphocytes, and natural killer (NK) cells. This is mediated through increased production of several cytokines (e.g., IL-2, IFN-γ, TNF-α), which play key roles in effectively targeting and destroying cancer cells (Shen et al. 2024). Additionally, these compounds exhibit pronounced antioxidant capacities, which, in turn, aid in the scavenging of free radicals and in reducing oxidative stress—factors known to cause DNA damage, mutation, and ultimately the initiation of cancer. Laminarin, for example, and ulvan have been shown to lower reactive oxygen species (ROS) levels intracellularly, protecting cells from oxidative damage (Michalak et al. 2022). In the context of chemotherapy, polysaccharides from marine algae exhibit chemo-sensitizing properties, enhancing the efficacy of traditional anticancer agents (e.g., cisplatin, doxorubicin, and paclitaxel). In some cases, they achieve this by lowering drug-resistance pathways, improving drug uptake in cancer cells, and downregulating multidrug resistance proteins. These effects allow for more efficacious treatment at reduced doses, thereby reducing side effects on normal components (Taghipour et al. 2025). In conclusion, polysaccharides extracted from marine algae induce anticancer effects through multiple mechanisms, including apoptosis induction, cell cycle arrest, inhibition of angiogenesis and metastasis, altered immune responses, decreasing oxidative stress, and synergistic effects on chemotherapeutic agents. Due to their natural origin, biocompatibility, and multi-targeted actions, they are ideal candidate agents for use or testing as part of a multimodal cancer treatment approach. Expanding research and numerous examples support the use of these unique marine-derived polysaccharides as integrative cancer therapies through the identification of additional applications and molecular targets.

3.2 Interaction with Cancer Cells: Apoptosis and Inhibition of Metastasis

Polysaccharides from marine algae engage in cancer cells via a number of molecular and cellular mechanisms that all contribute to their anticancer activity. These mechanisms include the induction of programmed cell death (apoptosis), inhibition of cell proliferation and metastasis, modulation of cell signaling pathways, and adjustment of the tumor microenvironment. The selective activity of marine polysaccharides to target tumor cells and non-normal cells makes them very attractive as chemopreventive and therapeutic agents in cancer.

3.3 Induction of Apoptosis

Programmed cell death is a highly regulated biological process that is often dysregulated by cancer cells, leading to uncontrolled proliferation and tumor progression. Several marine polysaccharides, especially fucoidan, laminarin, and carrageenan, have demonstrated their capacity to induce apoptosis through intrinsic (mitochondrial) and extrinsic (death receptor) pathways. Both intrinsic and extrinsic mechanisms can carry out the controlled cell-killing process known as apoptosis.

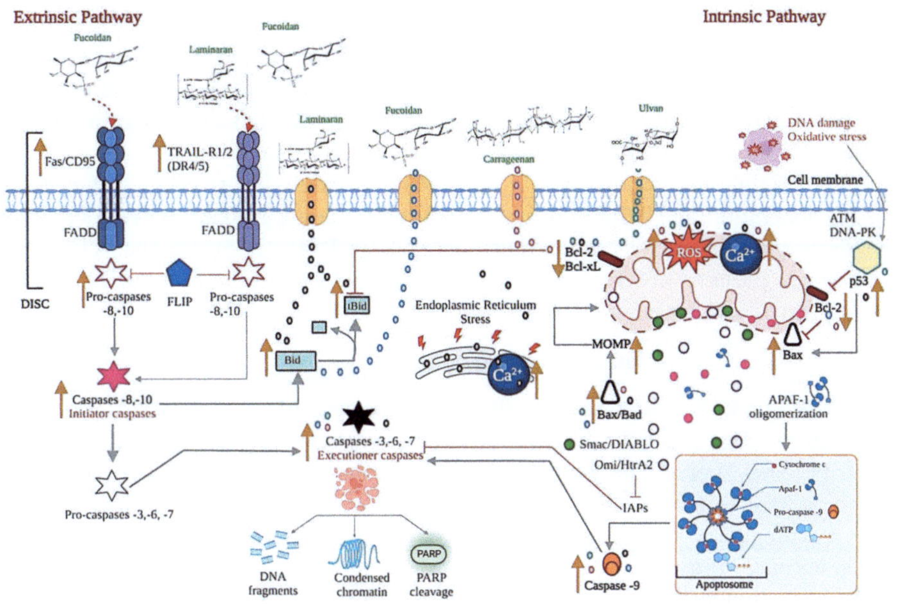

Fig. 2 The intrinsic and extrinsic apoptotic mechanisms are illustrated. (Reproduced from Agena et al. (2023) under the terms and conditions of the Creative Commons Attribution (CC BY) license http://creativecommons.org/licenses/by/4.0/)

However, one crucial molecular component of carcinogenesis is avoiding death through many means. Thus, one of the primary goals of cancer treatment is to induce apoptosis. The most important targets of both apoptosis pathways are thought to be death receptors, adaptor proteins, FLIP, NF-κB, pro- and anti-apoptotic proteins of the B cell lymphoma (Bcl)-2 family, intracellular ROS and Ca^{2+} levels, mitochondrial membrane permeability, p53, and initiator and effector caspases. In Fig. 2, The intrinsic and extrinsic apoptotic mechanisms. External stimuli or ligand molecules, especially those involving death receptors, initiate the extrinsic route. The creation of Bax/Bak pores in the mitochondrial membrane mediates the intrinsic route. Following its release, cytochrome cis joins forces with procaspase-9 and apoptotic protease activating factor-1 (Apaf-1) to form the apoptosome. In order to activate executioner caspases-3, -6, and -7, both pathways converge (Agena et al. 2023).

Intrinsic Pathway Activation

The intrinsic, also known as mitochondrial, apoptotic pathway is a primary apoptotic system by which polysaccharides derived from marine algae promote programmed cell death in cancer cells. The intrinsic apoptotic pathway is under the tight control of cellular signals mainly modulated by cellular damage (i.e., DNA damage, oxidative stress, activation of oncogenes, and other signals) that occurs inside the cell. Marine polysaccharides such as fucoidan, laminarin, and carrageenan have been well studied for their mechanisms of triggering intrinsic apoptosis specifically in tumor cells.

- Mitochondrial membrane permeabilization

A defining feature of the intrinsic apoptotic pathway is the Δψm loss of mitochondrial membrane potential, which results in the export of pro-apoptotic factors from the intermembrane space to the cytosol. Polysaccharides derived from marine algae, particularly fucoidan, are able to induce mitochondrial injury. This is achieved by depolarizing the mitochondrial membrane through reactive oxygen species (ROS) generation and inhibiting anti-apoptotic proteins. It also involves opening the mitochondrial permeability transition pore (mPTP), allowing the release of several key proteins involved in apoptosis such as cytochrome c, Smac/DIABLO, and apoptosis-inducing factor (AIF) (Yang et al. 2013).

- Regulation of Bcl-2 family proteins

Marine algae polysaccharides affect the balance of pro-apoptotic and anti-apoptotic proteins of the Bcl-2 family, which are primary regulators of mitochondrial integrity. They upregulate pro-apoptotic proteins, including Bax, Bak, and Bid, which promote mitochondrial outer membrane permeabilization (MOMP). They also downregulate anti-apoptotic proteins, including Bcl-2, Bcl-xL, and Mcl-1, which normally provide mitochondrial integrity and inhibit apoptosis. For example, it has been shown that treatment with fucoidan results in an increased Bax/Bcl-2 ratio, which favors apoptosis in several tumors (breast, lung, colon, and liver) (Matin et al. 2024).

- Cytochrome c release and apoptosome formation

When cytochrome c is released into the cytosol, it cooperates with apoptotic protease activating factor-1 (Apaf-1) and polymerizing dATP to form the apoptosome. This multiprotein complex leads to caspase-9 activation, which subsequently activates executioner caspases (including caspase-3 and caspase-7). Marine polysaccharides, such as laminarin and fucoidan, appear to increase caspase-9 and caspase-3 activity, leading to the execution phase of apoptosis characterized by DNA fragmentation, chromatin condensation, and cell membrane blebbing (Liu et al. 2016).

- Production of reactive oxygen species (ROS)

Many polysaccharides found in marine sources trigger intrinsic apoptosis via increased accumulation of intracellular ROS levels. Accumulation of excessive ROS leads to a dysregulation of redox homeostasis and damage to mitochondrial membranes. Consequences include the oxidation of cardiolipin, a mitochondrial lipid that tethers cytochrome c, thereby facilitating its release. The phosphorylation and activation of stress kinases JNK and p38 MAPK modify pro-apoptotic signaling proteins, such as Bax and Bcl-2. These changes enhance death signals that directly lead to neurologic dysfunction of mitochondria. The contribution of fucoidan to ROS accumulation and increased ROS levels has been observed in cancer models (HepG2, MCF-7, and HL-60 cells), thereby supporting an association between oxidative stress and fucoidan's anticancer efficacy (Fitton et al. 2015; Thinh et al. 2013).

- Caspase cascade activation

Activation of the caspase cascade is the endpoint of the intrinsic pathway and is a series of cysteine proteases that deconstruct cellular material into smaller proteins. Caspase-9 is the initiator caspase inside the apoptosome. Caspase-3 and caspase-7 are received downstream from caspase-9, wherein they cleave critical structural and repair proteins, such as poly(ADP-ribose) polymerase (PARP), DNA-PK, and lamins (Park et al. 2013).

Marine algae polysaccharides such as fucoidan, laminarin, and carrageenan initiate intrinsic apoptosis by interfering with mitochondrial function, modifying Bcl-2 family proteins, increasing intracellular ROS levels, and instigating the caspase cascade. Each of these processes leads to the selective elimination of cancer cells, making marine polysaccharides particularly appealing in the development of nontoxic anticancer therapeutic agents. Their use as direct agents in targeting the mitochondria—understood to be a known point of weakness in a number of tumors—makes them promising agents in an integrative approach to oncology.

Extrinsic Pathway Activation

- Death receptor upregulation

The extrinsic pathway starts by the binding of the extracellular death ligands to their respective transmembrane death receptors. Some examples of these death receptors are Fas (CD95/APO-1), tumor necrosis factor receptor 1 (TNFR1), and TRAIL receptors (DR4 and DR5). Some marine algae polysaccharides have been shown to increase the expression of death receptors on the surface of tumor cells, leading to increased apoptotic susceptibility. For instance, fucoidan enhanced the expression of Fas and DR5 in leukemia (HL-60), breast (MCF-7), and colon cancer (HCT-15) cells, sensitizing them to apoptosis through FasL or TRAIL. In some cancers, ulvan and carrageenan also show increased levels of the Fas receptor, where extrinsic apoptosis pathways can be triggered (Ercolano et al. 2019; Lin et al. 2020).

- Formation of death-inducing signaling complex (DISC)

After receptor engagement, the receptor's intracellular death domain (DD) recruits the adaptor protein FADD (Fas-associated death domain) which recruits procaspase-8 to form the DISC. Marine polysaccharides aid this process by: (1) enhancing the expression of FADD and facilitating the recruitment of procaspase-8 to promote DISC assembly and (2) causing conformational changes that promote the critical autocatalytic cleavage and activation of procaspase-8 to caspase-8, initiating the apoptotic signaling cascade. For example, fucoidan has modified and treated cancer cells to efficiently exhibit substantially increased levels of activated (cleaved) caspase-8, a key initiator caspase protein in downstream apoptotic signaling (Kim et al. 2010; Senthilkumar and Se-Kwon 2013).

- Activation of the caspase cascade

Activated caspase-8 leads to the execution phase of apoptosis through two key steps: (1) direct activation of executioner caspases (e.g., caspase-3 and caspase-7) that proteolytically cleave intracellular substrates and (2) interaction or cross-talk with the intrinsic pathway by cleaving Bid, a pro-apoptotic member of the Bcl-2 family, leading to truncated Bid (tBid) moving to the mitochondrial membrane, promoting cytochrome c release and amplifying the mitochondrial-mediated apoptotic pathway. Further, marine algae polysaccharides have been shown to facilitate Bid cleavage in cancer cells, encouraging a link between extra- and intrinsic apoptotic pathways and enhancing the death signal overall (Yamasaki et al. 2009).

- Strategies to overcome apoptotic resistance in cancer cells

Resistance to apoptosis has been a difficult barrier in cancer therapies and can arise from multiple causes, including reduced expression of death receptors; increased expression of FLIP (FLICE-like inhibitory protein), which prevents caspase-8 activation; and inhibition of caspases by IAP (inhibitor of apoptosis) proteins. Marine algae polysaccharides can overcome these resistances by restoring the expression of death receptors; downregulating/downmodulating anti-apoptotic proteins, i.e., FLIP and survivin; and sensitizing tumor cells to TRAIL and FasL, which are natural ligands that elicit death receptor-mediated apoptosis (Tamzi et al. 2024).

- Selective targeting of cancer cells

Selectivity is a noteworthy aspect of marine polysaccharide-mediated extrinsic apoptosis. They induce death receptor activation and promote caspase pathways in cancer cells, but generally, they have little effect on normal, healthy cells. This selective toxicity may be due to the enhanced expression of death receptors and decoy receptors in tumor and cancer cells, respectively, in addition to tumor cell's redox state that sensitizes them to death signaling (Kokoulin et al. 2025).

3.3.1 Inhibition of Cell Proliferation

Marine polysaccharides generate antiproliferative effects by blocking the cell cycle in different phases (G0/G1, S, or G2/M) and can do so according to the polysaccharide and the cancer cell type.

- *Cell cycle arrest*

Marine algae polysaccharides have had promising effects concerning cell cycle arrest, specifically in cancer research. It has been shown that sulfated polysaccharides derived from marine algae such as *Laurencia papillosa* can inhibit the proliferation of cancer cells by depositing the cells in the G1 phase. This involves the upregulation of Cip1/p21 and Kip1/p27 (predominant cell cycle regulators) as well as the downregulation of cyclins D1, D2, and E1 together with the ale cyclin-dependent kinases (Murad et al. 2016). Marine algae also contain bioactive compounds that can engage apoptosis and selective cytotoxicity toward cancer cell lines.

The unique chemical diversity of marine algae makes them candidates for anticancer drug development (Nurkolis et al. 2024).

- *Anti-telomerase activity*

The polysaccharides of marine algae have been proposed as a source of potential anti-telomerase activity, which is of particular relevance in cancer research. Cancer is a leading cause of death worldwide. Telomerase, an intracellular maintenance enzyme for telomeres, allows cancer cells to evade the natural aging process of a cell. In normal cells, telomeres shorten during replication until they reach a critical length. For this reason, telomerase activity is a hallmark of cancer cells, which can continue to replicate indefinitely. While there has only been limited investigation of marine algae extracts, the extract of *Caulerpa sertularioides* has shown telomerase inhibition in leukemia cells. Marine algae extracts are also being investigated for their antitumor effects. As an example, research has suggested that marine algae crude extracts can induce apoptosis in cancer cells while inhibiting growth or proliferation compared to control conditions. The distinct biophysical characteristics and unique repertoire of bioactive compounds found in marine algae make them promising candidates for the development of novel cancer therapies to combat cancer (Alves et al. 2018; Kanegawa et al. 2000).

3.3.2 Inhibition of Metastasis and Invasion

Marine-derived polysaccharides inhibit metastatic activity through multiple methods of action:

- *Suppression of matrix metalloproteinases (MMPs)*

Marine algae polysaccharides have exhibited encouraging potential for the suppression of matrix metalloproteinases (MMPs), with importance placed specifically on MMP-2 and MMP-9, as they are associated with cancer progression, inflammation, and tissue degradation. For example, *Sargassum horneri*, a type of brown seaweed, demonstrated anti-MMP activity by inhibiting the activity of MMPs against fibrosarcoma cells. *Sargassum horneri* algae extracts inhibited MMP-2 and MMP-9 enzymatic activities, reduced cell migration, and inhibited mRNA and protein expression. Another study reported an inhibitory heptameric peptide from the marine microalga *Pavlova lutheri*, which suppressed the secretion of MMP-9 by inactivating the JNK and p38 pathways with respect to NF-kB in fibrosarcoma cells (Karadeniz et al. 2018; Ko et al. 2018).

- *Inhibition of epithelial-mesenchymal transition (EMT)*

Marine algae polysaccharides have been shown to inhibit epithelial-mesenchymal transition (EMT), a significant process to cancer metastasis and progression. The change allows the epithelial cells to become mesenchymal-like cells which have greater mobility and capacity to invade. Polysaccharides derived from marine algae demonstrated anti-cellular features with respect to EMT by employing multiple types of signaling pathways, including TGF-β, Wnt/β-catenin, and NF-κB2. In one study, fucoidan, a sulfated polysaccharide derived from brown algae, was effective in reversing or inhibiting EMT by reducing the transcription factors Snail, Slug, and Twist. Various marine algae extracts also inhibited the activity of MMP-9, thereby inhibiting cancer cell migration (Kozak et al. 2021; Manfioletti and Fedele 2023).

3.3.3 Antiangiogenic Effects

Tumor proliferation and metastasis rely on the development of new blood vessels or angiogenesis. Some polysaccharides derived from marine organisms prevent angiogenesis by interrupting signaling pathways of angiogenic signaling molecules.

- *VEGF suppression*

Marine algae polysaccharides, especially fucoidan, exhibit the capacity to suppress VEGF which is an important component of antiangiogenic cancer therapies. VEGF (vascular endothelial growth factor) is a key factor in the growth of blood vessels, allowing the tumor to receive nutrients as it grows. Evidence suggests that fucoidan, extracted out of brown algae (*Fucus vesiculosus*), can slow down or inhibit the expression of VEGF and, in turn, inhibit angiogenesis and tumor growth (Kalimuthu Senthilkumar and Kim 2015). In addition, studies have developed enzyme-assisted exaction techniques that improve sanguineous extraction of marine algae polysaccharides, thereby enhancing anticancer and anti-inflammatory bioactivities (Lakmal H. H. Chamindaand Lee 2015). Other studies note a much broader category of anticancer mechanisms exhibited by marine polysaccharides, including, but not limited to, inducing apoptosis and preventing metastasis (Fedorov et al. 2013).

- *Inhibition of endothelial cell migration and tube formation*

Polysaccharides sourced from marine algae are capable of attenuating endothelial cell migration and tube formation, both of which are pivotal processes in the development of new blood vessels or angiogenesis. Some reports have demonstrated that carotenoids from marine algae such as fucoxanthin and siphonaxanthin inhibit fibroblast growth factor 2 (FGF-2) signaling, which diminishes migration and differentiation of endothelial cells into tube-like structures. Additionally, marine algae-derived compounds have been shown to exert antitumor effects by disrupting cell invasion and angiogenesis (Ganesan et al. 2013).

3.3.4 Modulation of Signaling Pathways

There are multiple intracellular signaling pathways that are routinely altered in cancer cells and are impacted by marine algae polysaccharides:

- *MAPK/ERK and PI3K/Akt pathways*

Polysaccharides from algae have the potential to modulate the MAPK/ERK and PI3K/Akt signaling pathways, both of which are key players in inflammation, cell survival, and cell proliferation. *Endarachne binghamiae*, a marine brown algae, may temporarily downregulate MAPK and PI3K/Akt and inhibit the inflammatory response. These pathways are of growing interest in the area of cancer treatment, and marine extracts have been documented to modulate MAPK signaling and inhibit tumor progression (Lee et al. 2025; Wei et al. 2021).

- *NF-κB pathway*

Polysaccharides derived from marine algae can regulate the NF-κB signaling pathway, which is important in inflammation and immunity; other evidence suggests that polysaccharides from *Enteromorpha prolifera* can inhibit the activation of NF-κB, alleviating oxidative stress and inflammatory responses. More specifically, animal studies have shown that supplementation with *Enteromorpha prolifera* polysaccharides resulted in lower levels of pro-inflammatory cytokines (Liu et al. 2022). Furthermore, marine algae-derived metabolites have shown potential for anticancer applications, modulating NF-κB signaling to suppress tumor progression (Sharma et al. 2023).

- *STAT3 inhibition*

Polysaccharides from marine algae are now being investigated for their ability to attenuate the STAT3 signaling associated with cancer progression and inflammation, as well regulation of the immune system. Some studies have suggested that marine algal compounds are able to reduce the risk of increased cancer risk and degree of inflammatory response by influencing STAT3 activation (De Jesus Raposo et al. 2015). For example, one study showed that sulfated polysaccharides from macroalgae were able to induce anti-inflammatory effects by targeting STAT3-mediated mechanisms (de Sousa et al. 2023). Marine algal nanoparticles have also been studied for their ability to facilitate site-specific drug delivery, suggesting that drugs delivered with marine algal nanoparticles could more effectively inhibit the activation of STAT3 in (1) cancer therapy and (2) inflammatory responses (Ramu Arunkumar and Ahmed 2021).

3.3.5 Tumor Microenvironment Modulation

The tumor microenvironment (TME) consists of stromal cells, immune cells, and elements from the extracellular matrix that help to support tumor progression. Marine polysaccharides modulate the TME in a variety of ways:

- *Immune activation*

Polysaccharides derived from marine algae have exhibited potential immune system-strengthening properties, especially in macrophage activation and cytokine regulation. The immune-enhancing effects of extracts from *Sargassum horneri*, *Sargassum fusiforme*, and *Undaria pinnatifida* have been investigated, demonstrating their ability to initiate macrophage proliferation under normoxic conditions and to increase the expression of immune-related cytokines, including IL-1β, TNF-α, and IL-6 (Sanjay et al. 2024). Furthermore, the polysaccharides derived from *Enteromorpha prolifera* have also altered the gut microbiota, contributing to immune health (Wassie et al. 2021).

- *Macrophage polarization*

Polysaccharides derived from certain marine algae can modulate macrophage polarization consequential to the regulation of immune response and the control of inflammation. In vitro experiments indicate that extracts of *Sargassum horneri*, *Sargassum fusiforme*, and *Undaria pinnatifida* may cause macrophage activation and cytokine expression, impacting the macrophage's polarization into either pro-inflammatory (M1) or anti-inflammatory (M2) macrophages (Sanjay et al. 2024). In addition, sulfated polysaccharides derived from red algae (*Gelidium crinale*) have been shown to exert anti-inflammatory effects by suppressing oxidative stress and the production of inflammatory cytokine in macrophages (Pei et al. 2021).

3.4 Synergistic Effects with Existing Therapies

Marine algae polysaccharides interact with cancer cells and their surrounding tissues, often called the tumor microenvironment (TME), through various mechanisms, including inducing apoptosis, preventing metastasis, suppressing angiogenesis, and modulating important intracellular pathways. Marine polysaccharides tend to interact selectively with cancer cells, which is favorable for potentially limiting the effects on normal tissues. As such, marine polysaccharides have the potential to become an adjunct or alternative treatment for solid tumors by improving therapeutic efficacy while lessening adverse effects. Marine algae polysaccharides have exhibited synergistic properties when used with current therapies. Their potential to enhance studies, particularly in cancer treatment, immune activation/modulation, and antimicrobial resistance, is particularly compelling. Specifically, evidence suggests that marine polysaccharides can improve the efficiency of chemotherapy and radiation therapy through mechanisms that reduce drug resistance and enhance tumor suppression (Lee et al. 2017; Qenawi et al. 2025). These marine polysaccharides, including fucoidan and carrageenan, have anti-inflammatory and immunomodulatory properties; as such, polysaccharides derived from marine algae can serve as useful adjuncts in the treatment of various autoimmune diseases and infections (Sharma et al. 2023). Moreover, marine algae offer diverse biomedical applications, including the use of marine algae-derived compounds in drug delivery systems that can improve the bioavailability of drugs administered through conventional methods (Negreanu-Pirjol et al. 2022; Qenawi et al. 2025). In the context of drug combinations, marine algae-derived polysaccharides demonstrate potential to act on common signaling pathways, such as NF-κB, STAT3, and PI3K/Akt, supporting their role in the development of combination therapy strategies.

4 Polysaccharides in Drug Delivery Systems

4.1 Role as Carriers for Anticancer Drugs

Polysaccharides derived from marine algae have strong potential as carriers for anticancer drugs due to their biodegradability, biocompatibility, and ability to enhance drug stability and delivery. Polysaccharides and their roles in tumor-targeted drug delivery systems include the following:

- Controlled release: Polysaccharides such as fucoidan, alginate, and carrageenan can influence/modulate the release of anticancer drug and sustain their delivery to tumor sites (Cui et al. 2024).
- Targeted drug delivery: Some polysaccharides from marine sources exhibit the ability to bind to receptors that are overexpressed on cancer cells, which can increase drug accumulation at the tumor site (Kuznetsova et al. 2020).
- Nanoparticle-based carriers: Nanoparticle drug carriers based on marine polysaccharides have been created to increase drug solubility and bioavailability while reducing side effects (Dalavi Pandurang Appana and Venkatesan 2020).
- Immunomodulation: Some marine algal polysaccharides have anti-inflammatory and/or immunomodulatory properties that could benefit cancer therapy by reducing inflammation associated with the tumor (Kuznetsova et al. 2020).

4.2 Types of Delivery Systems: Nanoparticles, Hydrogels, and Capsules

Marine algae-derived polysaccharides are being researched for advanced drug delivery systems due to their natural origin, versatile structures, biocompatibility, and functional properties. Their research value in drug delivery systems is especially pronounced in the direction of anticancer drug delivery because of their intrinsic ability to encapsulate therapeutic agents and target sites for controlled release. Figure 3 emphasizes the utilization of marine polysaccharides as building blocks for drug delivery systems (Cardoso et al. 2016).

- *Nanoparticles*

Nanoparticles synthesized from marine-derived polysaccharides such as alginate and fucoidan have been successful carriers for anticancer agents such as paclitaxel and doxorubicin. They can be synthesized through methods such as ionic gelation or polyelectrolyte complexation, often in combination with other polymers such as

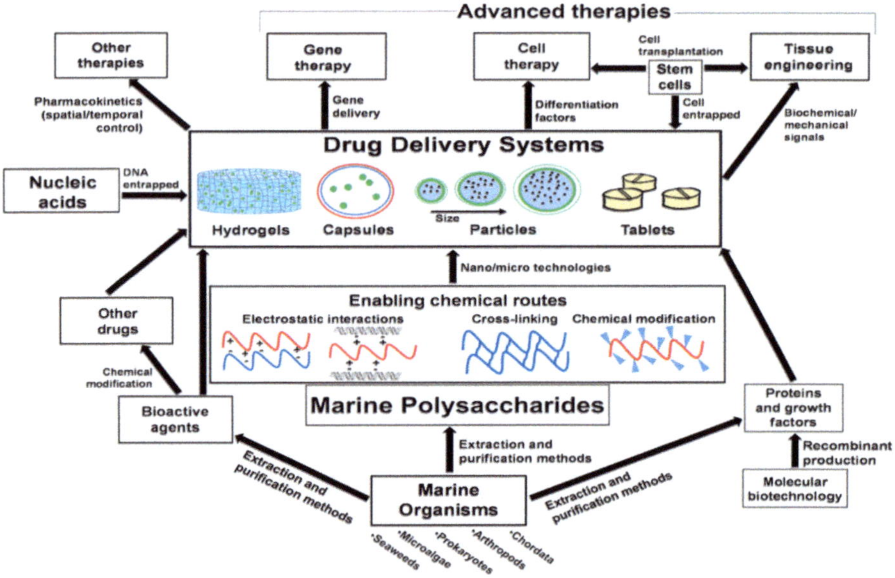

Fig. 3 Interactions between polysaccharides of marine origin in drug delivery systems for improved treatments and uses (seaweed polysaccharides). (Reproduced from Cardoso et al. (2016) under the terms and conditions of the Creative Commons Attribution (CC BY) license http://creativecommons.org/licenses/by/4.0/)

chitosan to improve stability and target specificity. Fucoidan is favored for drug delivery due to its anticancer and target-specific properties, particularly because P-selectin receptors are abundant in tumor environments. Nanoparticles will improve the bioavailability of poorly soluble drugs as well as target tumors passively with the assistance of the enhanced permeability and retention (EPR) effect (Venkatesan et al. 2016; Zhang et al. 2022).

- *Hydrogels*

Hydrogels of alginate, carrageenan, and ulvan can provide a moist 3D matrix for local and sustained delivery of anticancer drugs. Alginate hydrogels are formed through ionic cross-linking with calcium ions, allowing in situ gelation at the site, which makes them promising for post-surgical tumor treatments. Carrageenan hydrogels can offer temperature-sensitive and injectable characteristics, which are potentially useful in smart delivery release systems. This work focuses on minimizing the systemic toxicity of anticancer drugs by enabling their release specifically at tumor resection sites or through direct application to skin lesions (Stan et al. 2025).

- *Microspheres and microcapsules*

Microspheres and microcapsules, both of which are typically made of alginate or κ-carrageenan, are spherical delivery systems. These encapsulated delivery systems contain therapeutics designed to protect them from potentially harsh environments (e.g., gastric juices). Oral anticancer drug delivery is a promising application for these delivery systems, enabling the targeted release of drugs such as methotrexate or tamoxifen in the intestines rather than the stomach. Microspheres are formed through emulsification or ionic gelation and can be tailored to release their contents in response to pH or enzymatic triggers (Ramadan et al. 2025).

- *Films and coatings*

Films and coatings derived from marine polysaccharides such as alginate, carrageenan, and ulvan are thin and flexible delivery systems for localized anticancer delivery, particularly in the form of transdermal patches or wound-type applications. These films enable controlled delivery of bioactives while also acting as barriers against external contamination. For instance, carrageenan-based films have been utilized for the topical delivery of chemotherapeutics, while alginate-ulvan composites have been developed as bioadhesive patches for the sustained release of therapeutics on skin or mucosal surfaces (Cunha and Grenha 2016).

- *Emulsions and nanoemulsions*

Emulsions and nanoemulsions stabilized with marine polysaccharides (e.g., fucoidan, carrageenan, or agar) can encapsulate hydrophobic anticancer agents such as curcumin within a colloidal system. These emulsions improve the solubility and bioavailability of such drugs and are used in both oral and topical applications. Fucoidan-stabilized emulsions in particular showed enhanced stability and active delivery to tumor tissues via surface bioactivities (Geng et al. 2024).

4.3 Advantages of Marine-Derived Polysaccharides in Targeted Delivery

Marine algae polysaccharides (alginate, fucoidan, carrageenan, and agar) can be very helpful in creating drug delivery systems that can be targeted and delivered efficiently due to their high natural availability, different polysaccharide structures, their biocompatibility in the body, and their functional nature. They have particular potential in anticancer drug delivery because of their ability to encapsulate therapeutic agents and deliver to a location of interest, as well as drug release that can be controlled. Marine polysaccharides are biocompatible, biodegradable, and nontoxic, making them exceptionally well suited for biomedical applications. Because of their anionic properties, there can be ionic interactions with cationic drugs or polymers; thus, stable complexes and nanoparticles can form. Several of these polysaccharides exhibit various biological activities; for example, fucoidan exhibits antitumor, anti-inflammatory, and immunomodulatory properties—all of which can have additive effects alongside the action of encapsulated medicines. These polysaccharides possess mucoadhesive properties that help prolong retention time at mucosal sites, along with pH- and enzyme-responsiveness for site-specific drug release (e.g., an intestinal site or surrounding a tumor). Furthermore, polysaccharides are capable of binding to tumor-specific receptors (e.g., P-selectin or scavenger receptors), allowing for active targeting of cancer cells. These combined properties lower systemic toxicity and improve the therapeutic index of anticancer drugs, when using marine polysaccharide delivery vehicles (Kuznetsova et al. 2021; Sun et al. 2021).

5 Case Studies and Applications

5.1 *Examples of Successful Applications in Preclinical or Clinical Studies*

Polysaccharides derived from marine algae have gained much interest in the pharmaceutical field due to their great biocompatibility, biodegradability, and molecular bioactivities. Due to their diverse structures and ability to create many different types of drug delivery systems, such as nanoparticles, hydrogels, and microcapsules, natural polysaccharides have shown significant potential for targeted and controlled drug delivery. In the last decade, some studies have shown that polysaccharides can be used as therapeutic agents, while many preclinical studies, as well as clinical studies, have considered their use in the treatment of various disease models particularly for cancer therapy.

- *Fucoidan-based nanoparticles in the treatment of cancer*

  Fucoidan, a source of polysaccharides, has been researched heavily for its anticancer properties, particularly in the form of fucoidan-based nanoparticles. Studies have shown that these nanoparticles enhance the delivery of traditional chemotherapy agents such as paclitaxel and gemcitabine while also improving solubility, stability, and bioavailability. Fucoidan-based nanoparticles further offer advantage over drug delivery systems in terms of targeted delivery to tumor site, reducing systemic toxicity, and providing intrinsic anticancer activities, including the inhibition of angiogenesis and induction of apoptosis in cancer cells (Wang et al. 2024).

- *Alginate hydrogels for controlled drug release*

  Alginate is a polysaccharide from brown algae that has been used to create alginate hydrogels, with applications in controlled drug release. Alginate-based hydrogels can encapsulate a variety of drugs including anticancer drugs and release them in a controlled manner for extended periods of time. Biocompatibility and biodegradability make alginate a particularly appropriate material for sustained drug delivery systems with a local focus (Lin et al. 2019).

- *Carrageenan nanoparticles for mucosal drug delivery*

Carrageenan is a sulfated polysaccharide derived from red algae, and a number of studies have begun exploring the feasibility of using carrageenan in drug delivery systems. Carrageenan-based nanoparticles have been successfully used for the mucosal delivery of large drug macromolecules, providing a feasible alternative for oral administration by enhancing drug bioavailability of orally administered drugs. These delivery systems provide a pharmacokinetic pharmacology, enabling the delivery of oral biologics, botanicals, and other delicate drugs that might otherwise be compromised by the harsh gastrointestinal environment (Ahmad et al. 2022).

- *Ulvan-based nanoparticles for antibacterial applications*

Ulvan, a sulfated polysaccharide derived from green algae, has been used in the synthesis of silver nanoparticles (AgNPs) with enhanced antibacterial efficacies. Ulvan-coated AgNPs demonstrated strong antibacterial activity against a number of bacterial strains, including *Staphylococcus aureus* and *Escherichia coli*. The nanocomplexes formed by ulvan and AgNPs showed improved antibacterial efficacy than free ulvan alone, showing the potential of ulvan-based nanoparticles as carriers in antimicrobial drug delivery systems (Manlusoc et al. 2019).

- *Chlorella polysaccharides in neuroprotective drug delivery*

Polysaccharides derived from *Chlorella pyrenoidosa* have demonstrated neuroprotective effects in several preclinical Parkinson's disease models, including improved motor activity and increased dopamine expression. Additionally, these polysaccharides inhibited peripheral immunomodulatory responses and modulated oxidative stress. The neuroprotective effect of the drug is believed to result from its immunomodulatory action, thus showing the potential of *Chlorella polysaccharides* for targeted drug delivery in neurodegenerative diseases (Zhu et al. 2024).

The examples above are all effective uses of marine algae polysaccharides as drug delivery systems. Certainly, any drugs delivered using ulvan and *Chlorella*, as well as other marine algae polysaccharides, have potential to be used for effective therapeutic applications. The ability to develop diverse polysaccharide-based delivery systems with inherent biocompatibility and biodegradability is a key advantage in designing drug carriers—such as nanoparticles—for therapies targeting cancer, infections, and neurodegenerative diseases.

5.2 Specific Cancers Targeted (e.g., Breast, Lung, Colon)

To summarize case-based studies and applications of polysaccharides derived from marine algae in breast, lung, and colon cancers, the following sections illustrate their therapeutic promise and outcomes in vivo or clinical implementation.

- *Breast cancer: fucoidan-based nanoparticles*

Fucoidan, a sulfated polysaccharide that is largely found in brown algae such as *Fucus vesiculosus* and *Undaria pinnatifida*, has demonstrated impressive anticancer activity against breast cancer in several studies. Specifically, studies indicate that fucoidan caused cell death and inhibited proliferation, migration, and metastasis in breast cancer models including triple-negative types (MDA-MB-231 and 4T1) as well as estrogen-sensitive models like MCF-7. Also importantly, fucoidan has been shown to interact with immune checkpoints such as PD-L1 to augment the immune response against tumors. Despite promising preclinical efficacy and clinically relevant results, there have been few clinical trials specific to breast cancer. Interestingly fucoidan was approved by the FDA as a GRAS (Generally Recognized as Safe) substance, highlighting its safety and acceptability for further clinical studies in breast cancer treatment (Corso et al. 2021).

- *Lung cancer: alginate-based nanoparticles*

Alginate, which is a polysaccharide extracted from brown seaweed, has been researched for lung cancer therapy. Alginate-based nanoparticles encapsulating chemotherapeutic agents have been developed, which improved the stability, release, and circulation times of the drugs with targeted accumulation in tumor tissues. This type of drug delivery system improved the therapeutic action of the incorporated drugs. Moreover, alginate is biocompatible and biodegradable, making it an attractive agent for lung cancer treatment. While current research is promising, additional research and clinical trials are needed to define the clinical application for lung cancer-based delivery systems (Cai et al. 2025).

- *Colon cancer: ulvan and laminarin-based nanoparticles*

Ulvan is a sulfated polysaccharide derived from *Ulva lactuca* (green algae). The anticancer activity of ulvan has been reported in colon cancer models. Ulvan has been shown to decrease viability in colon cancer cells while leaving healthy cells unaffected. Ulvan extract can produce biogenic silver nanoparticles (AgNPs) that induce p53-dependent apoptosis in colon cancer HCT-116 cells. This would indicate a synergistic interaction with ulvan and AgNPs in targeting colon cancer cells. Researches on laminarin, a β-glucan from brown algae, have also evaluated its anticancer effects specifically against colon cancer. There is evidence that laminarin has enabled cell apoptosis in colon cancer cells. It has been also shown that sulfated derivatives of laminarin exhibited improved antitumor effects in comparison to unsulfated laminarin. Laminarin's anticancer activity is thought to be associated with increased levels of intracellular reactive oxygen species (ROS), decreased intracellular pH, and the activation of apoptosis, specifically through mitochondrial signaling and the receptor-induced pathway (Fu et al. 2022).

- *Colon cancer: Sargassum longifolium polysaccharide-based nanocarriers*

Polysaccharides extracted from *Sargassum longifolium*, a brown alga, were utilized in the form of nanocarriers, including nanoemulsions and nanostructured lipid carriers (NLCs), to improve the therapeutic efficacy against colon cancer. In vitro studies demonstrated that the polysaccharide-loaded nanocarriers showed controlled drug release and improved bioavailability. The polysaccharide NLC showed the highest cytotoxicity against HCT-116 colon cancer cells achieving 80% inhibition, whereas the nanoemulsions showed only 70% inhibition. This demonstrates the potential of seaweed-derived polysaccharides in nanomedicine for targeted colon cancer treatment (Shofia et al. 2018).

- *Gastric cancer: fucoidan from Fucus vesiculosus*

In a variety of cancer types, the sulfated polysaccharide fucoidan exhibits outstanding anticancer qualities with minimal toxicity. However, its precise pharmacological impact and mode of action in stomach cancer are still unknown. According to this study, fucoidan has the ability to inhibit the proliferation, migration, and invasion of gastric cancer (GC) cells. A cytokine expression screen showed that cells treated with fucoidan secreted less TGF-β1. According to our earlier research, upregulating CLEC-2 slowed the progression of GC. Fucoidan has also been demonstrated to be a platelet agonist for the C-type lectin-like receptor 2 (CLEC-2). Furthermore, it has been verified that fucoidan and CLEC-2, via the transcription factor CDX2—a key regulator of gut homeostasis—markedly enhance CLEC-2 expression in gastric cancer (GC) cells. Furthermore, silencing CLEC-2 restored fucoidan's inhibitory effects on the malignant phenotype of gastric cancer cells and reduced the production of TGF-β1. Based on these findings, fucoidan represents a promising therapeutic agent for gastric cancer, exerting antitumorigenic and anti-metastatic effects through its targeting of CLEC-2 to exert antitumorigenic and anti-metastatic effects (Xu et al. 2019).

- *Leukemia: polysaccharides from Sargassum latifolium*

A polysaccharide from the brown alga *Sargassum latifolium* showed selective cytotoxicity toward lymphoblastic leukemia cells. Specifically, fraction E3 induced cell cycle arrest in the S-phase and triggered apoptosis in 1301 cells without affecting the other tested cell lines. These results imply that polysaccharides from *S. latifolium* may have therapeutic potential against leukemia (Gamal-Eldeen et al. 2009).

- *Oral cancer: Gracilaria tenuistipitata extracts*

Ethanol and methanol extracts from the marine red algae *Gracilaria tenuistipitata* have demonstrated anti-proliferative activity in oral cancer cell lines, significantly inducing apoptosis and reducing cell viability and proliferative potential. This indicates that extracts from *G. tenuistipitata* may contain natural anticancer agents that will benefit oral cancer therapy (Yeh et al. 2012).

6 Challenges and Limitations

Structural complexity: Polysaccharides have various complex structures, making it difficult to standardize their properties and ensure consistent drug delivery.

Stability issues: They can degrade or lose activity based on variations to physiological conditions such as pH or enzymes.

Targeting limitations: As polysaccharides are biocompatible, targeted tissues or cells to the relevant tissues or cells usually require additional modifications.

Scalability and cost: Large-scale polysaccharide production with the targeted purity and function can be difficult and costly.

Immunogenicity: Some polysaccharides can elicit immune responses, which may limit their use in some patients.

Adherence to drug load and release: Efficient drug loading and controlled release can be a significant challenge, mostly with hydrophobic drugs.

These challenges and limitations emphasize how continued research and innovation will be important in optimizing polysaccharide-based drug delivery systems.

7 Future Perspectives

Marine algae polysaccharides offer great potential for future anticancer drug delivery systems. Here are just a few prospects:

Improved targeting: Marine polysaccharides, such as fucoidan and alginate, can be used to make targeted nanoparticles that recognize receptor sites on cancer cells. This could result in improved drug localization and limited toxic effects to the rest of the body.

Combined therapy: Marine polysaccharides can be used in combination with traditional chemotherapy agents and could increase the effectiveness of the drugs while lowering the side effects of traditional therapies.

Responsive systems: Marine polysaccharides can be individually adapted or adjusted with combinations of drugs for site-specific drug delivery, which is significant for personalized medicine as they exhibit both pH- and enzyme-based release characteristics.

Biocompatible nanocarriers: Marine polysaccharides can be utilized to build nanoparticles for the delivery of drugs, which stabilize the drug and control the drug release rate.

Immunomodulation: Some marine polysaccharides possess anticancer properties and can function both as drug carriers and as anticancer drugs.

8 Conclusion

Polysaccharides derived from marine algae could provide a valuable resource for anticancer drug delivery systems. Marine algae polysaccharides have appealing characteristics such as biocompatibility, biodegradability, and functional versatility. In addition to acting as passive carriers, they have intrinsic bioactive properties that can help formulate active drug delivery systems. Marine algae polysaccharides, such as alginate, fucoidan, carrageenan, ulvan, and agar, exhibit targeted delivery capabilities and responsiveness to extrinsic and intrinsic factors such as pH, enzymes, and tumor cell-specific receptors. Marine algae polysaccharides can also form hydrogels, nanoparticles, and capsules that enable controlled and sustained drug release, enhancing therapeutic effects while reducing systemic toxicity. Despite the current obstacles, such as scalability, structural complexity, and regulation, ongoing research is being done to maximize their benefits in combination therapies and personalized medicine. Marine algae polysaccharides not only offer a positive safety profile of anticancer agents but also provide anticancer, anti-inflammatory, and immunomodulatory attributes. As extraction methods and biotechnological inventions continue to progress, marine algae polysaccharides may play an important part in anticancer agent strategy.

References

Abka-khajouei, R., Tounsi, L., Shahabi, N., Patel, A.K., Abdelkafi, S., Michaud, P.: Structures, Properties and Applications of Alginates, (2022)

Agena, R., Cortés-Sánchez, A., Hernandez, H., Jaramillo-Flores, M.: Pro-Apoptotic Activity of Bioactive Compounds from Seaweeds: Promising Sources for Developing Novel Anticancer Drugs. Mar Drugs. 21, 182 (2023). https://doi.org/10.3390/md21030182

Ahmad, K., Khan, S., Afridi, M., Hassan, A., Shah, M.M., Rasheed, H., Ahmad, R., Ifqir, H.: Marine macroalgae polysaccharides-based nanomaterials: an overview with respect to nanoscience applications. Beni Suef Univ J Basic Appl Sci. 11, 156 (2022). https://doi.org/10.1186/s43088-022-00335-8

Alves, C., Silva, J., Pinteus, S., Gaspar, H., Alpoim, M.C., Botana, L.M., Pedrosa, R.: From marine origin to therapeutics: The antitumor potential of marine algae-derived compounds, (2018)

Atashrazm, F., Lowenthal, R.M., Woods, G.M., Holloway, A.F., Dickinson, J.L.: Fucoidan and cancer: A multifunctional molecule with anti-tumor potential, (2015)

Banerjee, R., Das, R., V.M, A., S, A., Sudhakaran, R.: Effect of algal metabolites in the inhibition of angiogenic channels for breast tumour. Aquaculture International. 31, 1–24 (2023). https://doi.org/10.1007/s10499-023-01110-x

Bhuyan, P.P., Nayak, R., Patra, S., Abdulabbas, H.S., Jena, M., Pradhan, B.: Seaweed-Derived Sulfated Polysaccharides; The New Age Chemopreventives: A Comprehensive Review, (2023)

Bilal, M., Iqbal, H.M.N.: Marine seaweed polysaccharides-based engineered cues for the modern biomedical sector, (2020)

Cai, J., Liao, W., Wen, J., Ye, F., Nie, Q., Chen, W., Zhao, C.: Algae-derived polysaccharides and polysaccharide-based nanoparticles: A natural frontier in breast cancer therapy. Int J Biol Macromol. 297, 139936 (2025). https://doi.org/10.1016/j.ijbiomac.2025.139936

Calvo, G.H., Cosenza, V.A., Sáenz, D.A., Navarro, D.A., Stortz, C.A., Céspedes, M.A., Mamone, L.A., Casas, A.G., Di Venosa, G.M.: Disaccharides obtained from carrageenans as potential antitumor agents. Sci Rep. 9, (2019). https://doi.org/10.1038/s41598-019-43238-y

Cardoso, M.J., Costa, R.R., Mano, J.F.: Marine origin polysaccharides in drug delivery systems, (2016)

Corso, C.R., de Oliveira, N.M.T., Cordeiro, L.M., da Silva, K.S., Soczek, S.H. da S., Rossato, V.F., Fernandes, E.S., Maria-Ferreira, D.: Polysaccharides with antitumor effect in breast cancer: A systematic review of non-clinical studies. Nutrients. 13, (2021). https://doi.org/10.3390/nu13062008

Cosenza, V.A., Navarro, D.A., Stortz, C.: Chemical modification of carrageenans and application of the modified products. In: Carrageenans: Sources and Extraction Methods, Molecular Structure, Bioactive Properties and Health Effects. pp. 189–227 (2016)

Cui, Z., Jiang, F., Li, L., Chi, Z., Liu, C.: Advances in Biomedical Applications of Hydrogels from Seaweed-Derived Sulfated Polysaccharides: Carrageenan, Fucoidan, and Ulvan. Journal of Ocean University of China. 23, 1329–1346 (2024). https://doi.org/10.1007/s11802-024-5988-z

Cunha, L., Grenha, A.: Sulfated seaweed polysaccharides as multifunctional materials in drug delivery applications, (2016)

Dalavi Pandurang Appana and Venkatesan, J. and R.V. and A.S.: Marine Polysaccharides Systems for Drug Delivery Applications. In: Nayak Amit Kumar and Hasnain, M.S. (ed.) Advanced Biopolymeric Systems for Drug Delivery. pp. 373–386. Springer International Publishing, Cham (2020)

Dalisay, D.S., Tenebro, C.P., Sabido, E.M., Suarez, A.F.L., Paderog, M.J. V., Reyes-Salarda, R., Saludes, J.P.: Marine-Derived Anticancer Agents Targeting Apoptotic Pathways: Exploring the Depths for Novel Cancer Therapies, (2024)

Duan, Y., Li, J., Jing, X., Ding, X., Yu, Y., Zhao, Q.: Fucoidan induces apoptosis and inhibits proliferation of hepatocellular carcinoma via the p38 MAPK/ERK and pi3k/akt signal pathways. Cancer Manag Res. 12, 1713–1723 (2020). https://doi.org/10.2147/CMAR.S243495

Elfeky, S., Qenawi, N.: Nanoformulations in Cancer Theranostics. Presented at the November (2024)

Elfeky, S., Qenawi, N., Tawfik, Prof.W., Loutfy, S., Subash, T.: Utilization of Nanographene Oxide-Folic Acid-Metal Chalcogen in Cancer Theranostics. NanoWorld J. 9, 206–214 (2024). https://doi.org/10.17756/nwj.2023-s5-041

Ercolano, G., De Cicco, P., Ianaro, A.: New drugs from the sea: Pro-apoptotic activity of sponges and algae derived compounds, (2019)

Fedorov, S.N., Ermakova, S.P., Zvyagintseva, T.N., Stonik, V.A.: Anticancer and cancer preventive properties of marine polysaccharides: Some results and prospects, (2013)

Ferreira, N., Ferreira, L., Miranda-Gonçalves, V., Reis, R., Seraphim, T., Borges, J., Baltazar, F., Gremiao, M.: Alginate hydrogel improves anti-angiogenic bevacizumab activity in cancer therapy. European Journal of Pharmaceutics and Biopharmaceutics. 119, (2017). https://doi.org/10.1016/j.ejpb.2017.06.028

Fitton, J.H., Stringer, D.N., Karpiniec, S.S.: Therapies from fucoidan: An update, (2015)

Flórez-Fernández, N., González Muñoz, M.J., Ribeiro, D., Fernandes, E., Domínguez, H., Freitas, M.: Algae polysaccharides' chemical characterization and their role in the inflammatory process. 24, 149–175 (2017). https://doi.org/10.2174/092986732366616102

Fu, Y., Xie, D., Zhu, Y., Zhang, X., Yue, H., Zhu, K., Pi, Z., Dai, Y.: Anti-colorectal cancer effects of seaweed-derived bioactive compounds. Front Med (Lausanne). Volume 9-2022, (2022). https://doi.org/10.3389/fmed.2022.988507

Gamal-Eldeen, A.M., Ahmed, E.F., Abo-Zeid, M.A.: In vitro cancer chemopreventive properties of polysaccharide extract from the brown alga, Sargassum latifolium. Food and Chemical Toxicology. 47, 1378–1384 (2009). https://doi.org/10.1016/j.fct.2009.03.016

Ganesan, P., Matsubara, K., Sugawara, T., Hirata, T.: Marine algal carotenoids inhibit angiogenesis by down-regulating FGF-2-mediated intracellular signals in vascular endothelial cells. Mol Cell Biochem. 380, 1–9 (2013). https://doi.org/10.1007/s11010-013-1651-5

Ganjoo, R., Sharma, S., Verma, C., Quraishi, M.A., Kumar, A.: Heteropolysaccharides in sustainable corrosion inhibition: 4E (Energy, Economy, Ecology, and Effectivity) dimensions. Int J Biol Macromol. 235, 123571 (2023). https://doi.org/10.1016/j.ijbiomac.2023.123571

Geng, H., Chen, M., Guo, C., Wang, W., Chen, D.: Marine polysaccharides: Biological activities and applications in drug delivery systems. Carbohydr Res. 538, 109071 (2024). https://doi.org/10.1016/j.carres.2024.109071

Hsu, C.Y., Allela, O.Q.B., Hussein, A.M., Mustafa, M.A., Kaur, M., Alaraj, M., Al-Hussainy, A.F., Radi, U.K., Ubaid, M., Idan, A.H., Alsaikhan, F., Narmani, A., Farhood, B.: Recent advances in polysaccharide-based drug delivery systems for cancer therapy: a comprehensive review, (2024)

Jazzara, M., Ghannam, A., Soukkarieh, C., Murad, H.: Anti-Proliferative Activity of λ-Carrageenan Through the Induction of Apoptosis in Human Breast Cancer Cells. Iran J Cancer Prev. In Press, (2016). https://doi.org/10.17795/ijcp-3836

De Jesus Raposo, M.F., De Morais, A.M.B., De Morais, R.M.S.C.: Marine polysaccharides from algae with potential biomedical applications, (2015)

Kadam, S.U., Tiwari, B.K., O'Donnell, C.P.: Extraction, structure and biofunctional activities of laminarin from brown algae. Int J Food Sci Technol. 50, 24–31 (2015). https://doi.org/10.1111/ijfs.12692

Kalimuthu Senthilkumar and Kim, S.-K.: Fucoidan, A Sulfated Polysaccharides from Brown Algae as Therapeutic Target for Cancer. In: Kim, S.-K. (ed.) Handbook of Anticancer Drugs from Marine Origin. pp. 145–164. Springer International Publishing, Cham (2015)

Kanegawa, K., Harada, H., Myouga, H., Katakura, Y., Shirahata, S., Kamei, Y.: Telomerase inhibiting activity in vitro from natural resources, marine algae extracts. Cytotechnology. 33, 221–227 (2000). https://doi.org/10.1023/A:1008179302906

Karadeniz, F., Lee, S.G., Oh, J.H., Kim, J.A., Kong, C.S.: Inhibition of MMP-2 and MMP-9 activities by solvent-partitioned Sargassum horneri extracts. Fish Aquatic Sci. 21, (2018). https://doi.org/10.1186/s41240-018-0093-0

Kim, E.J., Park, S.Y., Lee, J.-Y., Han, J., Park, Y.: Fucoidan present in brown algae induces apoptosis of human colon cancer cells. (2010)

Ko, S.-C., Heo, S.-Y., Choi, S.-W., Qian, Z.-J., Heo, S.-J., Kang, D.-H., Kim, N., Jung, W.-K.: A heptameric peptide isolated from the marine microalga Pavlova lutheri suppresses PMA-induced secretion of matrix metalloproteinase-9 through the inactivation of the JNK, p38, and NF-κB pathways in human fibrosarcoma cells. J Appl Phycol. 30, 2367–2378 (2018). https://doi.org/10.1007/s10811-018-1443-0

Kokoulin, M.S., Kuzmich, A.S., Filshtein, A.P., Prassolov, V.S., Romanenko, L.A.: Capsular polysaccharide from the marine bacterium Cobetia marina induces apoptosis via both caspase-dependent and mitochondria-mediated pathways in HL-60 cells. CarbohydrPolym. 347, 122791 (2025) https://doi.org/10.1016/j.carbpol.2024.122791

Komisarska, P., Pinyosinwat, A., Saleem, M., Szczuko, M.: Carrageenan as a Potential Factor of Inflammatory Bowel Diseases, (2024)

Kozak, J., Forma, A., Czeczelewski, M., Kozyra, P., Sitarz, E., Radzikowska-büchner, E., Sitarz, M., Baj, J.: Inhibition or reversal of the epithelial-mesenchymal transition in gastric cancer: Pharmacological approaches, (2021)

Kuznetsova, T.A., Andryukov, B.G., Besednova, N.N., Khotimchenko, Yu.S.: Polysaccharides from Marine Algae in Modern Technologies of Regenerative Medicine. Russ J Mar Biol. 47, 1–9 (2021). https://doi.org/10.1134/S1063074021010065

Kuznetsova, T.A., Andryukov, B.G., Besednova, N.N., Zaporozhets, T.S., Kalinin, A. V.: Marine algae polysaccharides as basis for wound dressings, drug delivery, and tissue engineering: A review, (2020)

Łabowska, M.B., Michalak, I., Detyna, J.: Methods of extraction, physicochemical properties of alginates and their applications in biomedical field - A review. Open Chem. 17, 738–762 (2019). https://doi.org/10.1515/chem-2019-0077

Lakmal H. H. Chaminda and Lee, J.-H. and J.Y.-J.: Enzyme-Assisted Extraction of a Marine Algal Polysaccharide, Fucoidan and Bioactivities. In: Ramawat Kishan Gopal and Mérillon, J.-M. (ed.) Polysaccharides: Bioactivity and Biotechnology. pp. 1065–1077. Springer International Publishing, Cham (2015)

Lee, H., Seyedian, R.: Fucoidan from Seaweed Fucus vesiculosus Inhibits Migration and Invasion of Human Lung Cancer Cell via PI3K-Akt-mTOR Pathways. PLoS One. 7, e50624 (2012). https://doi.org/10.1371/journal.pone.0050624

Lee, S.H., Lee, S.S., Lee, G.Y., Han, S.Y., Kim, D.S., Lee, B.H., Yoo, Y.C.: Endarachnebinghamiae Extract Ameliorates Inflammatory Responses in Macrophages Through Regulation of MAPK, NF-kB and PI3K/AKT Pathways, and Prevents Acute Lung Injury in Mice. Life. 15, (2025). https://doi.org/10.3390/life15010088

Lee, Y.-E., Kim, H., Seo, C., Park, T., Lee, K. Bin, Yoo, S.-Y., Hong, S.-C., Kim, J.T., Lee, J.: Marine polysaccharides: therapeutic efficacy and biomedical applications. Arch Pharm Res. 40, 1006–1020 (2017). https://doi.org/10.1007/s12272-017-0958-2

Li, Y., McGowan, E., Chen, S., Santos, J., Yin, H., Lin, Y.: Immunopotentiating Activity of Fucoidans and Relevance to Cancer Immunotherapy, (2023)

Lin, X., Ma, Q., Su, J., Wang, C., Kankala, R.K., Zeng, M., Lin, H., Zhou, S.F.: Dual-responsive alginate hydrogels for controlled release of therapeutics. Molecules. 24, (2019). https://doi.org/10.3390/molecules24112089

Lin, Y., Qi, X., Liu, H., Xue, K., Xu, S., Tian, Z.: The anti-cancer effects of fucoidan: A review of both in vivo and in vitro investigations, (2020)

Liu, F., Duan, G., Yang, H.: Recent advances in exploiting carrageenans as a versatile functional material for promising biomedical applications. Int J Biol Macromol. 235, 123787 (2023). https://doi.org/10.1016/j.ijbiomac.2023.123787

Liu, G., Kuang, S., Wu, S., Jin, W., Sun, C.: A novel polysaccharide from Sargassum integerrimum induces apoptosis in A549 cells and prevents angiogensis in vitro and in vivo. Sci Rep. 6, (2016). https://doi.org/10.1038/srep26722

Liu, W.C., Zhuang, D.P., Zhao, Y., Balasubramanian, B., Zhao, Z.H.: Seaweed-Derived Polysaccharides Attenuate Heat Stress-Induced Splenic Oxidative Stress and Inflammatory Response via Regulating Nrf2 and NF-κB Signaling Pathways. Mar Drugs. 20, (2022). https://doi.org/10.3390/md20060358

Manfioletti, G., Fedele, M.: Epithelial–Mesenchymal Transition (EMT), (2023)

Manlusoc, J.K.T., Hsieh, C.L., Hsieh, C.Y., Salac, E.S.N., Lee, Y.T., Tsai, P.W.: Pharmacologic application potentials of sulfated polysaccharide from marine algae, (2019)

Manzelat, S., Mufarrah, A., Hasan, A., Ali, N.: Macro algae of the Red Sea from Jizan , Saudi Arabia, (2018)

Matin, M., Koszarska, M., Atanasov, A.G., Król-Szmajda, K., Jóźwik, A., Stelmasiak, A., Hejna, M.: Bioactive Potential of Algae and Algae-Derived Compounds: Focus on Anti-Inflammatory, Antimicrobial, and Antioxidant Effects, (2024)

Matou-Nasri, S., Helley, D., Chabut, D., Bros, A., Fischer, A.-M.: Effect of fucoidan on fibroblast growth factor-2-induced angiogenesis in vitro. Thromb Res. 106, 213–221 (2002). https://doi.org/10.1016/S0049-3848(02)00136-6

McArdle, R., Hamill, R.: 10 - Utilisation of hydrocolloids in processed meat systems. In: Kerry, J.P. and Kerry, J.F. (eds.) Processed Meats. pp. 243–269. Woodhead Publishing (2011)

Mensah, E.O., Kanwugu, O.N., Panda, P.K., Adadi, P.: Marine fucoidans: Structural, extraction, biological activities and their applications in the food industry. Food Hydrocoll. 142, 108784 (2023). https://doi.org/10.1016/j.foodhyd.2023.108784

Michalak, I., Tiwari, R., Dhawan, M., Alagawany, M., Farag, M.R., Sharun, K., Emran, T. Bin, Dhama, K.: Antioxidant effects of seaweeds and their active compounds on animal health and production–a review, (2022)

Mo'o, F.R.C., Wilar, G., Devkota, H.P., Wathoni, N.: Ulvan, a polysaccharide from Macroalga Ulva sp.: A review of chemistry, biological activities and potential for food and biomedical applications, (2020)

Murad, H., Hawat, M., Ekhtiar, A., AlJapawe, A., Abbas, A., Darwish, H., Sbenati, O., Ghannam, A.: Induction of G1-phase cell cycle arrest and apoptosis pathway in MDA-MB-231 human breast cancer cells by sulfated polysaccharide extracted from Laurencia papillosa. Cancer Cell Int. 16, (2016). https://doi.org/10.1186/s12935-016-0315-4

Negreanu-Pirjol, B.S., Negreanu-Pirjol, T., Popoviciu, D.R., Anton, R.E., Prelipcean, A.M.: Marine Bioactive Compounds Derived from Macroalgae as New Potential Players in Drug Delivery Systems: A Review, (2022)

Nurkolis, F., Subali, D., Taslim, N., Mayulu, N., Hardinsyah, H., Tjandrawinata M, Frsph, R., Kim, B.: Unleashing the Potential of Marine Algae in Cancer Prevention and Treatment Through Combination of Tradition and Innovation. Presented at the April (2024)

Ouyang, Y., Qiu, Y., Liu, Y., Zhu, R., Chen, Y., El-Seedi, H.R., Chen, X., Zhao, C.: Cancer-fighting potentials of algal polysaccharides as nutraceuticals. Food Research International. 147, 110522 (2021). https://doi.org/10.1016/j.foodres.2021.110522

Pandya, Y.H., Bakshi, M., Sharma, A., Pandya, H.: Agar-agar extraction, structural properties and applications: A review. ~ 1151 ~ The Pharma Innovation Journal. 1151–1157 (2022)

Park, H.S., Hwang, J., Gi Young, K., Cha, H.-J., Kim, W.-J., Kim, N.D., Yoo, Y., Choi, Y.: Induction of Apoptosis by Fucoidan in Human Leukemia U937 Cells through Activation of p38 MAPK and Modulation of Bcl-2 Family. Mar Drugs. 11, 2347–2364 (2013). https://doi.org/10.3390/md11072347

Pei, Y., Yang, S., Xiao, Z., Zhou, C., Hong, P., Qian, Z.J.: Structural Characterization of Sulfated Polysaccharide Isolated from Red Algae (Gelidiumcrinale) and Antioxidant and Anti-Inflammatory Effects in Macrophage Cells. Front Bioeng Biotechnol. 9, (2021). https://doi.org/10.3389/fbioe.2021.794818

Ping-Hsiu, W., Onodera, Y., Recuenco, F.C., Giaccia, A.J., Quynh-Thu, L., Shimizu, S., Shirato, H., Jin-Min, N.: Lambda-carrageenan enhances the effects of radiation therapy in cancer treatment by suppressing cancer cell invasion and metastasis through racgap1 inhibition. Cancers (Basel). 11, (2019). https://doi.org/10.3390/cancers11081192

Pomin, V., Mourão, P.: Structure, biology, evolution, and medical importance of sulfated fucans and galactans. Glycobiology. 18, 1016–1027 (2008). https://doi.org/10.1093/glycob/cwn085

Qenawi, N., Abd-El aziz, A.M., Tawfik, W., Elfeky, S.: Innovative Graphene Oxide-Folic Acid-MoS2 Nanocomposite for Targeted Near-Infrared Photothermal Cancer Therapy. Egypt J Chem. (2025). https://doi.org/10.21608/ejchem.2025.358734.11274

Ramadan, N.E., Youssef, F.R., Alshishtawy, A.A.K., Elshikh, F.M., Newir, O., Abdelazeem, S.H., Ma'ruf, N.K., Shouman, H., Ali, S.S., El-Sheekh, M.M.: Marine algal polysaccharides for drug delivery applications: A review. Int J Biol Macromol. 295, 139551 (2025). https://doi.org/10.1016/j.ijbiomac.2025.139551

Ramu Arunkumar and Ahmed, B.A.: Marine Algal Products and Algal Nanoparticle Synthesis Against Cancer. In: Thangadurai Devarajan and Sangeetha, J. and P.R. (ed.) Bioprospecting Algae for Nanosized Materials. pp. 261–274. Springer International Publishing, Cham (2021)

Şahin, O.I.: 4 Seaweed Polysaccharides: Structure, Extraction and Applications. (2021)

Sanjay, Yoon, N.Y., Park, E.J., Lee, H.J.: Immune-Enhancing Effects of Marine Algae Extracts: Modulation of Macrophage Activation by Sargassum horneri, Sargassum fusiforme, and Undaria pinnatifida. Applied Sciences (Switzerland). 14, (2024). https://doi.org/10.3390/app14051794

Senthilkumar, K., Se-Kwon, K.: Cell Survival and Apoptosis Signaling as Therapeutic Target for Cancer: Marine Bioactive Compounds. Int J Mol Sci. 14, 2334–2354 (2013). https://doi.org/10.3390/ijms14022334

Sharma, A., Shahid, A., Banerjee, R., Kumar, K.J.: Emerging insights into the structure-activity relationship of water-soluble polysaccharides in antiviral therapy. European Journal of Medicinal Chemistry Reports. 10, 100122 (2024). https://doi.org/10.1016/j.ejmcr.2023.100122

Sharma, R., Mondal, A.S., Trivedi, N.: Anticancer potential of algae-derived metabolites: recent updates and breakthroughs. Futur J Pharm Sci. 9, (2023). https://doi.org/10.1186/s43094-023-00492-2

Shen, Y., Zhao, H., Wang, X., Wu, S., Wang, Y., Wang, C., Zhang, Y., Zhao, H.: Unraveling the web of defense: the crucial role of polysaccharides in immunity, (2024)

Shofia, S.I., Jayakumar, K., Mukherjee, A., Chandrasekaran, N.: Efficiency of brown seaweed (: Sargassum longifolium) polysaccharides encapsulated in nanoemulsion and nanostructured lipid carrier against colon cancer cell lines HCT 116. RSC Adv. 8, 15973–15984 (2018). https://doi.org/10.1039/c8ra02616e

de Sousa, A.K., Araujo, A.S.M.L., da Silva, T.M.L., de Sousa de Lima, F.M., dos Santos Ferreira, J., de Brito, T.V., dos Reis Barbosa, A.L.: Polysaccharides from macro algae: Anti-inflammatory actions against systemic inflammatory process and in the gastrointestinal tract. J Appl Phycol. 35, 381–395 (2023). https://doi.org/10.1007/s10811-022-02878-w

Stan, D., Mirica, A.C., Mocanu, S., Stan, D., Podolean, I., Candu, N., El Fergani, M., Stefan, L.M., Seciu-Grama, A.M., Aricov, L., Brincoveanu, O., Moldovan, C., Bocancia-Mateescu, L.A., Coman, S.M.: Hybrid Hydrogel Supplemented with Algal Polysaccharide for Potential Use in Biomedical Applications. Gels. 11, (2025). https://doi.org/10.3390/gels11010017

Stengel, D., Connan, S.: Natural Products from Marine Algae, Methods and Protocols. (2015)

Sun, Y., Ma, X., Hu, H.: Marine polysaccharides as a versatile biomass for the construction of nano drug delivery systems, (2021)

Synytsya, A., Čopíková, J., Kim, W., Park, Y.: Cell Wall Polysaccharides of Marine Algae. In: Springer Handbook of Marine Biotechnology. pp. 543–590 (2015)

Taghipour, R., Hassannia, H., Arabnozari, H., Enderami, S.E., Habibi, E.: Natural Polysaccharides in Breast Cancer: Fucoidan's Role in Enhancing Cisplatin Cytotoxicity and Reducing Chemotherapy Resistance. In: Monteiro, Prof.A.C. and Wang, D.Prof.L. (eds.) Latest Research on Breast Cancer. IntechOpen, Rijeka (2025)

Tamzi, N.N., Rahman, M.M., Das, S.: Recent Advances in Marine-Derived Bioactives Towards Cancer Therapy, (2024)

Thinh, P.D., Menshova, R. V., Ermakova, S.P., Anastyuk, S.D., Ly, B.M., Zvyagintseva, T.N.: Structural characteristics and anticancer activity of fucoidan from the brown alga Sargassum mcclurei. Mar Drugs. 11, 1453–1476 (2013). https://doi.org/10.3390/md11051456

Tusi, S.K., Khalaj, L., Ashabi, G., Kiaei, M., Khodagholi, F.: Alginate oligosaccharide protects against endoplasmic reticulum- and mitochondrial-mediated apoptotic cell death and oxidative stress. Biomaterials. 32, 5438–5458 (2011). https://doi.org/10.1016/j.biomaterials.2011.04.024

Vaikundamoorthy, R., Krishnamoorthy, V., Vilwanathan, R., Rajendran, R.: Structural characterization and anticancer activity (MCF7 and MDA-MB-231) of polysaccharides fractionated from brown seaweed Sargassum wightii. Int J Biol Macromol. 111, 1229–1237 (2018). https://doi.org/10.1016/j.ijbiomac.2018.01.125

Veluchamy, C., Palaniswamy, R.: A REVIEW ON MARINE ALGAE AND ITS APPLICATIONS. Asian Journal of Pharmaceutical and Clinical Research. 21–27 (2020). https://doi.org/10.22159/ajpcr.2020.v13i3.36130

Venkatesan, J., Anil, S., Kim, S.-K., Shim, M.: Seaweed Polysaccharide-Based Nanoparticles: Preparation and Applications for Drug Delivery. Polymers (Basel). 8, 1–25 (2016). https://doi.org/10.3390/polym8020030

Venkatesan, J., Lowe, B., Anil, S., Manivasagan, P., Kheraif, A.A.A., Kang, K.H., Kim, S.K.: Seaweed polysaccharides and their potential biomedical applications, (2015)

Vilaplana, F., Gilbert, R.G.: Characterization of branched polysaccharides using multiple-detection size separation techniques, (2010)

Wang, H., Hunter, R., Zhang, Q., Yu, H., Wang, J., Yue, Y., Geng, L., Wu, N.: The application of marine polysaccharides to antitumor nanocarriers. CarbohydrPolym. 342, 122407 (2024). https://doi.org/10.1016/j.carbpol.2024.122407

Wassie, T., Niu, K., Xie, C., Wang, H., Xin, W.: Extraction Techniques, Biological Activities and Health Benefits of Marine Algae Enteromorpha prolifera Polysaccharide, (2021)

Wei, J., Liu, R., Hu, X., Liang, T., Zhou, Z., Huang, Z.: MAPK signaling pathway-targeted marine compounds in cancer therapy. J Cancer Res Clin Oncol. 147, 3–22 (2021). https://doi.org/10.1007/s00432-020-03460-y

Xu, L., Liu, F., Li, C., Li, S., Wu, H., Guo, B., Gu, J., Wang, L.: Fucoidan suppresses the gastric cancer cell malignant phenotype and production of TGF-β1 via CLEC-2. Glycobiology. 30, (2019). https://doi.org/10.1093/glycob/cwz097

Yadav, N., Francis, A.P., Priya, V.V., Patil, S., Mustaq, S., Khan, S.S., Alzahrani, K.J., Banjer, H.J., Mohan, S.K., Mony, U., Rajagopalan, R.: Polysaccharide-Drug Conjugates: A Tool for Enhanced Cancer Therapy, (2022)

Yamasaki, Y., Yamasaki, M., Tachibana, H., Yamada, K.: Fucoidan Induces Apoptosis through Activation of Caspase-8 on Human Breast Cancer MCF-7 Cells. J Agric Food Chem. 57, 8677–8682 (2009). https://doi.org/10.1021/jf9010406

Yang, L., Wang, P., Wang, H., Li, Q., Teng, H., Liu, Z., Yang, W., Hou, L., Zou, X.: Fucoidan derived from Undaria pinnatifida induces apoptosis in human hepatocellular carcinoma SMMC-7721 cells via the ROS-mediated mitochondrial pathway. Mar Drugs. 11, 1961–1976 (2013). https://doi.org/10.3390/md11061961

Yeh, C.C., Tseng, C.N., Yang, J.I., Huang, H.W., Fang, Y., Tang, J.Y., Chang, F.R., Chang, H.W.: Antiproliferation and induction of apoptosis in Ca9-22 oral cancer cells by ethanolic extract of Gracilariatenuistipitata. Molecules. 17, 10916–10927 (2012). https://doi.org/10.3390/molecules170910916

Yu, Y., Jia, X., Wang, W., Jin, Y., Liu, W., Wang, D., Mao, Y., Xie, C., Liu, T.: Floridean Starch and Floridoside Metabolic Pathways of Neoporphyrahaitanensis and Their Regulatory Mechanism under Continuous Darkness. Mar Drugs. 19, (2021). https://doi.org/10.3390/md19120664

Zhang, S., Qamar, S.A., Junaid, M., Munir, B., Ain, Q.U., Bilal, M.: Algal Polysaccharides-Based Nanoparticles for Targeted Drug Delivery Applications. Starch - Stärke. 74, 2200014 (2022). https://doi.org/10.1002/star.202200014

Zheng, H., Pei, Y., He, Y.L., Liu, Y., Chen, M., Hong, P., Zhou, C., Qian, Z.J.: A Sulfated Polysaccharide from Red Algae (Gelidiumcrinale) to Suppress Cells Metastasis and MMP-9 Expression of HT1080 Cells. Foods. 11, (2022). https://doi.org/10.3390/foods11152360

Zhong, H., Gao, X., Cheng, C., Liu, C., Wang, Q., Han, X.: The Structural Characteristics of Seaweed Polysaccharides and Their Application in Gel Drug Delivery Systems, (2020)

Zhu, L., Ren, Y., Zhang, S., Guo, Y., Zong, J., Liu, Y.: Marine-derived polysaccharides: the potential agents against neurodegenerative diseases, (2024)

Marine Algal Polysaccharides in the Management of Liver Disease

Fatemeh Izadpanah Qeshmi, Saba Ghattavi, and Ahmad Homaei

Abstract Since marine algal polysaccharides have long presented a wide range of bioactivities, there has been an interest in them as possible remedies for liver diseases. Algal polysaccharides can be used as antioxidant, anti-inflammatory, anti-apoptotic, detoxifying, and anticancer in nature, and they act to counter oxidative stress, inflammation, apoptosis, and metabolic disturbances, especially in cases of NAFLD. Pairwise molecular interactions to semi-molecular interactions occur between marine algal polysaccharides and two or three key cell signaling pathways (such as Nrf2, NF-κB, and PI3K/Akt), regulating gene and enzyme activity related to hepatic metabolism, detoxification, and tumorigenesis. Because of their hepatobiliary properties, they can also modulate the gut-liver axis when algal polysaccharides interact with the gut microbiota and decrease the extent of translocation of endotoxins. Regardless of the strong evidence in preclinical studies, there are limited trials in human populations, primarily due to the heterogeneity of components and the lack of optimized standardization protocols, which precludes their complete clinical use. Future studies should focus on refining extraction protocols, ensuring product consistency, and demonstrating efficacy through human studies. Additionally, exploring the synergistic potential of marine algae with existing products/drugs, facilitated by advancements in algal biotechnology, could enable the production of custom polysaccharide profiles for targeted liver therapy. Given their promising nature, marine algal polysaccharides may lead to the development of safe and effective agents for the prevention and treatment of liver diseases.

Keywords Algal biotechnology · Marine algae · Polysaccharides · Liver disease

F. I. Qeshmi · A. Homaei (✉)
Department of Marine Biology, Faculty of Marine Science and Technology, University of Hormozgan, Bandar Abbas, Iran
e-mail: a.homaei@hormozgan.ac.ir

S. Ghattavi
Persian Gulf and Oman Sea Ecological Research Center, Iranian Fisheries Sciences Research Institute, Agricultural Research Education and Extension Organization (AREEO), Bandar Abbas, Hormozgan, Iran

S. Jana et al. (eds.), *Multifunctional Marine Polysaccharides*,
https://doi.org/10.1007/978-981-95-4126-3_8

1 Introduction

Algae are massive and diverse assemblages of organisms that grow mostly in aquatic environment and are able to transform CO_2 and minerals into biomass, photosynthetically, although some are heterotrophs. In marine environment algae can be found as microalgae and macroalgae, which differ from each other based on pigments, storage materials, cell walls, cell division, and morphology. Marine algae are fast-growing, multicellular, nonvascular algae that come in a variety of colors, contain chlorophyll, and can reach sizes of up to 60 m. Macrophytes can also be classified based on their pigments: Rhodophyceae (red algae), Chlorophyceae (green algae), and Phaeophyceae (brown algae) (Villarruel-López et al. 2017; Hira et al. 2019). Microalgae are the ancestors of present-day land flora and the first contributors of the aquatic ecosystem. Microalgae are unicellular microorganisms that require solar radiation to transform it into chemical energy. Microalgae can produce significant amounts of O_2 and are more efficient at biomass production in the atmosphere. These creatures exhibit rapid proliferation and produce more biomass rich in bioactive chemicals compared to superior flora. Microalgae have the most capacity to adapt to harmful environmental conditions. They do not compete with agricultural crops and can even thrive in sewage or saltwater. As early as the 1500s BC, algal biomass has served as both a fundamental dietary component and a therapeutic agent (Gamal and Ibrahim 2023). Seaweeds have benefited humans since antiquity, approximately 14,000 years, and have been consumed as food products in Japanese and Chinese cultures for millennia. The continued application of seaweeds in the food sector has not only developed, but more recently, seaweeds have gained wider applications in the textile, pharmaceuticals, cosmetics, and biotechnology sectors (Villarruel-López et al. 2017). The unprocessed components and bioactive components found in candidate algae demonstrate their potential to generate phytochemical compounds that fight modern noncommunicable diseases, including cardiovascular ailments, cancers, autoimmune conditions, neurodegenerative diseases, and metabolic disorders such as nonalcoholic fatty liver disease (NAFLD). Seaweeds possess exceptional polysaccharides that function as advantageous dietary fibers to manage energy consumption and nutrient uptake and metabolic equilibrium (El Rashed et al. 2022). The medicinal use of microalgae dates back over 2000 years, where they were used to combat famine-related diseases. Microalgae generate substantial quantities of valuable bioactive substances that serve numerous practical purposes. Both microalgae and macroalgae have rapid growth rates and possess beneficial bioactive compounds, making them valuable for applications in food, pharmaceuticals, cosmetics, and biofuels.

The liver is a vital organ that controls metabolic processes throughout the body. Inflammation of liver cells leads to hepatitis, which can progress to chronic liver disease if left untreated. The use of drugs to treat liver diseases has minimal success because these medications produce adverse effects during treatment. Therapies derived from natural substances maintain higher safety profiles compared to conventional medical drugs. Marine habitats provide an exceptional supply of bioactive natural compounds, which possess unique structural features that have never been identified in terrestrial plants (Hira et al. 2019).

Seaweed contains abundant polysaccharides, which make up half of its dry weight, serving as a natural storage system for these compounds (Hira et al. 2019). The activity of natural polysaccharides is determined by the covalent glycoside bonds that bind their constituent monosaccharides. The complex skeletal design includes various elements that store extensive biological information. Research demonstrates that polysaccharide biological functionality depends on its mono-polysaccharide composition and ratios, molecular weight, and the type of glycosidic bonds. These factors define the polysaccharide chain structure, which in turn determines its functional and structural outlines (Hira et al. 2019). Algal polysaccharides exist in abundance in diverse biomaterials and display antioxidant, anti-inflammatory, anticoagulant, and antithrombotic activities. The natural bioactive compounds found in marine algal species exhibit potential as anticancer, antioxidant, and anti-inflammatory agents, as free radicals generated by oxidative stress play a critical role in inflammatory responses and cancer development. Scientists have investigated marine algae in both laboratory and living organism experiments to demonstrate their antioxidative, anti-inflammatory, antimicrobial, and anticancer health benefits. Seaweed contains substantial amounts of complex carbohydrates that work as prebiotic agents. Additionally, marine algae have high levels of dietary fibers, minerals, lipids, proteins, omega-3 fatty acids, vital amino acids, polysaccharides, and vitamins A, B, C, and E. Research indicates that PLS (sulfated polysaccharides) have antioxidant and anti-inflammatory characteristics, making them extremely physiologically active (Nabil-Adam and Shreadah 2021) (Fig. 1).

2 Therapeutic Methods and Dietary Interventions for Liver Diseases

Functional food is food that has additional benefits or functions beyond its nutritive values. Nowadays, and as a new trend, eating functional food is being adopted by many people around the world and is seen as a complementary commitment to their healthy lifestyles. Given the continuous rise in global demand for functional foods, there will always be a growing need to develop novel functional food products (Devlina Das et al. 2010; Vicentini et al. 2016; Anil et al. 2022). Marine algae and plant-derived protein rank among the leading functional food components and have emerged as key trends in functional cuisine. Marine algae worldwide are perceived more positively as functional food because of their high levels of nutritional value and bioactive substances. They serve as abundant sources of iodine, glutathione, phlorotannin, and fucoxanthin, as well as carbohydrates like carrageenan, fucoidan, alginate, and agar (Quitral et al. 2012; Øverland et al. 2019). Consistent intake of marine algae biomass has improved the blood lipid profile in vivo. Marine algae contain numerous phytochemicals or bioactive substances, primarily in the form of pigments, such as chlorophyll, carotenoids, and phenolic compounds (Jiménez-Escrig et al. 2011) (Fig. 2).

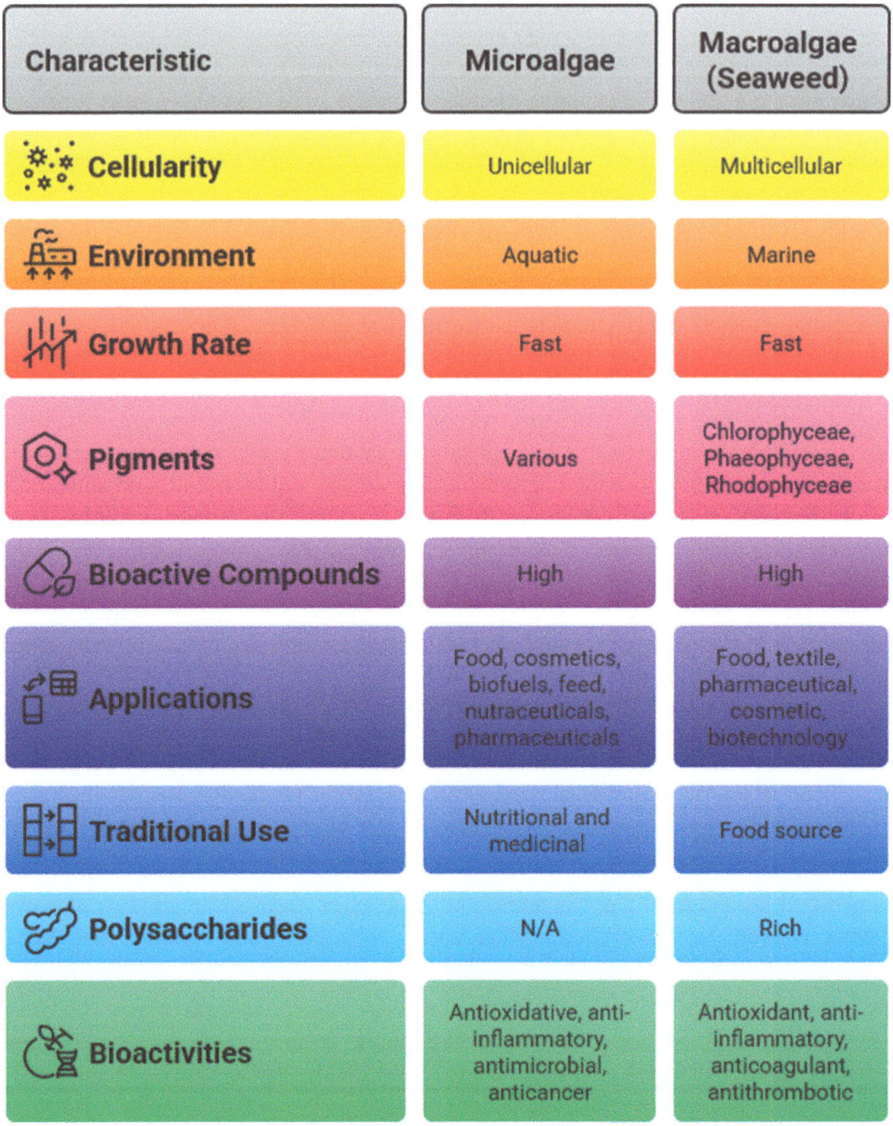

Characteristic	Microalgae	Macroalgae (Seaweed)
Cellularity	Unicellular	Multicellular
Environment	Aquatic	Marine
Growth Rate	Fast	Fast
Pigments	Various	Chlorophyceae, Phaeophyceae, Rhodophyceae
Bioactive Compounds	High	High
Applications	Food, cosmetics, biofuels, feed, nutraceuticals, pharmaceuticals	Food, textile, pharmaceutical, cosmetic, biotechnology
Traditional Use	Nutritional and medicinal	Food source
Polysaccharides	N/A	Rich
Bioactivities	Antioxidative, anti-inflammatory, antimicrobial, anticancer	Antioxidant, anti-inflammatory, anticoagulant, antithrombotic

Fig. 1 A comparative summary of microalgae and macroalgae (seaweed) in terms of their cell structure, growth environments, bioactive compounds, and applications in food, cosmetics, pharmaceuticals, and biofuels. Both exhibit significant bioactivities (antioxidative and anti-inflammatory) for nutritional, medicinal, and commercial use

Merging ingredients known for their health benefits can result in a unique functional food, characterized as food that offers specific advantages besides its nutritional benefits. The consumption of functional foods is currently accepted by numerous individuals globally, as it is seen as a trend and an extra element of a healthy lifestyle. Given the increasing worldwide demand for functional food, there

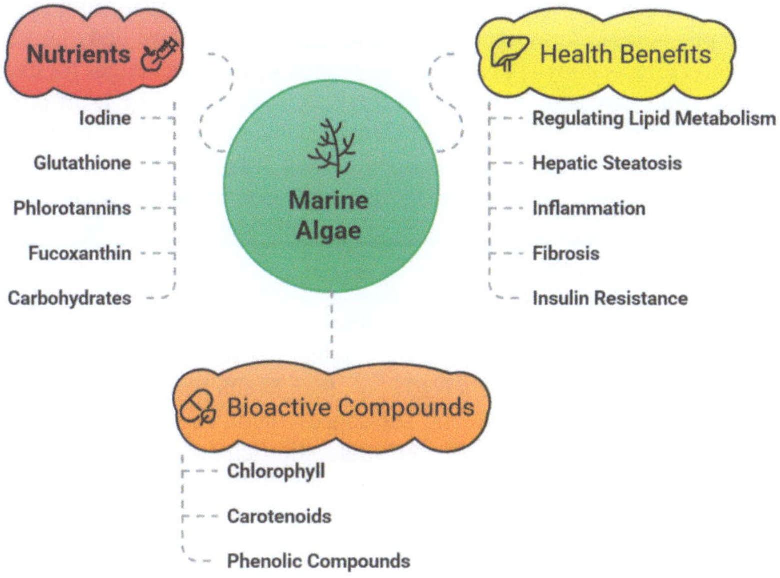

Fig. 2 Marine algae offer significant health benefits due to their rich content of essential nutrients

will always be a need for continuous innovation in the development of new functional foods (Bintari et al. 2021; Anil et al. 2022). Plant-based proteins as well as marine algae serve as functional food components that are becoming more and more well liked in the functional food sector. Marine algae have established themselves as a globally recognized functional food because they contain numerous beneficial compounds and nutrients. The composition of marine algae includes essential quantities of glutathione, phlorotannins, fucoxanthin, and carbohydrates such as carrageenan, fucoidan, alginate, and agar. Supplementation with marine algae biomass has enhanced the blood lipid profile in live subjects. Marine algae contain a wealth of different phytochemicals or bioactive substances, primarily in the form of pigments, such as chlorophyll, carotenoids, and phenolic compounds (Jiménez-Escrig et al. 2011). A fascinating and distinct way to formulate functional foods is to use known functionally food ingredients that provide good health benefits. Every functional ingredient can vary in its contribution to health enhancement and can enhance the advantageous qualities of the constituents, thereby boosting the advantages of new functional meals for general health. Moreover, these elements may work in concert to improve the functionality of novel functional meals. Therefore, we propose that combining marine algae could be an innovative way to create a novel functional meal (Assa et al. 2023). According to several studies, algal polysaccharides may be important in preventing cardiovascular disease, osteoarthritis, renal and liver problems, and underdiagnosed infectious diseases (Jiménez-Escrig et al. 2011).

Obesity represents a major health challenge. Nutrition describes both the pathological and physiological modifications that result from excessive body fat accumulation. Obesity affects body appearance and creates various challenges for everyday activities. Various diseases emerge from this condition, including heart problems, joint tissue damage, mental health problems, diabetes, and fatty liver. Existing pharmaceutical solutions for obesity concentrate on either blocking nutrient uptake or boosting metabolic functions. Drug treatments for obesity require thoughtful selection because they produce adverse effects and patients develop medication resistance according to Li et al. (2021).

Marine algae, considered a superfood, possess distinct bioactive elements, including polysaccharides, proteins, bioactive peptides, amino acids, polyunsaturated fatty acids, antioxidants, vitamins, and alkaloids, which serve various nutritional functions in food and supplement products to boost their health benefits. Polysaccharides are one of the fundamental metabolic substances found in marine algae. As prebiotics, marine algae polysaccharides generate short-chain fatty acids, which are then converted into energy sources, and increase feelings of fullness. They also decrease gluconeogenesis and lipid storage, which improves insulin sensitivity by activating AMP-activated protein kinase (Assa et al. 2023). The effectiveness of most MSPs in lipid metabolism has been demonstrated in several experimental investigations. By changing lipid absorption and boosting antioxidant capability, MSPs may have an impact on lipid metabolism (Li et al. 2021). Consequently, an innovative approach to promoting a healthy liver involves new functional foods. In individuals with nonalcoholic fatty liver disease, each function can improve the control of lipid metabolism, liver fat buildup, inflammation, scarring, and insulin resistance.

3 Liver Health and Algal Polysaccharide Relation

3.1 Antioxidant Effect of Marine Algal Polysaccharides

Oxygen is a vital element for aerobic biological organisms in their normal, metabolic processes. Residues will always be produced by organisms under high oxidative stress conditions. ROS can take part in a variety of physiological and metabolic processes in living things. Low to moderate levels of ROS can inhibit infectious agents from infecting host cells and may also prevent host cells from undergoing mitosis; however, if excessive ROS are produced, the balance between prooxidants and antioxidants in the organism's system is disrupted, leading to oxidative stress (Birben et al. 2012; Checa and Aran 2020). ROS may impair the nutrients available in food by causing oxidation after ingestion and may also damage cells' DNA, lipids, and proteins, contributing to aging, cancer, diabetes, inflammatory and neurological illnesses, and immune system damage. An imbalance between prooxidants and antioxidants in our systems is known as oxidative stress, and it may be considered a risk factor. The concept of oxidative stress assumes that the antioxidant defense system will normally remedy this imbalance. There are a number of antioxidant enzymes and nonenzymatic antioxidant systems that typically detect, control, and eliminate the generated free radicals (Birben et al. 2012; Rafieian-Kopaei et al. 2013). Unfortunately, once the amount of free radical exceeds its capacity to quench the oxidants, tissue damage and/or disease will begin to develop. The most simple and effective way to counter oxidative stress is the use of exogenous antioxidant supplements. Recent safety issues regarding synthetic antioxidants have led to increased interest in the study of naturally occurring antioxidants. Carotenoids, tocopherols, and flavonoids are naturally occurring antioxidants shown to have high capacities for scavenging unpaired electrons and reducing oxidative, inflammation-induced cellular damage. They have been used in medicine, food additives, and health supplements (Pham-Huy et al. 2008; Bouayed and Bohn 2010; Lobo et al. 2010; Anbudhasan et al. 2014). Polysaccharides are another class of naturally occurring compounds that have garnered a lot of interest due to their encouraging biological activity both in vitro and in vivo. Marine life has been considered a potential source of nutrients and chemicals with biological activity (Ruocco et al. 2016; Guan et al. 2024). Several publications in recent years have reported polysaccharides from marine organisms to have antioxidant activity (Zhong et al. 2019). Several publications in recent years have demonstrated that polysaccharides from marine sources exhibit antioxidant activity, including scavenging DPPH, hydroxyl, peroxyl, alkyl, H_2O_2, superoxide, and ABTS radicals, thereby reducing them. Polysaccharides with antioxidant activity derived from marine organisms could be used as therapeutic agents for oxidative stress-dependent disease states like liver injury, diabetes, obesity, neurodegenerative disease, colitis, and breast cancer. The reviewed polysaccharides were grouped by their provenance from marine algae, marine microorganisms, and marine animals. The pathways for antioxidant activity may involve three actions: scavenging of ROS, modulating the antioxidant system by secondary metabolites, and regulating the oxidative stress mechanisms. The results highlight the complexity of interactions involving antioxidant polysaccharides derived from marine organisms and demonstrate how their antioxidant activity modulates oxidative stress (Zhong et al. 2019). Figure 3 sums up the effect of ROS levels on cellular health from protective signaling to disease development and describes how marine algal polysaccharides restore redox balance by enhancing antioxidant efforts and regulating oxidative pathways.

3.2 Detoxifying Effects of Marine Algal Polysaccharides

Medicinal treatments aim to cure diseases, but excessive drug usage creates complications in the liver and multiple body organs. People show strong enthusiasm for investigating alternative medicine which uses natural elements that cause zero adverse reactions. The World Health Organization (also known as the WHO) reports that 80% of people rely on natural resources to meet their basic medical needs. The essential compounds that demonstrate effectiveness originate from plants together with microorganisms that live in both terrestrial and oceanic environments. The scientific community dedicates its attention to marine natural compounds with a

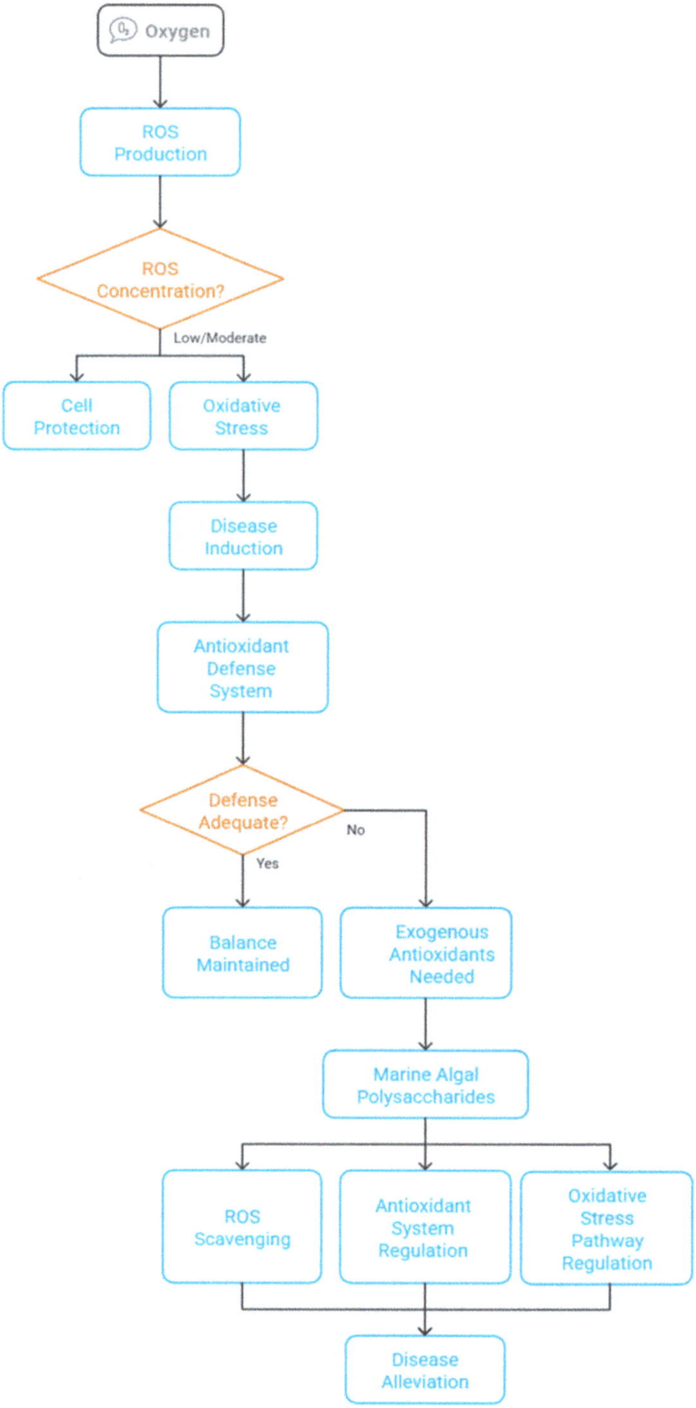

Fig. 3 Antioxidant effects of marine algal polysaccharides

special focus on eating seaweeds (Sohail and Farhat 2022). Various medications including acetaminophen (AAP) and methotrexate (Sohail and Farhat 2022) can cause liver toxicity, which results in liver damage. The liver operates as the central organ for drug and toxin conversion, allowing it to process carbohydrates, fats, and proteins. The liver is the most common site of drug-induced damage. Over many centuries the world has witnessed an increase in liver diseases. Hepatotoxicity remains a major concern for both the Food and Drug Administration (FDA) and pharmaceutical companies, as noted by Sohail and Farhat (2022).

The enzymes that make up liver markers include lactate dehydrogenase (LDH), aspartate aminotransferase (AST), alanine aminotransferase (ALAT), alkaline phosphatase (ALP), and bilirubin (both total and direct bilirubin). ALAT is found in the cytoplasm of the heart, kidneys, liver, and muscles, and it interferes with the transamination process. ALAT levels may increase as a result of any kind of liver damage. Hepatitis ischemic liver injury, which causes hepatic damage, may be the cause. Aspartate, a nitrogen byproduct of the urea cycle, is created when AST converts glutamate amino groups into oxaloacetate. Aspartate plays a role in the urea cycle, and its levels increase in individuals with cirrhosis and hepatic injuries that typically elevate ALAT (Hira et al. 2019; Sohail and Farhat 2022). In addition to these indicators, lipid profile (triglycerides and total cholesterol) and glucose are crucial biochemical markers for hepatotoxicity. Lipids undergo catabolic and anabolic processes in cells as part of metabolism, which can either break down or accumulate fat. These fats are either created in the livers of animals for energy use or obtained from the diet. Triglycerides and total cholesterol are examples of excess lipids in the human body (Sohail and Farhat 2022). Additionally, hepatic glutathione (GSH) and lipid peroxidation were measured to ascertain the state of the liver in liver tissue, while a number of biochemical markers, such as glucose, triglycerides, cholesterol, urea, and creatinine, were examined in the blood (Hira et al. 2019). For instance, the effects of NSAIDs are dependent on both the dose and duration, which makes liver involvement likely. In the UK and Australia, AAP is widely available as an over-the-counter (OTC) drug (Lau et al. 2016). It works well for mild to severe postpartum aching, headache, and muscular pain. It is one of the most often used medications, and reports from the USA indicate that acute liver failure (ALF) is caused by its toxicity. When drug toxicity increases in any organism, free radicals are generated, and oxidative stress plays a crucial role in AAP, leading to serious liver damage (Sohail and Farhat 2022). Cyclosporine A (CsA)-induced hepatotoxicity was shown by decreased liver marker enzyme activity. The degree of oxidative stress in rats treated with CsA is indicated by a significant increase in oxidant levels and a sharp decline in both enzymatic and nonenzymatic antioxidants. This subsequently resulted in increased lipid peroxidation, 8-hydroxy-2-deoxyguanosine, and protein carbonyls, as well as a reduction in ATPase activities and changes in lipid profile. The aforementioned abnormalities are also strongly supported by histopathological changes. However, concurrent treatment with *Sargassum wightii*-derived sulfate polysaccharides greatly reduced the morphological alterations and restored the aforementioned abnormalities to almost normal levels (Josephine et al. 2008). The detoxifying impact of various seaweeds in a Wistar rat model suggests that sulfate polysaccharides play an essential role in the liver-protecting benefits of

Characteristic	Drugs	Seaweed	Liver Markers
Use	Treat diseases	Alternative medicine source	Indicate liver health status
Side Effects	Overdosing causes side effects	Generally without side effects	Elevated levels indicate liver damage
Liver Impact	Can cause hepatotoxicity	Protects against liver toxicity	Assess liver status in tissue
Examples	Acetaminophen, Methotrexate	Sargassum Wightii, Laminaria	ALAT, AST, LDH, Bilirubin

Fig. 4 The comparative analysis of pharmaceutical drugs and seaweed-derived alternatives, focusing on liver health implications. Unlike hepatotoxic drugs (e.g., acetaminophen), seaweeds (e.g., *Laminaria*) exhibit hepatoprotective effects with minimal side effects. The diagram also identifies critical liver enzymes (ALAT, AST) and biomarkers commonly used to monitor hepatic function and damage

macroalgae. Further studies have shown that seaweeds protect against galactosamine-induced liver damage in a rat model, with the conclusion that fucoidan, a sulfated polysaccharide obtained from the brown algae *Laminaria*, largely mediates this protective action. A pig model has been used to show how eating seaweed affects glucose metabolism (Jiménez-Escrig et al. 2011). The presence of sulfate polysaccharides is necessary for the liver-protective properties of macroalgae, according to the detoxifying effects of different seaweeds in a Wistar rat model. Fucoidan, a sulfate polysaccharide obtained from the brown seaweed *Laminaria*, has been shown in further studies to partially mediate the protective effects of seaweeds against galactosamine-induced liver damage in a rat model. Seaweed consumption has been demonstrated to impact pigs' glucose metabolism (Kawano et al. 2007; Jiménez-Escrig et al. 2011). In Fig. 4 the comparison of therapeutic seaweed to pharmaceutical medications focuses on their effects on liver health. *Sargassum wightii* and other seaweed types not only protect the liver but also exhibit hepatoprotective effects, which is not the case for pharmaceutical drugs like acetaminophen which is known for its hepatotoxic effects. Key liver indicators—ALAT, AST, LDH, and bilirubin—are commonly used to assess liver condition.

3.3 Anticancer Effect of Marine Algal Polysaccharides

Liver cancer is one of the most deadly cancers, second only to lung cancer in terms of deaths. Together with viral hepatitis, hepatocellular carcinoma (HCC) is the sixth most frequent malignancy worldwide, accounting for an estimated 2 million fatalities per year. Eighty percent of liver cancer cases are HCC, the most common type of liver disease. Despite advancements in cancer detection, tumor identification, and chronic liver disease therapy, the prognosis for HCC is still much worse than that of other types of cancer. La carcinogénesis del HCC implica angiogénesis, inflamación crónica y tumores en macro y microambientes. Unfortunately, many patients miss the opportunity for resection because of late diagnosis (Abd-Elazeem et al. 2020).

The history of a cancer tumor, how much the disease has progressed, and the patient's history of interventions and preferences have a significant influence on the management plan. In general, the management plan is directed by either surgery, chemotherapy, or radiation. Surgery is still the best approach for most solid tumors. The survivorship post-cancer surgery is very dependent on the type of cancer and whether surgery is suitable. Some treatments, including chemotherapy and radiation therapy, have a high likelihood of being used alongside surgery. However, some treatments, such as surgery, come with considerable side effects, including fatigue, dry mouth, diarrhea, and, in some cases, outcomes contrary to the goals of cancer treatment, such as the development of additional tumors/future cancers (Abd-Elazeem et al. 2020).

Natural substances offer a trustworthy option when seeking medications that may assist in cancer prevention. Past studies have focused on natural compounds derived from marine life over recent decades, mainly due to their vast environment (encompassing approximately 70% of Earth's surface), remarkable biodiversity (95% of global biodiversity), and the unique conditions where these organisms thrive (such as pressure, salt, and extremely high temperatures). Among the examined marine substances, the anticancer capabilities of extracts and compounds sourced from marine algae are especially thrilling. Seaweeds contain a range of bioactive compounds that do not exist in the human diet or terrestrial plants. Recently introduced polysaccharides such as fucoidan, alginate, fucoxanthin, and others may exhibit unique or similar health-related or cancer-fighting properties beneficial to human health. Various extracts and cold-pressed products from different red, green, and brown seaweeds have been investigated for their antitumor potential (Abd-Elazeem et al. 2020).

Many seaweed compounds exhibit powerful anticancer activity. Seaweeds can respond and produce different kinds of unique secondary metabolites because of changing stresses in the environment (e.g., salinity, temperature, UV light, and light), making them a principal source of new medical materials for humans. Studies have shown that many different types of compounds from different marine algae can prevent cancer or slow cancer progression. Seaweeds possess strong anticancer properties. Extracts from seaweed caused cancer cells to undergo apoptosis. A growing body of evidence demonstrates that seaweed-derived bioactive chemicals have anticancer effects via a variety of mechanisms, including preventing tumor cell growth, invasion, and metastasis and causing cancer cells to undergo apoptosis. Consuming various seaweeds has been linked to a decreased incidence of cancer in Asian countries, where people have historically consumed substantial amounts of seaweeds (Abd-Elazeem et al. 2020) (Fig. 5).

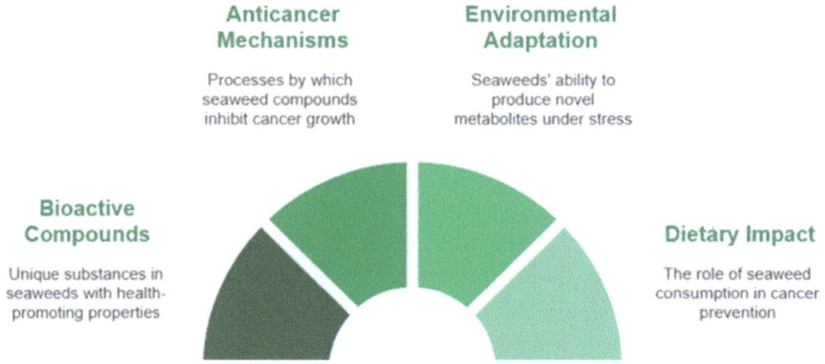

Fig. 5 The anticancer potential of seaweed-derived bioactive compounds

3.4 Anti-apoptotic Effects of Marine Algal Polysaccharides

Significant apoptosis or dysregulated apoptosis of hepatocytes will impair the liver and lead to advanced stages of the disease (Yang et al. 2013). Of the several types of algal polysaccharides, which are effective in reducing liver apoptosis and promoting hepatic cellular survival, marine polysaccharides stand out as unique, natural approaches due to their high potential in biomedical applications. Alterations in biological membranes during cell demise are characteristic of apoptosis, and one of the polysaccharides extensively researched in this type of cell death is fucoidan (El Rashed et al. 2022; Lu et al. 2023). Fucoidan is a brown seaweed polysaccharide obtained from species like *Fucus vesiculosus*, *Undaria pinnatifida*, and *Laminaria japonica* and possesses unexplored capabilities in addressing stress-induced apoptosis in cells (Boo et al. 2011; Senthilkumar et al. 2013; Yang et al. 2013). Recent investigations using metabolomic analysis have unveiled fascinating insights into how the parasite *S. japonicum* affects complex liver pathways, as cataloged in the Kyoto Encyclopedia of Genes and Genomes. This work highlights a remarkable intersection of parasitology and metabolic research with significant implications for understanding host-pathogen interactions. This affects mouse models of liver injury induced by carbon tetrachloride, a compound recognized for its potent metabolic effects on liver cells (Bai et al. 2020).

Some brown seaweeds have anti-apoptotic fucoidan which is able to act on the executed apoptotic signaling within the liver cells (Yang et al. 2013). For instance, it has been demonstrated that fucoidan, a sulfate polysaccharide present in brown seaweed, protects against liver damage brought on by apoptosis and increases the longevity of liver cells (Hira et al. 2019). Along with fucoidan, laminarin and alginate have also demonstrated anti-apoptotic activity in hepatic cells under stress. It is likely that all of these polysaccharides acted through antioxidant functions, downregulating ROS, a well-known initiator of apoptosis (Al Monla et al. 2022). By decreasing oxidative stress, fucoidan, laminarin, and alginate indirectly suppress specific stress-induced apoptotic signaling cascades, i.e., JNK and p38 MAPK (Chen et al. 2014) (Fig. 6).

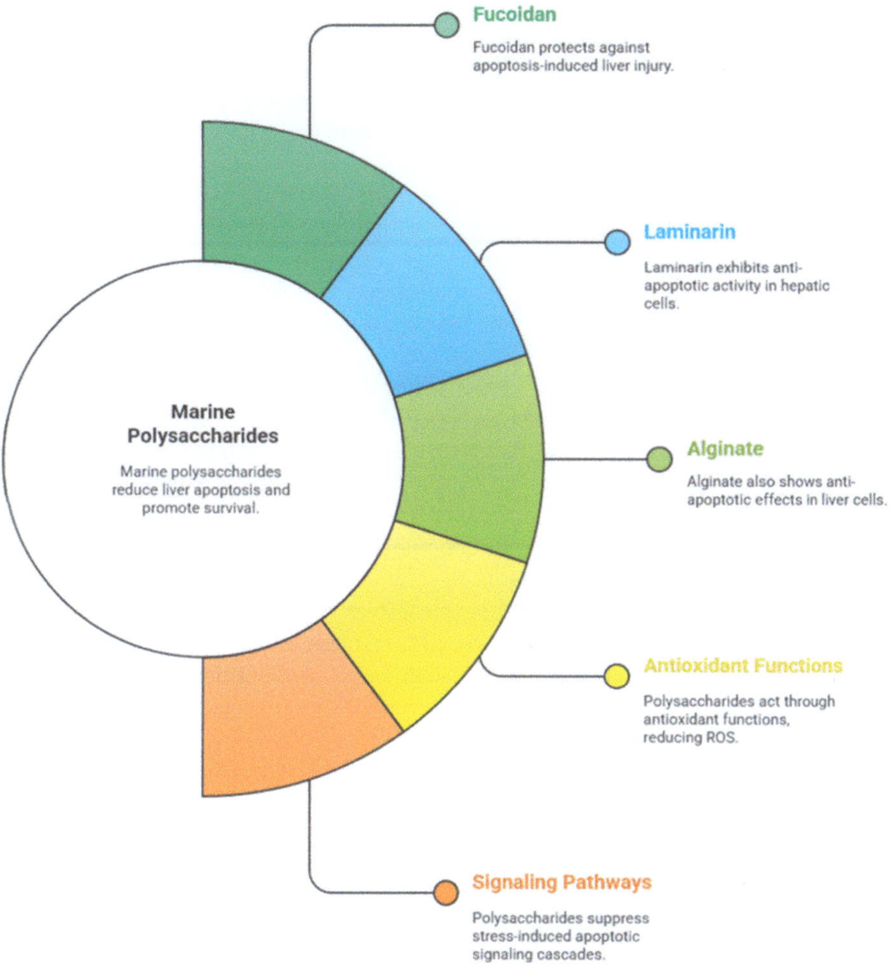

Fig. 6 The hepatoprotective effects of marine polysaccharides (fucoidan, laminarin, and alginate)

3.5 Anti-inflammation and Effects of Marine Algal Polysaccharides

The biological defense mechanism known as inflammation protects organisms from external threats and infections involving fungi viruses and bacteria. The physiological response activates leukocyte production and mediator synthesis. This decreases the expression of anti-inflammatory genes and increases the expression of pro-inflammatory genes. Acute inflammation causes five unique symptoms, including pain sensitivity, swelling, redness, temperature increase, and decreased function. Modern research demonstrates how inflammation exists as a multifaceted network that affects numerous bodily functions and the development of diseases in humans.

While the inflammatory response is crucial for safeguarding cellular physiological states, it is important that inflammation is adjusted according to the triggering stress and resolved promptly and systematically to prevent issues associated with chronicity. When the inflammatory response fails to cease promptly, prolonged inflammation may result in various health issues (Nabil-Adam and Shreadah 2021).

Liver inflammation caused by bacterial infection is among the most frequent pathological issues resulting in tissue injury or illness. Acute liver failure is the end result of a number of liver illnesses that are a major worldwide health concern with large economic ramifications. Oxidative stress-related inflammation and apoptosis are important pathogenic factors in these diseases. It is known that erythropoietin and its analogs influence the connection between hepatic inflammation and apoptosis (Nabil-Adam and Shreadah 2021).

By decreasing the inflammatory response and oxidative stress levels, as shown by lower levels of serum cytokines such as NFkB, MPO, and LPO, and by blocking the protein tyrosine kinase signaling pathway, *G. oblongata* demonstrated protective qualities against acute liver damage in mice. These findings suggested that the *G. oblongata* marine extract's detrimental effects on LPS-induced inflammation and organ damage may be related to its antioxidant qualities. These results suggested that the marine extract of *G. oblongata* may be used in biotechnological, nutraceutical, and pharmaceutical applications, most likely acting as potent therapeutic agents for acute liver damage caused by LPS through anti-inflammatory and antioxidant processes (Nabil-Adam and Shreadah 2021). Furthermore, ethanol-derived extracts of *S. fluitans* showed liver protective effects in rats against liver inflammation and fibrosis (Stiger-Pouvreau et al. 2023).

3.6 *Anti-NAFLD[1] Effects of Marine Algal Polysaccharides*

Nonalcoholic fatty liver disease or NAFLD is a worldwide issue acknowledged as the primary cause of more serious liver conditions. There is an urgent need to discover novel, efficient, safe, and simple preventive and treatment approaches (El Rashed et al. 2022). Scientific research has explored diverse algae species for their suitability as nutritional additives. Multiple scientific investigations have assessed various algae types to determine their suitability for human consumption. Biological active elements from algal polysaccharides show antioxidant activity, immune system regulation effects, anti-hyperlipidemic properties, antiviral effects, and antiradiation capabilities. Due to rising rates of obesity and metabolic disorders, nonalcoholic fatty liver disease (NAFLD) has become the most common chronic liver disease globally, with a current incidence of 25.2%. The population with NAFLD is expected to experience increasing rates of decompensated cirrhosis, hepatocellular carcinoma, and liver disease-related mortality due to the advanced

[1] Nonalcoholic fatty liver disease.

age of this population. At present, the primary approach to managing NAFLD involves lifestyle alterations, particularly through dietary modifications and exercise aimed at weight reduction. There remains a notable absence of approved pharmacological treatments for NAFLD. Several pharmaceutical compounds under research show promise through their effects on nuclear receptors and metabolic hormone derivatives and antifibrotic substances as well as combined medication approaches (Wan et al. 2022). Algae have become more popular recently because scientists are exploring their uses as functional foods and nutraceuticals beyond their established role in Asian culinary practices and nutritional benefits. The substantial variety of bioactive substances suggests that certain algae could provide phytochemicals with beneficial effects on modern noncommunicable diseases, including metabolic disorders such as NAFLD. Seaweeds contain specific polysaccharides that function as dietary fibers to affect how the body processes energy and absorbs nutrients and maintains metabolic equilibrium (El Rashed et al. 2022). Polysaccharides derived from *Ulva pertusa* enhance liver function metrics (AST, AST/ALT) and also prevent the abnormal growth of epididymal fat cells and excessive accumulation of lipids in the liver. Consequently, HU seems to have a safeguarding influence on the progression of NAFLD and the possibility of HU supplementation as a functional food for preventing NAFLD (Wan et al. 2022).

4 Mechanisms of Action of Marine Algal Polysaccharides

Polysaccharides from marine algae including fucoidan, laminarin, alginate, carrageenan, and ulvan modulated a number of pathways important to liver physiology and pathology (Besednova et al. 2014; El Rashed et al. 2022). The Nrf2 protein, known as nuclear factor erythroid 2-related factor 2, and its signaling pathway were the most frequently studied among all signaling entities. The pathway functions in liver cells to control oxidative stress and to activate enzymes involved in oxidative stress signaling. The pathway regulates essential phase II detoxification enzymes, including HO-1, GSTs, and NQO1, according to Ma (2013). These enzymes help reduce tissue damage caused by oxidative stress. The NF-κB pathway inhibition by algal polysaccharides results in decreased production of inflammatory cytokines, including TNF-α, IL-1β, and IL-6, according to Ku et al. (2013). Algal polysaccharides affect MAPK pathways, which control hepatocyte growth, cell death, and cellular adaptation to stress. Scientific evidence shows that algal polysaccharides affect both insulin resistance and autophagy mechanisms in liver cells via the PI3K/Akt and AMPK signaling pathways (Sajadimajd et al. 2019).

The gut-liver axis is now understood to function in a contemporary multitasking fashion in maintaining liver health. Marine algal polysaccharides act as prebiotics, modifying the gut microbiome and promoting the development of certain bitidinaria and lactobacillus, which produce short-chain fatty acids (SCFA) like butyrate, propionate, and acetate (Albillos et al. 2020; Guo et al. 2023). It is well known that butyrate and other SCFAs have both protective and hepatoprotective effects.

The gut microbiome plays an important role in moderating liver inflammation and injury. Cholecystokinin improves the antimicrobial balance and maintains gut barrier function, reducing the permeability to LPS and other endotoxins that are crucial in systemic inflammation as well as liver injury (Zhou et al. 2017; Ye et al. 2018; Pohl et al. 2022). Marine algal polysaccharides act to improve liver disease outcomes by protecting barrier functions and adjusting gut metabolites while strengthening the immune system and metabolic interactions according to El Rashed et al. (2022) and Lu et al. (2023). Various studies confirm that marine algal polysaccharides defend liver health through their effects on detoxification processes and metabolic functions while protecting hepatocytes from oxidative stress and increasing the levels of antioxidant enzymes SOD, CAT, and GPx (Wang et al. 2020). Polysaccharides modify lipid metabolism gene expression through their effects on PPARs and SREBPs and LXR receptors to decrease hepatic fat buildup and boost insulin sensitivity (Ding, Wang et al. 2021; Song, Lu et al. 2025). Some marine polysaccharides provide protection by inhibiting cytochrome P450 enzymes from transforming hepatotoxic agents into their active forms (Qu et al. 2020) (Fig. 7).

5 Overcoming Standardization and Clinical Evidence Gaps in Marine Algal Polysaccharides for Liver Disease Therapy

Algal polysaccharides derived from marine plants have great potential for the treatment of liver conditions. However, their therapeutic benefits are hindered by distinct challenges that need to be solved (El Rashed et al. 2022). Marine plant polysaccharides, such as starches, possess an incredible structural and functional variability from one type of algae to another, from one environment to another, and from one extraction method to the next (Xu et al. 2017). Additionally, variations in molecular weight, sulfate content, and sugar composition can also influence biological activity (Nishino et al. 1991; Qi and Kim 2018). Because of this, progression synthesis and analytical characterization focused on cultivation, extraction, and purification methods along policies defined for biological and clinical research, reproducibility trustable results is need for reasonable dependable outcomes (Reyes-Escogido et al. 2011; Patyra et al. 2022). Another gap that presents an issue is the lack of documented proof supporting the role of marine polysaccharides in the treatment of liver diseases in humans (Lu et al. 2023). The majority of research findings are based on animal experiments and living organism studies, which can only partially forecast human reaction patterns (El Rashed et al. 2022; Lu et al. 2023). Clinical investigations must urgently assess safety profiles, effectiveness, right dosing guidelines, and negative reactions in distinct patient groups over extended durations. Precision analysis of chronic liver diagnostic diseases such as NAFLD, viral hepatitis, or drug-induced liver injury would narrow the focus and provide specific insight, broadening the knowledge base of the health benefits of

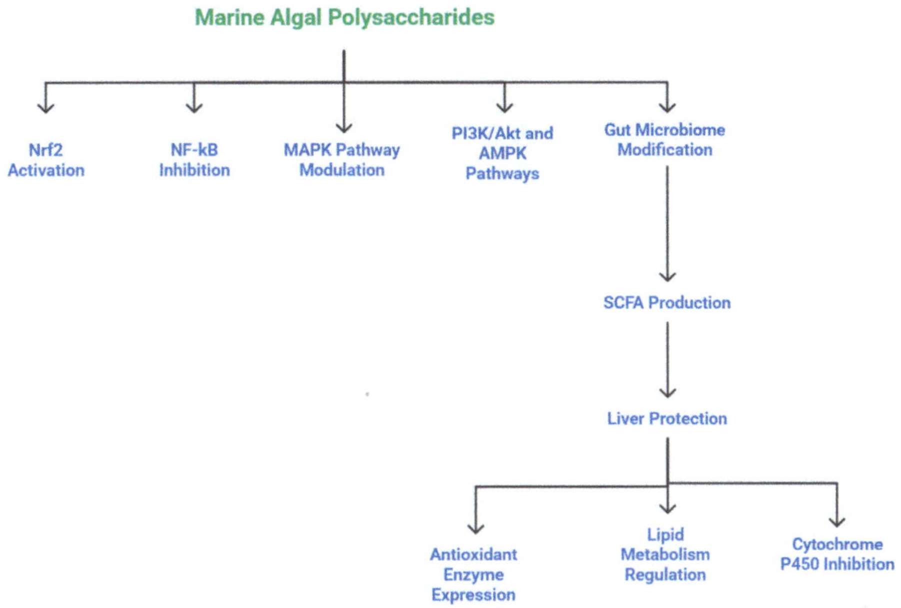

Fig. 7 Mechanisms of action of marine algal polysaccharides, showcasing their multi-target effects including Nrf2 activation, NF-κB inhibition, MAPK pathway modulation, PI3K/Akt/AMPK pathway regulation, and gut microbiome modification, leading to SCFA production, liver protection, lipid metabolism regulation, and cytochrome P450 inhibition

these compounds (Abenavoli et al. 2018; Foghis et al. 2023; Dhande et al. 2024). Additional research should look into how marine algal polysaccharides can act as supplements for various treatment approaches. Considering these compounds' nature and their anti-apoptotic, anti-inflammatory, and antioxidant qualities, it is possible that these polysaccharides would enhance the effectiveness of treatment and mitigate some of the adverse effects that would otherwise be present (Xu et al. 2017) (Fig. 8).

6 Conclusion and Future Prospects

Polysaccharide protocols derived from marine algae offer a multi-targeted strategy for liver disease prevention and therapy. These substances have antioxidizing, detoxifying, cancer-preventive, anti-apoptotic, anti-inflammatory, and anti-NAFLD biological actions that may help reduce damage that interferes with organ function. Fucoidan, laminarin, carrageenan, and ulvan are marine algae-derived substances that have shown encouraging outcomes in preclinical and limited observational clinical investigations. Although some progress has been made in the past few years, there is still a wide gap between lab results and actual clinical application.

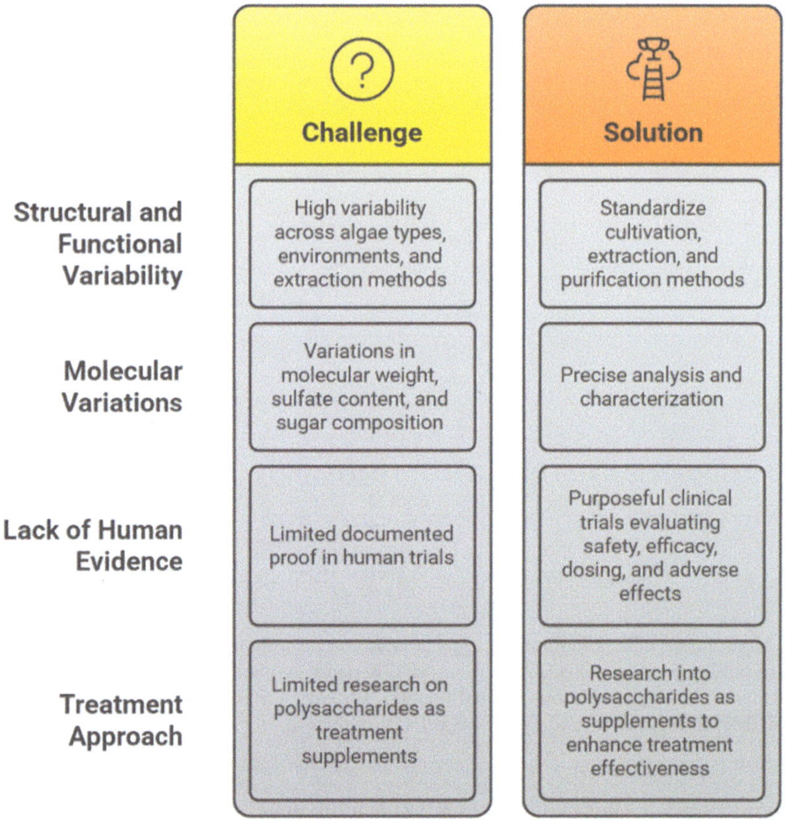

Fig. 8 Challenges and solutions for marine polysaccharides in liver disease treatment

The lack of large-scale human trials, standardization of polysaccharide composition, variability in biological effects, and many others remain unsolved. Quality control measures, unification of extraction and purification methodologies, cross-validation through rigorous clinical studies, and strong-to diverse liver diseases bolsters the require effort needed to eradicate these challenges.

Future research should prioritize the simultaneous study of marine algal polysaccharides alongside current therapeutic treatments to explore potential synergistic effects. Recent advancements in algal science together with genetic and metabolic engineering enable scientists to develop therapeutic polysaccharides that meet particular medical requirements. The development of natural algae-derived products as safe, noninvasive therapeutic options for liver diseases requires continued support and cross-disciplinary collaboration among marine biology experts, pharmacology and medicine professionals, and bioengineering specialists. In conclusion, despite current obstacles, this review highlights the emergence of a new area of investigation focused on the use of bioactive compounds with designated medicinal applications and complex marine algal polysaccharides, thereby supporting their use as supplements for liver health. Further exploration through clinical studies, alongside the research efforts invested, has the potential to significantly enhance liver disease management and improve therapeutic strategies based on functional nutrition.

References

Abd-Elazeem, O. M., N. A. Osman and N. S. El-Shenawy (2020). "Bioactive Compounds of Seaweeds and Their Effects on Certain Types of Cancer." Avicenna Journal of Medical Biochemistry**8**(2): 112–119.

Abenavoli, L., A. A. Izzo, N. Milić, C. Cicala, A. Santini and R. Capasso (2018). "Milk thistle (Silybum marianum): A concise overview on its chemistry, pharmacological, and nutraceutical uses in liver diseases." Phytotherapy research**32**(11): 2202–2213.

Al Monla, R., Z. Dassouki, N. Sari-Chmayssem, H. Mawlawi and H. Gali-Muhtasib (2022). "Fucoidan and alginate from the brown algae Colpomenia sinuosa and their combination with vitamin C trigger apoptosis in colon cancer." Molecules**27**(2): 358.

Albillos, A., A. De Gottardi and M. Rescigno (2020). "The gut-liver axis in liver disease: Pathophysiological basis for therapy." Journal of hepatology**72**(3): 558–577.

Anbudhasan, P., A. Surendraraj, S. Karkuzhali and P. Sathishkumaran (2014). "Natural antioxidants and its benefits." Int. J. Food Nutr. Sci**3**(6): 225–232.

Anil, P., K. Nitin, S. Kumar, A. Kumari and N. Chhikara (2022). "Food function and health benefits of functional foods." Functional foods: 419–441.

Assa, Y. A., N. Mayulu, R. Surya, N. A. Taslim, W. B. Gunawan, M. Samtiya, F. Kartawidjaja, A. A. Setiawan, A. Wijaya and F. Nurkolis (2023). "Soy and Algae Combination Using Tempe Fermentation Method: A Proposed Opinion for the Development of Functional Food." Nutrición clínica y dietética hospitalaria**43**(3).

Bai, X., M. Li, X. Wang, H. Chang, Y. Ni, C. Li, K. He, H. Wang, Y. Yang and T. Tian (2020). "Therapeutic potential of fucoidan in the reduction of hepatic pathology in murine schistosomiasis japonica." Parasites & vectors**13**: 1–14.

Besednova, N.N., Zaporozhets, T.S., Kuznetsova, T.A., Kryzhanovskiĭ, S.P., Kovalev, N.N. and Zviagintseva, T.N (2014). Hepatoprotective effects of extracts and polysaccharides from seaweed. Antibiotiki i Khimioterapiia= Antibiotics and Chemoterapy [Sic], 59(3-4), pp.30-37.

Bintari, S., M. Putri and D. Saputro (2021). Trends to the development of combined foods to create functional foods. Journal of Physics: Conference Series, IOP Publishing.

Birben, E., U. M. Sahiner, C. Sackesen, S. Erzurum and O. Kalayci (2012). "Oxidative stress and antioxidant defense." World allergy organization journal**5**: 9–19.

Boo, H. J., J. H. Hyun, S. C. Kim, J. I. Kang, M. K. Kim, S. Y. Kim, H. Cho, E. S. Yoo and H. K. Kang (2011). "Fucoidan from Undaria pinnatifida induces apoptosis in A549 human lung carcinoma cells." Phytotherapy Research**25**(7): 1082–1086.

Bouayed, J. and T. Bohn (2010). "Exogenous antioxidants—Double-edged swords in cellular redox state: Health beneficial effects at physiologic doses versus deleterious effects at high doses." Oxidative medicine and cellular longevity**3**(4): 228–237.

Checa, J. and J. M. Aran (2020). "Reactive oxygen species: drivers of physiological and pathological processes." Journal of Inflammation research: 1057–1073.

Chen, S., Y. Zhao, Y. Zhang and D. Zhang (2014). "Fucoidan induces cancer cell apoptosis by modulating the endoplasmic reticulum stress cascades." PloS one**9**(9): e108157.

Devlina Das, D. D., R. Vimala and N. D. Nilanjana Das (2010). "Functional foods of natural origin-an overview."

Dhande, D., A. Dhok, A. Anjankar, S. Nagpure and D. Dhande Jr (2024). "Silymarin as an Antioxidant Therapy in Chronic Liver Diseases: A Comprehensive Review." Cureus**16**(8).

Ding, M., Wang, G., Yuan, P., He, S., Shao, T., Liu, C. and Kong, X. (2021). Research progress in the role and mechanism of polysaccharides in regulating glucose and lipid metabolism. Nan Fang yi ke da xue xue bao= Journal of Southern Medical University, 41(3), pp.471-475.

El Rashed, Z., E. Grasselli, H. Khalifeh, L. Canesi and I. Demori (2022). "Brown-algae polysaccharides as active constituents against nonalcoholic fatty liver disease." Planta Medica**88**(01): 9–19.

Foghis, M., S. G. Bungau, A. F. Bungau, C. M. Vesa, A. L. Purza, A. G. Tarce, D. M. Tit, A. Pallag, T. Behl and S. S. ul Hassan (2023). "Plants-based medicine implication in the evolution of chronic liver diseases." Biomedicine & Pharmacotherapy**158**: 114207.

Guan, X., F. Wang, B. Zhou, X. Sang and Q. Zhao (2024). "The nutritional function of active polysaccharides from marine animals: A review." Food Bioscience**58**: 103693.

Guo, Q., Y. Li, X. Dai, B. Wang, J. Zhang and H. Cao (2023). "Polysaccharides: the potential prebiotics for metabolic associated fatty liver disease (MAFLD)." Nutrients**15**(17): 3722.

Hira, K., V. Sultana, N. Khatoon, J. Ara and S. Ehteshamul-Haque (2019). "Protective effect of crude sulphated polysaccharides from Sargassum Swartzii (Turn.) C. Ag. against acetaminophen induced liver toxicity in rats." Clinical Phytoscience**5**: 1–8.

Jiménez-Escrig, A., E. Gómez-Ordóñez and P. Rupérez (2011). "Seaweed as a source of novel nutraceuticals: sulfated polysaccharides and peptides." Advances in food and nutrition research**64**: 325–337.

Josephine, A., K. Nithya, G. Amudha, C. K. Veena, S. P. Preetha and P. Varalakshmi (2008). "Role of sulphated polysaccharides from Sargassum Wightii in Cyclosporine A-induced oxidative liver injury in rats." BMC pharmacology**8**: 1–9.

Kawano, N., Y. Egashira and H. Sanada (2007). "Effect of dietary fiber in edible seaweeds on the development of D-galactosamine-induced hepatopathy in rats." Journal of nutritional science and vitaminology**53**(5): 446–450.

Ku, C. S., T. X. Pham, Y. Park, B. Kim, M. S. Shin, I. Kang and J. Lee (2013). "Edible blue-green algae reduce the production of pro-inflammatory cytokines by inhibiting NF-κB pathway in macrophages and splenocytes." Biochimica et Biophysica Acta (BBA)-General Subjects**1830**(4): 2981–2988.

Lau, S. M., T. M. McGuire and M. L. Van Driel (2016). "Consumer concerns about paracetamol: a retrospective analysis of a medicines call centre." BMJ open**6**(6): e010860.

Li, Y., J. Qin, Y. Cheng, D. Lv, M. Li, Y. Qi, J. Lan, Q. Zhao and Z. Li (2021). "Marine sulfated polysaccharides: Preventive and therapeutic effects on metabolic syndrome: A review." Marine Drugs**19**(11): 608.

Lobo, V., A. Patil, A. Phatak and N. Chandra (2010). "Free radicals, antioxidants and functional foods: Impact on human health." Pharmacognosy reviews**4**(8): 118.

Lu, S.-Y., K. Tan, S. Zhong and K.-L. Cheong (2023). "Marine algal polysaccharides as future potential constituents against non-alcoholic steatohepatitis." International Journal of Biological Macromolecules**250**: 126247.

Ma, Q. (2013). "Role of nrf2 in oxidative stress and toxicity." Annual review of pharmacology and toxicology**53**(1): 401–426.

Nabil-Adam, A. and M. A. Shreadah (2021). "Red algae natural products for prevention of lipopolysaccharides (LPS)-induced liver and kidney inflammation and injuries." Bioscience Reports**41**(1): BSR20202022.

Nishino, T., Y. Aizu and T. Nagumo (1991). "The influence of sulfate content and molecular weight of a fucan sulfate from the brown seaweed Ecklonia kurome on its antithrombin activity." Thrombosis Research**64**(6): 723–731.

Øverland, M., L. T. Mydland and A. Skrede (2019). "Marine macroalgae as sources of protein and bioactive compounds in feed for monogastric animals." Journal of the Science of Food and Agriculture**99**(1): 13–24.

Patyra, A., M. Kołtun-Jasion, O. Jakubiak and A. K. Kiss (2022). "Extraction techniques and analytical methods for isolation and characterization of lignans." Plants**11**(17): 2323.

Pham-Huy, L. A., H. He and C. Pham-Huy (2008). "Free radicals, antioxidants in disease and health." International journal of biomedical science: IJBS**4**(2): 89.

Pohl, K., P. Moodley and A. Dhanda (2022). "The effect of increasing intestinal short-chain fatty acid concentration on gut permeability and liver injury in the context of liver disease: A systematic review." Journal of gastroenterology and hepatology**37**(8): 1498–1506.

Qi, J. and S. M. Kim (2018). "Effects of the molecular weight and protein and sulfate content of Chlorella ellipsoidea polysaccharides on their immunomodulatory activity." International Journal of Biological Macromolecules**107**: 70–77.

Quitral, V., C. Morales and M. Sepúlveda (2012) "Propiedades nutritivas y saludables de algas marinas y su potencialidad como ingrediente funcional Nutritional and health properties of seaweeds and its potential as a functional ingredient."

R. Gamal, M. E. E., H. Ibrahim (2023). "Curing Functions and Medical Applications of Microalgae." Egyptian Journal of Aquatic Biology & Fisheries**27**(5): 541–577.

Rafieian-Kopaei, M., A. Baradaran and M. Rafieian (2013). "Oxidative stress and the paradoxical effects of antioxidants." Journal of research in medical sciences: the official journal of Isfahan University of Medical Sciences**18**(7): 629.

Reyes-Escogido, M. D. L., E. G. Gonzalez-Mondragon and E. Vazquez-Tzompantzi (2011). "Chemical and pharmacological aspects of capsaicin." Molecules**16**(2): 1253–1270.

Ruocco, N., S. Costantini, S. Guariniello and M. Costantini (2016). "Polysaccharides from the marine environment with pharmacological, cosmeceutical and nutraceutical potential." Molecules**21**(5): 551.

Sajadimajd, S., S. Momtaz, P. Haratipour, F. F. El-Senduny, A. I. Panah, J. Navabi, Z. Soheilikhah, M. H. Farzaei and R. Rahimi (2019). "Molecular mechanisms underlying cancer preventive and therapeutic potential of algal polysaccharides." Current Pharmaceutical Design**25**(11): 1210–1235.

Senthilkumar, K., P. Manivasagan, J. Venkatesan and S.-K. Kim (2013). "Brown seaweed fucoidan: biological activity and apoptosis, growth signaling mechanism in cancer." International journal of biological macromolecules**60**: 366–374.

Sohail, N. and H. Farhat (2022). "Role of seaweeds in drug induced nephrotoxicity." Marine Science and Technology Bulletin**11**(4): 515–532.

Song, H., Lu, J. and Deng, R. (2025). Polysaccharides from Tremella Fuciformis Enhance Glucose and Lipid Metabolism in HepG2 Cells Through Activating the AMPK Signaling Pathway. Chemistry & Biodiversity, 22(2), p.e202401926.

Stiger-Pouvreau, V., L. Mattio, A. De Ramon N'Yeurt, S. Uwai, H. Dominguez, N. Flórez-Fernández, S. Connan and A. T. Critchley (2023). "A concise review of the highly diverse genus Sargassum C. Agardh with wide industrial potential." Journal of Applied Phycology**35**(4): 1453–1483.

Vicentini, A., L. Liberatore and D. Mastrocola (2016). "Functional foods: Trends and development of the global market." Italian Journal of Food Science**28**(2): 338.

Villarruel-López, A., F. Ascencio and K. Nuño (2017). "Microalgae, a potential natural functional food source–a review." Polish journal of food and nutrition sciences**67**(4).

Wan, Y., L. Liu, B. Zhang, S. Wang, X. Wang, K. Chen, Y. Li, T. Zhao and H. Qi (2022). "Structural characterization and anti-nonalcoholic fatty liver effect of high-sulfated Ulva pertusa Polysaccharide." Pharmaceuticals**16**(1): 62.

Wang, L., Yang, Y., Tan, H.Y., Li, S. and Feng, Y. (2020). Protective actions of acidic hydrolysates of polysaccharide extracted from mactra veneriformis against chemical-induced acute liver damage. Frontiers in Pharmacology, 11, p.446.

Xu, S.-Y., X. Huang and K.-L. Cheong (2017). "Recent advances in marine algae polysaccharides: Isolation, structure, and activities."Marine Drugs**15**(12): 388.

Yang, L., P. Wang, H. Wang, Q. Li, H. Teng, Z. Liu, W. Yang, L. Hou and X. Zou (2013). "Fucoidan derived from Undaria pinnatifida induces apoptosis in human hepatocellular carcinoma SMMC-7721 cells via the ROS-mediated mitochondrial pathway." Marine drugs**11**(6): 1961–1976.

Ye, J., L. Lv, W. Wu, Y. Li, D. Shi, D. Fang, F. Guo, H. Jiang, R. Yan and W. Ye (2018). "Butyrate protects mice against methionine–choline-deficient diet-induced non-alcoholic steatohepatitis by improving gut barrier function, attenuating inflammation and reducing endotoxin levels." Frontiers in microbiology **9**: 1967.

Zhou, D., Q. Pan, F.-Z. Xin, R.-N. Zhang, C.-X. He, G.-Y. Chen, C. Liu, Y.-W. Chen and J.-G. Fan (2017). "Sodium butyrate attenuates high-fat diet-induced steatohepatitis in mice by improving gut microbiota and gastrointestinal barrier." World journal of gastroenterology **23**(1): 60.

Zhong, Q., Wei, B., Wang, S., Ke, S., Chen, J., Zhang, H. and Wang, H. (2019). The antioxidant activity of polysaccharides derived from marine organisms: An overview. Marine drugs, 17(12), p.674.

Marine Polysaccharidic Matrix as Inhalational Drug Carrier

Muhammad Waseem Akram, Mohamed Effendi Mohamed Tenang, and Tin Wui Wong

Abstract Marine polysaccharides, due to their non-toxic, biocompatible and biodegradable nature, are considered as safe carrier materials for pulmonary drug delivery application. Marine polysaccharides, including fucoidan, alginate, agar, carrageenan, hyaluronic acid, chitosan and chondroitin sulphate, promote pulmonary drug delivery by minimizing protein corona formation; enhancing mucus diffusion, muco-adhesion and lung retention time; facilitating paracellular and transcellular drug transport via protein kinase pathway; increasing cell internalization; and reducing transepithelial electrical resistance. Marine polysaccharides, with molecular weights ranging from 10 to 3400 kDa, can deliver therapeutic agents into different regions of the lungs by modulating particle size for inhalation and targeting the macrophage or lung cell surface/P-selectin/CD44/hyaluronan receptors. Marine polysaccharides possess diverse functional groups, particularly sulphate, carboxyl, hydroxyl, acetamido and amino groups, which facilitate their formation into nano-/micro-complexes, enable hydrogen bond and hydrophilic character development

---

M. W. Akram
Non-Destructive Biomedical and Pharmaceutical Research Centre, Smart Manufacturing Research Institute, UniversitiTeknologi MARA Selangor, Puncak Alam, Malaysia

Particle Design Research Group, Faculty of Pharmacy, UniversitiTeknologi MARA Selangor, Puncak Alam, Malaysia

M. E. M. Tenang
Tenang Pharma SdnBhd, Nilai, Negeri Sembilan, Malaysia

T. W. Wong (✉)
Non-Destructive Biomedical and Pharmaceutical Research Centre, Smart Manufacturing Research Institute, UniversitiTeknologi MARA Selangor, Puncak Alam, Malaysia

Particle Design Research Group, Faculty of Pharmacy, UniversitiTeknologi MARA Selangor, Puncak Alam, Malaysia

Department of Industrial Pharmacy, Faculty of Pharmacy, Silpakorn University, Nakhon Pathom, Thailand
e-mail: wongtinwui@uitm.edu.my

S. Jana et al. (eds.), *Multifunctional Marine Polysaccharides*,
https://doi.org/10.1007/978-981-95-4126-3_9

and allow chemical modification into various functional derivatives to meet drug release and targeting functions. Thus far, the majority of research findings are obtained in vitro and in vivo. Its clinical translation requires human trials.

Keywords Aerosolization · Inhalation · Marine polysaccharide · Pulmonary drug delivery

1 Introduction

The inhalation route is considered as a more viable drug delivery option for the treatment of pulmonary disorders, offering distinct advantages over oral, skin and parenteral routes (Garcia-Fernandez et al. 2021). The enormous absorptive surface area of the lung (180 m^2), direct delivery of therapeutic agents into targeted region, avoidance of first-pass hepatic metabolism, higher deposition and bioavailability render inhalation route ideal for the treatment of lung disorders (Yue et al. 2023). However, pulmonary delivery system is also associated with various physiological barriers that impede the efficient deposition of drugs at the lung target site. These barriers include complex anatomical architect of the respiratory tract, mucociliary clearance, phagocytic clearance by alveolar macrophages and pulmonary mucus absorption barrier (Jin et al. 2023).

Pulmonary drug delivery systems are broadly available as aerosol, nebulized liquid and dry powder (Chaurasiya and Zhao 2021). The inhaled particles should possess an aerodynamic diameter ranging from 1 to 5 μm in order to effectively deposit into the lower lung (Alhajj et al. 2020). Inhaled particles (1–5 μm) tend to deposit in the large to small non-respiratory bronchioles, while particles <1 μm can efficiently reach the respiratory bronchioles and alveolar region. In contrast, particles around ~0.5 μm are more likely to be exhaled immediately after administration, whereas particles <0.5 μm are predominantly deposited in the peripheral lung regions (Akram and Wong 2024). Inhaled particles >6 μm are intercepted and cleared via mucus, whereas particles in the range of 1.5–3 μm are removed by alveolar macrophages through phagocytosis (Kumbhar et al. 2022). In recent years, targeted inhaled therapy utilizing microcarriers and nanocarriers has gained significant attention, offering the potential to enhance treatment strategies while significantly reducing systemic drug toxicity (Kumar et al. 2023). Currently, four devices are employed for pulmonary drug administration, namely, dry powder inhaler, metered-dose inhaler, nebulizer and soft mist inhaler (Kumar et al. 2022).

A variety of natural (e.g. albumin, gelatin), polysaccharide-based (e.g. chitosan, carrageenan, alginate) and synthetic (e.g. cyclodextrin, poly(lactic-co-glycolic) acid, polyethylene glycol, derivatives of acrylic acid) polymers have been explored as the matrix carrier for pulmonary drug delivery (Liu et al. 2020). Polysaccharides stand out among other polymers owing to their unique characteristics, such as excellent biocompatibility, biodegradability and processing adaptability (Tang et al. 2023). Polysaccharides are non-toxic carbohydrates composed of repeating units of

Table 1 Classification of polysaccharides derived from various sources

Source	Polysaccharide	References
Animal	Albumin, gelatine, collagen, silk etc.	Zaiki et al. (2023)
Plant	Pectin, starch, cellulose, glucomannan, *Ephedra sinica* Stapf etc.	Gopinath et al. (2018) and Nasrollahzadeh et al. (2020)
Marine algae	Fucoidan, alginate, agar, carrageenan, galactan, porphyran, laminarin, ulvan etc.	Barbosa et al. (2019)
Crustacean	Chitin, chitosan, chondroitin sulphate, hyaluronic acid etc.	Wang et al. (2024)
Microorganism	Xanthan gum, pullulan, dextran, exopolysaccharides, structural polysaccharides, intracellular polysaccharides etc.	Shen et al. (2021) and Zaiki et al. (2023)

monosaccharides [$C_n(H_2O)_n$] linked together by a glycosidic bond (Metaxa et al. 2021). Natural polysaccharides are derived from algae (e.g. fucoidan, carrageenan, ulvan), plants (e.g. pectin, glucomannan, *Ephedra sinica* Stapf), microbes (e.g. pullulan, dextran) and terrestrial and marine animals (e.g. chitosan, hyaluronic acid) (Table 1) (Gopinath et al. 2018; Nasrollahzadeh et al. 2020). Polysaccharides possess several unique physiochemical features—such as cationic, anionic or neutral charge; molecular weight ranging from few hundred to several thousand Daltons; and linear or branched structure—making them suitable candidates for the development of drug delivery carriers with varying drug release characteristics (Prasher et al. 2021). Chemical and biochemical modifications of the functional groups (–COOH, –OH, $-NH_2$) on polysaccharide structure lead to the generation of polysaccharide derivatives with inimitable properties tailored for specific therapeutic applications (Wu et al. 2020). The introduction of hydrophilic moieties, namely, carboxyl, amine and hydroxyl, enhances polysaccharide adhesion to cells and tissues, thereby improving the bioavailability of the therapeutic agents (Zhang et al. 2021). Further, polysaccharides have the ability to penetrate different physiological barriers in the body and deliver the drug cargo into the targeted region (Luo et al. 2023). In the past few years, the bioadhesive property of polysaccharides increase their appeal as muco-adhesive nano- and microcarriers in pulmonary drug delivery (Gopinath et al. 2018).

2 Marine Polysaccharides as Inhalational Carrier

Marine algae are a major source of bioactive natural compounds such as polyphenol and polysaccharides, which play vital functions in regulating biological activities, energy storage and cellular recognition process (Pradhan et al. 2023). Algal polysaccharides are typically classified into brown algae (alginate, fucoidan, laminarin), red algae (agar, carrageenan, galactan, porphyran) (Barbosa et al. 2019) and green algae (ulvan), while chitin, chitosan, chondroitin sulphate and hyaluronic acid are sourced from crustaceans (Wang et al. 2024). Exopolysaccharides, structural polysaccharides and intracellular polysaccharides can be derived from marine microorganisms (Shen et al. 2021). Marine polysaccharides, due to their non-toxic, biocompatible and biodegradable nature, are considered as safe carrier materials for drug delivery application (Pushpamalar et al. 2016).

3 Marine Algal Polysaccharide

3.1 *Fucoidan*

Fucoidan, a hydrophilic marine polysaccharide having molecular weight between 10,000 and 100,000 Da, primarily originates from brown algae and few sea cucumbers (Pradhan et al. 2020). Fucoidans are anionic and mainly composed of sulphated groups and L-fucose, while several other sugar molecules are also present in trace amounts (<10%), such as xylose, galactose, rhamnose, glucose, arabinose, mannose, glucuronic acid and acetyl groups (Usoltseva et al. 2019; Jiang et al. 2024). Fucoidan is composed of a backbone made up of sulphated L-fucose, which can be categorized into two main types: one type consists of repeating (1 → 3)-linked α-L-fucopyranose units, while the other type features a chain with alternating (1 → 3)- and (1 → 4)-linked α-L-fucopyranose units (Ramos-de-la-Peña et al. 2022). Fucoidan originating from the *Fucales* family of brown algae consists of alternating (1 → 3)-α-L-fucose and (1 → 4)-α-L-fucose linkages (Lahrsen et al. 2018). Fucoidan, owing to the presence of sulphate groups and sugar molecule residues, can interact with alveolar macrophage surface receptors and cytokines, and this interaction promotes cellular internalization and facilitates the delivery of drugs into specific lung cells or targets (Wang et al. 2024).

Cunha et al. (2018) prepared spray-dried fucoidan (derived from *Laminaria japonica*) microparticles encapsulating two anti-tubercular drugs, namely, isoniazid and rifabutin (Cunha et al. 2018). These microparticles exhibited good inhalation profiles (mass median aerodynamic diameter (MMAD) = 3.90–3.64 μm; fine particle fraction (FPF) = 50.2–45.4% of isoniazid and rifabutin, respectively). In vitro uptake study showed that 23% and 68% of the microparticles were taken up by macrophage like-cells, such as THP-1 human monocytic leukaemia cells and NR8383 rat pulmonary macrophages, respectively. Fucoidan-based (molecular weight = 20~200 kDa, originated from *Fucus vesiculosus*) nanoparticles (particle size = 217 nm; zeta potential = −33.60 mV) delivered more epigallocatechin-3-gallate into lipopolysaccharide (LPS)-stimulated RAW 267.4 macrophages and reduced the pro-inflammatory cytokines including nitric oxide (NO) and interleukin (IL)-6 (Ho et al. 2020). The uptake of nanoparticles by LPS-stimulated RAW 264.7 macrophages also increased with time (initial = 64.6%; after 20 min of exposure = 82.6%). Fucoidan (*Undaria pinnatifida*)-encapsulated bosutinib nanocrystals (particle size = 150 nm; zeta potential = −43.30 ± 2.5 mV), designed for lung cancer treatment, demonstrated a sixfold increase in mucus permeation within 6 h of incubation compared to neat bosutinib, and their inhalation efficiency was characterized by a FPF of 40.66 ± 2.51% (Kumar et al. 2024a). In another study by Kumar et al. (2024a, b), paclitaxel nanocrystals stabilized by fucoidan (*Undaria pinnatifida*) were developed (Kumar et al. 2024b). The nanocrystals had a particle size of 350 ± 50 nm and zeta potential of −37 ± 2.74 mV. In vitro cascade impactor study showed that a high FPF (60.15%) was attained. The fucoidan-stabilized nanocrystal displayed a high mucus diffusion (29.45 μg/ml) in contrast to neat-paclitaxel (4.3 μg/ml) within an hour of contact with cancer cells, and this gave rise to a relatively high drug bioavailability in the lungs. Chitosan-/fucoidan-based (*Fucus vesiculosus*) nanoparticles (particle size = 270–300 nm; zeta potential = 0.11–1.05 mV in phosphate buffer saline) are engineered for pulmonary delivery of gentamicin to treat pneumonia (Huang et al. 2016). An in vivo pharmacokinetic study indicated that intratracheal administration of chitosan/fucoidan nanoparticles (dose of gentamicin: 0.27 mg/kg) resulted in a higher ratio of area under concentration-time curve/minimum inhibitory concentration in comparison to intravenous administration of free gentamicin in Sprague Dawley rats at a dose of 0.5 mg/kg, highlighting improved anti-microbial efficacy and reduced systemic toxicity. Fucoidan is selective towards P-selectin, which is highly expressed in human lung cancer cells (Don et al. 2024). This translates to fucoidan being suitable as an inhalation carrier for lung cancer treatment. In vitro and in vivo studies highlight that fucoidan is not cytotoxic to healthy cells and does not induce unwanted side effects (Don et al. 2024; Atashrazm et al. 2015).

3.2 Alginate

Alginate is a linear copolymer heteropolysaccharides, mainly derived from the cell wall of brown algae also known as brown seaweed and extracellular matrices of *Azotobacter* and *Pseudomonas* species of bacteria (Raus et al. 2021). The molecular weight of alginate lies between 32,000 and 400,000 g/mol (Kirti and Khora 2022). Structurally, alginate is composed of β-d-mannuronic acid (M) and α-L-guluronic acid (G) units connected through 1,4-glycosidic linkage (Alfatama et al. 2021). The concentration and arrangement of M and G residues vary based on the source from which alginate is derived (Gomez d'Ayala et al. 2008). Alginate derived from *Laminaria digitata* showed a M/G ratio of 1.16, while alginate from *Ascophyllum nodosum* expressed a M/G ratio of 1.82 (Hariyadi and Islam 2020). The carboxyl group in alginate becomes charged at pH above 3–4, rendering it soluble in alkaline and neutral environment (Cardoso et al. 2016). Alginate occurs as a composite salt with various cations such as Na^{+}, Ca^{+2}, Mg^{+2}, Ba^{+2} and Sr^{+2} (Piras and Smith 2020). Alginate interacts with other biomaterials and form nano-/micro-complexes via different mechanisms, such as cross-linking, electrostatic interaction and chemical modification (Wang et al. 2023). Biocompatibility, muco-adhesion and non-toxic characteristics make alginate a successful biopolymer in the pulmonary drug delivery field (Ching et al. 2017).

Alipour et al. (2010) highlighted that the sodium alginate (250 cps of 2% solution)-encapsulated paclitaxel microparticles (particle size = 3.0 ± 0.7 μm; drug loading = 7.8–19.5%), designed for lung cancer treatment, show acceptable inhalation profiles with an MMAD of 5.9 ± 0.33 μm and FPF of 13.9 ± 0.57% (Alipour et al. 2010). In addition, alginate-based microparticles showed no cytotoxicity profile when investigated at different concentrations of paclitaxel (0.025–25 μg/ml) in human lung cancer A549 and Calu-6 cells. Mobus et al. (2012) prepared Zn^{2+}-cross-linked alginate microparticles loaded with protein bovine serum albumin for lower lung deposition (Möbus et al. 2012). The spray-dried microparticles showed a mean volume diameter in the range of 3–5 μm and a FPF up to 40%. In vitro release study indicated that the protein release from microparticles was dependent on alginate and zinc sulphate content of a formulation. In another study, sodium alginate was employed as a microcarrier-forming matrix, using calcium beta-glycerophosphate as the source of calcium ion to form cross-linkage (Mahmoud et al. 2018). The alginate-loaded roflumilast microparticles, prepared by emulsification-spray drying method, exhibited a better inhalation performance (MMAD = 2.47 ± 0.008 μm; FPF = 42.7 ± 1.1%; inhaled dose = 75.9 ± 6.5%) than neat-roflumilast (MMAD = 3.22 ± 0.49 μm; FPF = 22.5 ± 9.2%; inhaled dose = 41.4 ± 1.9%). These microparticles inhibited the expression of pro-inflammatory cytokines (IL-6, IL-10 and tumour necrosis factor (TNF-α)) inA549 human lung cancer cells. Inhaled spray-dried alginate-loaded colistin sulphate microparticles (particle size = 4.45 ± 1.40 μm; drug loading = 8.5 ± 1.50%) inhibited the growth of *Pseudomonas aeruginosa* via porosifying the cell wall of bacteria, as visualized using the scanning electron microscopy technique (Arauzo et al. 2022). No cytotoxicity was however observed when alginate-based microparticles were tested on human cells such asA549 and Calu3 cells. Hybrid alginate-hyaluronic acid aerogel microspheres, prepared via emulsion gelation followed by drying using supercritical CO_2, were characterized by inhaled aerodynamic diameter of 5 μm, low density value of 0.035–0.063 g/cm^3 and high porosity at 97.6–98.7% (Athamneh et al. 2019). These attributes suggested that the hybrid microspheres are suitable for use as an inhalation carrier for the treatment of pulmonary disorders. Sodium alginate-based inhalable spray-dried microparticles (particle size: 2–5 μm) showed sustained release of sildenafil citrate up to 24 h and a FPF of 24–30% (Shahin et al. 2019). Alginate-based (molecular weight = 403 kDa; M/G ratio = 30/70) aerogel microparticles, prepared by supercritical fluid technology, demonstrated powder compressibility of 15.8 ± 1.6%, specific surface area of 299 ± 15 m^2/g, high surface roughness, amorphous nature, aerodynamic diameter of 1–5 μm, high FPF of 68–72%, sustained drug release, non-cytotoxic against the fibroblast and high lung tissue permeability (Duong et al. 2024). These physical and biological characteristics of aerogel microparticles made them an ideal candidate for pulmonary drug delivery. Alizadeh et al. (2024) investigated the inhalation profile of sodium alginate-based microparticles loaded with anti-microbial agent (levofloxacin) for targeting *Pseudomonas aeruginosa* (Alizadeh et al. 2024). Spray-dried engineered microparticles (particle size = 2–5 μm; drug loading = 89%; amorphous nature;

morphology = round) had favourable aerodynamic parameters (FPF = 46.2–60.6%; emitted dose = 66.67–87.75%) required for pulmonary drug delivery.

Inhalable alginate nanoparticles (235.5 nm) could control the release of anti-tubercular drugs, such as isoniazid, rifampicin and pyrazinamide, and displayed a respirable fraction of 80.5% (Zahoor et al. 2005). Clinical trial (NCT02157922) by the Food and Drug Administration (FDA) highlighted that low molecular weight alginate is safe and well tolerated in humans after inhalation (van Koningsbruggen-Rietschel et al. 2020). Intratracheal administration of alginate-loaded (M/G ratio = 1: 1; viscosity = 200 ± 20 MPa) curcumin nanogel (particle size = 77 nm; polydispersity index = 0.242; zeta potential = −59.17 mV; morphology = spherical) via nebulization was associated with the suppression of pro-inflammatory markers such as TNF-α, IL-6 and IL-1β and acute lung injury reversal (Cai et al. 2024). Alginate, cross-linked with zinc ion into nanogel particles (particle size = 55.22 ± 2.43 nm; polydispersity index = 0.154 ± 0.030; zeta potential = −15.9 ± 0.92 mV) and directly administered to the trachea via ultrasonic aerosol inhalation, was found to remain in the lungs for a prolonged duration due to good bioadhesion in the bronchus that enhanced the therapeutic response (Chen et al. 2024). These nanoparticles suppressed the expression of asthmatic markers such as IL-4, IL-5, IL-6, IL-13 and interferon gamma (INF-γ) as well as decreased the number of lymphocyte, monocyte, neutrophil, eosinophil and basophil counts.

3.3 Agar

Agar originates from the cell wall of red algae, particularly from the genera *Gelidium* and *Gracilaria*. In terms of composition, it is mainly composed of agarose and agaropectin (Padmesh and Singh 2021). Agarose (molecular weight = 100 kDa; water-soluble) is the major component of agar. Structurally, it consists of repeating units of β-D-galactose and 3,6-anhydro-α-L-galactose, with traces of sulphate (Yazdi et al. 2020). Agaropectin comprises the basic disaccharide repeating units of agarose, in addition to having some hydroxyl groups on the 3,6-anhydro-α-L-galactose residues substituted with sulpho, methoxy and pyruvate groups (Bertasa et al. 2020). Agar could form composite with other materials such as inorganic (e.g. silver, gold), marine-based (e.g. chitosan, alginate) and lipid-based materials, and generally these composites are formed by utilizing supercritical technology, free radical-polymerization, microwave-aided formation, gel-casting process, 3D printing technique, thermophysicomechanical processing and chemical cross-linking (Shah et al. 2024; Arfat et al. 2017).

Varshosaz et al. (2016) developed agar-based nanospheres (particle size = 320 ± 90 nm; polydispersity index = 0.85; zeta potential = −29.6 mV; drug loading = 43.1 ± 0.28%; morphology = spherical) for pulmonary delivery of ibuprofen (Varshosaz et al. 2016). In vitro drug release findings showed that 66.7 ± 25% of ibuprofen were released from the nanospheres at 5 h, while in vivo pharmacokinetic study via pulmonary administration showed that these nanospheres were characterized by a higher plasma concentration (1927.93 ng/ml) in contrast to simple solution (9.93 ng/ml). The agar-based nanospheres were deemed suitable for systemic drug delivery via pulmonary route. Agarose remains neutral in charge across different pHs, and this property minimizes protein corona formation and enhances mucus permeation of particles that are essential in drug delivery (Yazdi et al. 2020; Nguyen and Lee 2017).

3.4 Carrageenan

Carrageenan is a high molecular weight, linear, anionic sulphated polysaccharide that is generally derived from the red seaweed species belonging to the Rhodophyceae class (Li et al. 2014). Chemically, carrageenan is primarily composed of two units (galactose and anhydro-galactose) that are linked by glycosidic bond (Jiao et al. 2011). Carrageenan, on the basis of ester sulphate content (15–40%), solubility and extraction source, can be further classified into seven types, namely, *kappa* (κ-), *iota* (ι-), *lambda* (λ-), *mu* (μ-), *nu* (ν-), *beta* (β-) and *Theta* (θ-) (Pacheco-Quito et al. 2020). Among them, *kappa* (ester sulphate content = 25–30%), *iota* (ester sulphate content = 28–30%) and *lambda* (ester sulphate content = 32–39%) carrageenan are mostly commonly utilized in the pharmaceutical sector (Pacheco-Quito et al. 2020). Carrageenan is considered a suitable carrier matrix for drug delivery owing to its (a) glycosidic bond, making it susceptible to cleavage by hydrolase enzymes and biodegradation; (b) negative charge due to the presence of sulphate group, which promotes polyelectrolyte behaviour that can be exploited in cross-linking and complexation, along with dosage form development; and (c) the presence of hydroxyl group in structure, which allows hydrogen bond formation and enhances hydrophilic character (Cunha and Grenha 2016).

Rodrigues et al. (2020a) engineered inhalable starch-/kappa-carrageenan-based microparticles containing isoniazid and rifabutin (particle size = 7.0 ± 0.7 μm; span = 2.5 ± 0.2; drug loading = 96.3 ± 3.4% (isoniazid) and 74.4 ± 11.9% (rifabutin)) for targeting the macrophages to treat pulmonary tuberculosis (Rodrigues et al. 2020a). These microparticles were characterized by satisfactory inhalation parameters (MMAD = 3.9 ± 0.3 μm and 3.3 ± 0.4 μm; FPF = 32.1 ± 9.4% and 37.9 ± 8.0% for isoniazid and rifabutin, respectively). They showed no cytotoxic effect in A549 human lung cancer cells, while mild cytotoxicity was observed in THP-1 differentiated macrophages cells, with microparticles exhibiting a dose-dependent uptake by the cells. κ-Carrageenan-encapsulated ciprofloxacin hydrochloride microspheres were formulated as a dry powder inhalation product using the ionic gelation method (Hariyadi et al. 2019). These carrageenan-based microspheres (drug loading = 13.49–18.90%; encapsulation efficiency = 10.54–28.69%; morphology = spherical) had particles sizes of 1.41–1.67 μm suitable for lung inhalation. Rifampicin-loaded liposomes were coated with polyelectrolyte complex of chitosan/kappa-carrageenan and spray dried to obtain dry powder for inhalation (Manca et al. 2014). These particles were 1 μm in size and spherical and positively charged, with drug encapsulation efficiency of ~70%, MMAD of 2 μm and FPF of ~50%. They gradually decreased A549 human lung cancer cell viability over 48 h and exhibited enhanced internalization efficiency with time. Inhalable kappa-carrageenan microspheres containing ciprofloxacin hydrochloride (particle size = 1.34–1.70 μm; morphology = spherical; drug loading = 15.63–38.72%; muco-adhesion capacity = 0.0059–0.0096 kg; in vitro release at 24 h = 74.38–81.02%) were fabricated to treat lung infection (Hariyadi et al. 2021). Owing to possessing inhalable sizes, they were found to remain in deep lung by in vivo fluorescence microscopy evaluation. Similar studies with inhaled kappa-carrageenan and alginate-based microspheres encapsulating ciprofloxacin hydrochloride (particles size = 1.24–1.72 μm; entrapment efficiency = 52.86–76.29%; muco-adhesion capacity = 0.009–0.032 kg; in vitro drug release at 2 h = 69.58–82.20%) demonstrated that the carrageenan-alginate microspheres were capable of depositing the drug in the lungs (Hariyadi et al. 2023). With reference to iota- and kappa-carrageenan, they could effectively regulate the absorption rate of fluticasone propionate and theophylline without causing inflammation and tissue damage to pulmonary tissues (Yamada et al. 2005).

4 Marine Animal Polysaccharide

4.1 Hyaluronic Acid

Hyaluronic acid, also known as hyaluronan or sodium hyaluronate, is a non-sulphated and non-protein polysaccharide of the glycosaminoglycan family and is generally derived from marine sources such as sharks (skin and cartilage), zebrafish, fish eyes, swordfish, shellfish, stingrays (liver) and mollusc bivalve (Abdallah et al. 2020). The structure of hyaluronic acid consists of repeated disaccharide units of D-glucuronic acid and D-N-acetylglucosamine which are connected by glucuronidic β-1,3 bond (Bhattacharyya et al. 2023). Marine and mammalian hyaluronic acids share an identical structure and biological activities. However, what sets marine hyaluronic acid apart is its lower molecular size, which may enhance its ability to penetrate more effectively into cell targets compared to mammalian hyaluronic acid (Abdel-Rahman and Abdel-Mohsen 2023).

Hyaluronic acid presents in three molecular weight ranges: (a) low molecular weight, 50–150 kDa (immune-stimulant properties); (b) medium molecular weight, 500–700 kDa (wound healing and embryonic development bioactivity); and (c) high molecular weight, 1 million Da (anti-inflammatory, anti-angiogenic, anti-microbial) (Fouda et al. 2016; Matějková et al. 2024). The presence of various functional groups, namely, hydroxyl, acetamido and carboxyl, enhances the hydrophilic character of hyaluronic acid. Meanwhile, the hydrophobic domain arises from its axial hydrogen atom (C-H), imparting amphiphilic behaviour that facilitates the formation of nanoparticles and micelles (Luo et al. 2019). Hyaluronic acid-coated nanoparticles exhibited 2.5 times less protein adsorption in contrast to chitosan-coated nanoparticles and lower protein corona effect than the commonly utilized polyethylene glycol (Luo et al. 2019). Hyaluronic acid, owing to its cell surface receptor binding affinity, particularly with CD44 (overexpressed in cancerous cells, immune cells and stem cells), is used as a targeting ligand for carriers used in the treatment of various disorders (Hussain et al. 2024). In the lungs, hyaluronic acid impacts the inflammatory mediators and triggers the clustering of alveolar macrophages, which delay phagocytosis, extend drug retention in the lungs and facilitate sustained drug absorption into the lungs (Nikjoo et al. 2021). Low toxicity, excellent targeting ability and the ability to degrade in the lungs after drug release render hyaluronic acid a promising candidate for pulmonary drug delivery (Yan et al. 2021).

In contrast to high molecular weight counterparts, low molecular weight hyaluronic acid-based (50 kDa) inhaled plasmid DNA powder (particle size = 10 μm; FPF = 20.8–68.6%) exhibited good aerosol performance and expressed high transfection efficiency upon intratracheal administration in mice and in A549 human lung cancer cells in vitro (Ito et al. 2025). Mucin 1 (MUC-1) peptide, encapsulated in hyaluronic acid-decorated polyethylene glycol-linked poly(D,L-lactide-co-glycolide) nanoparticles (particle size = 136.2 ± 18.38 nm; zeta-potential = −28.34 ± 6.77 mV; peptide release at 24 h = 97.95%), targeted the CD44 receptors presented on antigen-presenting cells and generated mucosal immune response (Jyoti et al. 2023). Its cellular uptake was high (86.2%) in RAW 264.7 macrophages, and mice immunized through inhalation generated a strong immunoglobulin A (IgA) antibody titre. Fukushige et al. (2020) engineered inhalable hyaluronic acid-coated liposomes containing small interfering RNA (siRNA) (particle size = 207.8 ± 16.7 nm; zeta potential = −13.1 ± 4.5 mV) and later dispersed the nanoparticles into mannitol solution and spray freeze-dried into microparticles (particle size = 32.3 ± 12.7 μm; FPF = 39.2 ± 5.4%) (Fukushige et al. 2020). The nano-in-microparticle formulation showed lower cytotoxicity in human umbilical vein endothelial cells due to the hyaluronic acid coating, and it demonstrated significant gene silencing effect of Bcl-2 siRNA in A549 human lung cancer cells due to the targeting ability of hyaluronic acid at CD44 receptors. Functionalization of chitosan-encapsulated ferulic acid nanoparticles (particle size = 164.2 ± 9.7 nm; zeta-potential = 24.0 ± 0.5 mV; encapsulation efficiency = 65.0 ± 1.5%; MMAD = 1.81 ± 0.15 μm) with hyaluronic acid enhanced their in vivo thermal stability and therapeutic effectiveness (Dhayanandamoorthy et al. 2020). This was attributed to improved interaction and transport across mucus, when these nanoparticles were nebulized in BALB/c mice. An inhalable reconstituted nanosuspension of dexamethasone-loaded hyaluronic acid nanoparticles, with a size range of 200–250 nm, is suitable for macrophage engulfment in combating lung inflammation (Camara et al. 2021). The nebulized nanosuspension exhibited a high level of aerosolization (FPF: 75 ± 0.2%), with the drug being delivered into the deeper regions of the lungs. High molecular weight hyaluronic acid tends to form a hydrogel upon contact with the body fluid, enabling sustained release of drugs from a matrix (Xu et al. 2012). Intratracheal administration of inhaled budesonide-loaded hyaluronic acid microparticles (particle size = 6.3 ± 0.1 μm; span = 4.0 ± 0.1; drug loading = 21.0 ± 0.3%; FPF = 35.6 ± 3.3%) in rats showed sustained anti-inflammatory response, and this was attributed to muco-adhesion property of hyaluronic acid (Liu et al. 2018). Li et al. (2017) reported that hyaluronic acid-based microparticles possessed good muco-adhesion, and this led to prolonged lung retention (Li et al. 2017). Polymyxin B-loaded hyaluronic acid (molecular weight = 8 kDa)-poly(lactic-co-glycolic-acid) (PLGA)-based nanoparticles (particle size = 220 nm; zeta-potential = −50 mV) penetrated the lung mucus barrier upon nebulization and entered infected alveolar cells via targeting the CD44 receptor (Wu et al. 2022). Within the cells, both hyaluronic acid and PLGA were degraded through the action of hyaluronidase and lysozymes. Vascular endothelial growth factor (Flt1) peptide-hyaluronic acid conjugate nanoparticles (particle size = 110.2 ± 17.4 nm; zeta potential = −20 mV) showed efficient cell uptake into A549 human lung epithelial cells via hyaluronan (HA) receptor-mediated endocytosis (Kim et al. 2013). Mukhtar et al. (2022) reported that isoniazid-loaded hyaluronic acid-mannose conjugate-decorated chitosan nanoparticles (particle size = 303 ± 16 nm; zeta potential = 34.3 ± 6.03 mV; drug loading = 25.9 ± 2.11%) exhibited good aerosolization performance (MMAD = 2.7 μm; FPF = 35%) and expressed high cellular internalization in RAW 264.7 macrophages (Mukhtar et al. 2022). These characteristics made inhalable dry powder-based hyaluronic acid nanoparticles a promising drug carrier for the treatment of tuberculosis. Hyaluronic acid-vancomycin dry powder complex (particle size = 2.90 ± 0.02 μm) designed for the treatment of cystic fibrosis demonstrated good aerosolization performance (MMAD = 4.29 ± 0.03 μm; FPF = 42.9 ± 0.2%), and it was suitable for delivering the drug into the deeper regions of the lungs (Magi et al. 2024).

4.2 *Chitosan*

Chitosan is a linear, cationic polysaccharide obtained through the N-deacetylation of chitin with hot alkali (Rasul et al. 2020). After cellulose, chitin is the second most abundant biopolymer and generally originates from marine crustacean shells, insects and invertebrate exoskeleton (Joseph et al. 2021). Chitosan, sourced from the N-deacetylation of chitin, exhibits lower crystallinity in contrast to chitin (Liang et al. 2022). It dissolves readily in most aqueous acidic solutions with a pH below its pKa value (approximately 6.5), including acetic, formic, lactic and citric acids (Zaiki et al. 2023). Chitosan exhibits a degree of deacetylation ranging from 40% to 98%, with its molecular weight varying between 2×10^6 and 5×10^4 Da (Antonino et al. 2017). Chemical modification of hydroxyl and amino groups in the chitosan structure gives rise to generations of chitosan derivatives such as cationic chitosan, N-acyl chitosan, O-acyl chitosan, N-carboxyalkyl chitosan, O-carboxyalkyl chitosan, thiolated chitosan, sulphated chitosan and sugar-linked chitosan, with each derivative possessing a wide range of physicochemical and pharmacological properties (Rasul et al. 2020; Islam et al. 2019). Thiolated chitosan derivative forms disulphide linkages with mucus glycoproteins like mucin (Ways et al. 2018). In addition, ionic interactions occur between the primary amine groups in chitosan and the sulphonic acid groups in mucus, while hydrogen bonds form between the hydroxyl and amine moieties of chitosan and mucin (Ali et al. 2020). These combined interactions enhance the retention time and facilitate the transport of drugs through mucus and mucosal barriers to achieve targeted delivery. Chitosan can be engineered into nano- and microcarrier systems through precise modulation of its molecular weight and degree of deacetylation (Mao et al. 2010). Non-toxic, biocompatible, biodegradable, muco-adhesive, mucus permeation and ease of chemical modification and transformation into nano- or microcarriers make chitosan a suitable polymer for inhalational drug delivery (Mura et al. 2022). Upon contact with mucosal interface, cationic chitosan interacts with negatively charged glycoprotein of mucin, and this electrostatic interaction facilitates muco-adhesion and promotes mucus permeation phenomenon (Menchicchi et al. 2014). Chitosan lessens transepithelial electrical resistance through modulating tight junctions between epithelial cells (Aibani et al. 2021). It increases paracellular and transcellular drug transport by inducing the translocation of tight junction proteins from the membrane to the cytoskeleton via the Protein Kinase C pathway (Patil and Nanduri 2017). Chitosan has been considered as a safe biomaterial for human consumption and has been utilized as food additive in multiple countries such as Italy, Japan, Finland and the USA (Morin-Crini et al. 2019). Table 2 summarizes the potential use of chitosan as a nano- or microparticulate inhaled drug carrier for the treatment of various pulmonary disorders.

4.3 Chondroitin Sulphate

Chondroitin sulphate is obtained from marine animals, particularly shark cartilage, fish bones and fins (Yuan et al. 2024). Functional groups such as hydroxyl, carboxyl and amino are present on chondroitin sulphate chain, which facilitate its modification with other hydrophobic agents or drugs (Khan et al. 2020). Esterification and amidation reactions are mostly performed to synthesize new derivatives (Zhao et al. 2015). The molecular weight of chondroitin sulphate lies between 10^4 and 10^5 Da (Abdallah et al. 2020). Chondroitin sulphate consists of alternating sulphated N-acetylgalactosamine and glucuronic acid units, which are identified by

Table 2 Chitosan as an inhalational nano- or microcarrier for pulmonary drug delivery

Chitosan attribute	Lung delivery characteristic	Nano-microparticle design	Remark	References
Molecular weight: 120–350 kDa Degree of deacetylation: 95%	**Formulation type:** solid **Targeted disease:** lung cancer **Cell/animal model:** A549 human lung cancer cells and 4-(methylnitrosamino)-1-(3-pyridyl)-1-butanone (NNK)-induced lung cancer in Sprague Dawley rats	**Drug**: silibinin **Inhaled nanoparticle attribute:** Particle size: 275 ± 1.20 nm Zeta-potential: 32.50 ± 0.21 mV Encapsulation efficiency: 75.52 ± 0.87% MMAD:2.75 ± 1.02 μm	Following 24-h treatment, folate receptor-targeted chitosan-based nanoparticles showed higher cell uptake in vitro and exhibited IC_{50} value of 24.5 g/mL In vivo reduction in tumour volume and a high content of silibinin were retained in lung tissue	Patel et al. (2024)
–	**Formulation type:** liquid **Target disease:** infectious acute pneumonia **Cell/animal model:** A549-H460 cell lines derived from human lung tumour tissues and acute lung infection in BALB/c mice model	**Drug:** polymyxin B **Inhaled nanoparticle attribute:** Particle size: 365.5 ± 4.7 nm Zeta-potential: 21.3 ± 0.8 mV Encapsulation efficiency: ~36.5%	In vivo findings revealed that interaction between chitosan and negatively charged mucin in tracheal region enabled the sustained release of polymyxin B in the lungs for up to 24 h post-inhalation In vitro antibacterial activity showed that >99.9% bacteria were killed when treated with nanoparticles (polymyxin B-equivalent dosage of at 8 μg/mL)	Fang et al. (2025)
Degree of deacetylation: ≥75%	**Formulation type:** solid **Target disease:** tuberculosis **Cell/animal model:** Wistar rats	**Drug:** linezolid **Inhaled microparticle attribute:** Particle size: 3.9–4.8 μm Zeta potential: 27 mV Encapsulation efficiency: 82.67–87.97% Morphology: spherical MMAD: 4.2 μm	Dry powder inhalation formulation showed 1.25 times higher bioavailability compared to oral tablet	Meravanige et al. (2025)

(continued)

Table 2 (continued)

Chitosan attribute	Lung delivery characteristic	Nano-microparticle design	Remark	References
Degree of deacetylation: 95% Viscosity: 100–200 mPa·s	**Formulation type:** solid **Target disease:** organ transplantation **Cell/animal model:** A549 human lung cancer cells and Sprague Dawley rat	**Drug:** cyclosporine **Dry powder inhalation formulation attribute:** MMAD: 1.58 ± 0.04–1.94 ± 0.02 μm FPF: 79.22 ± 2.12–81.55 ± 0.43% Emitted fraction: 77.15 ± 1.46–78.29 ± 2.10%	Dry powder inhalation formulation showed no cytotoxicity in A549 cells The in vivo bioavailability of cyclosporine was promoted by dry powder inhalation in contrast to orally available Neoral®	Huang et al. (2023)
Molecular weight: 3400 kDa	**Formulation type:** solid **Target disease:** non-small cell lung cancer **Cell/animal model:** A549 human lung cancer cells and NKK mouse model	**Drug:** niclosamide **Dry powder inhalation formulation attribute:** Particle size: ~1–6 μm MMAD: 4.28 ± 1.29 μm Geometric standard deviation (GSD): 1.31 μm FPF: 72.89 ± 11.37%	Inhalable niclosamide-loaded hybrid chitosan-poly(ε-caprolactone)-based nano-assemblies (NIC-CS-PCL-NA) expressed higher fluorescence intensities in human lung cancer A549 cells indicating higher cellular uptake In vivo inhalation of NIC-CS-PCL-NA was translated to higher lung deposition, retention and metabolic stability than positive control (neat cisplatin)	Ray et al. (2024)
Molecular weight: 190,000–310,000 Da	**Formulation type:** liquid **Target disease:** respiratory infection **Cell/animal model:** A549 human lung cancer cells and NCI-H358 non-small cell lung cancer cells	**Drug:** colistin sulphate **Metered-dose inhalation formulation attribute:** MMAD: 2.34 ± 1.01 μm GSD: 0.21 ± 0.02 μm FPF: 61.08% ± 2.03	Colistin-containing chitosan-coated gold nanoparticles (Col-CS-AuNP) effectively killed *Escherichia coli* after 6- and 12-h incubations at 5× and 10× the minimum inhibitory concentration Col-CS-AuNPs exhibited lower toxicity compared to free colistin when investigated on human A549 and NCI-H358 cells	Changsan et al. (2024)
–	**Formulation type:** liquid **Target disease:** asthma	**Drug:** baicalein **Inhaled nanoparticle**	Nebulized chitosan-encapsulated baicalein nanoparticles suppressed the expression of	Wang et al. (2021)

	Cell/animal model: ovalbumin-induced asthmatic BALB/c mice	**attribute:** Particle size: 285 ± 25 nm Zeta-potential: −2.5 mV Encapsulation efficiency: 96.1% Drug loading: 72.4%	IL-5 and decreased the goblet cell hyperplasia and peri-bronchial inflammation	
Molecular weight: 90–310 kDa Degree of deacetylation: 75–85%	**Formulation type:** solid **Target disease:** asthma **Cell/animal model:** ovalbumin-induced asthmatic BALB/c mice	**Drug:** naringenin and doxofylline **Inhaled microparticle attribute:** Particle size: 2.1 μm Zeta-potential: 31.2 mV Entrapment efficiency: >79% FPF: 62 ± 0.41%	Inhaled chitosan-based microspheres significantly reduced the serum bicarbonate level and eosinophil count in murine asthmatic model In vitro release study found that cumulative drug releases was about 78% for doxofylline and 72% for naringenin after 6 and 12 h	Pareek et al. (2024)
–	**Formulation type:** solid **Target disease:** tuberculosis **Cell/animal model:** J774 macrophages and Wistar rat	**Drug:** rifampicin **Inhaled nanoparticle attribute:** Particle size: 124.1 nm Entrapment efficiency: 72% MMAD: 3.3 ± 0.18 μm FPF: 33.27% ± 0.87	No cytotoxicity of chitosan-based nanoparticles was observed both in vitro and in vivo	Rawal et al. (2017)
Molecular weight: 50,000–190,000 Da	**Formulation type:** liquid **Target disease:** tuberculosis **Cell/animal model:** A549 human lung cancer cells	**Drug:** rifampicin **Nanoparticle attribute:** Particle size: 524 ± 39 nm Zeta-potential: 30.85 ± 2.7 mV Encapsulation efficiency: 90.2%	Chitosan-coated rifampicin-loaded solid lipid nanoparticles attained the higher mucoadhesion and cellular permeability in A549 cells	Vieira et al. (2021)

(continued)

Table 2 (continued)

Chitosan attribute	Lung delivery characteristic	Nano-microparticle design	Remark	References
Molecular weight: 50–200 kDa Degree of deacetylation: ≥85%	**Formulation type:** solid **Target disease:** asthma **Cell/animal model:** ovalbumin-induced asthmatic BALB/c mice	**Drug:** budesonide **Inhaled microparticle attribute:** Particle size: 3.2–3.7 μm MMAD: 3.41–3.70 μm FPF: 43–47% For microparticles/lactose physical blend: 64 ± 6%	Inhaled microparticles reduced the level of IL-4 and IL-5 in bronchoalveolar lavage fluid and the infiltration of macrophages, eosinophils, lymphocytes, neutrophil and overall inflammation	Zhang et al. (2018)

macrophage receptors, providing a crucial benefit for strategies aimed at targeting the macrophages (Rodrigues and Grenha 2015). Abdelaziz et al. (2020) found that inhalable nanocomposite coated with chondroitin sulphate demonstrated superior tumour targeting for CD44 receptors, which led to decreased expression of vascular endothelial growth factor and increased levels of caspase-3, in contrast to the spray-dried free drug (Abdelaziz et al. 2020). In another study, the chondroitin sulphate-coated nanocomposite exhibited higher cellular internalization in A549 human lung cancer cells, mediated through CD44 receptors (Abd Elwakil et al. 2018). Rodrigues et al. (2020b) demonstrated that the spray-dried isoniazid and rifabutin-loaded chondroitin sulphate microparticles (particle size: 4.1 μm; span: 3.1; morphology: spherical) for macrophage targeting exhibited good aerosolization and inhalation performances (MMAD = ~4 μm; FPF = approximately 44%) (Rodrigues et al. 2020b). The macrophage uptake of spray-dried microparticles was mediated in a dose-dependent manner in J744A.1 cell line (derived from ascites of an adult female mouse with reticulum cell sarcoma). The high targeting affinity of chondroitin sulphate for overexpressed CD44 receptors on lung cancer cells and macrophages makes it a promising carrier for delivering drugs to treat different pulmonary disorders. Table 3 listed all the marine polysaccharides and summarized their functional properties suitable for pulmonary drug delivery.

5 Conclusion

To address pulmonary delivery challenges, polysaccharides have emerged as superior candidates among natural and synthetic polymers. Polysaccharides have the tendency to penetrate different physiological barriers and deliver drug cargo to targeted regions. Particularly, marine polysaccharides derived from brown algae (alginate, fucoidan), red algae (agar, carrageenan) and crustacean (chitosan, chondroitin sulphate and hyaluronic acid) are considered as safe carrier materials for pulmonary drug delivery application. Results from clinical trial exhibit that low molecular weight alginate is safe for inhalation. By tailoring the aerodynamic characteristics of marine polysaccharides, they can be effectively delivered to the lungs via aerosol, nebulization and dry powder inhalers. Findings from both in vitro and in vivo studies highlight the potential of marine polysaccharides to deliver therapeutic agents to different regions of the lungs for the treatment of various lung disorders.

Table 3 Overview of marine polysaccharides and their functional properties for pulmonary drug delivery

Marine polysaccharide	Source of origin	Molecular weight	Structural attribute	Targeted receptor	References
Fucoidan	Brown algae; *Laminaria japonica*, *Undaria pinnatifida*, *Fucus vesiculosus*	10,000–100,000 Da	L-fucose and other sugars $< 10\%$ Sulphate, acetyl groups	Macrophage surface receptor P-selectin	Wang et al. (2024), Pradhan et al. (2020), and Don et al. (2024)
Alginate	Brown algae; *Laminaria digitata*, *Ascophyllum nodosum*	32–400 kDa	β-D-mannuronic acid (M) and α-L-guluronic acid (G) Carboxyl, hydroxyl groups	Macrophage surface receptor	Kirti and Khora (2022) and Bi et al. (2017)
Agar	Red algae; *Gelidium* and *Gracilaria*	100 kDa	Agarose and agaropectin Sulpho, methoxy, hydroxyl, pyruvate groups	–	Padmesh and Singh (2021) and Yazdi et al. (2020)
Carrageenan	Red algae; Rhodophyceae class	100–1000 kDa	Galactose and anhydrogalactose Sulphate, hydroxyl groups	–	Jiao et al. (2011) and Neamtu et al. (2022)
Hyaluronic acid	Marine animal; glycosaminoglycan family	50–1000 kDa	D-Glucuronic acid and D-N-acetylglucosamine Hydroxyl, acetamido, carboxyl groups	CD44, hyaluronan receptor	Bhattacharyya et al. (2023), Hussain et al. (2024), and Kim et al. (2013)
Chitosan	Marine animal, crustacean shells, insects and invertebrate exoskeleton	50–2000 kDa	Degree of deacetylation ranging from 40 to 98% Hydroxyl, amino groups	Macrophage surface receptor	Antonino et al. (2017)
Chondroitin sulphate	Marine animal; shark cartilage, fish bones and fins	10–100 kDa	Sulphated N-acetylgalactosamine and glucuronic acid Hydroxyl, carboxyl, amino groups	CD44	Abdallah et al. (2020) and Abdelaziz et al. (2020)

References

Garcia-Fernandez, A., F. Sancenon, and R. Martinez-Manez, *Mesoporous silica nanoparticles for pulmonary drug delivery.* Advanced Drug Delivery Reviews, 2021. **177**: p. 113953.

Yue, L., et al., *Inhaled drug delivery: Past, present, and future.* Nano Today, 2023. **52**: p. 101942.

Jin, Z., et al., *Harnessing inhaled nanoparticles to overcome the pulmonary barrier for respiratory disease therapy.* Advanced Drug Delivery Reviews, 2023: p. 115111.

Chaurasiya, B. and Y.-Y. Zhao, *Dry powder for pulmonary delivery: a comprehensive review.* Pharmaceutics, 2021. **13**(1): p. 31.

Alhajj, N., et al., *Critical physicochemical attributes of chitosan nanoparticles admixed lactose-PEG 3000 microparticles in pulmonary inhalation.* Asian journal of pharmaceutical sciences, 2020. **15**(3): p. 374–384.

Akram, M.W. and T.W. Wong, *Translational hurdles in anti-asthmatic nanomedicine development.* 2024, Taylor & Francis. p. 987–989.

Kumbhar, P., et al., *Inhalation delivery of repurposed drugs for lung cancer: approaches, benefits and challenges.* Journal of Controlled Release, 2022. **341**: p. 1–15.

Kumar, M., et al., *Micro and nano-carriers-based pulmonary drug delivery system: Their current updates, challenges, and limitations–A review.* JCIS Open, 2023. **12**: p. 100095.

Kumar, R., et al., *Nanotechnology-assisted metered-dose inhalers (MDIs) for high-performance pulmonary drug delivery applications.* Pharmaceutical research, 2022. **39**(11): p. 2831–2855.

Liu, Q., et al., *Physicochemical properties affecting the fate of nanoparticles in pulmonary drug delivery.* Drug discovery today, 2020. **25**(1): p. 150–159.

Tang, W., et al., *Application of chitosan and its derivatives in medical materials.* International Journal of Biological Macromolecules, 2023. **240**: p. 124398.

Metaxa, A.-F., et al., *Drug delivery systems based on modified polysaccharides: synthesis and characterization.* Supramolecules in Drug Discovery and Drug Delivery: Methods and Protocols, 2021: p. 151–161.

Gopinath, V., et al., *A review of natural polysaccharides for drug delivery applications: Special focus on cellulose, starch and glycogen.* Biomedicine & Pharmacotherapy, 2018. **107**: p. 96–108.

Nasrollahzadeh, M., et al., *Recent progresses in the application of cellulose, starch, alginate, gum, pectin, chitin and chitosan based (nano) catalysts in sustainable and selective oxidation reactions: A review.* Carbohydrate Polymers, 2020. **241**: p. 116353.

Prasher, P., et al., *Current-status and applications of polysaccharides in drug delivery systems.* Colloid and Interface Science Communications, 2021. **42**: p. 100418.

Wu, D., et al., *Chitosan-based colloidal polyelectrolyte complexes for drug delivery: a review.* Carbohydrate polymers, 2020. **238**: p. 116126.

Zhang, J., P. Zhan, and H. Tian, *Recent updates in the polysaccharides-based Nano-biocarriers for drugs delivery and its application in diseases treatment: A review.* International Journal of Biological Macromolecules, 2021. **182**: p. 115–128.

Luo, W., et al., *Polysaccharides-based nanocarriers enhance the anti-inflammatory effect of curcumin.* Carbohydrate polymers, 2023. **311**: p. 120718.

Pradhan, B., P.P. Bhuyan, and J.-S. Ki, *Immunomodulatory, antioxidant, anticancer, and pharmacokinetic activity of Ulvan, a seaweed-derived sulfated polysaccharide: An updated comprehensive review.* Marine drugs, 2023. **21**(5): p. 300.

Barbosa, A.I., et al., *Marine polysaccharides in pharmaceutical applications: Fucoidan and chitosan as key players in the drug delivery match field.* Marine Drugs, 2019. **17**(12): p. 654.

Wang, H., et al., *The application of marine polysaccharides to antitumor nanocarriers.* Carbohydrate Polymers, 2024: p. 122407.

Shen, S., et al., *Marine polysaccharides for wound dressings application: An overview.* Pharmaceutics, 2021. **13**(10): p. 1666.

Pushpamalar, J., et al., *Biodegradable polysaccharides for controlled drug delivery.* ChemPlusChem, 2016. **81**(6): p. 504–514.

Zaiki, Y., A. Iskandar, and T.W. Wong, *Functionalized chitosan for cancer nano drug delivery.* Biotechnology Advances, 2023. **67**: p. 108200.
Pradhan, B., et al., *Multifunctional role of fucoidan, sulfated polysaccharides in human health and disease: A journey under the sea in pursuit of potent therapeutic agents.* International Journal of Biological Macromolecules, 2020. **164**: p. 4263–4278.
Usoltseva, R.V., et al., *Fucoidans from brown algae Laminaria longipes and Saccharina cichorioides: Structural characteristics, anticancer and radiosensitizing activity in vitro.* Carbohydrate polymers, 2019. **221**: p. 157–165.
Jiang, Y., et al., *Roles and mechanisms of fucoidan against dermatitis: A review.* International Journal of Biological Macromolecules, 2024: p. 135268.
Ramos-de-la-Peña, A.M., et al., *Structural and bioactive roles of fucoidan in nanogel delivery systems. A review.* Carbohydrate Polymer Technologies and Applications, 2022. **4**: p. 100235.
Lahrsen, E., I. Liewert, and S. Alban, *Gradual degradation of fucoidan from Fucus vesiculosus and its effect on structure, antioxidant and antiproliferative activities.* Carbohydrate polymers, 2018. **192**: p. 208–216.
Cunha, L., et al., *Inhalable fucoidan microparticles combining two antitubercular drugs with potential application in pulmonary tuberculosis therapy.* Polymers, 2018. **10**(6): p. 636.
Ho, C.-H., et al., *The development of hyaluronan/fucoidan-based nanoparticles as macrophages targeting an epigallocatechin-3-gallate delivery system.* International Journal of Molecular Sciences, 2020. **21**(17): p. 6327.
Kumar, M., et al., *Fucoidan-based bosutinib nanocrystals for pulmonary drug delivery: Solid state characterization and in-vitro assessment.* Chemical Physics Impact, 2024a. **8**: p. 100644.
Kumar, M., et al., *Lipid-coated nanocrystals of paclitaxel as dry powder for inhalation: Characterization, in-vitro performance, and pharmacokinetic assessment.* Colloids and Surfaces B: Biointerfaces, 2024b. **237**: p. 113865.
Huang, Y.-C., et al., *Biphasic release of gentamicin from chitosan/fucoidan nanoparticles for pulmonary delivery.* Carbohydrate polymers, 2016. **138**: p. 114–122.
Don, T.-M., et al., *Improved camptothecin encapsulation and efficacy by environmentally sensitive block copolymer/chitosan/fucoidan nanoparticles for targeting lung cancer cells.* International Journal of Biological Macromolecules, 2024. **277**: p. 133901.
Atashrazm, F., et al., *Fucoidan and cancer: A multifunctional molecule with anti-tumor potential.* Marine drugs, 2015. **13**(4): p. 2327–2346.
Raus, R.A., W.M.F.W. Nawawi, and R.R. Nasaruddin, *Alginate and alginate composites for biomedical applications.* Asian Journal of Pharmaceutical Sciences, 2021. **16**(3): p. 280–306.
Kirti and S.S. Khora, *Alginate: a promising biopolymer in drug delivery system*, in *Marine Biomaterials: Drug Delivery and Therapeutic Applications*. 2022, Springer. p. 61–95.
Alfatama, M., L.Y. Lim, and T.W. Wong, *Chitosan oleate-tripolyphosphate complex-coated calcium alginate bead: Physicochemical aspects of concurrent core-coat formation.* Carbohydrate Polymers, 2021. **273**: p. 118487.
Gomez d'Ayala, G., M. Malinconico, and P. Laurienzo, *Marine derived polysaccharides for biomedical applications: chemical modification approaches.* Molecules, 2008. **13**(9): p. 2069–2106.
Hariyadi, D.M. and N. Islam, *Current status of alginate in drug delivery.* Advances in pharmacological and pharmaceutical sciences, 2020. **2020**(1): p. 8886095.
Cardoso, M.J., R.R. Costa, and J.F. Mano, *Marine origin polysaccharides in drug delivery systems.* Marine drugs, 2016. **14**(2): p. 34.
Piras, C.C. and D.K. Smith, *Multicomponent polysaccharide alginate-based bioinks.* Journal of Materials Chemistry B, 2020. **8**(36): p. 8171–8188.
Wang, Y., et al., *Marine biomaterials in biomedical nano/micro-systems.* Journal of Nanobiotechnology, 2023. **21**(1): p. 408.
Ching, S.H., N. Bansal, and B. Bhandari, *Alginate gel particles–A review of production techniques and physical properties.* Critical reviews in food science and nutrition, 2017. **57**(6): p. 1133–1152.

Alipour, S., H. Montaseri, and M. Tafaghodi, *Preparation and characterization of biodegradable paclitaxel loaded alginate microparticles for pulmonary delivery.* Colloids and Surfaces B: Biointerfaces, 2010. **81**(2): p. 521–529.

Möbus, K., J. Siepmann, and R. Bodmeier, *Zinc–alginate microparticles for controlled pulmonary delivery of proteins prepared by spray-drying.* European Journal of Pharmaceutics and Biopharmaceutics, 2012. **81**(1): p. 121–130.

Mahmoud, A.A., N.A. Elkasabgy, and A.A. Abdelkhalek, *Design and characterization of emulsified spray dried alginate microparticles as a carrier for the dually acting drug roflumilast.* European Journal of Pharmaceutical Sciences, 2018. **122**: p. 64–76.

Arauzo, B., et al., *Engineering alginate-based dry powder microparticles to a size suitable for the direct pulmonary delivery of antibiotics.* Pharmaceutics, 2022. **14**(12): p. 2763.

Athamneh, T., et al., *Alginate and hybrid alginate-hyaluronic acid aerogel microspheres as potential carrier for pulmonary drug delivery.* The journal of supercritical fluids, 2019. **150**: p. 49–55.

Shahin, H.I., et al., *Design and evaluation of novel inhalable sildenafil citrate spray-dried microparticles for pulmonary arterial hypertension.* Journal of Controlled Release, 2019. **302**: p. 126–139.

Duong, T., et al., *Alginate aerogels by spray gelation for enhanced pulmonary delivery and solubilization of beclomethasone dipropionate.* Chemical Engineering Journal, 2024. **485**: p. 149849.

Alizadeh, H., et al., *Evaluating the effect of sodium alginate and sodium carboxymethylcellulose on pulmonary delivery of levofloxacin spray-dried microparticles.* DARU Journal of Pharmaceutical Sciences, 2024: p. 1–15.

Zahoor, A., S. Sharma, and G. Khuller, *Inhalable alginate nanoparticles as antitubercular drug carriers against experimental tuberculosis.* International journal of antimicrobial agents, 2005. **26**(4): p. 298–303.

van Koningsbruggen-Rietschel, S., et al., *Inhaled dry powder alginate oligosaccharide in cystic fibrosis: a randomised, double-blind, placebo-controlled, crossover phase 2b study.* ERJ open research, 2020. **6**(4).

Cai, J., et al., *Inhalable multi-stimulus sensitive curcumin-alginate nanogels for scavenging reactive oxygen species and anti-inflammatory co-ordination to alleviate acute lung injury.* International Journal of Biological Macromolecules, 2024: p. 137816.

Chen, Y.-B., et al., *A bio-adhesion nanogel particle as an anti-inflammation agent for efficient aerosol inhalation therapy to asthma.* Materials & Design, 2024. **239**: p. 112734.

Padmesh, S. and A. Singh, *Agars: Properties and applications.* Polysaccharides: Properties and Applications, 2021: p. 75–93.

Yazdi, M.K., et al., *Agarose-based biomaterials for advanced drug delivery.* Journal of Controlled Release, 2020. **326**: p. 523–543.

Bertasa, M., et al., *Agar gel strength: A correlation study between chemical composition and rheological properties.* European Polymer Journal, 2020. **123**: p. 109442.

Shah, M., et al., *Advances in agar-based composites: a comprehensive review.* Carbohydrate Polymers, 2024: p. 122619.

Arfat, Y.A., J. Ahmed, and H. Jacob, *Preparation and characterization of agar-based nanocomposite films reinforced with bimetallic (Ag-Cu) alloy nanoparticles.* Carbohydrate polymers, 2017. **155**: p. 382–390.

Varshosaz, J., et al., *In vitro/in vivo evaluation of agar nano spheres for pulmonary delivery of bupropion HCl.* Drug Delivery, 2016. **23**(6): p. 1948–1954.

Nguyen, V.H. and B.-J. Lee, *Protein corona: a new approach for nanomedicine design.* International journal of nanomedicine, 2017: p. 3137–3151.

Li, L., et al., *Carrageenan and its applications in drug delivery.* Carbohydrate polymers, 2014. **103**: p. 1–11.

Jiao, G., et al., *Chemical structures and bioactivities of sulfated polysaccharides from marine algae.* Marine drugs, 2011. **9**(2): p. 196–223.

Pacheco-Quito, E.-M., R. Ruiz-Caro, and M.-D. Veiga, *Carrageenan: drug delivery systems and other biomedical applications.* Marine Drugs, 2020. **18**(11): p. 583.

Cunha, L. and A. Grenha, *Sulfated seaweed polysaccharides as multifunctional materials in drug delivery applications.* Marine drugs, 2016. **14**(3): p. 42.

Rodrigues, S., et al., *Carrageenan from red algae: an application in the development of inhalable tuberculosis therapy targeting the macrophages.* Drug Delivery and Translational Research, 2020a. **10**: p. 1675–1687.

Hariyadi, D.M., E. Hendradi, and N. Sharon, *Development of carrageenan polymer for encapsulation of ciprofloxacin HCL: In vitro characterization.* International Journal of Drug Delivery Technology, 2019. **9**(1): p. 89–93.

Manca, M.L., et al., *Fabrication of polyelectrolyte multilayered vesicles as inhalable dry powder for lung administration of rifampicin.* International journal of pharmaceutics, 2014. **472**(1–2): p. 102–109.

Hariyadi, D.M., et al., *Performance and drug deposition of kappa-carrageenan microspheres encapsulating ciprofloxacin HCl: Effect of polymer concentration.* Journal of Advanced Pharmaceutical Technology & Research, 2021. **12**(3): p. 242–249.

Hariyadi, D.M., et al., *Influence of Polymer Combination Concentration on the Characteristics, In Vitro Release, and In Vivo Lung Deposition of Alginate-Carrageenan Microspheres Encapsulating Ciprofloxacin HCl.* Indonesian Journal of Pharmacy/Majalah Farmasi Indonesia, 2023. **34**(1).

Yamada, K., et al., *Carrageenans can regulate the pulmonary absorption of antiasthmatic drugs and their retention in the rat lung tissues without any membrane damage.* International journal of pharmaceutics, 2005. **293**(1–2): p. 63–72.

Abdallah, M.M., et al., *Hyaluronic acid and Chondroitin sulfate from marine and terrestrial sources: Extraction and purification methods.* Carbohydrate Polymers, 2020. **243**: p. 116441.

Bhattacharyya, M., H. Jariyal, and A. Srivastava, *Hyaluronic acid: More than a carrier, having an overpowering extracellular and intracellular impact on cancer.* Carbohydrate Polymers, 2023. **317**: p. 121081.

Abdel-Rahman, R.M. and A. Abdel-Mohsen, *Marine Biomaterials: Hyaluronan.* Marine Drugs, 2023. **21**(8): p. 426.

Fouda, M.M., et al., *Wound healing of different molecular weight of hyaluronan; in-vivo study.* International journal of biological macromolecules, 2016. **89**: p. 582–591.

Matějková, N., et al., *Hyaluronic Acid Nanoparticles with Parameters Required for In Vivo Applications: From Synthesis to Parametrization.* Biomacromolecules, 2024. **25**(8): p. 4934–4945.

Luo, Z., Y. Dai, and H. Gao, *Development and application of hyaluronic acid in tumor targeting drug delivery.* Acta Pharmaceutica Sinica B, 2019. **9**(6): p. 1099–1112.

Hussain, Z., et al., *Hyaluronic Acid Based Functionalization of Nanodelivery Systems: A Promising Strategy for CD44-Receptors-Mediated Targeted Therapy of Lung Cancer.* Journal of Drug Delivery Science and Technology, 2024: p. 106183.

Nikjoo, D., et al., *Hyaluronic acid hydrogels for controlled pulmonary drug delivery—a particle engineering approach.* Pharmaceutics, 2021. **13**(11): p. 1878.

Yan, Y., et al., *Zinc ions coordinated carboxymethyl chitosan-hyaluronic acid microgel for pulmonary drug delivery.* International Journal of Biological Macromolecules, 2021. **193**: p. 1043–1049.

Ito, T., et al., *Development of naked pDNA inhalation powder formulation with high transfection efficiency using hyaluronic acid and phenylalanine as excipients.* Advanced Powder Technology, 2025. **36**(1): p. 104750.

Jyoti, K., et al., *Hyaluronate decorated polyethylene glycol linked poly (lactide-co-glycolide) nanoparticles encapsulating MUC-1 peptide augmented mucosal immune response in Balb/c mice through inhalation route.* Biochimica et Biophysica Acta (BBA)-General Subjects, 2023. **1867**(4): p. 130317.

Fukushige, K., et al., *Developing spray-freeze-dried particles containing a hyaluronic acid-coated liposome–protamine–DNA complex for pulmonary inhalation.* International Journal of Pharmaceutics, 2020. **583**: p. 119338.
Dhayanandamoorthy, Y., et al., *Aerosolized hyaluronic acid decorated, ferulic acid loaded chitosan nanoparticle: A promising asthma control strategy.* International Journal of Pharmaceutics, 2020. **591**: p. 119958.
Camara, C.I., et al., *Hyaluronic acid—dexamethasone nanoparticles for local adjunct therapy of lung inflammation.* International Journal of Molecular Sciences, 2021. **22**(19): p. 10480.
Xu, X., et al., *Hyaluronic acid-based hydrogels: from a natural polysaccharide to complex networks.* Soft matter, 2012. **8**(12): p. 3280–3294.
Liu, T., et al., *Budesonide nanocrystal-loaded hyaluronic acid microparticles for inhalation: In vitro and in vivo evaluation.* Carbohydrate polymers, 2018. **181**: p. 1143–1152.
Li, Y., et al., *Inhaled hyaluronic acid microparticles extended pulmonary retention and suppressed systemic exposure of a short-acting bronchodilator.* Carbohydrate polymers, 2017. **172**: p. 197–204.
Wu, J., et al., *Mucus-permeable polymyxin B-hyaluronic acid/poly (lactic-co-glycolic acid) nanoparticle platform for the nebulized treatment of lung infections.* Journal of Colloid and Interface Science, 2022. **624**: p. 307–319.
Kim, H., et al., *Bioimaging and pulmonary applications of self-assembled Flt1 peptide–hyaluronic acid conjugate nanoparticles.* Biomaterials, 2013. **34**(33): p. 8478–8490.
Mukhtar, M., et al., *Dry powder comprised of isoniazid-loaded nanoparticles of hyaluronic acid in conjugation with mannose-anchored chitosan for macrophage-targeted pulmonary administration in tuberculosis.* Pharmaceutics, 2022. **14**(8): p. 1543.
Magi, M.S., et al., *Novel Dry Hyaluronic Acid–Vancomycin Complex Powder for Inhalation, Useful in Pulmonary Infections Associated with Cystic Fibrosis.* Pharmaceutics, 2024. **16**(4): p. 436.
Rasul, R.M., et al., *A review on chitosan and its development as pulmonary particulate anti-infective and anti-cancer drug carriers.* Carbohydrate polymers, 2020. **250**: p. 116800.
Joseph, S.M., et al., *A review on source-specific chemistry, functionality, and applications of chitin and chitosan.* Carbohydrate Polymer Technologies and Applications, 2021. **2**: p. 100036.
Liang, X., et al., *Functionalized chitosan as a promising platform for cancer immunotherapy: A review.* Carbohydrate Polymers, 2022. **290**: p. 119452.
Antonino, R., et al., *Preparation and characterization of chitosan obtained from shells of shrimp (Litopenaeus vannamei Boone).* Mar. Drugs, 2017. **15**(5): p. 1–12.
Islam, N., I. Dmour, and M.O. Taha, *Degradability of chitosan micro/nanoparticles for pulmonary drug delivery.* Heliyon, 2019. **5**(5).
M. Ways, T.M., W.M. Lau, and V.V. Khutoryanskiy, *Chitosan and its derivatives for application in mucoadhesive drug delivery systems.* Polymers, 2018. **10**(3): p. 267.
Ali, M.S., et al., *Chitosan-coated nanodiamonds: Mucoadhesive platform for intravesical delivery of doxorubicin.* Carbohydrate polymers, 2020. **245**: p. 116528.
Mao, S., W. Sun, and T. Kissel, *Chitosan-based formulations for delivery of DNA and siRNA.* Advanced drug delivery reviews, 2010. **62**(1): p. 12–27.
Mura, P., et al., *Multiple roles of chitosan in mucosal drug delivery: an updated review.* Marine Drugs, 2022. **20**(5): p. 335.
Menchicchi, B., et al., *Structure of chitosan determines its interactions with mucin.* Biomacromolecules, 2014. **15**(10): p. 3550–3558.
Aibani, N., et al., *Chitosan nanoparticles at the biological interface: implications for drug delivery.* Pharmaceutics, 2021. **13**(10): p. 1686.
Patil, S.V. and L.S. Nanduri, *Interaction of chitin/chitosan with salivary and other epithelial cells—An overview.* International journal of biological macromolecules, 2017. **104**: p. 1398–1406.
Morin-Crini, N., et al., *Fundamentals and applications of chitosan.* Sustainable agriculture reviews 35: chitin and chitosan: history, fundamentals and innovations, 2019: p. 49–123.

Patel, P., et al., *Formulation of Folate Receptor-Targeted Silibinin-Loaded Inhalable Chitosan Nanoparticles by the QbD Approach for Lung Cancer Targeted Delivery.* ACS omega, 2024. **9**(9): p. 10353–10370.

Fang, Z., et al., *Muco-adhesive chitosan-coated polyphenol nanoparticle for treatment of infectious acute pneumonia through sustained pulmonary delivery of polymyxin B.* International Journal of Biological Macromolecules, 2025. **284**: p. 138233.

Meravanige, G., et al., *Chitosan-Based Linezolid Dry Powder Inhalers: A Novel Approach for Targeted Pulmonary Delivery in Tuberculosis Treatment.* Ind. J. Pharm. Edu. Res, 2025. **59**(1): p. 1–13.

Huang, Y., et al., *Cyclosporine A-loaded chitosan extra-fine particles for deep pulmonary drug delivery: In vitro and in vivo evaluation.* Journal of Controlled Release, 2023. **362**: p. 243–256.

Ray, E., et al., *Inhalable chitosan-coated nano-assemblies potentiate niclosamide for targeted abrogation of non-small-cell lung cancer through dual modulation of autophagy and apoptosis.* International Journal of Biological Macromolecules, 2024. **279**: p. 135411.

Changsan, N., et al., *In Vitro Evaluation of Colistin Conjugated with Chitosan-Capped Gold Nanoparticles as a Possible Formulation Applied in a Metered-Dose Inhaler.* Antibiotics, 2024. **13**(7): p. 630.

Wang, D., E.M. Nasab, and S.S. Athari, *Study effect of Baicalein encapsulated/loaded Chitosan-nanoparticle on allergic Asthma pathology in mouse model.* Saudi Journal of Biological Sciences, 2021. **28**(8): p. 4311–4317.

Pareek, A., et al., *Development of a new inhaled swellable microsphere system for the dual delivery of naringenin-loaded solid lipid nanoparticles and doxofylline for the treatment of asthma.* European Journal of Pharmaceutical Sciences, 2024. **193**: p. 106642.

Rawal, T., et al., *Rifampicin loaded chitosan nanoparticle dry powder presents an improved therapeutic approach for alveolar tuberculosis.* Colloids and Surfaces B: Biointerfaces, 2017. **154**: p. 321–330.

Vieira, A.C., et al., *Lipid nanoparticles coated with chitosan using a one-step association method to target rifampicin to alveolar macrophages.* Carbohydrate polymers, 2021. **252**: p. 116978.

Zhang, L., et al., *Sustained therapeutic efficacy of budesonide-loaded chitosan swellable microparticles after lung delivery: Influence of in vitro release, treatment interval and dose.* Journal of Controlled Release, 2018. **283**: p. 163–174.

Yuan, Q., et al., *Recent progress in marine chondroitin sulfate, dermatan sulfate, and chondroitin sulfate/dermatan sulfate hybrid chains as potential functional foods and therapeutic agents.* International Journal of Biological Macromolecules, 2024: p. 129969.

Khan, A.R., et al., *Chondroitin sulfate derived theranostic and therapeutic nanocarriers for tumor-targeted drug delivery.* Carbohydrate polymers, 2020. **233**: p. 115837.

Zhao, L., et al., *Chondroitin sulfate-based nanocarriers for drug/gene delivery.* Carbohydrate polymers, 2015. **133**: p. 391–399.

Rodrigues, S. and A. Grenha, *Activation of macrophages: Establishing a role for polysaccharides in drug delivery strategies envisaging antibacterial therapy.* Current pharmaceutical design, 2015. **21**(33): p. 4869–4887.

Abdelaziz, H.M., et al., *Inhalable lactoferrin/chondroitin-functionalized monoolein nanocomposites for localized lung cancer targeting.* ACS Biomaterials Science & Engineering, 2020. **6**(2): p. 1030–1042.

Abd Elwakil, M.M., et al., *Inhalable lactoferrin–chondroitin nanocomposites for combined delivery of doxorubicin and ellagic acid to lung carcinoma.* Nanomedicine, 2018. **13**(16): p. 2015–2035.

Rodrigues, S., et al., *Inhalable spray-dried chondroitin sulphate microparticles: Effect of different solvents on particle properties and drug activity.* Polymers, 2020b. **12**(2): p. 425.

Bi, D., et al., *Alginate enhances Toll-like receptor 4-mediated phagocytosis by murine RAW264. 7 macrophages.* International journal of biological macromolecules, 2017. **105**: p. 1446–1454.

Neamtu, B., et al., *Carrageenan-based compounds as wound healing materials.* International Journal of Molecular Sciences, 2022. **23**(16): p. 9117.

Part II
Biomedical Applications

Antioxidant Potentials of Marine-Derived Polysaccharides

Sowmiya Govindaragavan, Anandhi Anandaraj, and Rajasekar Thirunavukkarasu

Abstract Marine life produces a vast array of bioactive substances with great potential for various industrial and medicinal uses. Marine species have evolved protection mechanisms to thrive in a variety of frequently hostile environments. This has led to the production of distinct primary and secondary metabolites, including polyunsaturated fatty acids (PUFAs), vitamins, proteins, pigments, enzymes, polysaccharides and polyphenols. These substances have strong antioxidant activity in addition to a variety of biologically beneficial qualities, such as antibacterial, anticancer, anti-inflammatory, neuroprotective, and gut microbiota-regulating capabilities. As chronic infections and drug-resistant pathogens become more prevalent, the demand for dual-active compounds that combine antioxidant and antibacterial functionalities continues to grow. The pharmaceutical, nutraceutical, and cosmeceutical sectors now use more innovative marine-derived substances, thanks to advancements in marine biotechnology that have made it easier to discover and extract them. However, challenges such as sustainability, cost-effectiveness, and consumer acceptance, particularly in Western markets, remain barriers to commercial success. Unlocking the full potential of marine-derived bioactive chemicals for business and health will require ongoing research into marine bioresources and state-of-the-art extraction techniques.

Keywords Polysaccharides · Marine creatures · Antioxidants · Marine organisms

1 Introduction

Global research is focused on marine creatures and their metabolites in an effort to discover new physiologically active substances recognized as crucial for the development of potential medications and the future bioeconomy. The bioactivity of distinct, structurally varied compounds originating from marine sources can

S. Govindaragavan · A. Anandaraj · R. Thirunavukkarasu (✉)
Centre for Drug Discovery and Development, Sathyabama Institute of Science and Technology, Chennai, Tamil Nadu, India

S. Jana et al. (eds.), *Multifunctional Marine Polysaccharides*,
https://doi.org/10.1007/978-981-95-4126-3_10

occasionally outperform that of molecules originating from terrestrial habitats (Balasa et al. 2020).

Marine biota has developed defense mechanisms in response to environmental stressors and fluctuations, which has led to the synthesis of secondary metabolites and macromolecules with established antioxidant qualities. The resilience and biological variety of marine ecosystems are enhanced by these bioactive chemicals, which are essential for defense, adaptation, and survival (Angiolella et al. 2018).

There is significant interest in the investigation of marine antioxidants and their possible uses in the cosmetic, pharmaceutical, and nutraceutical sectors (Vuong 2021). Numerous bioactive substances of marine origin, including peptides, polyphenols, polysaccharides, and carotenoids, have a number of other biological benefits, such as skin-protective, neuroprotective, lipid-lowering, antimicrobial, antifibrotic, anticancer, anti-Alzheimer's, sleep-enhancing, wound-healing, and antidiabetic properties. This multifunctionality enhances their appeal for therapeutic and commercial applications, driving ongoing innovations in marine biotechnology (Hosseini et al. 2020)

Recent years have seen a major advancement in the study of substances originating from marine sources, such as dietary supplements and nutraceuticals (Senadheera et al. 2023). In spite of these advancements, According to Barzkar et al. (2022), the ocean's enormous biodiversity continues to serve as a vast reservoir for the identification of new bioactive compounds and even completely unique substances. The effective extraction of marine sources has been made possible by ongoing technological advancements, which have encouraged their commercial use in a variety of businesses (Sun et al. 2018).

Microorganisms, seaweeds, vertebrates, and marine invertebrates are among the leading sources of bioactive compounds, distinguished by their diverse biochemical attributes. Nevertheless, consumer skepticism—especially in Europe and North America—continues to hinder widespread adoption. To overcome these barriers, it is imperative to develop products that align with consumer expectations, offering affordability, sustainability, nutritional value, and visual appeal (Wijesekara and Kim 2015). Because of the harsh and changing environmental circumstances they face, marine creatures are rich in bioactive chemicals. Because biotic and abiotic variables, including salinity, pH, temperature, pressure, contaminants, and light exposure, can change quickly, marine life must evolve adaptive survival strategies. A wide variety of primary and secondary metabolites are produced as a result, some of which are species-specific (Suleria et al. 2015).

Polyphenols, vitamins, pigments, PUFAs, enzymes, and proteins are some examples of these metabolites (Simat et al. 2020). Recent studies demonstrate their pharmacological and physiological advantages, exhibiting properties including immunomodulatory, wound healing, anti-inflammatory, antibacterial, antitumor, antidiabetic, and gut microbiota modulation (Hosseini et al. 2022). As a result, these bioactive substances are highly valued in the pharmaceutical, cosmeceutical, and nutraceutical sectors, encouraging further research and use (Sun et al. 2018).

2 Antioxidant Activity

Oxygen is essential to the regular metabolic processes of aerobic organisms (Li et al. 2017a, b, c). Hydroxyl radicals (OH), superoxide anion (O_2^-), hydrogen peroxide (H_2O_2), nitric oxide (NO), and peroxyl radicals (ROO^-) are examples of reactive oxygen species (ROS), which are unavoidably produced by organisms in an environment with high redox potential (Wu et al. 2015). Because cellular antioxidant mechanisms are unable to fight excessive ROS/RNS, oxidative stress results (Valko et al. 2007). Increased oxidative stress in biological systems can have negative consequences, such as molecular harm to lipids, proteins, and nucleic acids, which may seriously impair one's health (Carocho and Ferreira 2013).

ROS are important for many bodily physiological and metabolic processes in living things. In addition to degrading food's nutritional value through oxidation, too much ROS before ingestion, but can impair the normal operation of cell proteins, lipids, and DNA to induce illnesses such as diabetes, cancer and inflammatory diseases (Acharya et al. 2010) immune system impairment, aging and neurological illnesses (Gandhi and Abramov 2012; Pisoschi and Pop 2015).

According to Rahal et al. (2014), oxidative stress is defined as a disruption between the body's prooxidants and antioxidants, which is typically eliminated by the antioxidant defense system, which includes a variety of antioxidant enzymes and nonenzymatic antioxidants. Antioxidants (Aos) are crucial components of these defensive mechanisms (Forman and Zhang 2021). The efficient antioxidant system of cells, which is composed of enzymes and other nonenzymatic compounds, reduces the negative effects of free radicals, which are continuously produced by cells. Antioxidants can stop or reduce the interactions of biomolecules with free radicals by providing electrons to free radicals and inhibiting the oxidative process. This can aid in the prevention and/or treatment of chronic diseases (Rudrapal et al. 2022).

Unfortunately, tissue damage and even diseases begin to manifest when the body's antioxidant defense mechanism is unable to neutralize the excess free radicals. Most exogenous antioxidants are a popular and efficient means to combat oxidative stress (Poljsak et al. 2013). Antioxidant defense generally involves a variety of processes, including (1) slowing down or preventing the generation of free radicals; (2) free mechanisms; (3) converting free radicals into less harmful substances; (4) postponing the development of secondary toxic active species; (5) blocking the chain propagation reaction (chain breaking antioxidants); (6) strengthening the body's defenses against free radicals by working in concert with other antioxidants; and (7) chelating metal ions (Adwas et al. 2019; Costa et al. 2021a, b). The bioactive polysaccharides displayed antioxidant activity, generally due to (Zhong et al. 2019):

ROS (reactive oxygen species) scavenging capacity: ability to hunt highly reactive molecules such as super oxides (O_2^-), hydrogen peroxides (H_2O_2), and hydroxyl groups (OH^-), which cause cellular damage.

Controlling the antioxidants system's levels: cellular redox balance and oxidative system protection depend on the maintenance of superoxide dismutase (SOD), catalase (CAT), and glutathione (GSH) levels. Mediating through pathways generated by oxidative stress: SIRT1, AMPK, MAPK, and PGC-1α are important pathways that help cells respond to oxidative damage and regulate metabolism, thereby reducing oxidative stress. It was discovered that the molecular weight of the compound, the kind of monosaccharide involved, the degree of sulfation and position, and the type of glycosidic linkages all affect how well polysaccharides work by donating hydrogen atoms to free radicals.

2.1 Molecular Weight of the Compound

According to a recent study, low molecular weight polysaccharides have more antioxidant activity than those with higher molecular weights because they include more reducing ends that interact with free radicals (Peasura et al. 2015). However, it has been demonstrated that excessive breakdown of marine polysaccharides into smaller molecular weights results in a lower level of activity than the original polymer.

2.2 Monosaccharide Involved

The chemical composition of marine polysaccharides varies greatly depending on the season, region, and place of origin. It was discovered that the antioxidant potential of marine polysaccharides may be impacted by the same type of monosaccharide in varying amounts. High galactose and polysaccharide content is associated with increased antioxidant activity. However, the mechanism is still unknown.

2.3 Degree of Sulfation and Position

According to studies, the location and amount of sulfate have a significant impact on a polysaccharide's antioxidant activity by activating the hydrogen atoms on the anomeric carbon, thereby improving the polysaccharide's capacity to supply hydrogen. If the sulfation level is changed to a greater degree, it disrupts the polysaccharide's triple helical structure, lowering its antioxidant capacity. As a result, polysaccharides with higher levels of sulfation have stronger antioxidant properties, provided that the triple helical structures are preserved. Likewise, it appears that the polysaccharide's sulfation location affects the antioxidant activity's potential. Research revealed that the antioxidant activity of sulfate derivatization at the C-4 and C-6 positions was higher than at the C-2 position (Sellimi et al. 2014).

3 Antioxidant Action Mechanisms

Numerous in vitro models have been created in order to assess the antioxidant activities and identify which antioxidants would be advantageous for food and biological systems (Halliwell et al. 1995; Sanchez-Moreno 2002) Techniques for evaluating antioxidant activity can be broadly categorized into two groups based on their reaction mechanisms: methods based on hydrogen atom transfer (HAT) and methods based on single electron transfer (SET). The HAT-based methods include total radical adsorption capacity (ORAC) or oxygen radical absorbance capacity (ORAC). The ability to quench free radicals by hydrogen donation is commonly evaluated using the total radical trapping antioxidant parameter (TRAP), suppression of induced low-density lipoprotein (LDL) oxidation, total oxyradical scavenging capacity assay, and others (O).

But SET-based methods, such as the ferric ion reducing antioxidant power (FRAP) assay, 2,2-diphenyl-1-picrylhydrazyl radical (DPPH) scavenging (Table 1), and the Trolox equivalent antioxidant capacity (TEAC) assay, determine the ability to transfer a single electron to reduce any compound, including metals,

Table 1 Antioxidant mechanisms

Reaction mechanisms	Method	Characteristics	References
SET or HAT The antioxidants are able to donate a hydrogen to reduce the stable radical DPPH to the yellow-colored no radical diphenylpicrylhydrazine (DPPH-H)	Inhibition of 2,2-diphenyl1-picrylhydracyl radical (DPPH*) DPPH *AH → DPPH-H + A* DPPH* + R* → DPPH-R	Colorimetric method based on the measurement of the scavenging capacity of antioxidants toward DPPH	Lu et al. (2010)
SET or HAT ABTS*· radicals involve a single-electron transfer process. Bleaching of a preformed solution of the blue-green radical cation ABTS*	Inhibition of 2,2′-azino-bis- (3-ethylbenzothiazoline-6-sulfonic acid) (ABTS$^{\bullet+}$) radical	Colorimetric method to evaluate the decay of ABTS$^{\bullet+}$ in the presence of an antioxidant agent ABTS*assay was based on the activation of metmyoglobin with hydrogen peroxide in the presence of ABTS to produce the radical cation, in the presence or absence of antioxidants	Lu et al. (2010)
Total phenols assay by Folin Ciocalteu reagent	SET	A mixture of phosphomolybdate and phosphotungstate in highly basic medium oxidized phenolic compounds	Vl et al. (1999)

(continued)

Table 1 (continued)

Reaction mechanisms	Method	Characteristics	References
Ferric-reducing antioxidant power (FRAP)	SET	Colorimetric method that evaluates the reduction of Fe^{3+} -tripyridyltriazine complex (Fe^{3+} -TPTZ) by turning it into a ferrous form (Fe^{2+} -TPTZ)	Benzie et al. (1996)
Total antioxidant capacity (TAC)	SET	This method is used to measure the peroxide level during the initial stage of lipid oxidation. Peroxides are formed during the linoleic acid oxidation, which reacts with Fe^{2+} to form Fe^{3+} and later these ions form a complex with thiocyanate	Roginsky et al. (2005)
Total radical-trapping antioxidant parameter (TRAP)	HAT The production of peroxyl radicals from 2,2′-azobis(2-amidinopropane) hydrochloride (AAPH) is the basis for this technique	TRAP assay involves the initiation of lipid peroxidation by generating water-soluble $ROO^{\bullet}$ and is sensitive to all known chain-breaking antioxidants	Wayner et al. (1985)
Total oxyradical scavenging capacity total assay (TOSCA)	HAT	Evaluates inhibition oxidation of α-keto-γ methiolbutyric acid (KMBA) by ROS. The antioxidant activity is measured through ethylene concentration, generated during decomposition of KMBA, relative to a control reaction monitored by headspace gas chromatography (HS-GC)	Winston et al. (1998)
Crocin-bleaching assays (CBAs)	HAT	CBA is based on the abstraction of hydrogen atoms and/or addition of radical to the polyene structure of crocin and results in a disruption of the conjugated system accounting for crocin bleaching	Bors et al. (1984)
Oxygen radical absorbance capacity (ORAC)	HAT	ORAC assay is based upon the inhibition of peroxyl radical induced oxidation initiated by thermal decomposition of azo compounds such as AAPH	Cao et al. (1997)

carbonyls, and radicals, and induce a color shift when the compound is reduced. Additional experiments include hydrogen peroxide scavenging, superoxide radical scavenging, and singlet oxygen quenching (Gülcin et al. 2012; Tan and Lim 2015).

1. Numerous fucoidans, which range from 1.15 to 4.50 mg Trolox/g fucoidan, are discovered in brown algae, such as *Sargassum filipendula*, *Cladosiphon okamuranus*, *Sargassum horneri*, *Kjellmaniella crassifolia*, *Nemacystus decipiens*, and *Fucus vesiculosus*. These fucoidans have a high antioxidant potential. According to Ajisaka et al. (2016), the free radical scavenging activity of fucoidan varies due to fluctuations in the sulfate content of the extracted fucoidan (Laeliocattleya et al. 2020). Fucoidan from *Saccharina japonica* showed notable levels of sulfate and total sugar but only moderate amounts of polyphenols. The results showed that the fucoidan with a higher sulfate level had a noticeable antioxidant action. According to El Rashed et al. (2021), fucoidans exhibit a potent ability to scavenge ABTS radical cations. Fucoidans in *S. japonica* showed better antioxidant activity in the FRAP test compared to the ABTS test.
2. Following hydrogen peroxide treatment, MRC-5 cells in kelp (brown seaweed) showed noticeably greater MDA levels and dramatically reduced levels of SOD, GSH, and CAT. In addition to SOD, MDA, GSH, and CAT's previously documented roles in oxidative damage consequently, the results of this investigation indicated that MRC-5 cells clearly increased the levels of SOD, GSH, and CAT while simultaneously decreasing MDA levels, suggesting that laminarin protects against oxidative damage (Liu et al. 2017)
3. Many chemical antioxidants, including butyl hydroxyanisole, butylated hydroxytoluene, and tertiary butyl hydroquinone, have been shown to be carcinogenic and toxic (Soubra et al. 2007). The well-known ROS scavenger fucoidan is a naturally occurring polymer that is active. *Laminaria japonica* (*L. japonica*) is the source of fucoidan, an antioxidant that has been demonstrated to be effective in treating diseases caused by free radical damage. Likewise, there is notable antioxidant activity in fucoidan that was isolated from *U. pinnatifida*. It has been demonstrated that fucoidan can prevent amyloid-β-induced toxicity by lowering the buildup of ROS and amyloid-β. After fucoidan administration, glutathione and superoxide dismutase activities were similarly increased. Accordind to Wang et al. (2019) fucoidan is frequently utilized in skin care products and neuro-health foods as a natural antioxidant polysaccharide.
4. According to Wang et al. (2018), *L. japonica* exhibited significantly greater superoxide radical scavenging activity compared to *P. haitanesis* and *U. pertusakjellm*. In vitro, the majority of *L. japonica* fractions exhibited more antioxidant activity than fucoidan. Sulfate content and superoxide radical scavenging capacity have been found to be positively correlated. Additionally, the metal-ion-chelation and hydroxyl radical scavenging activities were shown to be related to the ratio of sulfate concentration to fucose.

3.1 Detection of Antioxidant Property

The antioxidant property of marine-derived bioactive compounds such as polysaccharides can be assessed by several in vitro and in vivo methods. In vivo method includes animal studies, where the compound is administered to the animal, which is later sacrificed for analysis of tissue or blood samples. ABTS, DPPH, ferric reducing antioxidant power (FRAP), and superoxide radical scavenging activity (SOD) are in vitro tests frequently used to evaluate the antioxidant activity of polysaccharides (Alam et al. 2013).

3.2 ABTS (2,2′-Azinobis-(3-Ethylbenzothiazoline-6-Sulfonate))

It is a stable target molecule that can be dissolved in both organic and aqueous solvents and is used to assess a sample's antioxidant activity when peroxides are present. The antioxidant content is determined by the sample's reduction of ABTS and the degree of discoloration. Given that ABTS and DPPH have the ability to take up electrons from antioxidants, there is a close association between DPPH's capacity to scavenge radicals and its ability to block ABTS (Santos et al. 2019).

3.3 DPPH Assay for Radical Scavenging (1,1-Diphenyl-2-Picrylhydrazil)

An organic compound containing stable free radicals can compensate for electron defeciency and act as antioxidants. This approach measures how much free radicals are reduced by substances with antioxidant activity (Santos et al. 2019).

3.4 Assay for Total Antioxidant Capacity

It is described as a compound's capacity to prevent or reduce the oxidative breakdown of lipids. The peroxide value is frequently measured using the ferric thiocyanate method. To improve the compound's antioxidant activity, the peroxidation of a fatty acid emulsion must be prevented. Typically employed as a model, the hydroperoxide from linoleic acid reacts with Fe^{2+} to form Fe^{3+} by ion oxidation. The peroxide value, which has a maximum absorbance at 500 nm, is measured by the complexation of these Fe^{3+} ions with thiocyanate. To find the ideal peroxide value, it is preferable to conduct the reaction without oxygen (Santos et al. 2019).

3.5 FRAP or Ferric Reducing Antioxidant Power

Through the reduction of ferric ion (Fe^{3+}) to ferrous ion (Fe^{2+}), a blue color complex is formed, which is how the overall antioxidant activity of the sample is measured. A significant decrease in absorbance at 700 nm indicates the sample's reducing power, and the reaction should be conducted in an acidic environment to maintain Fe solubility (Santos et al. 2019).

3.6 Scavenging Activity of Super Radicals (SOD)

It refers to the ability of a compound to neutralize or eliminate superoxide radicals (O_2^-), which are highly reactive. They are produced as byproducts of cellular metabolism. Nitroblue tetrazolium (NBT) is a dye that is reduced to a blue formazan. The color change occurs when NBT reacts with a superoxide radical, and the amount of formazan formed indicates the scavenging capacity of the substance (Santos et al. 2019).

4 Sources of Marine-Derived Polysaccharides

4.1 Marine Macroalgae

The term "macroalgae" refers to multicellular algae that are visible to the human eye, whereas "microalgae" refers to less visible forms. The taxonomically varied group of macroalgae exhibits variation in both shape and color. In addition to being classified by color into green (Chlorophyta), red (Rhodophyta), and brown (Phaeophyta), they can also be divided by size into macroalgae and microalgae (Khan et al. 2018; Baweja and Sahoo 2015). The different hues of algae are believed to be brought on by the pigments phycobilins, fucoxanthin, and chlorophyll a and b, which were isolated from red, green, and brown algae, respectively (Kadam et al. 2013).

5 Brown Seaweeds

Brown algae are a group of algae that belong to the class Phaeophyceae. Brown seaweeds are the second-largest group of marine macroalgae, after red seaweeds (Ghaliaoui et al. 2020). Their color ranges from brown to olive green indicating variations in pigmentation. The majority of brown algae inhabit marine environments. Approximately 1,500 species of brown algae exist, exhibiting wide variations in size and shape. The protein content of seaweeds varies according to their taxonomic class. Brown seaweeds often have lower protein levels (4.5–16.8% dw), while red seaweeds contain the highest levels (12.5–32% dw), followed by green seaweeds (9.6–23.3% dw). Although some species are native to fresh and brackish environments, brown seaweeds, also known as *Ochrophyta* or *Phaeophyceae*, are common macroalgae that grow abundantly in marine cold seas at northern latitudes. Fucoxanthin, a carotenoid pigment found in brown algae, gives the plant its distinctive brown hue by inhibiting the production of other pigments. Brown algae plant bodies vary in size, from a few millimeters to around 70 m, demonstrating that different species within the same algal class have different structures and compositions (Jonsson et al. 2020). Numerous studies have demonstrated the strong DPPH free radical scavenging and reduction properties of sulfated polysaccharides derived from brown algae (Table 2) (Lu et al. 2018). Fucoidan, which is derived from brown

Table 2 Antioxidant activity of marine-derived polysaccharides from brown seaweeds

SSS S. no	Scientific name	Locality	Polysaccharides	Antioxidant activity	References
1	*Ecklonia stolonifera*	Busan, Republic of Korea	Phlorotannins and oxylipins	DPPH: IC_{50} = 1.57 ± 0.08 and 3.56 ± 60.22 μM	Manandhar et al. (2019
2	*Hizikia fusiforme*	Jeju Island, South Korea	Fucoidan	DPPH: IC_{50} = 18.33% at 1 mg/ mL OH: 32.98% at 1 mg/ mL	Wang et al. (2020)
3	*Ecklonia maxima*	University of Cape Town, South Africa	Fucoidan	Invitro in Vero cells: low ROS levels; in vivo in zebrafish: high survival rate	Wang et al. (2020)
4	*Laminaria japonica*	China coast	Heterofucan	DPPH: IC_{50}= 4.64 at 4.50 mg/mL	Dong et al. (2019)
5	*Dictyota dichotoma*	Hodeida city, Yemen	Diterpenes	DPPH: IC_{50} = 204.6 at 8.3 μg/mL	El-Shaibany et al. (2020)
6	*Dictyota mertensii*	Pirambuzois Beach, Brazil	Fucan, fucoidan, and diterpenes	RP: 60% at 0.5 mg/mL FRAP: 40% at 0.5 mg/ mL OH: 10.2% at 0.5 mg/ mL superoxide: 14% at 0.5 mg/mL	Nunes Pinheiro et al. (2019)
7	*Sargassum fulvellum*	Jejuisland, South Korea	Sulfated polysaccharides	Alkyl radical: IC_{50} = 0.86 at 0.01 mg/mL DPPH: IC_{50} = 6.9 at 0.66 mg/mL OH: 1.14 at 0.12 mg/ mL	Wang et al. (2020)

(continued)

Table 2 (continued)

SSS S. no	Scientific name	Locality	Polysaccharides	Antioxidant activity	References
8	*Cystoseira amentacea*	Ligurian Sea, Mediterranean	*Cystoseira amentacea* extracts	DPPH:EC_{50} = 0.34 μg/mL OH: EC_{50} = 292.9 μg/mL NO:EC_{50} = 546.2 μg/mL	De La Fuente et al. (2021)
9	*Fucus spiralis*	Peniche Coast, Portugal	Phlorotannins	DPPH:2.79,2.82 μg/mL	Francisco et al. (2020)
10	*Colpomenia sinuosa*	North Lebanese Coast, Mediterranean	Polyphenolics	In vitro in HCT-116 cells: high ROS in cancer cells	Al Monla (2020)

algae, has been shown in numerous in vivo antioxidant studies to reduce oxidative stress-induced bodily damage by controlling the body's antioxidant defense mechanism. For example, by increasing superoxide dismutase (SOD) and decreasing malondialdehyde (MDA) levels, fucoidan from *Costaria costata* shields the liver from oxidative stress in mice treated with CCL4 (Wang et al. 2014).

5.1 The Polysaccharide (Fucoidan)

The class of fucose-containing sulfated polysaccharide (FCPs), comprises polysaccharides with varying branching patterns, chain lengths, and degree of sulfation, including fucoidan. In addition to galactose, mannose, xylose, and glucuronic acid residues, fucose is the primary component of fucoidan (Lim et al. 2016; Ale et al. 2011). Two subgroups of fucoidans exist: one group's backbone is made up of 1,3-l-fucopyranose residues, while the other group's l-fucopyranose residues alternate 1,3- and 1,4-linked groups. The variation among fucoidans is reflected in the broad range of reported molecular weights, which range from about 40 to 1600 KDa (Fletcher et al. 2017).

5.2 Alginate

Alginates are linear anionic polysaccharides composed of 1,4- linked salts of alginic acid, which consist of β-D-mannuronic acid (M) and α-L-guluronic acid (G) residues. As a result, alginic acids could have three structural components. Patterns include homo-polymeric sections of successive G blocks, b homo-polymeric sections of consecutive M blocks, and hetero-polymeric portions of randomly connected G and M block residues, usually with a 1:1 (Gs:Ms) ratio. Alginates are produced when alginic acid combines with preexisting metal ions such as calcium, sodium, or magnesium. Calcium alginate gels are insoluble in water; however, the sodium and magnesium ions of alginic acid change into water- soluble gels (Domozych et al. 2019). When the glycosidic bonds tying the sugar monomers of alginate polymers are subjected to breakage in both alkaline and acidic conditions, the substance breaks down.

Temperature has an impact on the copolymer's stability as well as free radicals generated by contaminants such as polyphenol. The size, M/G ratio, and integrated G- block features of copolymers affect the compound's mechanical strength, biocompatibility, physical properties, and functionalities (Lim et al. 2016). Harvest time, algal species, and variations in the age and repeating structure of algal tissue all affect the M/G ratio (mannuronic acid to guluronic acid) of alginates. The chelating properties of alginate are determined by the length of the compounds' G-blocks, which are the repeating structure of guluronic acid (Zhao et al. 2012). (1–4) These two conformational isomer residues are joined by glycosidic linkages (Tanna and Mishra 2019). Due to the numerous theological characteristics of these polysaccharides, they are extensively utilized in a variety of industries, including pharmaceuticals, medical technology, cosmetics, food, agriculture, textiles, and paper (Lim et al. 2016).

5.3 *Laminarin*

Laminarin is a significant low molecular weight storage carbohydrate present in brown algae. Laminarian (also known as laminaran) and its derived oligosaccharides are structurally related polysaccharides. Oswald Schmiedeberg discovered the *Laminariaceae* family in 1885 (Kadam et al. 2013). The short polymer known as storage glucan laminarin is composed of 25–50 glucose units joined by β-1,3 glycosidic bonds. In some cases, it has also branches at the O-6 position and β-1,6-glycosidic bonds. The fibrillar cell walls of brown algae include laminarins, and the reducing end of these laminarins can differ in intercellular spaces. This is analogous to a mannitol residue in M-type laminarins and a glucose residue in G-type laminarins, resulting in different solubilities. In particular, D-mannitol is present at the reducing end of an M-chain structure but not at the reducing end of a G-chain. According to Rioux et al. (2007), a laminarin with more branches dissolves in cold water, whereas one with fewer branches is only soluble in warm water. Although laminarin is rarely present in *Ascophyllum*, *Fucus*, and *Undaria* species, it is commonly present in *Saccharina* and *Laminaria* species. The molecular weight (MW) of laminarin is approximately five kDa, which is substantially lower than that of the vast majority of other seaweed polysaccharides. Actually, the degree of polymerization has a significant impact on the molecular weight. Laminarin, which makes up 22–49% of seaweed's dry matter, is the primary energy source of macroalgae (Kadam et al. 2013). After building up polysaccharides throughout the hot months, seaweeds mostly use it in the winter. Since the human body cannot digest it, one of the most pertinent advantages of this molecule is its capacity to function as dietary fiber (Sterner et al. 2021). However, because it can efficiently stimulate cell activity and encourage tissue regeneration, both of which are crucial for the healing process, laminarin has been recognized as a wonderful asset in the fields of medication delivery and tissue engineering (Zargarzadeh et al. 2020).

6 Red Algae

Rhodophyta, a group of primarily multicellular photosynthetic eukaryotic organisms, includes more than 7000 species of red seaweed. Warmer climates are home to more species, even if up to 5% of them can thrive in freshwater environments. They mainly develop in seawater habitats. Because phycocyanin and phycoerythrin are more prevalent than other pigments like carotene and chlorophyll A, the color red is the outcome. Red algae store sugars as floridean starch, which is a highly branched amylopectin that lacks amylose, which accumulates in the cytoplasm of the cell outside the plastid. Cellulose and carrageenan, the main constituents of seaweed cell walls, serve a variety of purposes. Protein level varies by seaweed taxonomic class, with brown seaweeds often having lower protein levels (4.5–16.8% dw) and red (12.5–32% dw) and green (9.6–23.3% dw) seaweeds having higher levels (Table 3) (Jönsson et al. 2020).

Table 3 Antioxidant activity of marine-derived polysaccharides from red seaweeds

S. no	Scientific name	Locality	Polysaccharides	Antioxidant activity	References
1	*Gloiopeltis furcata*	Nanji Archipelago coast of China	Furonan (sulfated polysaccharides)	Superoxide (64.37% at 90 g/mL) DPPH (23.49% at 0.1 mg/mL)	Shao et al. (2013)
2	*Gracilaria rubra*	Dayang Food stuff Co.; Ltd	Sulfated polysaccharides	DPPH (41.59% at 2.5 mg/mL) Superoxide (64.78% at 2.5 mg/mL) ABTS (59.01% at 2.5 mg/mL)	Di et al. (2017)
3	*Sarcodia ceylonensis*	Antarctic algae Co. (Xiamen, China)	Water-soluble polysaccharides (SCP 60)	Hydroxyl (83.33% at 4 mg/mL) ABTS (IC_{50} = 3.99 mg/mL)	He et al. (2016)
4	*Solieria filiformis*	Atlantic coast, northeast of Brazil	Sulfated polysaccharides, (specifically carrageenan)	TAC (86.6 ± 10.8 mg) DPPH (88.93% at 4.0 mg/mL); ABTS (IC_{50} = 2.01 mg/mL)	Sousa et al. (2016)

(continued)

Table 3 (continued)

S. no	Scientific name	Locality	Polysaccharides	Antioxidant activity	References
5	*Kappaphycus alvarezii*	Pekan, East coastal region, Malaysia	Kappa-carrageenan	DPPH (IC_{50}=0.6451 ± 0.12 mg/mL); ABTS (7.859 ± 0.09 mg/mL);	Bhuyar et al. (2021)
6	*Gracilaria intermedia*	Atlantic coast of Brazil (Taiba beach, São Gonçalo - Ceará)	Sulfated polysaccharides	TAC (28.98 ± 1.86 mg/g); Ion Chelation (11.64 ± 0.83% at 0.1%) and 28.19 ± 0.97% at 1.5%); DPPH 9.89 ± 1.32% (at a concentration of 0.1%) and 41.83 ± 0.97% (at a concentration of 1.5%)	Castro et al. (2018)
7	*Pyropia yezoensis*	Wando Island coast of South Korea	Porphyran (sulfated polysaccharides)	Alkyl (IC_{50} = 191.4 g/mL) H_2O_2 (IC_{50} = 91.0 g/mL)	Lee et al. (2016)

6.1 *Carrageenan*

The cell wall of red seaweed contains carrageenan, a high molecular weight, anionic, sulfated polymer that interacts with other bioactive materials such as proteins, lipids, pigments, and other polysaccharides. It is composed of alternating units of 3,6-anhydro-α-D-galactose and β-D-galactose. Glycosidic linkages α-(1,3) and β-(1,4) bind anhydro-α-D-galactose. The three main commercial forms of carrageenan are kappa (κ), iota, and lambda (λ). Carrageenans, which vary in the amount of 3,6-anhydrogalactose residues as well as in the number and position of sulfate ester groups, exhibit different chemical and functional properties. There are 25–30% sulfate ester groups and 28–35% anhydrogalactose in carrageenan. Carrageenan's sulfate ester concentration is similar to that of carrageenan (28–30%), but its anhydrogalactose unit proportion is lower (25–30%). Carrageenan has a comparatively significant sulfate substitution (32–39%) but no anhydrogalactose residues (Campo et al. 2009). Pyruvate ketal, which is only known to occur in the carrageenan family, can substitute the backbone (Amimi et al. 2001).

6.2 *Agar*

Agar is a polysaccharide-based hydrocolloid seaweed with a potent gelling ability. In the middle of the seventeenth century, an innkeeper named Tarozaemon Minoya discovered agar by accident in what is now Kyoto, Japan. The story that was recorded states that the residual food particles on the plate transformed into a white, squash-like substance, now known as agar, when a high-ranking officer was served the seaweed *Gelidium* spp. during dinner in the cold season (Pandya et al. 2022). Seaweeds are also known as the "Medical Food of the Twenty-First Century" (Khan and Satam 2003).

In India, natural seaweed beds and seaweed-based liquid fertilizer provide the majority of raw materials required to make agar, alginates, and other goods. About 25 agar and 10 algin producers are dispersed throughout the coastal states of Gujarat, Andhra Pradesh, Karnataka, Kerala, and Tamil Nadu. Red algae such as *Gelidiella acerosa*, *Gracilaria edulis*, *G. crassa*, *G. filicina*, and *G. verrucosa* are currently used to make agar, whereas brown algae like *Sargassum* spp., *Turbinaria* spp., and *Cystoseira indica* are used to produce alginates and liquid seaweed fertilizers. Among these agarophytes, *G. acerosa* generates bacteriological-grade agar, whereas *Gracilaria species* produce food-quality agar (Hernandez-Carmona et al. 2013). Agar, a mixture of agarose and agaropectin, contains agarose which possesses the most desirable properties (Olatunji 2020).

Sattar et al. (2018) stated that agar-agar is a polymer of agarobiose made up of 3,6-anhydro-L-galactopyranose and D-galactose repeating units, β which are alternatively linked by β-(1→4) and α-(1→3). Link L-galactoses, D-galactoses, and 3,6-anhydro-L-galactose make up the majority of the heterogeneous galactans in agar (Chi et al. 2012). Agar-derived oligosaccharides, also known as monosugars, produced by various agarases, have emerged as a potentially interesting area of study due to their distinct biological properties, which include anti-fatigue, anticariogenic, immunomodulatory, antitumor, antioxidant, and skin-whitening and skin-moisturizing properties (Park et al. 2020). The galactose-based backbone of both agarose and agaropectin is neutrally charged, but agaropectin has undergone significant modification with acidic side groups such as pyruvate and sulfate (Raphael et al. 2010). The main structure has been examined by Araki and his group. when agarophyte red algae are treated with alkali, a linear polymer called agarose can be recovered from them (Nishinari and Fang 2017).

7 Green Algae

Within each seaweed taxonomic class, the protein content varies, with green (9.6–23.3% dw) and red (12.5–32% dw) seaweeds containing more protein than brown seaweeds (4.5–16.8% dw). Most polysaccharides are water-soluble sulfated polysaccharides found in green algae's interstitium and cell wall. Green algae polysaccharides have a complicated chemical composition that varies depending on the type of green algae utilized for extraction, the growing conditions, and the harvest period, according to Li et al. (2017a, b, c) and Zhong et al. (2020). The main components of ulvan, a polysaccharide derived from green algae, are glucuronic acid (GlcA), iduronic acid (IdoA), 3-sulfated rhamnose (Rha3S), and trace amounts of xylose (Xyl) (Ulaganathan et al. 2017), as well as mannose, galactose, and arabinose (Jmel et al. 2019). When Kidgella et al. (2021) examined ulva's monosaccharide compositions from multiple sources, they discovered that there were notable differences between the polysaccharides from leafy and filamentous ulva. In particular, it was discovered that rhamnose made up the majority of the polysaccharides derived from these sources, albeit glucuronic acid was also detected. Interestingly, iduronic acid content of filamentous ulva's polysaccharide was typically lower (about 7 mol%) than that of leafy ulva (about 14 mol%). Additionally, in contrast to other species of *Ulva*, the polysaccharides of U. ralfsiis showed a much higher concentration of 16 mol% (Table 4).

Table 4 Antioxidant activity of marine-derived polysaccharides from green seaweeds

S. no	Scientific name	Locality	Polysaccharide	Antioxidant activity	Reference
1	*Ulva fasciata*	Coast of Nanji Archipelago (Zhe-jiang province, China)	Sulfated heteropolysaccharide	Superoxide (81.45% at 90 μg/mL); hydroxy radical assay: 62.08% at 100 μg/mL: DPPH: 37.63% at 100μg/mL	Shao et al. (2013)
2	*Kappaphycus striatus*	Pekan, East coastal region, Malaysia	Carrageenan, a sulfated polysaccharide	DPPH: 1.522 ± 0.08 mg/mL at IC_{50} 0.31 ± 0.03 mg/mL ABTS: 15.56±0.12 mg/mL	Bhuyar et al. (2021)
3	*Caulerpa racemosa*	Malaysian seaweeds	Sulfated polysaccharide	DPPH; (EC_{50} at 0.65 ± 0.03 mg/mL),	Yap et al. (2019)
4	*Ulva intestinalis*	Pattani Bay, Thailand	Sulfated polysaccharides	DPPH (the highest 82.23%)	Peasura et al. (2016)
5	*Caulerpa racemosa*	Coastal area of Sambai, Ramanadhapuram (9°31′15.3″ N 78° 56′08.1″ E) Tamil Nadu, India.	Sulfated polysaccharide	DPPH; 54.21 ± 1.39% and ABTS: 76.62 ± 1.08%	Palaniyappan et al. (2023)

(continued)

Table 4 (continued)

S. no	Scientific name	Locality	Polysaccharide	Antioxidant activity	Reference
6	*Caulerpa lentillifera*	Malaysian seaweeds	Sulfated polysaccharide	DPPH; EC_{50} at 81.55 ± 4.22 mg/mL	Yap et al. (2019)
7	*Codium fragile*	Çanakkale located on the western coast and Antalya on the southern coast in Turkey	Sulfated polysaccharide	CUPRAC; 7.80 ± 0.04, ABTS; 2.85 ± 0.01	Yalçın et al. (2021)

7.1 Ulvan

One of the main polysaccharides found in *Ulva* sp. is ulvan (Morelli et al. 2017). Reports state that ulvan accounts for 9–36% of *Ulva* sp. cells' dry weight biomass (Kidgell et al. 2019). Lahaye et al. (2007) state that based on the extraction and depending on the purifying method, the ulvan yield could range from 8% to 29% of the algae's dry weight. It is based on two main repeating disaccharides: type A ulvanobiuronic acid 3-sulfate (A3S) and type B ulvanobiuronic acid 3-sulfate (B3S) (Olasehinde et al. 2019; Kammoun et al. 2019; Kammoun et al. 2017; Chiellini et al. 2011; Lakshmi et al. 2020). Ulvan is a common food ingredient, and numerous research have looked into its potential medical uses (Chiellini et al. 2011; Lakshmi et al. 2020; Alves et al. 2013). Cellulose, xyloglucan, and glucuroran make up the majority of ulvan, along with other kinds of sugars. Mannose, galactose, and arabinose are present in trace amounts. Ulvan is mostly composed of a repeating series of disaccharides, such as xylose, uronic acid, iduronic acid, or rhamnose sulfate. Stability and physiological effects are linked to the physicochemical characteristics of ulvan's active ingredients, which include hydration, polarity, swelling, and viscosity. The extraction procedure will determine these characteristics (Cindana et al. 2020).

8 Microalgae

De Jesus Raposo et al. (2013) state that the review focuses on microalgal polysaccharides as bio-antioxidant agents. These substances counteract free radicals. They shield cells from harm because they are either gathered within or released from cells in reaction to stresses. In literature, polysaccharides of different sources constitute a class of extremely useful compounds used in cosmetics, food, and medicine. The three groups of polysaccharides found in photosynthetic microorganisms are (i) internal storage polysaccharides, (ii) cell wall structural polysaccharides, and (iii) exopolysaccharides, which are categorized according to their functions.

Table 5 Antioxidant activity of marine-derived polysaccharides from microalgae

S. no	Scientific name	Polysaccharide	Antioxidant activity	References
1	*Chlorella minutissima*	Both homopolysaccharides and heteropolysaccharides	DPPH: 10–70% inhibition (extracts at 200 μg mL^{-1})	Aremu et al. (2015)
2	(i) *Chlorella zofingiensis* (ii) *Chlorella vulgaris*	(i) Exopolysaccharides (ii) Heteropolysaccharides	DPPH: (i) 71.5% (ii) 59.6% at the concentration of 3.0 mg/mL	Zhang et al. (2019)
3	*Enteromorpha linza*	Sulfated polysaccharides	DPPH: 83±7% at the concentration of 3.61 mg/mL	Zhang et al. (2013)
4	*C. pyrenoidosa*	Heteropolysaccharides	DPPH: 54.16 ± 4.49%(Crude) at concentration of 10 mg/mL In sPs: 55.2% at 2.0 mg/ ml	Zhang et al. (2019)
5	*Graesiella* sp.	Sulfated polysaccharides	Hydroxyl (IC50 = 0.87 mg/mL); Ferrous ion-chelating (IC50 = 0.33 mg/mL)	Trabelsi et al.
6	*Arthrospira platensis*	Extracellular polysaccharides (EPS)	DPPH: 68.29% at 300 μg ABTS: 71.12% at 400 μg	El-Baky et al. (2013)
7	Nostoc commune	Extracellular polysaccharides (EPS)	Superoxide: 65% Hydroxide: 51%, Increase of: Survival rate of *Caenorhabditis elegans*, and antioxidant enzymes (SOD)	Li et al. (2011)
8	*Anabaena* sp.	Extracellular polysaccharides (EPS)	DPPH: no response, ABTS: 30 μmol TE g^{-1} DW	Vega et al. (2020)
9	*Lyngbya* sp.	Extracellular polysaccharides (EPS)	DPPH: 12 mmol TE g^{-1} DW ABTS: 18 mmol TEg^{-1} DW	Vega et al. (2020)
10	*Spirullina* sp.	Extracellular polysaccharides (EPS)	DPPH: 31,0% ± 4.0 at 90 °C	Chaiklahan et al (2013)
11	*Scytonema* sp.	Extracellular polysaccharides (EPS)	DPPH: 25 μmol TE g^{-1} DW ABTS: 35 μmol TEg^{-1} DW	Vega et al. (2020)

These organisms are capable of producing substances having antiviral, antibacterial, and antioxidant qualities, such as polysaccharides. The production of polysaccharides by *Chlorella* sp., *Nostoc* sp., *Spirulina* sp., *and Porphyridium* sp. has been investigated (Table 5).

9 Exopolysaccharides

Exopolysaccharides can be categorized as extracellular polysaccharides or extracellular polymeric substances if they are completely released into the external environment or as capsular polysaccharides or cell-bound polysaccharides if they remain attached to the cell (Delattre et al. 2016; Gaignard et al. 2019). All varieties of the polysaccharides that were described in this paper were referred to as "polysaccharide (PS)." The main microalgae species known to synthesize polysaccharides include *Porphyridium* sp., *Chlamydomonas reinhardtii*, *Chlorella vulgaris*, *Scenedesmus quadricauda*, and *Spirulina* sp. Because of their antioxidant qualities, PSs from *Porphyridium cruentum* and other species have attracted a lot of attention (De Jesus Raposo et al. 2013; Galasso et al. 2019; Ferdous and Yusof 2021; Rani et al. 2021). Microalgae have the ability to extrude several enzymes and extracellular polymeric substances (EPSs) into the growth medium (Lv et al. 2019). Appreciatively, those EPSs and enzymes, as well as microalgal co-metabolism, catalyzed the contaminant. As a result, microalgae may degrade long-chain organic pollutants more efficiently.

Both intracellular and extracellular actions are possible for the enzymatic and nonenzymatic antioxidants utilized for ROS detoxification. Metal-chelating agents, hydrogen and electron donors, peroxide decomposers, enzyme inhibitors, and regulators of gene expression are a few examples of radical scavengers and singlet O_2 quenchers. Enzymes like oxidases and peroxidases, electron transport chains in mitochondria and chloroplasts, and photosensitizers like chlorophyll all contribute to the production of ROS in microalgae (Saed-Moucheshi et al. 2014). As a result, reactive oxygen species are primarily produced in the chloroplasts, mitochondria, and peroxisomes (Cirulis et al. 2013). ROS, in a broader sense, are O_2 derivatives that are more reactive than O_2. This comprises nonradical compounds and free radicals with at least one unpaired electron (Demidchik 2015).

Red microalgae PSs scavenge free radicals, boost the activity of antioxidant enzymes, and stop lipid oxidation, according to a number of studies done recently (Ferdous and Yusof 2021; Chen et al. 2016). *Porphyridium* sp. is a spherical, unicellular marine microalga that belongs to the *Porphyridiales* group and is the most frequently recorded red microalga. The negatively charged mucilaginous polysaccharide that encases *Porphyridium* sp. cells is typically made up of roughly ten proteins, sulfate, monosugars, and maybe phenols. The polysaccharide's negative charge is caused by glucuronic acid and half-ester sulfate groups.

10 Polysaccharide from Marine Bacteria

Compared to terrestrial bacteria, marine microorganisms have not been as thoroughly studied for antioxidant chemicals. Usually consisting of high molecular weight polymers, polysaccharides are composed of glycosidic bonds connecting ten or more monosaccharide units (Khan et al. 2022). Depending on whether they contain one or more forms of monosaccharides, they can be classified as either homopolysaccharides or heteropolysaccharides (Mahmoud et al. 2021; Zeidan et al. 2017). They may also be branched or linear in structure. Although D-glucose is usually the most common component in the latter case, other sugars (such as D-xylose, D-mannose, D-galactose, L-galactose, L-arabinose, and D-fructose) may also be present, as well as derivatives like simple sugar acids (glucuronic and iduronic acids) or amino sugars (D-glucosamine and D-galactosamine). Last but not least, in addition to the previously listed sugars, nonorganic moieties including sulfates, phosphates, pyruvates, and acetates are frequently seen (Khan et al. 2022; Ibrahim et al. 2022).

Microbial polysaccharides display a broad variety of structural and compositional variation due to different combinations of these changeable properties. Among marine microorganisms, bacteria and phytoplanktons, such as diatoms, cyanobacteria, and dinoflagellates, are the main suppliers of extracellular polymeric substances (EPSs). Numerous microbes that generate extracellular polysaccharides (EPSs) have been found in marine environments, such as saltwater, sea ice, sediment, and deep-sea hydrothermal vents (Zhang et al. 2015). Researchers have looked into how marine bacteria, such as *Acinetobacter*, *Arthrobacter*, *Pseudomonas*, *Halomonas*, *Myroides*, *Corynebacterium*, *Bacillus*, and *Alteromonas* sp., produce EPSs (Satpute et al. 2010). During famine, some polysaccharides, such as glycogen, which are present inside the cells, serve as molecules that store energy (Khan et al. 2022; Zeidan et al. 2017; Zeitz et al. 2019). Others can be found in the capsules or cell walls of fungus and bacteria. In addition to shielding cells from environmental stressors and regulating membrane permeability, structural polymers also mediate interactions with the environment, which in the case of pathogenic microorganisms may involve initiating immunological responses (Garcia-Rubio et al. 2020; Gow et al. 2017; Agustinho et al. 2018). Finally, polysaccharides that are secreted outside of microbial cells are called exopolysaccharides or extracellular polysaccharides (EPSs). The bioactive metabolites isolated from seaweed, sponges, and bacteria were examined and found to have strong antioxidant properties that require a great deal of focus in terms of drug discovery.

11 Seaweed Associated of Marine Bacteria

Since the late 1980s, more than 50,000 naturally occurring bioactive chemicals have been discovered in marine microorganisms. Over 8000 of these substances exhibited bactericidal action. Bactericidal chemicals are frequently produced by marine bacteria to preserve the connections between epiphytic bacterial communities as well as prevent microbial infections. Associated bacteria are bacterial communities characterized by direct or indirect interactions with their host. Certain bacterial species exhibit bactericidal activity and host specificity against particular diseases; these traits include intricate metabolic interactions between bacteria and seaweed (Newman and Cragg 2012). The bioactive chemicals produced by the bacteria associated with seaweed may find utility in biomedical applications.

Table 6 Antioxidant activity of marine-derived polysaccharides from marine bacteria

Fractions	Phosphomolybdenum assay (IC_{50}) value	DPPH(IC_{50}) value assay
F1	103.03	5.420
F2	30.80	1.008
F3	105.43	7.140
F4	90.01	2.517
Ascorbic acid	20.15	0.521

12 Antioxidant Activity of Marine Bacteria

Guo et al. (2010) stated that the DPPH radical, hydroxyl radical, and lipid peroxidation inhibition scavenging capacities of ETW1 and ETW2 (two water-soluble extracellular polysaccharides of *Edwardsiella tarda*) were 87.66–76.54%, 88.96–76.85%, and 78.93–71.48%, respectively, at 8.0 mg/mL. Two common antioxidants, ascorbic acid and BHT, were used to compare their antioxidant properties. The antioxidant activities of BHT and ascorbic acid were marginally higher than those of ETW1 and ETW2 at 8.0 mg/mL.

Following the extraction of the *Bacillus* strain from the sea sponge *Spongia officinalis* and its regular maintenance in marine broth, the extract was purified using vacuum liquid chromatography with four fractions (F1, F2, F3, and F4) (Table 6).

The potent antioxidant activity of the extract and its VLC fractions was evidenced by low IC50 values (1.008–7.140 mg/mL) in the DPPH experiment. BF2 had the highest antioxidant activity, with an IC50 value of 1.008 mg/mL, while BF3 had the lowest, with an IC50 value of 7.140 mg/mL. The extract and BF2 exhibited greater overall antioxidant activity, with IC50 values of 44.55 and 30.80 mg/mL, respectively (Odekina et al. 2020).

A study reported that *Nitratireductor* sp. (family *Phyllobacteriaceae)* is known for being nitrate-reducing bacteria (IC_{50} 0.49 mg·mL1), *Alteromonas* sp. (IC_{50} 0.61 mg.mL1), specifically Gram-negative, aerobic bacteria found in various marine environments and *Enterobacter* sp. within the genus Enterobacter, which is a a group of rod-shaped bacterium, Gram-negative, facultatively anaerobic produced EPS that was more effective against the DPPH radical (IC_{50} 0.44 mg·mL1).

The goal of this project is to isolate and enrich marine soil from the North-West coastal region of India in order to identify prospective microorganisms that produce antioxidants. A total of 156 bacterial isolates were acquired, and they were examined for their potential to generate antioxidants outside the cells. There were a number of pigmented and nonpigmented isolates that have shown strong antioxidant production ability. The percentage of radical scavenging activity ranged from 30% to 51% in nonpigmented isolates, compared to 28–69% in pigmented isolates. The highest radical scavenging activity was shown by isolates 6-3 and 8-1, which were 69% and 63%, respectively. In addition, both isolates produced pigment (Shivale et al. 2018).

The *Bacillus subtilis* strain, from which the novel EPS (EPSR4) was isolated and extracted, demonstrated a 64.8 ± 2.1% scavenging capacity against hydrogen peroxide. Antioxidant activity testing further showed 97.6 ± 1.5% scavenging activity against DPPH free radicals at concentration of 1500 μg/mL after 120 min and 86.3 ± 1.8% after 30 min (Abdel-Wahab et al. 2022).

Mohamed et al. (2015) reported that 50 isolates obtained from marine environments and 30 isolates from soil samples were used in this study to extract crude exopolysaccharides and examined using the DPPH (1,1-diphenyl-2-picrylhydrazyl) assay. A total of 22 isolates from marine environments and 7 seven isolates from soil exhibited shown antioxidant activity. The top nine isolates demonstrating antioxidant activity were M7 (*Bacillus circulans*) (98.10%), M8 (*Bacillus licheniformis*) (97.34%), S1 (*Bacillus alvei*) (95.83%), M3 (*Bacillus insolitus*) (85.01%), S22 (Bacillus polymyxa) (84.31%), M9 (*Bacillus marinus*) (83.26%), M6 (*Bacillus anthracis*) (81.00%), M5 (*Staphylococcus sp.*) (80.42%), and M4 (*Bacillus brevis*) (76.90%).

13 Antioxidant Activity of Polysaccharides Derived from Marine Fungi

Polysaccharides derived from marine fungi may be classified as exopolysaccharides or endopolysaccharides based on their origin and location within the cell. Comprehensive analysis have revealed that exopolysaccharides exhibit stronger antioxidant activity than endopolysaccharides; however, their mechanisms of action remain unclear and need further investigation. Although the factors affecting antioxidants are not fully understood, the occurrence of sulfation and the presence of certain compounds, such as glucuronic acid and its derivatives, have been reported as highly relevant. Studies conducted in several locations across China, including the Yellow Sea and South China Sea, have reported that fungi from different marine habitats produce extracellular polysaccharides with strong antioxidant activity. These include species such as *Alternaria* sp., *Aspergillus terreus*, *Aspergillus versicolor*, and *Fusarium oxysporum*, which exhibited DPPH, hydroxyl, and superoxide antioxidant activity (Table 7). Prominently, the monosaccharides involved are glucose, mannose, and galactose in various proportions. It was found that extracellular polysaccharides derived from these fungi seem to have lower molecular weights and are composed of simple monosaccharides, making them more promising for strong antioxidant activities. The two exopolysaccharides (ENP1 and ENP2) from the marine fungus *Epicoccum nigrum* JJY40 showed moderate antioxidant activity against DPPH, hydroxyl, and superoxide radicals, with EC50 values of 0.43 and 0.38 mg/mL, respectively, as well as peroxidation inhibition. Reports suggest that the increased antioxidant activity may be due to increased uronic acid content (Sun et al. 2011).

Table 7 Antioxidant polysaccharides derived from different marine habitat fungi

Fungi	Monosaccharides in extracellular polysaccharides	Marine habitat	Antioxidant activity scavenging	Origin	References
Aspergillus terreus	Mannose and galactose	Fish associated *(Barracuda* sp)	DPPH and scavenging	Yellow Sea, China	Wang et al. (2013)
Aspergillus versicolor LCJ-5-4	Glucose and mannose	Coral associated (*Cladiella sp)*	Hydroxyl and superoxide	Lingao, Hainan Province of China	Wang et al. (2013)
Fusarium oxysporum	Galactose and furanose	Mangrove associated	DPPH, Hydroxyl and superoxide	South Sea, China	Chen et al. (2015)
Aspergillus versicolor N[2]bc	Mannose, glucose, and galactose	mud of deep waters	DPPH and Superoxide	South Sea, China	Yan et al. (2016)
Alternaria sp	Mannose, glucose, and galactose	Sponge endophyte	DPPH and hydroxyl	South Sea, China	Chen et al. (2016)
Fusarium equiseti ANP2	Mannose and glucose	Mangrove endophyte	Hydroxyl	Krishna River Delta, India	Prathyusha et al. (2018)
Penicillium sp F23-2	Mannose, glucose, and galactose	Marine fungus	Superoxide and hydroxyl	Jiaozhou Bay, in China	Sun et al. (2009)

Marine fungal species such as *Keissleriella* sp., *Penicillium* sp., and *Aspergillus* sp. are known for producing exopolysaccharides (EPSs) that contain fewer and less diverse monosaccharides, yet exhibit higher antioxidant capacity compared to bacteria. *Aureobasidium melanogenum* SCAU-266 has been reported to secrete EPS AUM-1, which is speculated to have higher ROS level and possess potential ferroptosis-related immunomodulatory properties (Lin et al. 2022).

The first report on EPS isolation from *Fusarium equiseti* ANP2, a mangrove endophytic fungus from the Krishna River Delta, revealed that this strain exhibited stronger in vitro hydroxyl radical scavenging than *Aspergillus versicolor* LCJ-5-5, but lesser activity compared to the marine fungus *Fusarium oxysporum* (Prathyusha et al. 2018). A recent study in 2021 identified a novel fungal isolate *Aspergillus* sp. DHE6, as the best producer of exopolysaccharide under submerged fermentation, with a yield of 7.2 g/L. The EPS showed strong antioxidant activity, with an EC50 value of 573.6 μg/mL in the DPPH radical scavenging assay, along with other antibacterial activity against human pathogens, making it a promising candidate for medical and food industry applications (Ghonemy et al. 2021).

The marine filamentous fungus *Phoma herbarum* YS4108 is the source of a novel CPS, YCP, which was extracted and found to contain a polymer of glucose and glucuronic acid. There are very few studies on endopolysaccharides (CPS) from fungi that have been published. The crude polymer is produced through a number of more potent techniques, including hot water extraction (80 °C), filtration, dialysis, and successive solvent washes, followed by purification using anion exchange and gel filtration chromatography. It has been shown that endopolysaccharide sulfation greatly boosts its antioxidant ability, including lipid peroxidation, metal chelation, superoxide scavenging, and hydroxyl scavenging (Yang et al. 2005).

13.1 The Antioxidative Properties of Polysaccharides Obtained from Marine Organisms

In addition to marine microorganisms and seaweeds, marine creatures such as crustaceans and invertebrates also possess antioxidant potential. The common group of polysaccharides found in marine animals are chitosan and glycosaminoglycans.

13.2 Chitosan

These are chitin-derived linear polysaccharides obtained by chitin deacetylation, forming a randomly disturbed glucosamine residue. Chitin is a water-insoluble compound, mainly found as an exoskeleton component of crustacean and arthropods, such as lobsters, shrimps, and crabs. It is also present in fungi and some nematodes. This water-insoluble form is converted into soluble derivatives, such as chitosan and carboxymethyl chitosan, by dissolving in a wide range of acidic and alkaline solutions. Chitosan has been demonstrated to have antioxidant, antibacterial, anti-inflammatory, and antitumor properties.

The degree of deacetylation in chitosan affects the mechanisms behind its antioxidant action (DDA), molecular weight, and NH2 groups. By adding functional groups and polyphenols to the chitosan skeleton, several modifications to its molecular structure have produced synergistic effects that increase the chitosan derivatives' capacity to scavenge radicals. Further enhancing the scavenging capacity was the N-methylation of 1,2,3-triazole groups. According to their level of deacetylation, a study on various crustacean sources revealed that they have potent antioxidant activity (Hajji et al. 2015) (Table 8).

Table 8 Degree of deacetylation in various Crustacean species

Source from marine crustaceans	Degree of deacetylation
Waste of Tunisian marine shrimp (*Penaeus kerathurus*)	88%
Shells of crab (*Carcinus mediterraneus*)	83%
Bones of cuttle fish (*Sepia officinalis*)	95%

According to a study, chitosan isolated from the exoskeletal chitin of the lobster *Thenus unimaculatus* exhibited antioxidant activity and was nontoxic, making it a viable option for pharmaceutical business (Arasukumar et al. 2019). Dietary chitosan derived from crabs was found to have in vivo antioxidant properties against oxidative stress caused by hyperlipidemia in the kidneys and livers of male albino rats, which demonstrated elevated activities of glutathione peroxidase, catalase, SOD, and malondialdehyde (MDA). This makes it a viable regimen in the management of complications related to obesity (Ugbaja et al. 2020). In Indonesia, chitosan extracted from the marine *Penaeus indicus* (white shrimp) has been reported to have strong antioxidant activity against DPPH scavenging than commercial chitosan, which is attributed to its higher degree of deacetylation (78.60%) compared to that of commercial chitosan (73.46%). The IC50 value of DPPH was 4.25.2 mg/mL (Purgiyanti et al. 2022).

Chito-oligosaccharides are one of the recent trending chitosan derivatives highly recommended compounds as natural oxidants in biological importance obtained with degree of polymerization with average molecular weight. The biological importance of chito-oligosaccharides includes lowering blood pressure and cholesterol, protecting against infections, increasing calcium uptake, and exhibiting antitumour properties (Mourya et al. 2011).

An investigation into the extraction of water-soluble polysaccharides from the body wall of the edible marine organism *Sipunculus nudus* L. revealed significant antioxidant capacity and hematopoietic activity. These properties play an important role in preventing irradiation-induced damage, making the polysaccharides a promising candidate for antiradiation hematopoiesis therapy (Li et al. 2016).

13.3 Glycosaminoglycan (GAG)

Glycosaminoglycans are linear heteropolysaccharides with a negative charge, formed by repeating disaccharide units consisting of N-acetylated hexosamine and uronic acid. Several types of glycosaminoglycans with varying bioactivities are present, among which hyaluronan and chondroitin sulfate are the most common. Other types, such as dermatan sulfate, heparan sulfate, keratan sulfate, and sulfated glycosaminoglycans, have lower bioavailability. The antioxidant property seems to be stronger in chondroitin sulfate, while other types exhibit important biological activities such as anticoagulation, cell proliferation, tissue regeneration, and anticancer activity.

According to reports, a polysaccharide called GAGs isolated from the sea snail *Rapana venosa* demonstrated promising antioxidant activity in ferric ion reduction and free radical scavenging tests. Chondroitin, the primary constituent, was identified as a sulfated type of GAG, which requires further analysis and characterization to reach its full potential (Gaspar et al. 2024). Polysaccharides (LSP3 and LMP3) extracted from the skin and meat of the sea snake *Lapemis curtus* exhibited notable antioxidant properties, including potent radical scavenging, which is attributed to their high content of uronic acid and sulfate (Bai et al. 2018).

13.4 Chondroitin Sulfate

A homogeneous polysaccharide found in the skate cartilage of the marine fish *Raja porosa*, chondroitin sulfate (CS) was shown in a study to have a stronger ability to scavenge free radicals than shark CS. The polysaccharide functions as an antioxidant agent because it has been demonstrated to increase resistance to oxidative stress (Zhou et al. 2020). According to a recent study, fucosylated chondroitin sulfate (FCS) isolated from three edible sea cucumbers—*Apostichopus japonicus*, *Stichopus chloronotus*, and *Acaudina molpadioides*—collected from various marine regions of China exhibited strong antioxidant activities, including scavenging of DPPH and nitric oxide radicals and inhibition of lipid peroxidation. The antioxidant potentials are also significantly influenced by fucose's sulfation pattern (Mou et al. 2018a, b) (Table 9).

Table 9 Antioxidant activities of polysaccharides derived from sea cucumber

Sea cucumber	Polysaccharides	Polysaccharideextraction methods	Rate of antioxidant activity	References
Holothuria mexicana	Glycosaminoglycans (HmG)	Hydrogen peroxide/ ascorbic acid	Moderate scavenging of superoxide and hydroxyl radicals	Mou et al. (2018a)
Holothuria fuscogliva	Polysaccharide (HfP)	Enzymatic hydrolysis	Stronger superoxide radical scavenging	Li et al. (2017)
Thelenota ananas	Novel polysaccharide (TA-FUC)	Enzymatic hydrolysis	Strong super-oxide radical scavenging	Yu et al. (2014)
Sipunculus nudus	Polysaccharide (SNP)	Alkali extraction	Strong hydroxyl and superoxide scavenging ability and also prevent radiation damage	Li et al. (2016)

14 Applications

14.1 Antioxidant Therapy

Anraku et al. (2011) reported that a high molecular weight chitosan supplement (HMCS) inhibits the development of oxidative stress in the systemic circulation in the gastrointestinal tract by lowering levels of pro-oxidants such as cholesterol and uremic toxins, which are protein antioxidants in renal failure.

14.2 Bone Tissue Engineering

Chitosan nanofibers fabricated from crab shells have been used in ultrasonication for mechanical disruption, and chitin nanofibers have been reported for applications in inflammatory bowel disease. Several composites prepared with alginate, hydroxyapatite, or calcium phosphate combined with chitosan have been used in bone tissue engineering (Martino et al. 2005).

14.3 Hyaluronans

Hyaluronan is a linear, polysaccharide structure that is mostly present in the cartilage of marine animals and the vitreous humor of several fish species. It plays a significant role in tissue regeneration, cell proliferation, differentiation, and migration in humans and is a key component of the synovial fluid found in joints and cartilages. Because of its high viscoelasticity and biocompatibility, hyaluronan finds extensive usage in tissue engineering applications and the production of wound-healing structures (Chen and Abatangelo 1999).

14.4 Neuroprotection Activity

The invertebrate *Phallusia nigra* contains dermatan sulfate, a kind of glycosaminoglycan that has been shown to have neuroprotective and antioxidant properties in addition to reducing ROS cell line neuroblastoma-2A. It can be utilized as a stabilizing agent for cytokines and other growth factors and is also isolated from the skin of ray fish. According to a recent study, dermatan sulfates are an excellent substitute for heparin because they don't affect factor X of the coagulation cascade (Vitale et al. 2013). In food and nutraceutical industries, dermatan sulfates are used as gelling agents, emulsifiers, and stabilizers to improve the texture and longevity of food items as well as nutraceuticals.

References

Abdel-Wahab, B. A., F. Abd El-Kareem, H., Alzamami, A., A. Fahmy, C., H. Elesawy, B., Mostafa Mahmoud, M., Ghareeb, A., El Askary, A., H. Abo Nahas, H., G. M. Attallah, N., Altwaijry, N., & M. Saied, E. (2022). Novel Exopolysaccharide from Marine *Bacillus subtilis* with Broad Potential Biological Activities: Insights into Antioxidant, Anti-Inflammatory, Cytotoxicity, and Anti-Alzheimer Activity. *Metabolites*, *12*(8), 715. https://doi.org/10.3390/metabo12080715

Acharya, A., Das, I., Chandhok, D., & Saha, T. (2010). Redox regulation in cancer: a double-edged sword with therapeutic potential. *Oxidative medicine and cellular longevity*, *3*(1), 23–34. https://doi.org/10.4161/oxim.3.1.10095

Adwas, A. A., Elsayed, A., Azab, A. E., &Quwaydir, F. A. (2019). Oxidative stress and antioxidant mechanisms in human body. *J. Appl. Biotechnol. Bioeng*, *6*(1), 43–47. https://doi.org/10.15406/jabb.2019.06.00173

Agustinho, D. P., Miller, L. C., Li, L. X., & Doering, T. L. (2018). Peeling the onion: the outer layers of Cryptococcus neoformans. *Memórias do Instituto Oswaldo Cruz*, *113*(7), e180040.

Ajisaka, K., Yokoyama, T., & Matsuo, K. (2016). Structural characteristics and antioxidant activities of fucoidans from five brown seaweeds. *Journal of Applied Glycoscience*, *63*(2), 31–37.

Al Monla, R., Dassouki, Z., Kouzayha, A., Salma, Y., Gali-Muhtasib, H., & Mawlawi, H. (2020). The Cytotoxic and Apoptotic Effects of the Brown Algae *Colpomeniasinuosa* are Mediated by the Generation of Reactive Oxygen Species. *Molecules*, *25*(8), 1993. https://doi.org/10.3390/molecules25081993

Alam, M.N.; Bristi, N.J.; Rafiquzzaman, M. Review on in vivo and in vitro methods evaluation of antioxidant activity. *Saudi Pharm. J.* 2013, *21*, 143–152

Ale, M. T., Mikkelsen, J. D., & Meyer, A. S. (2011). Important determinants for fucoidan bioactivity: a critical review of structure-function relations and extraction methods for fucose-containing sulfated polysaccharides from brown seaweeds. *Marine drugs*, *9*(10), 2106–2130. https://doi.org/10.3390/md9102106

Alves, A., Sousa, R. A., & Reis, R. L. (2013). A practical perspective on ulvan extracted from green algae. Journal of Applied Phycology, 25(2), 407–424.

Amimi, A., Mouradi, A., Givernaud, T., Chiadmi, N., &Lahaye, M. (2001). Structural analysis of Gigartina pistillatacarrageenans (Gigartinaceae, Rhodophyta). Carbohydrate Research, 333(4), 271–279.AGAR

Angiolella L., Sacchetti G., Efferth T. Antimicrobial and Antioxidant Activities of Natural Compounds. Evid.-Based Complement. Altern. Med. 2018;2018:1945179

Anraku, M., Fujii, T., Kondo, Y., Kojima, E., Hata, T., Tabuchi, N., ... &Tomida, H. (2011). Antioxidant properties of high molecular weight dietary chitosan in vitro and in vivo. *Carbohydrate Polymers*, *83*(2), 501–505.

Arasukumar, B.; Prabakaran, G.; Gunalan, B.; Moovendhan, M. Chemical composition, structural features, surface morphology and bioactivities of chitosan derivatives from lobster (Thenusunimaculatus) shells. *Int. J. Biol. Macromol.* 2019, *135*, 1237–1245

Aremu, A. O., Neményi, M., Stirk, W. A., Ördög, V., & van Staden, J. (2015). Manipulation of nitrogen levels and mode of cultivation are viable methods to improve the lipid, fatty acids, phytochemical content, and bioactivities in Chlorella minutissima. *Journal of Phycology*, *51*(4), 659–669

Bai M, Han W, Zhao X, Wang Q, Gao Y, Deng S. Glycosaminoglycans from a Sea Snake (*Lapemiscurtus*): Extraction, Structural Characterization and Antioxidant Activity. *Marine Drugs*. 2018; 16(5):170. https://doi.org/10.3390/md16050170

Balasa A.F., Chircov C., Grumezescu A.M. Marine Biocompounds for Neuroprotection—A Review. Mar. Drugs. 2020;18:290. https://doi.org/10.3390/md18060290.

Barzkar N., Babich O., Das R., Sukhikh S., Tamadoni Jahromi S., Sohail M. Marine Bacterial Dextranases: Fundamentals and Applications. Molecules. 2022;27:5533

Baweja, P., & Sahoo, D. (2015). Classification of algae. *The algae world*, 31–55.

Benzie, I. F., & Strain, J. J. (1996). The ferric reducing ability of plasma (FRAP) as a measure of "antioxidant power": the FRAP assay. *Analytical biochemistry*, *239*(1), 70–76.

Bhuyar, P., Sundararaju, S., Rahim, M. H. A., Unpaprom, Y., Maniam, G. P., & Govindan, N. (2021). Antioxidative study of polysaccharides extracted from red (Kappaphycusalvarezii), green (Kappaphycus striatus) and brown (Padina gymnospora) marine macroalgae/seaweed. *SN Applied Sciences*, *3*, 1–9.

Bors, W., Michel, C., & Saran, M. (1984). Inhibition of the bleaching of the carotenoid crocin a rapid test for quantifying antioxidant activity. *Biochimica et Biophysica Acta (BBA)-Lipids and Lipid Metabolism*, *796*(3), 312–319.

C. Sanchez-Moreno, "Review: methods used to evaluate the free radical scavenging activity in foods and biological systems," Food Science and Technology International, vol.8, no.3, pp.121 137, 2002.

Campo, V. L., Kawano, D. F., da Silva Jr, D. B., & Carvalho, I. (2009). Carrageenans: Biological properties, chemical modifications and structural analysis–A review. *Carbohydrate polymers*, *77*(2), 167–180.

Cao, G., Sofic, E., & Prior, R. L. (1997). Antioxidant and prooxidant behavior of flavonoids: structure-activity relationships. *Free radical biology and medicine*, *22*(5), 749–760

Carocho, M., & Ferreira, I. C. (2013). A review on antioxidants, prooxidants and related controversy: natural and synthetic compounds, screening and analysis methodologies and future perspectives. *Food and chemical toxicology: an international journal published for the British Industrial Biological Research Association*, *51*, 15–25. https://doi.org/10.1016/j.fct.2012.09.021

Castro, J. P. L. D., Costa, L. E. C., Pinheiro, M. P., Francisco, T. D. S., Vasconcelos, P. H. M. D., Funari, L. M., … & Freitas, A. L. P. (2018). Polysaccharides of red alga Gracilaria intermedia: structure, antioxidant activity and rheological behavior. *Polímeros*, *28*(2), 178–186.

Chaiklahan, R., Chirasuwan, N., Triratana, P., Loha, V., Tia, S., & Bunnag, B. (2013). Polysaccharide extraction from Spirulina sp. and its antioxidant capacity. *International journal of biological macromolecules*, *58*, 73–7.

Chen Y.L., Mao W.J., Tao H.W., Zhu W.M., Yan M.X., Liu X., Guo T.T., Guo T. Preparation and characterization of a novel extracellular polysaccharide with antioxidant activity, from the mangrove-associated fungus Fusarium oxysporum. Mar. Biotechnol. 2015;17:219–228. https://doi.org/10.1007/s10126-015-9611-6.

Chen, W.Y.; Abatangelo, G. Functions of hyaluronan in wound repair. Wound Repair Regen. 1999, 7, 79–89.

Chen, Y.; Mao, W.-J.; Yan, M.-X.; Liu, X.; Wang, S.-Y.; Xia, Z.; Xiao, B.; Cao, S.-J.; Yang, B.-Q.; Li, J. Purification, Chemical Characterization, and Bioactivity of an Extracellular Polysaccharide Produced by the Marine Sponge Endogenous Fungus *Alternaria* sp. SP-32. *Mar. Biotechnol.* 2016, *18*, 301–313.

Chi, W. J., Chang, Y. K., & Hong, S. K. (2012). Agar degradation by microorganisms and agar-degrading enzymes. Applied microbiology and biotechnology, 94, 917–930.

Chiellini, F., & Morelli, A. (2011). Ulvan: A versatile platform of biomaterials from renewable resources. Biomaterials—physics and chemistry, 75–98.

Cindana Mo'o, F. R., Wilar, G., Devkota, H. P., & Wathoni, N. (2020). Ulvan, a polysaccharide from macroalga Ulva sp.: a review of chemistry, biological activities and potential for food and biomedical applications. Applied Sciences, 10(16), 5488.

Cirulis, J. T., Scott, J. A., & Ross, G. M. (2013). Management of oxidative stress by microalgae. *Canadian journal of physiology and pharmacology*, *91*(1), 15–21.

Costa, J. A. V., Lucas, B. F., Alvarenga, A. G. P., Moreira, J. B., & de Morais, M. G. (2021a). Microalgae polysaccharides: an overview of production, characterization, and potential applications. *Polysaccharides*, *2*(4), 759–772.

Costa, M., Losada-Barreiro, S., Paiva-Martins, F., & Bravo-Díaz, C. (2021b). Polyphenolic Antioxidants in Lipid Emulsions: Partitioning Effects and Interfacial Phenomena. *Foods (Basel, Switzerland)*, *10*(3), 539. https://doi.org/10.3390/foods10030539

De Jesus Raposo, M. F., De Morais, R. M. S. C., & de Morais, A. M. M. B. (2013). Bioactivity and applications of sulphated polysaccharides from marine microalgae. *Marine drugs*, *11*(1), 233–252.

De La Fuente, G., Fontana, M., Asnaghi, V., Chiantore, M., Mirata, S., Salis, A., Damonte, G., & Scarfì, S. (2021). The Remarkable Antioxidant and Anti-Inflammatory Potential of the Extracts of the Brown Alga *Cystoseiraamentacea* var. *stricta*. *Marine Drugs*, *19*(1), 2. https://doi.org/10.3390/md19010002

Delattre, C., Pierre, G., Laroche, C., & Michaud, P. (2016). Production, extraction and characterization of microalgal and cyanobacterial exopolysaccharides. *Biotechnology advances*, *34*(7), 1159–1179.

Demidchik, V. (2015). Mechanisms of oxidative stress in plants: from classical chemistry to cell biology. *Environmental and experimental botany*, *109*, 212–228.

Di, T., Chen, G., Sun, Y., Ou, S., Zeng, X., & Ye, H. (2017). Antioxidant and immunostimulating activities in vitro of sulfated polysaccharides isolated from Gracilaria rubra. *Journal of Functional Foods*, *28*, 64–75.

Domozych, D. et al. (2019) Algal Cell Wall. In Encyclopedia of Life Sciences, 4th ed.; John Wiley & Sons Ltd.: Chichester, UK, 2019; pp. 1–11.

Dong, X., Bai, Y., Xu, Z., Shi, Y., Sun, Y., Janaswamy, S., et al., 2019. Phlorotannins from Undaria pinnatifida sporophyll: extraction, antioxidant, and anti-inflammatory activities. Mar. Drugs 17 (8) 10.3390/md17080434

El Rashed, Z., Lupidi, G., Kanaan, H., Grasselli, E., Canesi, L., Khalifeh, H., & Demori, I. (2021). Antioxidant and Antisteatotic activities of a new Fucoidan extracted from Ferulahermonis roots harvested on Lebanese mountains. *Molecules*, *26*(4), 1161.

El-Baky, H. A., El-Baz, K. H., & El-Latife, S. A. (2013). Induction of sulfated polysaccharides in Spirulina platensis as response to nitrogen concentration and its biological evaluation.

El-Ghonemy, D. H. (2021). Antioxidant and antimicrobial activities of exopolysaccharides produced by a novel Aspergillus sp. DHE6 under optimized submerged fermentation conditions. *Biocatalysis and Agricultural Biotechnology*, *36*, 102150.

El-Shaibany, A., Al-Habori, M., Al-Maqtari, T., & Al-Mahbashi, H. (2020). The Yemeni brown algae Dictyota dichotoma exhibit high in vitro anticancer activity independent of its antioxidant capability. *BioMed Research International*, *2020*(1), 2425693.

Ferdous, U. T., & Yusof, Z. N. B. (2021). Medicinal prospects of antioxidants from algal sources in cancer therapy. *Frontiers in Pharmacology*, *12*, 593116.*Marine drugs*, *18*(1), 28.

Fletcher, H. R., Biller, P., Ross, A. B., Adams, J. M. M. (2017). The seasonal variation of fucoidan iwithin three species of brown macroalgae. Algal research, 22, 79–86.

Forman, H. J., & Zhang, H. (2021). Targeting oxidative stress in disease: promise and limitations of antioxidant therapy. *Nature Reviews Drug Discovery*, *20*(9), 689–709

Francisco, J., Horta, A., Pedrosa, R., Afonso, C., Cardoso, C., Bandarra, N. M., & Gil, M. M. (2020). Bioaccessibility of Antioxidants and Fatty Acids from *Fucus Spiralis*. *Foods*, *9*(4), 440.

Gaignard, C., Gargouch, N., Dubessay, P., Delattre, C., Pierre, G., Laroche, C., … & Michaud, P. (2019). New horizons in culture and valorization of red microalgae. *Biotechnology advances*, *37*(1), 193–222.

Galasso, C., Gentile, A., Orefice, I., Ianora, A., Bruno, A., Noonan, D. M., … & Brunet, C. (2019). Microalgal derivatives as potential nutraceutical and food supplements for human health: A focus on cancer prevention and interception. *Nutrients*, *11*(6), 1226.

Gandhi, S., & Abramov, A. Y. (2012). Mechanism of oxidative stress in neurodegeneration. *Oxidative medicine and cellular longevity*, *2012*, 428010. https://doi.org/10.1155/2012/428010

Garcia-Rubio, R., de Oliveira, H. C., Rivera, J., & Trevijano-Contador, N. (2020). The fungal cell wall: Candida, Cryptococcus, and Aspergillus species. *Frontiers in microbiology*, *10*, 2993.

Gaspar-Pintiliescu, A.; Stefan, L.M.; Mihai, E.; Sanda, C.; Manoiu, V.S.; Berger, D.; Craciunescu, O. Antioxidant and antiproliferative effect of a glycosaminoglycan extract from Rapanavenosa marine snail. *PLoS ONE* 2024, *19*, e0297803.

Ghaliaoui, N., Mokrane, H., Hazzit, M., Hadjadj, M., Saidotmani, F., Touati, S., &Seridi, H. (2020). Impact of freezing and drying preprocessing on pigments extraction from the brown seaweed «Phyllariareniformis» collected in Algerian coast.

Ghonemy, M. M., et al. (2021). Characterization and bioactivity of exopolysaccharides produced by marine bacteria: Antioxidant and antibacterial potential. Published in: International Journal of Biological Macromolecules, Volume 183, Pages 1894–1904.

Gow, N. A., Latge, J. P., & Munro, C. A. (2017). The fungal cell wall: structure, biosynthesis, and function. *Microbiology spectrum*, *5*(3), 10–1128.

Guo, S., Mao, W., Han, Y., Zhang, X., Yang, C., Chen, Y., … & Xu, J. (2010). Structural characteristics and antioxidant activities of the extracellular polysaccharides produced by marine bacterium Edwardsiellatarda. *Bioresource Technology*, *101*(12), 4729–4732.

Gülcin, I. (2012). Antioxidant activity of food constituents: an overview. Archives of toxicology, 86 (3), 345–391.

Hajji, S.; Younes, I.; Rinaudo, M.; Jellouli, K.; Nasri, M. Characterization and in vitro evaluation of cytotoxicity, antimicrobial and antioxidant activities of chitosans extracted from three different marine sources. *Appl. Biochem. Biotech.* 2015,

Halliwell, B., Aeschbach, R., Löliger, J., &Aruoma, O. I. (1995) The characterization of antioxidants. *Food and Chemical Toxicology*, *33*(7), 601–617.

He, J., Xu, Y., Chen, H., & Sun, P. (2016). Extraction, Structural Characterization, and Potential Antioxidant Activity of the Polysaccharides from Four Seaweeds. *International journal of molecular sciences*, *17*(12), 1988. https://doi.org/10.3390/ijms17121988

Hernandez-Carmona, G., Freile-Pelegrín, Y., & Hernández-Garibay, E. (2013). Conventional and alternative technologies for the extraction of algal polysaccharides. In Functional ingredients from algae for foods and nutraceuticals (pp. 475–516). Woodhead Publishing.

Hosseini S.F., Rezaei M., McClements D.J. Bioactive Functional Ingredients from Aquatic Origin: A Review of Recent Progress in Marine-Derived Nutraceuticals. Crit. Rev. Food Sci. Nutr. 2020;62:1242–1269.

Hosseini S.F., Rezaei M., McClements D.J. Bioactive functional ingredients from aquatic origin: A review of recent progress in marine-derived nutraceuticals. Crit. Rev. Food Sci. Nutr. 2022;62: 1242–1269.

I. G¨ulc ¸in, "Antioxidant activity of food constituents: an overview," Archives of Toxicology, vol. 86,no.3,pp. 345–391, 2012.

Ibrahim, H. A., Abou Elhassayeb, H. E., & El-Sayed, W. M. (2022). Potential functions and applications of diverse microbial exopolysaccharides in marine environments. *Journal of Genetic Engineering and Biotechnology*, *20*(1), 151.

J. B. L. Tan and Y. Y. Lim, "Critical analysis of current methods for assessing the in vitro antioxidant and antibacterial activity of plant extracts," Food Chemistry,vol.172, pp.814–822,2015.

Jmel, M. A., Anders, N., Messaoud, G. B., Marzouki, M. N., Spiess, A., & Smaali, I. (2019). The stranded macroalga Ulva lactuca as a new alternative source of cellulose: Extraction, physico-chemical and rheological characterization. Journal of Cleaner Production, 234, 1421–1427.

Jönsson, M., Allahgholi, L., Sardari, R. R., Hreggviðsson, G. O., & Nordberg Karlsson, E. (2020). Extraction and modification of macroalgal polysaccharides for current and next-generation applications. *Molecules*, *25*(4), 930

Kadam, S. U., Tiwari, B. K., & O'Donnell, C. P. (2013). Application of novel extraction technologies for bio actives from marine algae. *Journal of agricultural and food chemistry*, *61*(20), 4667–4675. https://doi.org/10.1021/jf400819p

Kammoun, I., Sellem, I., Ben Saad, H., Boudawara, T., Nasri, M., Gharsallah, N., ... & Amara, I. B. (2019). Potential benefits of polysaccharides derived from marine alga Ulva lactuca against hepatotoxicity and nephrotoxicity induced by thiacloprid, an insecticide pollutant. Environmental toxicology, 34(11), 1165–1176.

Kammoun, I., Bkhairia, I., Ben Abdallah, F., Jaballi, I., Ktari, N., Boudawara, O., ... & Ben Amara, I. (2017). Potential protective effects of polysaccharide extracted from Ulva lactuca against male reprotoxicity induced by thiacloprid. Archives of physiology and biochemistry, 123(5), 334–343.

Khan, M. I., Shin, J. H., & Kim, J. D. (2018). The promising future of microalgae: current status, challenges, and optimization of a sustainable and renewable industry for biofuels, feed, and other products. *Microbial cell factories*, *17*, 1–21.

Khan, R., Shah, M. D., Shah, L., Lee, P. C., & Khan, I. (2022). Bacterial polysaccharides—A big source for prebiotics and therapeutics. *Frontiers in Nutrition*, *9*, 1031935.

Khan, S. I., & Satam, S. B. (2003). Seaweed mariculture: scope and potential in India. Aquaculture asia, 8(4), 26–29.

Kidgell, J. T., Magnusson, M., de Nys, R., & Glasson, C. R. (2019). Ulvan: A systematic review of extraction, composition and function. Algal research, 39, 101422.

Kidgell, J. T., Carnachan, S. M., Magnusson, M., Lawton, R. J., Sims, I. M., Hinkley, S. F., ... & Glasson, C. R. (2021). Are all ulvans equal? A comparative assessment of the chemical and gelling properties of ulvan from blade and filamentous Ulva. Carbohydrate Polymers, 264, 118010.

Laeliocattleya, R. A., Suloi, A. F., Gayatri, P. P., Putri, N. A., &Anggraeni, Y. C. (2020). Fucoidan content from brown seaweed (Sargassum filipendula) and its potential as radical scavenger. In *Journal of Physics: Conference Series* (Vol. 1430, No. 1, p. 012023). IOP Publishing.

Lahaye, M., & Robic, A. (2007). Structure and functional properties of ulvan, a polysaccharide from green seaweeds. Biomacromolecules, 8(6), 1765–1774.

Lakshmi, D. S., Sankaranarayanan, S., Gajaria, T. K., Li, G., Kujawski, W., Kujawa, J., & Navia, R. (2020). A short review on the valorization of green seaweeds and ulvan: Feedstock for chemicals and biomaterials. Biomolecules, 10(7), 991.

Lee, J. H., Kim, H. H., Ko, J. Y., Jang, J. H., Kim, G. H., Lee, J. S., Nah, J. W., & Jeon, Y. J. (2016). Rapid preparation of functional polysaccharides from Pyropiayezoensis by microwave-assistant rapid enzyme digest system. *Carbohydrate polymers*, *153*, 512–517. https://doi.org/10.1016/j.carbpol.2016.07.122

Li J, Chi Z, Yu L, Jiang F, Liu C (2017a) Sulfated modification, characterization, and antioxidant and moisture absorption/retention activities of a soluble neutral polysaccharide from Enteromorpha prolifera. Int J BiolMacromol 105:1544–1553

Li N., Shen X.R., Liu Y.M., Zhang J.L., He Y., Liu Q., Jiang D.W., Zong J., Li J.M., Hou D.Y., et al. Isolation, characterization, and radiation protection of Sipunculusnudus L. polysaccharide. Int. J. Biol. Macromol. 2016; 83:288–296. https://doi.org/10.1016/j.ijbiomac.2015.11.071

Li, H., Ding, F., Xiao, L., Shi, R., Wang, H., Han, W., & Huang, Z. (2017b). Food-Derived Antioxidant Polysaccharides and Their Pharmacological Potential in Neurodegenerative Diseases. *Nutrients*, *9*(7), 778. https://doi.org/10.3390/nu9070778

Li, H., Xu, J., Liu, Y., Ai, S., Qin, F., Li, Z., ... & Huang, Z. (2011). Antioxidant and moisture-retention activities of the polysaccharide from Nostoc commune. *Carbohydrate Polymers*, *83*(4), 1821–1827.

Li, R.F.; Yu, H.H.; Yue, Y.; Liu, S.; Xing, R.E.; Chen, X.L.; Li, P.C. Sulfated polysaccharides with antioxidant and anticoagulant activity from the sea cucumber *Holothuria fuscogliva*. *Chin. J. Oceanol. Limnol.* 2017c, *35*, 763–769

Lim, S. J., Mustapha, W. A. W., Maskat, M. Y., Latip, J., Badri, K. H., & Hassan, O. (2016). Chemical properties and toxicology studies of fucoidan extracted from Malaysian *Sargassum binderi. Food science and biotechnology*, *25*(Suppl 1), 23–29. https://doi.org/10.1007/s10068-016-0094-7

Lin, Y.; Yang, J.; Luo, L.; Zhang, X.; Deng, S.; Chen, X.; Li, Y.; Bekhit, A.E.A.; Xu, B.; Huang, R. Ferroptosis Related Immunomodulatory Effect of a Novel Extracellular Polysaccharides from Marine Fungus Aureobasidiummelanogenum. *Mar. Drugs* 2022, *20*, 332.

Liu, X., Liu, H., Zhai, Y., Li, Y., Zhu, X., & Zhang, W. (2017). Laminarin protects against hydrogen peroxide-induced oxidative damage in MRC-5 cells possibly via regulating NRF2. *PeerJ*, *5*, e3642.

Lu, J. M., Lin, P. H., Yao, Q., & Chen, C. (2010). Chemical and molecular mechanisms of antioxidants: experimental approaches and model systems. *Journal of cellular and molecular medicine, 14*(4), 840–860. https://doi.org/10.1111/j.1582-4934.2009.00897.x

Lu, J., Shi, K. K., Chen, S., Wang, J., Hassouna, A., White, L. N., Merien, F., Xie, M., Kong, Q., Li, J., Ying, T., White, W. L., & Nie, S. (2018). Fucoidan Extracted from the New Zealand *Undaria pinnatifida*—Physicochemical Comparison against Five Other Fucoidans: Unique Low Molecular Weight Fraction Bioactivity in Breast Cancer Cell Lines. *Marine Drugs, 16*(12), 461. https://doi.org/10.3390/md16120461

Lv, J., Zhao, F., Feng, J., Liu, Q., Nan, F., & Xie, S. (2019). Extraction of extracellular polymeric substances (EPS) from a newly isolated self-flocculating microalga Neocystis mucosa SX with different methods. *Algal research, 40*, 101479.

Mahmoud, Y. A. G., El-Naggar, M. E., Abdel-Megeed, A., & El-Newehy, M. (2021). Recent advancements in microbial polysaccharides: Synthesis and applications. *Polymers, 13*(23), 4136.

Manandhar, B., Wagle, A., Seong, S. H., Paudel, P., Kim, H.-R., Jung, H. A., & Choi, J. S. (2019). Phlorotannins with Potential Anti-Tyrosinase and Antioxidant Activity Isolated from the Marine Seaweed *Ecklonia stolonifera. Antioxidants, 8*(8), 240. https://doi.org/10.3390/antiox8080240

Martino, A.D.; Sittinger, M.; Risbud, M.V. Chitosan: A versatile biopolymer for orthopaedic tissue-engineering. *Biomaterials* 2005, *26*, 5983–5990.

Mohamed, S., Shimaa, R., El Awady, M., & El Sayed, O. (2015). Screening of bacterial antioxidant exopolysaccharides isolated from Egyptian habitats. *J. Chem. Pharm. Res, 7*, 980–986.

Mohammed, A. S. A., Naveed, M., & Jost, N. (2021). Polysaccharides; classification, chemical properties, and future perspective applications in fields of pharmacology and biological medicine (a review of current applications and upcoming potentialities). *Journal of Polymers and the Environment, 29*, 2359–2371.

Morelli, A., Puppi, D., & Chiellini, F. (2017). Perspectives on biomedical applications of ulvan (pp. 305–330). Amsterdam, The Netherlands: Elsevier.

Mou, J., Li, Q., Qi, X., & Yang, J. (2018a). Structural comparison, antioxidant and anti-inflammatory properties of fucosylated chondroitin sulfate of three edible sea cucumbers. *Carbohydrate Polymers, 185*, 41–47.

Mou, J.; Wang, C.; Li, Q.; Qi, X.; Yang, J. Preparation and antioxidant properties of low molecular holothurian glycosaminoglycans by H_2O_2/ascorbic acid degradation. *Int. J. Biol. Macromol.* 2018b, *107*, 1339–1347

Mourya, V.K.; Inamdar, N.N.; Choudhari, Y.M. Chitooligosaccharides: Synthesis, characterization and applications. *Polym. Sci. Ser. A* 2011, *53*, 583–612.

Newman, D. J., & Cragg, G. M. (2012). Natural products as sources of new drugs over the 30 years from 1981 to 2010. *Journal of natural products, 75*(3), 311–335.

Nishinari, K., & Fang, Y. (2017). Relationship between structure and rheological and thermal properties of agar. A mini-review on the effect of alkali treatment and the role of agaropectin. Food structure, 13, 24–34.

Nunes Pinheiro, A. D., Pereira Lopes-Filho, E. A., De-Paula, J. C., Pereira Netto, A. D., & Teixeira, V. L. (2019). *Diterpenes from the brown alga Dictyotamertensii. Biochemical Systematics and Ecology, 86, 103926* https://doi.org/10.1016/j.bse.2019.103926

Odekina, P. A., Agbo, M. O., & Omeje, E. O. (2020). Antimicrobial and antioxidant activities of novel marine bacteria (Bacillus 2011SOCCUF3) isolated from marine sponge (Spongia officinalis). *Pharmaceutical Sciences, 26*(1), 82–87.

Olasehinde, T. A., Mabinya, L. V., Olaniran, A. O., & Okoh, A. I. (2019). Chemical characterization of sulfated polysaccharides from Gracilaria gracilis and Ulva lactuca and their radical scavenging, metal chelating, and cholinesterase inhibitory activities. International Journal of Food Properties, 22(1), 100–110.

Olatunji, O. (2020). Aquatic biopolymers: understanding their industrial significance and environmental implications. Springer Nature.

Palaniyappan, S., Sridhar, A., Kari, Z. A., Téllez-Isaías, G., & Ramasamy, T. (2023). Evaluation of Phytochemical Screening, Pigment Content, In Vitro Antioxidant, Antibacterial Potential and GC-MS Metabolite Profiling of Green Seaweed *Caulerpa racemosa*. *Marine Drugs*, *21*(5), 278. https://doi.org/10.3390/md21050278

Pandya, Y. H., Bakshi, M., Sharma, A., Pandya, Y. H., & Pandya, H. (2022). Agar-agar extraction, structural properties and applications: A review. The Pharma Innovation Journal, 6, 1151–1157.

Park, S. H., Lee, C. R., & Hong, S. K. (2020). Implications of agar and agarase in industrial applications of sustainable marine biomass. Applied microbiology and biotechnology, 104, 2815–2832.

Peasura N., Laohakunjit N., Kerdchoechuen O., Wanlapa S. Characteristics and antioxidant of Ulva intestinalis sulphated polysaccharides extracted with different solvents. Int. J. Biol. Macromol. 2015;81:912–919. https://doi.org/10.1016/j.ijbiomac.2015.09.030

Peasura, N., Laohakunjit, N., Kerdchoechuen, O., Vongsawasdi, P., & Chao, L. K. (2016). Assessment of biochemical and immunomodulatory activity of sulphated polysaccharides from Ulva intestinalis. *International journal of biological macromolecules*, *91*, 269–277.

Pisoschi, A. M., & Pop, A. (2015). The role of antioxidants in the chemistry of oxidative stress: A review. *European journal of medicinal chemistry*, *97*, 55–74.

Poljsak, B., Šuput, D., &Milisav, I. (2013). Achieving the balance between ROS and antioxidants: when to use the synthetic antioxidants. *Oxidative medicine and cellular longevity*, *2013*(1), 956792.

Prathyusha, A. M. V. N., Sheela, G. M., & Bramhachari, P. V. (2018). Chemical characterization and antioxidant properties of exopolysaccharides from mangrove filamentous fungi Fusarium equiseti ANP2. *Biotechnology Reports*, *19*, e00277.

Priyanka, P., Arun, A. B., Young, C. C., & Rekha, P. D. (2015). Prospecting exopolysaccharides produced by selected bacteria associated with marine organisms for biotechnological applications. *Chinese Journal of Polymer Science*, *33*, 236–244.

Purgiyanti, P., Kumoro, A. C., & Legowo, A. M. (2022). The antioxidant and antibacterial activities of chitosan extract from white shrimp shell (Penaeus indicus) in the waters north of Brebes, Indonesia. *Biodiversitas Journal of Biological Diversity*, *23*(3).

Rahal, A., Kumar, A., Singh, V., Yadav, B., Tiwari, R., Chakraborty, S., &Dhama, K. (2014). Oxidative stress, prooxidants, and antioxidants: the interplay. *BioMed research international*, *2014*(1), 761264.

Rani A, Saini KC, Bast F et al (2021) Microorganisms: a potential source of bioactive molecules for antioxidant applications. Molecules 26:1142

Raphael, E., Avellaneda, C. O., Manzolli, B., & Pawlicka, A. (2010). Agar-based films for application as polymer electrolytes. Electrochimica Acta, 55(4), 1455–1459.

Rioux, L. E., Turgeon, S. L., & Beaulieu, M. (2007). Characterization of polysaccharides extracted from brown seaweeds. Carbohydrate polymers, 69(3), 530–537.

Roginsky, V., & Lissi, E. A. (2005). Review of methods to determine chain-breaking antioxidant activity in food. *Food chemistry*, *92*(2), 235–254.

Rudrapal, M., Khairnar, S. J., Khan, J., Dukhyil, A. B., Ansari, M. A., Alomary, M. N., & Devi, R. (2022). Dietary polyphenols and their role in oxidative stress-induced human diseases: Insights into protective effects, antioxidant potentials and mechanism (s) of action. *Frontiers in pharmacology*, *13*, 806470.

Saed-Moucheshi, A., Shekoofa, A., &Pessarakli, M. (2014). Reactive oxygen species (ROS) generation and detoxifying in plants. *Journal of Plant Nutrition*, *37*(10), 1573–1585.

Santos-Sánchez, N. F., Salas-Coronado, R., Villanueva-Cañongo, C., & Hernández-Carlos, B. (2019). *Antioxidant compounds and their antioxidant mechanism*. IntechOpen.

Satpute, S. K., Banat, I. M., Dhakephalkar, P. K., Banpurkar, A. G., &Chopade, B. A. (2010). Biosurfactants, bioemulsifiers and exopolysaccharides from marine microorganisms. *Biotechnology advances*, *28*(4), 436–450.

Sattar, H., Aman, A., & Qader, S. A. U. (2018). Agar-agar immobilization: An alternative approach for the entrapment of protease to improve the catalytic efficiency, thermal stability and recycling efficiency. International journal of biological macromolecules, 111, 917–922.

Sellimi, S.; Kadri, N.; Barragan-Montero, V.; Laouer, H.; Hajji, M.; Nasri, M. Fucans from a Tunisian brown seaweed Cystoseirabarbata: Structural characteristics and antioxidant activity. Int. J. Biol. Macromol. 2014, 66, 281–288.

Senadheera T.R.L., Hossain A., Shahidi F. Marine Bioactives and Their Application in the Food Industry: A Review. Appl. Sci. 2023;13:12088.

Shao, P., Chen, X., & Sun, P. (2013). In vitro antioxidant and antitumor activities of different sulfated polysaccharides isolated from three algae. *International Journal of Biological Macromolecules*, *62*, 155–161.

Shivale, N., Marar, T., Samant, M., &Harmalkar, M. (2018). Screening of Antioxidant Activity of marine bacteria isolated from marine soil obtained from North-West coastal region of India. *Int. J. Biol. Pharm. Allied Sci*, *7*.

Simat V., Elabed N., Kulawik P., Ceylan Z., Jamroz E., Yazgan H., Čagalj M., Regenstein J.M., Özogul F. Recent advances in marine-based nutraceuticals and their health benefits. Mar. Drugs. 2020;18:627

Soubra, L., Sarkis, D., Hilan, C., & Verger, P. (2007). Dietary exposure of children and teenagers to benzoates, sulphites, butylhydroxyanisol (BHA) and butylhydroxytoluen (BHT) in Beirut (Lebanon). *Regulatory toxicology and pharmacology,RTP*, *47*(1),68–77. https://doi.org/10.1016/j.yrtph.2006.07.005

Sousa, W. M., Silva, R. O., Bezerra, F. F., Bingana, R. D., Barros, F. C. N., Costa, L. E., … & Freitas, A. L. P. (2016). Sulfated polysaccharide fraction from marine algae Solieriafiliformis: Structural characterization, gastroprotective and antioxidant effects. *Carbohydrate polymers*, *152*, 140–148.

Sterner, M., & Gröndahl, F. (2021). Extraction of laminarin from Saccharina latissima seaweed using cross-flow filtration. Journal of Applied Phycology, 33(3), 1825–1844.

Suleria H.A.R., Osborne S., Masci P., Gobe G. Marine-based nutraceuticals: An innovative trend in the food and supplement industries. Mar. Drugs. 2015;13:6336–6351.

Sun Z., Dai Z., Zhang W., Fan S., Liu H., Liu R., Zhao T. Bioactive Seaweeds for Food Applications: Natural Ingredients for Healthy Diets. Elsevier; Amsterdam, The Netherlands: 2018. Antiobesity, Antidiabetic, Antioxidative, and Antihyperlipidemic Activities of Bioactive Seaweed Substances; pp. 239–253.

Sun, H. H., Mao, W. J., Chen, Y., Guo, S. D., Li, H. Y., Qi, X. H., … & Xu, J. (2009). Isolation, chemical characteristics and antioxidant properties of the polysaccharides from marine fungus Penicillium sp. F23-2. *Carbohydrate polymers*, *78*(1), 117–124.

Sun, H.-H.; Mao, W.-J.; Jiao, J.-Y.; Xu, J.-C.; Li, H.-Y.; Chen, Y.; Qi, X.-H.; Chen, Y.-L.; Xu, J.; Zhao, C.-Q.; et al. Structural Characterization of Extracellular Polysaccharides Produced by the Marine Fungus Epicoccum nigrum JJY-40 and Their Antioxidant Activities. *Mar. Biotechnol.* 2011, *13*, 1048–1055

Tanna, B., & Mishra, A. (2019). Nutraceutical potential of seaweed polysaccharides: Structure, bioactivity, safety, and toxicity. *Comprehensive Reviews in Food Science and Food Safety*, *18*(3), 817–831.

Ugbaja, R. N., Akinloye, D. I., James, A. S., Ugwor, E. I., Kareem, S. E., David, G., … &Oyebade, O. E. (2020). Crab derived dietary chitosan mollifies hyperlipidemia-induced oxidative stress and histopathological derangements in male albino rats. *Obesity Medicine*, *20*, 100300.

Ulaganathan T, Boniecki MT, Foran E, Buravenkov V, Mizrachi N, Banin E, Helbert W, Cygler M (2017) New Ulvan-degrading polysaccharide lyase family: structure and catalytic mechanism suggests convergent evolution of active site architecture. ACS Chem Biol 12(5):1269–1280.

Valko, M., Leibfritz, D., Moncol, J., Cronin, M. T., Mazur, M., &Telser, J. (2007). Free radicals and antioxidants in normal physiological functions and human disease. *The international journal of biochemistry & cell biology*, *39*(1), 44–84. https://doi.org/10.1016/j.biocel.2006.07.001

Vega, J., Bonomi-Barufi, J., Gómez-Pinchetti, J. L., & Figueroa, F. L. (2020). Cyanobacteria and red macroalgae as potential sources of antioxidants and UV radiation-absorbing compounds for cosmeceutical applications. *Marine Drugs*, *18*(12), 659.
Vitale, C.; Berutti, S.; Bagnis, C.; Soragna, G.; Gabella, P.; Fruttero, C.; Marangella, M. Dermatan sulfate: An alternative to unfractionated heparin for anticoagulation in hemodialysis patients. J. Nephrol. 2013, 26, 158–163
Vl, S. (1999). Analysis of total phenols and other oxidation substrates and antioxidants by means of Folin-Ciocalteu reagent. *Methods in Enzymology*, *299*, 152–178
Vuong T.V. Natural Products and Their Derivatives with Antibacterial, Antioxidant and Anticancer Activities. Antibiotiotic. 2021;10:70.
Wang C.Y., Mao W.J., Chen Z.Q., Zhu W.M., Chen Y.L., Zhao C.Q., Li N., Yan M.X., Liu X., Guo T.T. (2013). Purification, structural characterization and antioxidant property of an extracellular polysaccharide from Aspergillus terreus. Process Biochem. 48:1395–1401.https://doi.org/10.1016/j.procbio.2013.06.029.
Wang, J., Zhang, Q., Zhang, Z., & Li, Z. (2008). Antioxidant activity of sulfated polysaccharide fractions extracted from Laminaria japonica. *International journal of biological macromolecules*, *42*(2), 127–132.
Wang, L., Jayawardena, T., U., Yang, H., Lee, H., 2020. The potential of sulfated polysaccharides isolated from the brown seaweed Ecklonia maxima in cosmetics: antioxidant, antimelanogenesis and photoprotective activities. Antioxidants 9, 724 https://doi.org/10.3390/antiox9080724
Wang, Q., Song, Y., He, Y., Ren, D., Kow, F., Qiao, Z., … & Yu, X. (2014). Structural characterisation of algae Costariacostata fucoidan and its effects on CCl4-induced liver injury. *Carbohydrate polymers*, *107*, 247–254.
Wang, J., Zhang, Q., Zhang, Z., & Li, Z. (2018). Antioxidant activity of sulfated polysaccharide fractions extracted from Laminaria japonica. International journal of biological macromolecules, 42(2), 127–132. https://doi.org/10.1016/j.ijbiomac.2007.10.003
Wang, Y., Xing, M., Cao, Q., Ji, A., Liang, H., & Song, S. (2019). Biological activities of fucoidan and the factors mediating its therapeutic effects: A review of recent studies. *Marine Drugs*, *17*(3), 183.
Wayner, D. D. M., Burton, G. W., Ingold, K. U., & Locke, S. (1985). Quantitative measurement of the total, peroxyl radical-trapping antioxidant capability of human blood plasma by controlled peroxidation: The important contribution made by plasma proteins. *FEBS letters*, *187*(1), 33–37.
Wijesekara I., Kim S.K. Application of Marine Algae Derived Nutraceuticals in the Food Industry. Mar. Algae Extr. Process. Prod. Appl. 2015;2:627–638. https://doi.org/10.1002/9783527679577.ch35
Winston, G. W., Regoli, F., Dugas Jr, A. J., Fong, J. H., & Blanchard, K. A. (1998). A rapid gas chromatographic assay for determining oxyradical scavenging capacity of antioxidants and biological fluids. *Free Radical Biology and Medicine*, *24*(3), 480–493.
Wu, R., Wu, C., Liu, D., Yang, X., Huang, J., Zhang, J., … & Li, H. (2015). Overview of antioxidant peptides derived from marine resources: The sources, characteristic, purification, and evaluation methods. *Applied biochemistry and biotechnology*, *176*, 1815–1833.
Yalçın, S., Karakaş, Ö., Okudan, E. Ş., Başkan, K. S., Çekiç, S. D., & Apak, R. (2021). HPLC detection and antioxidant capacity determination of brown, red and green algal pigments in seaweed extracts. *Journal of Chromatographic Science*, *59*(4), 325–337.
Yan M.X., Mao W.J., Liu X., Wang S.Y., Xia Z., Cao S.J., Li J., Qin L., Xian H.L. Extracellular polysaccharide with novel structure and antioxidant property produced by the deep-sea fungus Aspergillus versicolor N(2)bC. Carbohydr. Polym. 2016;147:272–281. https://doi.org/10.1016/j.carbpol.2016.03.090
Yang, X.; Gao, X.; Han, F.; Tan, R. Sulfation of a polysaccharide produced by a marine filamentous fungus Phomaherbarum YS4108 alters its antioxidant properties in vitro. Biochim. Et Biophys. Acta 2005, 1725, 120–127

Yap, W. F., Tay, V., Tan, S. H., Yow, Y. Y., & Chew, J. (2019). Decoding antioxidant and antibacterial potentials of Malaysian green seaweeds: Caulerpa racemosa and Caulerpa lentillifera. *Antibiotics*, *8*(3), 152.

Yu, L.; Xue, C.H.; Chang, Y.G.; Xu, X.Q.; Ge, L.; Liu, G.C.; Wang, Y.C. Structure elucidation of fucoidan composed of a novel tetrafucose repeating unit from sea cucumber *Thelenota ananas*. *Food Chem.* 2014, *146*, 113–119.

Zargarzadeh, M., Amaral, A. J. R., Custódio, C. A., & Mano, J. F. (2020). Biomedical applications of laminarin. Carbohydrate polymers, 232, 115774. https://doi.org/10.1016/j.carbpol.2019.115774

Zeidan, A. A., Poulsen, V. K., Janzen, T., Buldo, P., Derkx, P. M., Øregaard, G., & Neves, A. R. (2017). Polysaccharide production by lactic acid bacteria: from genes to industrial applications. *FEMS microbiology reviews*, *41*(Supp_1), S168–S200.

Zeitz, M. A., Tanveer, Z., Openshaw, A. T., & Schmidt, M. (2019). Genetic regulators and physiological significance of glycogen storage in Candida albicans. *Journal of Fungi*, *5*(4), 102.

Zhang, J., Liu, L., Ren, Y., & Chen, F. (2019). Characterization of exopolysaccharides produced by microalgae with antitumor activity on human colon cancer cells. *International Journal of Biological Macromolecules*, *128*, 761–767.

Zhang, Z., Chen, Y., Wang, R., Cai, R., Fu, Y., & Jiao, N. (2015). The fate of marine bacterial exopolysaccharide in natural marine microbial communities. *PLoS One*, *10*(11), e0142690.

Zhang, Z., Wang, X., Zhao, M., Yu, S., & Qi, H. (2013). The immunological and antioxidant activities of polysaccharides extracted from Enteromorpha linza. *International journal of biological macromolecules*, *57*, 45–49.

Zhao, X., Li, B., Xue, C., & Sun, L. (2012). Effect of molecular weight on the antioxidant property of low molecular weight alginate from Laminaria japonica. *Journal of Applied Phycology*, *24*, 295–300.

Zhong, Q.; Wei, B.; Wang, S.; Ke, S.; Chen, J.; Zhang, H.; Wang, H. The Antioxidant Activity of Polysaccharides Derived from Marine Organisms: An Overview. *Mar. Drugs* 2019, *17*, 674.

Zhong, H., Gao, X., Cheng, C., Liu, C., Wang, Q., & Han, X. (2020). The structural characteristics of seaweed polysaccharides and their application in gel drug delivery systems. Marine Drugs, 18(12), 658.

Zhou, C.; Mi, S.; Li, J.; Gao, J.; Wang, X.; Sang, Y. Purification, Characterisation and Antioxidant Activities of Chondroitin Sulphate Extracted from Raja porosa Cartilage. Carbohydr. Polym. 2020, 241, 116306

Marine Polysaccharides in Wound Healing

M. R. Divya, Reshma Anns Raju, and M. R. Rekha

Abstract Marine polysaccharides, particularly alginate and chitosan, have gained importance attention in biomedical field due to properties like biocompatibility, biodegradability, and inherent biological properties. Among their diverse uses, wound healing represents a critical field where these materials demonstrate remarkable efficacy. Wound dressings of different types are made using these polysaccharides, such as films, sponges, and hydrogels, by the application they are intended to be used. This chapter reviews the structural characteristics of alginate and chitosan, their role in wound healing, different forms and modifications of alginate and chitosan-based materials as wound dressings, and their application in clinical studies.

Keywords Alginate · Chitosan · Wound Healing · Biomolecules · Drug Delivery

1 Introduction

The biological process of wound healing is intricate and dynamic, with multiple overlapping stages: hemostasis, inflammation, proliferation, and remodelling. Chronic wounds and delayed healing remain major health concerns, prompting the need for advanced wound care strategies. Marine-derived biopolymers, particularly chitosan and alginate, have become viable options for wound care management because of the favorable biological activities and ability to form a variety of functional biomaterials (Rajinikanth et al. 2024).

Alginate is a class of anionic polysaccharide isolated and extracted from brown seaweeds. Alginate is biocompatible and biodegradable. Its ability to promote cell proliferation and tissue regeneration makes it particularly valuable in wound healing applications. Alginate dressings can be tailored into various forms, such as films and sponges, to suit different wound types and healing stages (Hay et al. 2013).

M. R. Divya · R. A. Raju · M. R. Rekha (✉)
Division of Biosurface Technology, Biomedical Technology Wing, Sree Chitra Tirunal Institute for Medical Sciences and Technology, Thiruvananthapuram, Kerala, India
e-mail: rekhamr@sctimst.ac.in

S. Jana et al. (eds.), *Multifunctional Marine Polysaccharides*,
https://doi.org/10.1007/978-981-95-4126-3_11

Chitosan is cationic marine polysaccharide obtained by deacetylation from chitin. The characteristics like excellent biocompatibility and biodegradability make it a versatile and multipotent biomaterial. It has proven good physico-chemical characteristics, like high specific surface, porosity, and tensile strength. It is synthesized and fabricated into several forms (such as films, fibers, sponges, powders, gels, etc.) which are used in clinical applications (Abourehab et al. 2022a).

1.1 Alginate in Wound Healing

Alginate is a naturally occurring linear water soluble anionic polysaccharide extracted from the cell wall of brown seaweed/algae belonging to the class Pheophyceae (Hay et al. 2013) such as *Ascophyllum nodosum*, *Laminaria hyperborea*, *Laminaria digitata*, *Laminaria japonica*, and *Macrocystis pyrifera* and some bacterial species like *Acetobacter* and *Pseudomonas* species (Lee and Mooney 2012). Alginate is of great importance due to its natural origin, excellent biocompatibility, simplicity in handling, non-toxicity, non-immunogenic nature, and economic affordability (Tomić et al. 2023). Sodium alginate is one of the commercially marketed form of alginate (Remminghorst and Rehm 2006). When it comes to terminology, alginate is usually referred as alginic acid and its derivatives (Barbu et al. 2021). The alginate in the form of hydrogel mimics structurally to extracellular matrix of living tissues opening up a variety of applications in the field of dermatology and tissue regeneration (Tomić et al. 2023).

1.1.1 Structure and Properties of Alginate

Alginate is a versatile copolymer containing linearly ordered hexauronic acid monomers, namely, 1,4 linked β-D-mannuropyranosyl (M block) and 1,4 linked α-L- glucopyranosyl units (Yang et al. 2011). The monomer units are grouped in a block-like sequence which can be homogeneous (such as poly M, poly G) or heterogeneous (such as MG) blocks (Barbu et al. 2021). The mechanical characteristics of alginate also depend on the molecular weight and G-block length (Lee and Mooney 2012). Alginate is hydrophilic in nature and forms stable hydrogel with multivalent cations (Tomić et al. 2023). The factors that affect solubility of alginate attribute to its structure, protonated/deprotonated state of carboxylic groups, ionic strength, pH, solvents, temperature and concentration of "gelling ions" like calcium and sodium ions, presence of aromatic groups, etc. (Barbu et al. 2020; Szekalska et al. 2016). Alginate exhibits pH-dependent anionic properties and interacts with cationic polyelectrolytes, thus making it a suitable system for loading of cells (Lee and Mooney 2012). Alginate polymer precipitates at pKa below 3.28–3.68. The sodium alginate aqueous solution with 1% w/v concentration possesses a viscosity ranging between 20 and 400 mPa at a temperature of 20 °C (Barbu et al. 2021). The alginate solution shows maximum viscosity at pH range 3.0–3.5 (Lee and Mooney 2012).

Alginate possesses excellent mucoadhesive character due to the presence of carboxyl functional group (Abourehab et al. 2022b). Alginate possesses unique capability of formation of two different types of gel which depend on the pH—namely, acid gel at low pH and ionotropic gel at high pH (Tønnesen and Karlsen 2002). The divalent cations like Ba^{2+} and Ca^{2+} and G-block of alginate construct egg-box systems to form alginate hydrogels through gelation (Tavakoli et al. 2019). These gelling ions trigger the cross-linking process of alginate chains and subsequent gelation (Barbu et al. 2020; Szekalska et al. 2016). A high concentration of Ca^{2+} causes better water resistance and swelling behavior (Lee and Mooney 2012). Alginate is reported to have antioxidant and anti-inflammatory properties. According to previously published research work, alginate oligosaccharides help reduce NO, ROX, eicosanoids such as prostaglandin E2, and C0X-2 production (Zhou et al. 2015).

Unlike neutral polysaccharides, alginate is abundant in free hydroxyl and carboxyl groups distributed in polymeric chain backbone, which can be modified to change the properties of parent compounds (Yang et al. 2011). Due to its inherent prominent properties such as biocompatibility, biodegradability, marginal toxicity, chemical versatility, exceptional stable gel forming property in aqueous solutions, and sol-gel transition capability, alginate is exploited for various biomedical applications. Alginate can be modified so as to fulfill the needs of pharmaceutical and biomedical applications (Abourehab et al. 2022b).

1.1.2 Extraction of Alginate

The commercial form of alginate is derived from brown algae using aqueous solution of NaOH. The NaOH-treated extract is filtered, and Ca^{2+}/Na^{+} is added to the filtrate and alginate is precipitated. The salt of alginate so formed is converted to alginic acid by dilute HCl, and water-soluble powdered form of sodium alginate is purified. On commercial extraction, alginate content is about 22–30% for *Ascophyllum nodosum* and 25–44% for *Laminaria digitata* (Sahoo and Biswal 2021). The molecular weight of commercially marketed alginate ranges 32,000–4,00,000 g/mol (Lee and Mooney 2012).

1.1.3 Alginate in Wound Management

The design of biologically interactive biopolymer-based advanced wound dressing materials with superior characteristics is one of the key concerns for successful outcome in the healing of wounded tissues (Tomić et al. 2023).

Alginate has proved to be an excellent biopolymer when modified and in combination with other natural/synthetic polymers or by loading therapeutic molecules to achieve wound healing properties (Tomić et al. 2023). Alginate finds widespread use in wound dressing, owing to its increased water uptake, sustained drug release, enhanced non-immunogenicity, and porosity (Aderibigbe and Buyana 2018).

The calcium alginate and sodium alginate are most commonly explored alginate types in wound care, depending on the wound type and desired dressing form (Barbu et al. 2021). The alginate-based wound dressing has the potential to exchange the gelling ions with wound exudate when directly administered on the wound site. A reliable and non-woven type wound dressing based on calcium alginate has capability to exchange sodium ions exuding from infected wounds. This property prevents wound dressing from adhering to the wound bed, facilitating a painless removal of wound dressing. The newly formed tissue is unaffected by the removal of alginate fibers. In addition to this, a self-adherence property in the peri-wound region with a good cover of the injured area is observed (Lee and Mooney 2012). The concentration of alginate employed in commercial wound dressing is 0.001–95% depending on dressing type (Barbu et al. 2021).

This section of this chapter details the multifunctional biomedical application of alginate-based wound healing material—such as hydrogels, scaffolds, foam, electrospun membranes, nanocomposites, etc.—highlighting the key properties of alginates and its influence on essential features of a wound dressing material.

1.2 Alginate-Based Foams for Wound Healing Applications

Biopolymer-based foams represent an innovative technological platform for wound healing. The versatility of foam lies in its ability to mold its structure, with respect to its density, pore nature, formulation and composition, shape, and the multiple phases in the system. These foams can be developed as a favorable sterile dressing material for both hemostatic and secondary applications (Trucillo and Di Maio 2021). The order of requirements of an ideal dressing is protection of wound from microorganisms, necrosis, mechanical protection, wettability, movable/removable property, stiffness, strength, wound pain relief, and economic affordability (Rezvani Ghomi et al. 2019). Foam dressing is attractive nowadays due to a protective cushioning effect on the wound, due to its sufficient thickness (Gheorghita Puscaselu et al. 2020).

Foam exhibit macroporous architecture when polymer strands are organized as interconnecting network. Compared to hydrogels, foams support anchorage-dependent cell lines and help activate nutrient transport and avert formation of necrotic center (Tomić et al. 2023). Foams act as solid porous matrices which can be administered to wounds, after sterilization, without causing any damage to patients. Properties of foam such as thickness, density, and mechanical characters—such as tensile strength and elongation of freeze-dried foam—have to be taken into consideration. Otherwise, an application of wound dressing to a patient may cause discomfort and skin maceration around the periphery of the wound (Aderibigbe and Buyana 2018).

As per previous literatures, the foam-based wound dressing materials are developed with hydrophobic as well as hydrophilic foams possessing adhesive or non-adhesive borders for proper positioning (Trucillo and Di Maio 2021). The hydrophobic part of the wound dressing guides the materials from liquid, permit gas exchange, and water vapor. The hydrophilic portion helps maintain moist environment (Varaprasad et al. 2020). Foam-based wound dressings are applicable to the treatment of traumatic wounds, burns, diabetic ulcers, etc. (Aderibigbe and Buyana 2018).

In recent years, foams based on alginate have gained attention in wound dressing applications owing to its high porosity, surface area, and pore volume and water uptake capacity. Alginate-based foams are biocompatible, absorb wound exudate, accelerate exchange of gases, prevent maceration of wound, and maintain wound in moist environment (Varaprasad et al. 2020). Alginate-based foam is gaining popularity as artificial extracellular matrix, in vitro, for maintenance of an interface with in vivo biological system in tissue engineering research (Tomić et al. 2023). Alginate-based foam dressing promotes epithelialization and healing via inducing cell migration. Alginate-based forms are characterized by prolonged hydration time and can be withdrawn from wound area without significant damage to the tissue. But, they are not ideal for low exudate and dry wounds, as these dressings require frequent changing (Dhivya et al. 2015).

Alginate-based foam dressings are prepared by rapid homogenization of mixture of sodium alginate in aqueous solution along with a plasticizing agent, a sequestering agent, an active surface agent, and di- or trivalent metal ion in order to obtain water-insoluble hydrogel. The mixture so obtained is poured in a tray and placed in a freezer, and a frozen form of alginate hydrogel is obtained. The hydrogel is then subjected to lyophilization to remove moisture. This results in alginate foam dressings with interconnected three-dimensional structures (Gheorghita Puscaselu et al. 2020; Nayak et al. 2020a).

A new wound care material with rapid hemostatic and antibacterial property was introduced by Xie et al. (2022). This innovative foam gel dressing was formulated using calcium alginate foam substrate and chito-oligosaccharide-modified graphene oxide (CG). The CG is found to have potent interaction with platelets facilitating hemostasis and show sufficient antibacterial properties. The chito-oligosaccharide-modified graphene oxide loaded foam gel dressings exhibit healing properties within 12 days. Moreover, these wound dressings promote vascular remodeling and lower inflammatory response. These wound dressings exhibited seamless skin contact, and CG loading improved the thermal stability, porosity, mechanical property, and water absorption as well as retention rate and antibacterial, hemostatic, and healing properties of the modified foam. Overall, a soft and flexible type foam wound care material is reported to have increased absorption rate and wound fluid exudate and help to prevent festering wound.

Various systems for biomedical application have been developed using alginate/pectin, due to their synergistic interaction. In a study led by Oh et al. (2020), alginate/pectin composite foams for wound dressing application were synthesized using calcium ion cross-linking method. Alginate/pectin was blended in different ratios

(9:1, 10:0, 7:3, and 5:5) to fabricate composite foams. The direct/indirect cytotoxic studies of these modified foams on NHDF-neo and keratinocyte cells proved its nontoxic nature. Composite foams with higher pectin level exhibited better swelling properties. Moreover, with increasing pectin content in composite foams, release ability of BSA is enhanced. In addition, the control of pectin concentration in this composite foam increases mechanical strength, swelling, as well as drug release property. Thus alginate/pectin composite foams are a potential wound dressing material.

Another approach by Hegge et al. (2011) was to develop curcumin-loaded alginate foams for application in antimicrobial photodynamic therapy (aPDT) of infected wounds. These drug-loaded foams were fabricated such that it aided in a burst release of the curcumin when foams are hydrated. The foams remained intact even after hydration and exhibited extended hydration. It could be removed from wound area before irradiation, causing no damages to the tissues, thereby reducing light attenuation in PDT. Different tests were carried out to test the efficiency of these foams in wound healing. For example, in a model physiological fluid, both the curcumin loaded/unloaded alginate foams get hydrated within 1 minute and could absorb 12–16 times water than its dry weight. As curcumin exhibits low solubility in water, cyclodextrins (CDs) and PEG 400 were used as solubilizing medium and aided in the burst release of the photosensitizer. According to antimicrobial assay, exposure to these foams in combination with visible light irradiation (9.7 J/cm^2) resulted in >6 log reduction of population of *Enterococcus faecalis*. An 81% reduction in viable population of *Escherichia coli* was observed after treatment with the modified foams containing PEG 400 as the only solubilizer of curcumin combined with irradiation by visible light (29 J/cm^2).

In a similar study by Bergh et al. (2018), alginate-based dry foams intended for the use in antibacterial photodynamic therapy (aPDT) of infected wounds were developed. Antibacterial photodynamic therapy (aPDT) is a therapeutic modality that involves the use of suitable wavelength, a photosensitizer (PS), and oxygen. aPDT generates radicals that can destroy bacteria by a fast and unspecific route, and hence there are less chances of development of bacterial resistance, and so aPDT is a promising approach for topical treatment of infected wounds. A model photosensitizer, 5,10,15,20-tetrakis(4-hydroxyphenyl)porphyrin (THPP)-loaded alginate foams, was developed. THPP exhibits low solubility at the range of physiological pH which leads to aggregation and hence reduces aPDT effect. The foams contained poloxamer such as pluronic F127 and/or different derivatives of b-cyclodextrin. The poloxamers and cyclodextrin derivatives were used to induce disaggregation of the porphyrin and increase aqueous solubility of drug, thus facilitating efficient loading of THPP into alginate foams. Moreover, b-cyclodextrin has the capability to form inclusion complexes when combined with hydrophobic drugs.

The foams exhibited sufficient mechanical strength for clinical use. The foams are easy to handle due to its thin and pliable nature and could cut to fit a wound. Foams disintegrated in water and PBS, while remained intact in Hank's balanced salt solution. The THPP loading was compared in all foams, and it accounts for about 0.12–0.13% w/w. The THPP release was improved due to the presence of bCD derivatives. Thus alginate-based dry foams loaded with PF127 and bCD derivative along with THPP are a promising delivery vehicle for photosensitizer in aPDT wounds (Valerón Bergh et al. 2018).

Active ingredients such as asiaticoside, a plant-derived wound healing agent, and silver, used as an antibacterial, can be incorporated to alginate foam dressing. In this formulation, alginate helps generate the release of silver and asiaticoside, enhances foam properties by increasing compressive strength and absorption property, and displays nontoxicity and a similar antimicrobial effect in disc diffusion test (Namviriyachote et al. 2019).

In a research conducted by Wang et al., the influence of alginate in bleeding control was studied. Double cross-linking method was employed for fabrication of PVA/alginate composite foams (PACFs) with varying alginate concentration and followed by lyophilization. According to the findings, the incorporation of alginate led to a marginal decrease in water absorption property and porosity of the PVA/alginate foams. On the other hand, PACF enhanced hemostatic performance—help trigger intrinsic pathway of blood coagulation, thereby aiding blood coagulation and rapid plasma absorption to increase concentration of RBC and platelets in the wound area. An increased ability to stimulate thrombus generation, blood clotting, blood cell adhesion, and aggregation was observed to be a property of PACF with high alginate content. Interestingly, PACF showed 20-fold volume expansion, high flexibility, and unique shape-adaptive capability, facilitating the property to expand and fill the irregular and deep penetrating wounds. These properties of PACF were further demonstrated in a hemorrhaging liver mouse model and gunshot swine artery injury model. The in vivo hemostatic studies supported potential ability of PACFs to accelerate hemostasis. These findings suggested that these composite foams are strong hemostatic materials (Wang et al. 2018).

1.3 Alginate-Based Films/Membranes for Wound Healing Applications

Alginate-based films/membrane are gaining attention as a potential wound dressing material. Studies have shown that alginate films stimulate wound healing process, increase permeability (water vapor, carbon dioxide, oxygen), protect wound area from pathogenic bacteria and subsequent infections, allows easy wound area monitoring, etc. The properties of alginate film in terms of mechanical strength and wound healing are enhanced by combining it with other polymeric substances, with or without incorporating bioactive molecules, therapeutic drugs, nanoparticles, antibacterial drugs, ions, etc. (Aderibigbe and Buyana 2018).

There are different techniques used for film production in laboratory scale. The technique of film preparation basically depends on physicochemical properties of the desired final film. In solvent casting method, polymer solutions are spread on a uniform surface and subjected to oven drying or room temperature to evaporate the solvent part, and the film is obtained. Other methods are electrospinning and electrodrying. Electrospinning is used to generate fibers of nanoscale diameters or thin porous membranes. Electrospraying employs high tension to polymer droplets generated by spraying technique, imparting an electric charge, and generating coulomb forces, change in surface tension, and eventually formation of micro-/nano-droplets. In the past few decades, different attempts have been reported to develop alginate-based films as wound care materials (Varaprasad et al. 2020; Saraiva et al. 2023).

Medicated films of alginate were successfully developed. In a study carried out by George et al., silver sulfadiazine was incorporated into films made up of sodium alginate and gelatin employing a method of solvent casting. The films were transparent and flexible with smooth surface. The SA/gelatin formulations were subjected to different physico-chemical assessment such as weight variation, surface pH, moisture evaluation tests, folding endurance, biodegradability, and in vitro drug release, and all these parameters were found satisfactory. The folding endurance of the modified films ranged between 337 ± 0.96 and 459 ± 0.69, revealing the ability of SA/gelatin films to withstand sufficient mechanical pressure and exhibit good flexibility. The drug entrapment of silver sulfadiazine in SA/gelatin film was studied, and about 93–97% of encapsulation percentage, an acceptable range for all formulations, was observed indicating uniform distribution of the drug molecule. The in vitro drug release profile demonstrated that films released silver in a sustained pattern for a period of 1 week. In vitro degradation study of these medicated films in PBS 7.4 containing 1.5 μg/ml of lysozyme at 37 °C was carried out. The weight loss assay showed 70–86% biodegradability after 10 days, indicating its controllable biodegradability. The silver sulfadiazine-loaded modified SA/gelatin wound dressing system could be developed as a novel polymeric membrane-based dressing for wound management (George et al. 2017).

In another study, Shao et al. have incorporated silver sulfadiazine (AgSD particles), a topical antibacterial agent, employed as a topical cream for burn wounds, into a novel bacterial cellulose/sodium alginate (BC/SA) composite matrix. The SEM, FTIR, and TG characterization analysis indicated successful impregnation of silver sulfadiazine into BC/SA matrix. The BC/SA/AgSD matrix displayed pH-responsive swelling properties in different ranges of pH. These matrices exhibited a pattern of increase in swelling ratio on increasing pH. The antibacterial efficiency of BC/SA/AgSD composites was tested with cultures of *E. coli*, *S. aureus*, and *C. albicans*. The experimental reports showed BC/SA/AgSD matrices have improved antibacterial properties. Moreover, in vitro cytotoxicity assays revealed non-toxic effect on HEK 293 cell line. Hence BC/SA/AgSD composite showed good biocompatibility, promising its use as a potential wound dressing material (Shao et al. 2015).

Different studies have demonstrated that the topical application of simvastatin can promote wound healing in diabetic mice model through augmentation of angiogenesis and lymphangiogenesis. Resvanian et al. formulated simvastatin-loaded alginate composite film-based wound dressings via solvent casting technique. These composite films were a blend of sodium alginate/pectin as well as sodium alginate/

gelatin. According to the pre-formulation studies, SA/PC blended films exhibited superior properties with respect to mechanical properties, expansion profile, and drug release. The WVTR was found to be 1455, 1385, and 1394 g/m^2/day, respectively for simvastatin-loaded SA film, simvastatin-loaded SA/pectin film, and simvastatin-loaded gelatin film. This reflects the permissibility of these modified films to water vapor and its property to maintain humid environment on wound area in exudating wounds without much dehydration. The gel and rehydrated film was evaluated for its rheological properties. An apparent viscosity of sodium alginate/gelatin gel loaded with simvastatin at 250^{s-1} was significantly reduced as compared to other similar gel compositions. In vitro drug release profile was investigated, and the rate of simvastatin release was influenced by the ratio of the polymer content. The rate of simvastatin release from SA/pectin films loaded with simvastatin, SA film loaded with simvastatin, and SA/gelatin film loaded with simvastatin was 0.826 ± 0.069 mg/cm^2, 0.929 ± 0.101 mg/cm^2, and 1.736 ± 0.134 mg/cm^2, respectively. The cell viability assay indicated drug-loaded SA/PC film is non-toxic to human dermal fibroblast cells with a cell viability of 83.20% with respect to untreated cells. To conclude observations of the study, simvastatin-incorporated alginate/pectin composite film is an appropriate wound dressing material (Rezvanian et al. 2016).

Han et al. (2014) and team designed and developed ciprofloxacin hydrochloride-incorporated alginate/chitosan bilayer composite membrane wound dressing. The in vitro antimicrobial properties, drug permeation study, morphology, cytotoxicity, skin irritation, and in vivo pharmacodynamics were evaluated. The alginate/chitosan bilayer membranes showed high sensitivity to bacterial cultures such as *Staphylococcus aureus*, *Escherichia coli*, and *Pseudomonas aeruginosa* and hence potentially inhibit growth of microorganisms for more than a week. When treated with these membranes, no significant change in metabolic activity of HaCaT fibroblast cell lines was noted. In primary skin irritation test in rabbits, ciprofloxacin-loaded alginate/chitosan bilayer membrane exhibited no notable irritation, edema, and erythema even after 14 days of treatment. In vivo pharmacodynamics studies showed that the bilayer membrane was more efficient in wound healing progression. In summary, alginate/chitosan bilayer composite membrane could possibly reduce wound infection, improve compliance, and could act as a drug carrier for sustained release dressings.

In a recent study, Li and colleagues (2017) designed films based on strontium-loaded silk fibroin (SF)/sodium alginate (SA) blend films as wound care material. The strontium-incorporated SF/SA films with 5 mg/ml strontium could satisfactorily fulfill the requirements of an ideal wound dressing in terms of its water absorption capacity, water vapor transmission rate, mechanical properties, cytocompatibility to fibroblast, etc. Furthermore, films fabricated with 5 mg/ml strontium stimulated the secretion of vascular bFGF and VEGF for 4 days in in vitro conditions, indicating its ability to induce angiogenesis benefits in wound dressing. The current study indicated that strontium-loaded SF/SA blend films could be developed as a good biomaterial for wound care applications.

A study conducted by Dantas et al. evaluated the healing of wounds caused by burns using sodium alginate/chitosan-based films combined with laser therapy. Studies were carried out in 60 Wistar albino rats assigned into 6 study groups, namely, control untreated, dressed with cellulose films only, dressed with films based on sodium alginate and chitosan, undressed but laser irradiated wounds, laser irradiated wounds with cellulose dressing, and laser irradiated wounds with sodium alginate as well as chitosan-based film dressing. The animals underwent laser therapy for a period of 7 days, followed by euthanasia on 8th or 14th day. Prominent inflammatory reactions were observed in the control groups than laser irradiated groups after a period of 8 days and 2 weeks. Moreover, the laser therapy induced differentiation of myofibroblasts within 8 days of the study period, with and without the use of dressing films. A combination of wound dressing and laser therapy proved to improve epithelialization, formation of blood vessel, and collagenization, stimulate rapid replacement of type III for type I collagen, and promote better arrangement of newly synthesized collagen fibers. Hence laser arrays could potentially accelerate the healing and repair injuries in soft tissue (Dantas et al. 2011).

Nanoparticle-loaded alginate-based wound dressings have been developed. Sharma et al. reported a new, facile, simple, and ecofriendly method for development of silver nanoparticle-loaded sodium alginate blended with chitosan to form PEC complex and which was successfully casted into stable films. The sodium alginate acts as both reducing and stabilizing agent. The Alg-AgNPs were about 14 ± 3 nm in size and displayed an antibacterial property. The films developed with sodium alginate/chitosan in 1:1 ratio showed superior mechanical properties, increased percentage of water uptake, and smooth texture. The films were efficient in inhibiting gram-positive bacteria and were promising as a wound dressing material (Sharma et al. 2012).

Curcumin was incorporated as a model drug owing to its significant contribution in wound healing due to its antimicrobial, antifungal, and anti-inflammatory properties. The curcumin was incorporated into polycaprolactone nanoparticles using emulsification-diffusion technique. SA, PVA, and PVP were combined with plasticizers. The sodium alginate membrane containing PVP and PEG exhibited superior mechanical and swelling characteristics and was chosen to develop film with curcumin nanoparticles. This novel alginate-based membrane showed diverse functional features, necessary to be used as a substitute to synthetic skin, such as high swelling capacity, adherence to the skin, presence of pores to control the loss of transdermal water, easy wound monitoring, and controlled drug release by addition of nanoparticles. The incorporation of these nanocarriers helps drug permeation into various layers of the skin, overcoming the solubility problem of curcumin. The clinical application of this innovative wound dressing is to cover areas of first- and second-degree wounds without the requirement for removal of wound dressing and thereby reduces discomfort of patient. In vivo studies in rat model demonstrated that prolonged and sustained analgesic and anti-inflammatory effects of curcumin were released from these wound dressings (Guadarrama-Acevedo et al. 2019).

In an approach by Oliveira et al. (2020), a double-layer biomembrane for delivery of two potential drugs was developed for treatment of wounds. The bilayer is composed of chitosan/hydroxypropyl methylcellulose and lidocaine chloride (anesthestic drug) in the first layer and sodium alginate-polymyxin B sulfate (antibiotic) in the second layer. These double layer membranes demonstrated adequate mechanical properties, excellent biocompatibility, low cytotoxicity, and antibacterial properties as imparted by polymyxin B. The healing ability of membrane was proved by in vivo studies revealing promising outcomes to be applied in clinical trials.

Tarusha et al. (2018) reported an innovative wound dressing material which incorporates lactose-modified chitosan (chitlac) and silver nanoparticles into a blend of alginate and hyaluronic acid membrane. The membrane was synthesized by gelling, foaming, and freeze casting of alginate, hyaluronic acid, and chitlac-silver nanoparticles, and the cross-linking agent used was calcium ions. In vitro studies reported that hyaluronic acid released from the wound dressing stimulates wound healing and metal silver possesses antibacterial property against biofilms and planktonic bacteria.

Various bioactive materials with wound care properties have been added to alginate-based films/membrane. In a study conducted by Moreira et al. (2020), papain, a proteolytic enzyme from *Carica papaya* latex, was immobilized on calcium-alginate membrane wound dressing. The enzyme-incorporated modified alginate-based wound dressing compiles therapeutic properties of both alginate and papain. The immobilization process was effective—papain remained active after immobilization, resulting in lower rate of deactivation of enzyme with storage. The papain-incorporated alginate membranes were non-hemolytic, indicating these membranes to be a bioactive dressing for healing of wounds. In another approach, alpha tocopherol-nanocellulose-loaded alginate-based membrane and pluronic F-127 hydrogels were developed to treat diabetic wounds. Full-thickness skin wound in diabetic rat model was healed by the application of both the membrane and hydrogel, indicating enhanced angiogenesis with rapid wound healing with no observable toxicity (Shefa et al. 2022). Similarly, root extract of *Capparis sepiaria*-loaded innovative SA-based single and double layer membrane was developed as a potential wound dressing. The fabricated membranes demonstrated high wound exudate absorption, blood clotting capability, biocompatibility, hemocompatibility, biodegradability, antibacterial efficacy, and non-toxicity toward HaCaT cell lines (Ndlovu et al. 2024).

Pacheto et al. (2020) reported a combination of several biopolymers in the formulation of silk fibroin/chitosan/sodium alginate multilayer membrane for wound healing applications. In this context, the aim of the study was to merge the synergistic properties, in a composite biomaterial, such as biocompatibility and mechanical strength of silk fibroin, and wound exudate absorption capability of sodium alginate and antimicrobial characteristics of chitosan. The drug diclofenac sodium was loaded into this modified multilayer membrane. The mechanical barrier as well as microbiological permeation properties was not changed by the incorporation of the drug moiety. Drug release was in a controlled manner and followed

Fickian diffusion behavior. These results supported the idea that the bilayer membrane could serve as high-performance wound dressings.

Wang et al. (2002) reported calcium chloride cross-linked flexible cast of chitosan/alginate polyelectrolyte complex film as potential wound dressing. These PEC membranes were non-cytotoxic and supported cell proliferation in mouse and human fibroblast cell line. As compared to the conventional gauze-based wound dressing, these chitosan/alginate/PEC membranes accelerated the healing of incisional wound in rat model, indicating potential application as wound care material. Moreover, the handling ease, cost-effectiveness, biodegradability, ease of formulation, storage stability, and increased batch-to-batch reproducibility are advantages of this wound dressing.

1.4 Alginate-Based Hydrogels for Wound Healing

Hydrogels are cross-linked 3D network made from water-soluble polymeric systems capable to absorb and hold aqueous fluids in high volume and swell but without dissolving in water demonstrating their exceptional networking properties (Nayak et al. 2020b). Hydrogels can be fabricated in different forms such as slabs, microparticles, nanoparticles, coatings, as well as films. Due to its unique attributes, hydrogels are used in different healthcare domains like diagnostics, drug delivery, regenerative medicine, and cellular immobilization (Nayak et al. 2020b). The properties of hydrogel such as porosity, water absorbing capacity, swelling property, drug loading and release, tensile strength, etc. differ with different types of biopolymer used and type and density of cross-linking (Hoare and Kohane 2008).

Hydrogels can be synthesized using different strategies. The structure of hydrogel includes the covalent junction among the polymeric structure that could be developed by different cross-linking techniques such as physical/chemical/enzymatic method, high energy irradiation, photochemical reaction, and grafting (Nayak et al. 2020b). The cross-linking mechanism can be physical such as ionic interactions or chemical such as covalent bonding or interaction with reactive species or cross-linking agents (Hoare and Kohane 2008).

The mechanical and compositional characteristics of hydrogels are comparable to those of the extracellular matrix. Hydrogel-based wound dressings have the advantage of absorbing the wound exudate while keeping the wound moist, which encourages fibroblast proliferation and keratinocyte migration—both of which are critical for the epithelialization process and wound healing. The mesh-like structure formed by hydrogel covers the surface of the wound, thereby preventing the entry of microorganisms and subsequent infections (Markovic et al. 2024).

The wound site is alkaline in nature, so the alginate gets swollen causing gel formation and then disintegration. An electrostatic repulsion occurs among carboxyl anions, due to ion exchange process between calcium released from dressing and sodium released from exudate. This stimulates the swelling as well as erosion of alginate gel systems (Barnett et al. 1987). Alginate dressing is helpful in stopping bleeding from wounds as calcium ions help aid in the hemostatic property of wound bed. According to studies conducted by Barnett et al. (1987), non-woven calcium alginate wound dressing was found to be effective in healing of partial and full-thickness wounds, where no additional dressing material layer was used. These materials help to reduce dehydration and exhibited excellent hemostatic property.

Wet films based on alginate hydrogel are effective in the treatment of dry and painful wounds. The films are applied to the wound region after being hydrated first by immersion in suitable solvents like water and saline (Pereira et al. 2013a). Then the films cause the release of previously absorbed water, thus maintaining a moist environment that can rehydrate the dry wound. For improved therapeutic efficiency, the entrapped or impregnated therapeutics such as proteins, drugs, and growth factors are gradually released into the wound area in both dry and wet films (Pereira et al. 2013b).

Alginate-based hydrogels have the capability to aid sustained release of loaded small and large drug moieties, proteins, growth factors, and other chemical substances, in a steady state over a long time. Another effective method for curing inflammatory and infected wounds that require tissue regeneration for appropriate wound healing is the loading of therapeutics into an alginate-based hydrogel dressing. The hydrogel acts as a supporting matrix for tissue regeneration and aids in better drug delivery. Currently, this makes alginate-based hydrogel as a popular dressing material for wound healing applications (Sezer and Cevher 2011).

Many factors affect the rate of drug release from alginate hydrogel wound dressings. Chemical composition of alginate, its degree of swelling, density of cross-linking, porosity, entrapment of drugs, exchange of calcium ions with sodium ions, kinetics of degradation of alginate, nature of wound exudate, and its perfusion nature of diffusion of drug loaded and the presence of enzymes as well as infectious microorganisms colonized at the wound site (Lee and Mooney 2012; Aderibigbe and Buyana 2018). The systemic method of delivery of drugs is relatively inefficient as compared to localized delivery. The latter aids in the topical release of drugs, growth factors, etc. at the localized wound. Accordingly, different alginate-based hydrogel wound dressings have been developed for localized delivery of drugs (Leise 2018).

Straccia et al. (2015) synthesized chitosan-coated alginate hydrogel using internal gelation method, with a dual aim of delaying the release of hydrophilic drug molecules from alginate matrix and imparting antimicrobial characteristics to the hydrogel. In this modified hydrogel, the carboxyl group of alginate interacts with $-NH_3$ group of chitosan resulting in polyelectrolyte complexation. This complexation was used to formulate alginate/chitosan hydrogel system for release of therapeutic drug, rhodamine B. The coated hydrogels exhibited good homogeneity and higher water content. The water uptake of hydrogels was 200–450%, which helps prevent accumulation of exudates in wound bed and excessive dehydration. These hydrogels possessed enhanced mechanical strength and reduced porosity. Structural analysis of the coated hydrogels using cryogenic scanning electron microscopy analysis revealed a regular and compact surface. The coated hydrogels are found to exhibit antibacterial activity against *E. coli*. In vitro cytotoxicity studies on mesenchymal stem cells revealed non-toxic nature of these modified hydrogels. A low molecular weight hydrophilic drug, rhodamine B, exhibited a sustained release from the hydrogel at the wound region, making it a potential candidate for wound dressing application.

In a recent research by Bagher et al. (2020), hesperidin-loaded alginate/chitosan hydrogel was developed for wound healing applications. Different concentration of hesperidin was loaded into the hydrogel, and each was tested for its porosity, release profile, weight loss, cytocompatibility, antibacterial and toxicity properties, etc. SEM studies revealed the highly porous microstructure of alginate/chitosan hydrogel with interconnected pores with a porosity of $91.2 \pm 5.33\%$. The in vitro drug release of hesperidin from the formulated hydrogel system indicated the release of hesperidin in a sustained manner for a period of 2 weeks. The percentage weight loss assay depicted 80% biodegradability of the modified hydrogel after 14 days. The hydrogel exhibited non-toxic effect on murine fibroblast 3T3 cell lines. The in vivo study pertaining to the wound healing potential of the developed hydrogel with 10% hesperidin was evaluated using a full-thickness dermal wound in rat model. The hydrogel exhibited good wound closure properties in comparison to that of gauze-treated control group. Moreover, study group administered with alginate/chitosan hydrogel with 10% hesperidin exhibited maximum wound closure. The hydrogel was found to help reduce inflammation and promote proliferation of fibroblast causing rapid formation of epidermal layer formation, tissue granulation, and remodeling.

A similar study by Ehterami et al. (2019) investigated the activity of vitamin E (α-tocopherol)-loaded alginate/chitosan hydrogels for the treatment of skin injury in rat model. This modified alginate/chitosan/α-tocopherol hydrogel was fabricated by using covalent cross-linker (100 ul glutaraldehyde) and ionic cross-linker (100 mM $CaCl_2$). The resultant hydrogel was porous with numerous interconnected pores and exhibited a biodegradability of 80% within 14 days. In vitro tocopherol release profile indicated rapid initial release up to 12 h and sustained pattern for 2 weeks. As per the results of in vitro cell culture investigations, the maximum cell proliferation was observed in cells treated with alginate/chitosan hydrogel loaded with 400 IU α-tocopherol. The therapeutic efficacy of α-tocopherol-loaded alginate/chitosan hydrogel was studied in full-thickness excisional wound model. A prominent wound closure was observed in animal groups treated with modified hydrogel dressings in comparison with that of gauze-treated control group. A highest wound closure was noted with 400 IU α-tocopherol-loaded hydrogel-treated animal group. The outcome of this experiment suggests that the alginate/chitosan/α-tocopherol-loaded hydrogel-based wound dressing is promising for successful skin injury treatment.

To develop clindamycin, an antibiotic-loaded wound dressing, cross-linked hydrogel films based on PVA and SA were developed. Different ratios of 10% polyvinyl alcohol and 3% sodium alginate were blended. Three consecutive freeze-thaw cycles were performed with freezing at −20 °C for 18 h followed by thawing at room temperature for 6 h. The hydrogels were dried for 6 h at 50 °C to obtain hydrogel films. Upon increasing the sodium alginate content in hydrogel composition, a reduction in gelation capacity, mechanical strength, and break elongation was observed. However, it caused augmentation in swelling properties, elastic parameters, and thermal stability of the clindamycin-loaded hydrogel film. This modified hydrogel demonstrated an improved wound healing efficacy of artificial wound in experimental rat model. Thus a clindamycin-loaded wound dressing material containing sodium alginate/PVA can be developed as a candidate for wound care (Kim et al. 2008).

In a study conducted by Balakrishnan et al. (2006), a dibutyryl cyclic adenosine monophosphate (DBcAMP), a lipophilic analog of cAMP, was introduced into in situ hydrogel based on periodate-oxidized alginate and gelatin, and the hydrogel was studied for wound healing applications. The in vitro release profile of DBcAMP from the hydrogel into PBS was demonstrative of a slow release and was gradually increased with time. Over a period of 2 days, 50–60% of DBcAMP was released into the medium in a sustained manner. The DBcAMP-incorporated dressing promoted re-epithelialization of wounds in 10 days, in a full-thickness wound in rat model.

Kamoun et al. (2015) developed sodium ampicillin-loaded PVA/SA hydrogel-based wound dressing membranes. Different ratios of PVA/SA solutions were cross-linked using freeze-thaw method. In this modified hydrogel, upon increasing the sodium alginate concentration with PVA, the gel fraction, elasticity, and elongation at break of the hydrogel were decreased. However, sodium alginate content enhanced swelling properties; exhibited high protein adsorption, roughness of membrane surface, pore size, and pore area distribution; and increased hydrolytic degradation. The high content of sodium alginate was found to have feasible effect on ampicillin release from PVA/SA hydrogel. In addition, the PVA/SA hydrogel wound dressing membrane loaded with ampicillin can be developed as a potential wound dressing material with sufficient blood compatibility as indicated by hemocompatibility studies.

Xerogels are a type of biopolymer that forms dried and porous polymeric networks and show highly advanced and diverse functional characteristics. Xerogels can be fabricated with organic or inorganic substances and demonstrate high drug loading capabilities. A different type of hybrid wound dressing material was presented by Rajalekshmi et al. Alginate-based xerogel was grafted using g-poly (methacrylic acid) chains for delivery of insulin for wound healing applications. The modified xerogel exhibited good physical stability, swelling properties, and low rate of degradation. A sustained release of insulin, about 70%, from the xerogel was observed within 2 days, which in turn modulated the wound healing process (Rajalekshmy and Rekha 2021a).

Alginate-based hydrogel systems used for wound dressing applications are summarized in Table 1.

Table 1 Alginate-based hydrogel developed for wound dressing applications

Material	Method of cross-linking	Active ingredient	Properties	Type of study	References
Alginate/Zinc oxide	Ionic cross-linking	–	Antibacterial properties Improved wound healing	Full-thickness skin wound in rats	Wang et al. (2019a)
Oxidized alginate/N,O-carboxymethyl chitosan	Covalent cross-linking	Curcumin	Controlled release of nano-curcumin	In vivo: full-thickness open excision wound on Sprague-Dawley mouse	Li et al. (2012)
Alginate/Chitosan	Ionic cross-linking	Alpha-tocopherol	Highly porous Biodegradable hydrogel Wound closure	In vitro: full-thickness excisional wound on Wistar rats In vitro: L929 murine fibroblast cell line	Ehterami et al. (2019)
Alginate/PVP/chitosan	Photo cross-linking	Silver nanoparticles	Antibacterial properties Absorbs wound exudate	In vitro: human keratinocytes, mouse fibroblasts, human dermal fibroblast	Khampieng et al. (2018)
Alginate/carboxymethyl cellulose	Molecular entanglements	–	Composite hydrogel with good water vapor permeability Promote wound healing	In vivo: deep second-degree burn wounds in Sprague-Dawley rats	Liang et al. (2019)
Oxidized sodium alginate/ dopamine	Hydrogen bonds and Schiff cross-linking	–	High tensile strength Ultra stretchability	In vitro: NIH-3T3 fibroblast cell line, In vivo: circular wounds on rats	Chen et al. (2018)
Alginate/PVA/Laponite nanoplatelets	Ionic cross-linking with divalent ion	–	Blood coagulation	In vitro: human dermal fibroblasts, MG63 cell line	Golafshan et al. (2017)
Alginate/gelatin	Photo cross-linking and ionic cross-linking	–	Cell adhesion and proliferation	In vitro: HFF-1 foreskin fibroblast cell line	Stubbe et al. (2019)
Alginate	Ionic cross-linking	Cefazolin	Thermo responsive	Adult normal human epidermal keratinocyte cells	Mostafalu et al. (2018)

1.5 *Alginate-Based Nanofibers for Wound Healing Applications*

Studies have reported sodium alginate-based nanofibers for wound healing applications. Nanofibers promote the growth of epithelial cells and the synthesis of new tissue by mimicking the ECM. The nanosize range diameter and nanofibrous mesh-like structure help induce hemostasis of the wounded tissues, increase the absorption of wound exudate, and promote drug delivery through the skin, cell respiration, and increased gas permeation by prevention infection caused by pathogenic bacteria (Aderibigbe and Buyana 2018).

Nanofibrous mats based on ZnO-loaded sodium alginate (SA)/poly (vinyl alcohol) (PVA) was developed by electrospinning technique. ZnO nanoparticles with an average diameter of about 160 nm were synthesized, and SA/PVA/ZnO nanofibrous mats incorporating 0.5, 1.0, 2.0, and 5% ZnO concentration were prepared. According to the in vitro cytotoxic studies, 0.5 and 1% ZnO-loaded SA/PVA fibers were found to be less toxic, whereas those with high concentration of ZnO were toxic. The antibacterial activity of SA/PVA/ZnO was evaluated with *Staphylococcus aureus* and *Escherichia coli*, and it was found that these nanofibers were effective against the bacterial strains which could be potentially due to the presence of ZnO nanoparticles. In cell adhesion studies in L929 cell lines, SA/PVA/ZnO nanofibrous mats with low concentrations of ZnO show comparatively better spreading, but on increasing ZnO concentrations, cells showed more rounded morphology, and this nature was further confirmed by DAPI staining of nucleus (Shalumon et al. 2011).

In a study, Hajiali et al. (2016) fabricated sodium alginate-polyethylene oxide (SA/PEO)-based nanofibers loaded with lavender essential oil with about 93 ± 22 nm in size. The incorporation of PEO and pluronic F-127 aided in the electrospinnability of sodium alginate. The fabricated fibers were hydrophilic, indicating wound exudate absorption property of the fibers. They showed sufficient mechanical properties—nanofibers were flexible and easy to handle without breaking and adapt to skin wounds. The lavender oil-loaded SA/PEO fibers were effective against *S. aureus* culture. In vivo studies of nanofibers on burn wound indicated the ability of nanofibers to prevent inflammation which was evident by complete disappearance of erythema within 48 h. Moreover, the fibers exhibited anti-inflammatory property which was evident by the decreased level of anti-inflammatory cytokines such as IL-6, IL-1β, and TNF-α in mice model.

Ustundag and team (2010) developed sodium alginate-based nanofibers for wound dressing application by electrospinning technique. 1% sodium alginate and PVA were blended in the ratio of 2:1. The electrospun fibers displayed a uniform and continuous form and average diameter of 100.35 ± 12.79 nm. In in vivo studies, the wound healing efficiency of SA/PVA nanofibers mat was compared macroscopically with that of drug containing cotton gauze, antibacterial Bactigras, and Suprasorb A (a commercial alginate-based wound dressing). The electrospun mat showed better healing potential than that of drug loaded cotton gauze and antibacterial Bactigras.

The results demonstrated that the PVA/SA electrospun nanofibrous mat as a potential wound dressing exhibited wound healing properties.

In a research conducted by Fu et al. (2016), moxifloxacin hydrochloride sodium alginate-poly(vinyl alcohol) nanofibrous membrane was synthesized using electrospinning technique. The diameter of the modified nanofiber was 175 ± 75 nm. The nanofiber exhibited adequate antibacterial property against *Staphylococcus aureus* and *Pseudomonas aeruginosa*. The antibacterial property of nanofibers was found to increase in proportion with increased concentration of moxifloxacin hydrochloride in the nanofiber. The drug release pattern of the drug was investigated, and about 80% moxifloxacin hydrochloride is released from electrospun after an incubation period of 10 h at 37 °C. The outcome of the experiment suggests that moxifloxacin hydrochloride PVA/SA nanofiber is a potential bioactive wound dressing for biomedical applications.

1.6 Commercially Available Alginate-Based Wound Dressings

The market value commercially available wound dressing based on alginate is growing in a fast pace. The most recent FDA-approved alginate-based wound dressing is Luofucon® Extra Silver Alginate Dressing and Luofucon® Antibacterial Alginate Wound Dressing. The scientists state that the dressings have proven antibacterial activity against *E. coli*, *E. faecalis*, *K. pneumoniae*, methicillin-resistant *S. aureus* (MRSA), *P. aeruginosa*, *S. aureus*, *S. pyogenes*, and vancomycin-resistant *Enterococcus* (VRE) (Barbu et al. 2021).

Enzymes were incorporated into a polyethylene glycol-alginate hydrogel called Flaminal® Forte that underwent clinical trials in humans for treating burns of partial thickness and exhibited good results than the silver sulfadiazine-based hydrogel marketed as Flamazine®, comparing to the number of times the dressing needs to be changed. Alginate-based wound dressing for pressure ulcers is developed. A honey-loaded alginate-based product, named Algivon®, was used for this purpose. An improved, modified version of this dressing, named Algivon® Plus, displayed better clinical results when applied on chronic wounds. Algivon® Ribbon or Plus is also useful in the treatment of diabetes, pressure, and leg ulcers, fungating lesions, and chronic or complicated surgical wounds and abrasions. Calcium alginate wound dressing incorporated with Manuka honey marketed as Activon® Tube is administered to treat diabetes and leg ulcers, pressure sores, and wounds which are malodorous, infected, dry, and necrotic (Barbu et al. 2021).

Hyalogran® is a commercial wound dressing made of sodium alginate and Hyaff®, which is a three-dimensional matrix of a hyaluronic acid ester. The eschar resection, wound debridement, was followed by 21 days of the first dressing period, second dressing was applied for a period of 2 weeks, and the third dressing for an unmentioned period. It was observed that after 2 months from the initial treatment, the wound was found to be completely healed, with minimal scaring and thus revealing the benefits of wound treatments involving hyaluronic acid in combination with sodium alginate. Silvercel® is another commercially available alginate-based non-adherent wound dressing, which was used in a wound healing experiment, when it was applied on a diabetic patient, with a frequency of 2 days per week, on a repetitive non-infected venous leg ulcer, and the wound healed in about 2 weeks (Barbu et al. 2021).

Other commercially available dressings that contain both alginate and silver, like Aquacel™ Ag EXTRA™ Hydrofiber™ or ALGS6 Ag Alginate wound dressing, possess similar wound healing properties. Other different commercially available alginate-based dressings that were involved in multiple comparative studies were Suprasorb® A (100% alginate), Suprasorb® A-Ag (alginate, ionic Ag), and LG-nano Ag ® Acticoat Absorbent with SILCRYST™, investigated for its antimicrobial property, binding to elastase capacity, antioxidant capacity, cytotoxicity, and effect on HaCaT keratinocytes, which showed promising results (Barbu et al. 2021). Some of the commercially marketed alginate-based wound dressings are listed in Table 2.

2 Chitosan in Wound Healing

Chitosan is a cationic biopolysaccharide derived from chitin by deacetylation. Chitin is present in shells of crustaceans. Chitosan is present with β-(1 → 4)-linkage of D-glucosamine and N-acetyl-D-glucosamine. Its unique physico-chemical characteristics and biological characteristics give a versatile biomaterial for biomedical applications (Feng et al. 2021a).

2.1 Characteristics of Chitosan

Chitosan, a partially deacetylated form of chitin, is the most abundant natural polysaccharides, second only to cellulose. It is present with β-(1 → 4)-linked D-glucosamine and N-acetyl-D-glucosamine units. The chitosan is made by deacetylation of chitin, which is obtained from crustacean shells such as shrimp and crab and results in a copolymer that possesses unique structural characteristics valuable in biomedical applications, particularly wound healing (Kozma et al. 2022).

2.1.1 Structure of Chitosan

Chemically chitosan is composed of $(C_6H_{11}NO_4)$ n consisting of linear chains of deacetylated and acetylated units of β-(1 → 4)-linked D-glucosamine and N-acetyl-D-glucosamine. The degree of deacetylation (DD) of chitosan is the proportion of amino $(-NH_2)$ groups present compared to the total number of acetylated and

Table 2 Alginate-based commercially available pharmaceutical products for wound healing

Alginate-based pharmaceutical products	Composition	Target	Study type/ effects	Reference
Fibracol 10% Ca ALG in Fibracol Plus dressing	90% collagen 10% calcium alginate	Exuding full- and partial-thickness wounds Second-degree burns Diabetic and venous ulcers	Clinical trial/ healing time of diabetic foot ulcers	Szekalska et al. (2016) and Donaghue et al. (1998)
Aquacel™ Ag EXTRA™ Hydrofiber™	Bilayer sodium alginate Carboxylethylcellulose and silver	Effective against minor cuts and burns, surgical, traumatic, exuding, wounds	Absorption of wound exudate, inhibition of bacterial growth	Barbu et al. (2021)
Flaminal® gel	Alginate-polyethylene matrix, lactoperoxidase, notatin, guaiacol	Used to treat diabetic ulcers, leg and pressure ulcers, burns, wounds caused by surgery	Bacteriostatic property, absorbs wound exudate, act as surface moisturizer for wound, debrides necrotic tissues, antimicrobial property	Rashaan et al. (2016)
Medihoney® gel	Calcium alginate, Manuka honey	Applied for ulcers, diabetic foot, pressure ulcers, burns, surgical and traumatic wounds	Antibacterial properties	Das and Baker (2016)
Lucofucon® antibacterial wound dressing	Calcium alginate, silver	Effective for minor cuts, abrasions, burns	Promotes wound healing, antibacterial effect	Barbu et al. (2021)

deacetylated units, which indicates how much chitosan has been deacetylated from its acetylated state (Wang et al. 2016). The degree of deacetylation (DD) typically ranges between 50% and 95%. It significantly influences the solubility, charge density, and biological activity of chitosan. A higher DD increases the number of unbound amino groups, enhancing solubility in acidic environments and boosting bioactivity. Chitosan is available in different molecular weights (50–2000 kDa), influencing its viscosity, degradation rate, and mechanical properties.

Under acidic conditions the amine groups in chitosan get protonated and give a positive charge to chitosan, which is critical for its interaction with oppositely charged biological membranes, bacterial cell walls, and extracellular matrix components (Kołodziejska et al. 2021).

2.1.2 Physico-chemical Characteristics

Chitosan has several different physico-chemical characteristics which make it suitable for biomedical purposes: some of the physico-chemical properties are solubility, biodegradability, film-forming ability, mucoadhesive property, viscosity, and polyelectrolytic complex formation, which give chitosan a versatile nature in the biomedical field (Alemu and Mondal 2023). The protonation $-NH_2$ groups make chitosan dissolvable in dilute acidic solutions such as acetic acid, HCl, and citric acid while remaining insoluble in water and alkaline environments (Roy et al. 2017). This pH-dependent solubility is a critical factor in designing chitosan-based formulations for biomaterial development for applications such as controlled delivery of drugs for wound healing and tissue engineering.

Chitosan is biodegradable. Its enzymatic breakdown by lysozyme and other glycosidases converts it into harmless oligosaccharides that can be easily metabolized by the body (Matica et al. 2017). The film-forming ability of chitosan makes it useable to create translucent, flexible films that are applicable in transdermal administration systems and wound dressings. In addition to this, chitosan has mucoadhesive properties that allow it to adhere in mucosal surfaces and can enhance localized drug delivery. Viscosity of chitosan varies with concentration, molecular weight, and degree of deacetylation; this property is important for hydrogel formation. These characteristics can be modified through chemical modifications (e.g., carboxymethylation, sulfation, quaternization) to tailor chitosan for specific applications (Dash et al. 2011).

2.1.3 Mechanical and Thermal Properties

Chitosan's mechanical strength and thermal stability are critical parameters in designing wound healing scaffolds and films. Molecular weight (MW) and thickness of the chitosan scaffold influence the parameters such as tensile strength and modulus. Compared with chitosan of low molecular weight, better mechanical property is observed in chitosan of high molecular weight. Degradation occurs typically around 200–250 °C, which is acceptable for most biomedical applications. The semi-crystalline nature of chitosan influences degradation rate and water uptake modified via processing methods such as freeze-drying and cross-linking (Dong et al. 2020).

2.1.4 Biological Properties

Chitosan is a versatile polymer which makes it especially attractive for wound healing. Chitosan's unique biological properties make it an acceptable material in wound healing applications. Its biocompatibility, hemostatic activity, antimicrobial properties, immunomodulatory effects, and capability to support cell adhesion and proliferation contribute notably to its effectiveness in promoting wound healing.

Chitosan exhibits high cytocompatibility in both in vitro and in vivo studies, making it acceptable for medical applications. Its non-toxic nature gives less opposite reactions when used as wound dressings (Singh et al. 2017; Aduba and Yang 2017).

Chitosan promotes platelet adhesion and aggregation through electrostatic interactions, which aids in rapid clot formation. This is particularly advantageous in the management of open wounds and preventing excessive bleeding (Liu et al. 2023; Biranje et al. 2020). It also has antibacterial activity against a variety of bacterial species, such as *Escherichia coli* and *Staphylococcus aureus* (Confederat et al. 2021). Its mechanism involves disrupting microbial membranes, which enhances its effectiveness as a wound dressing (Biranje et al. 2020).

Chitosan modulates inflammatory responses, enhancing macrophage function and promoting a favorable healing environment (Liu et al. 2023). This immunomodulatory effect can reduce chronic inflammation, facilitating faster recovery. Chitosan supports the adhering and growth of keratinocytes, fibroblasts, and endothelial cells, essential for tissue regeneration (Singh et al. 2017). Its properties enable the formation of a conducive scaffold for new tissue development (Aduba and Yang 2017). These properties can be amplified by introducing functional groups or incorporating active agents such as growth factors, antibiotics, and stem cells. Minocycline and gentamycin sulfate-loaded chitosan-PVA hydrogel showed good antibacterial activity. Chitosan-based hydrogels have been loaded with different therapeutic molecules to develop antibacterial function for promoting the formation of granulation tissue, reducing infection, and accelerating wound healing (Liu et al. 2018).

2.2 *Chemical Modifications of Chitosan*

Chitosan has been chemically altered to enhance its functionality, such as poor solubility in neutral pH. Modified chitosan derivatives include carboxymethyl chitosan (CMC), quaternized chitosan, hydroxypropyl chitosan, phosphorylated, and sulfated chitosan (Chen et al. 2022). These derivatives give the scope of chitosan in wound healing by improving its bioavailability, stability, and functional delivery. Bioavailability pertains to the proportion of a digested substance that enters the systemic circulation and is absorbed for physiological activity. So, bioavailability determines how much of the ingested fractions can be absorbed and used by the body. The bioavailability of chitin and chitosan is greatly influenced by their particle size. Particles with reduced size may have higher surface area for enzyme action and absorption, influencing their overall availability for physiological effects (Baharlouei and Rahman 2022). The degree of deacetylation (DA) of chitosan influences its solubility and charge density. An increased degree of deacetylation can enhance the bioavailability of chitosan by enhancing its interaction with the intestinal epithelium. Etherification and amine quaternization are used to modify the chitosan matrix at the amino group in the C-2 position and at the hydroxyl group in the C-3 position/C-6 carbon (Wang et al. 2020; Cai et al. 2009):

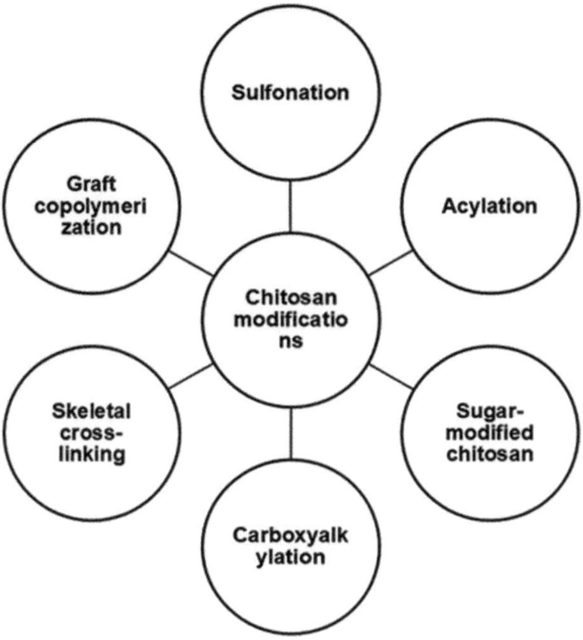

Carboxylation in chitosan is the introduction of carboxyl (–COOH) groups into the chitosan. One active group or two active groups can undergo the carboxylation process in the amino or hydroxyl group simultaneously. Glyoxylic acid and chloroacetic acid are reagents used for modification reactions. The glyoxylic acid oxidizes chitosan's hydroxyl group to carboxyl groups without any intermediate step. In the case of chloroacetic acid, chloroacetic acid reacts with reactive amino group in C2 position (C2-NH2) and C6-NH2 on chitosan to produce N, O-carboxymethyl chitosan. The addition of carboxyl groups improves the hydrophilicity, antibacterial, and biocompatible characteristics (Abreu and Campana-Filho 2005). For biomedical purposes such as dressings for wounds, bacteriostatic agents, and blood anticoagulants, carboxyalkylation at O-/N of chitosan provides the amphoteric polyelectrolyte nature required (Wijesekara and Xu 2024). Carboxyl and amino chitosan functionality helps for regulated therapeutic delivery, such as hydrophilic O-carboxy methylchitosan microspheres for controlled antibiotic delivery (Cao et al. 2021).

The acylation of chitosan (CS) involves the introduction of acyl groups through reactions with anhydrides and acyl chlorides, primarily targeting the amino groups because of the increased reactivity compared to hydroxyl groups. This process improves the hydrophobic properties and water solubility of chitosan, resulting in the generation of N-acylated chitosan (N-ACCS) and O-acylated chitosan

(O-ACCS) under specific conditions. The acylation disrupts hydrogen bonding, facilitating solubilization, particularly at the C6 position of the chitosan structure (Selvan 2017). Chitosan is naturally cationic (positively charged), and acetylation introduces acetyl groups that can alter the overall charge distribution. This change can enhance the binding affinity of chitosan to negatively charged microbial surfaces, leading to increased antimicrobial action.

Sugar-modified chitosan is synthesized through reductive N-alkylation using sodium cyanoborohydride and sugar-aldehyde derivative (glycolaldehyde, DL-glyceraldehyde, D-ribose, D-xylose, 2-deoxyD-ribose, 2-deoxy-D-glucose, 3-O-Me-D-glucose, D-galactose, D-mannose, GlcNAc). These derivatives act as a liver-specific therapeutic molecule carrier by particularly binding at sialo glycoprotein receptors (Varshosaz 2007). These NH2-alkylated chitosan derivatives are soluble in both basic and neutral pH ranges, whereas lactose, maltose, and cellobiose sugars were soluble in a broad pH range. Hepatocyte adhesion is facilitated by the synthetic extracellular matrix of galactosylated chitosan derivatives (Wijesekara and Xu 2024).

Combinations of sulfating agents, such as concentrated sulfuric acid, oleum, sulfur trioxide, pyridine, sulfur trioxide/trimethylamine, sulfur trioxide/sulfur dioxide, chlorosulfonic acid-sulfuric acid, DMF-dichloroacetic acid, tetrahydrofuran, and formic acid, are used to sulfonate chitosan. The reaction media have been used in a range of temperatures (Mourya and Inamdar 2008). However, depolymerization and polymer degradation are challenging when sulfuric acid and microwave radiation are present. Chitosan sulfates derived are often N,O-disubstituted or be partially N,O,O-tri-substituted. Selective O-sulfonation happens when N-acyl or N-alkyl chitosan is used as the starting polysaccharide, whereas selective N or N, O-sulfonation happens when O-substituted chitosan is used (Jain et al. 2013). By reacting with 5-formyl-2-furansulfonic acid sodium salt using the Schiff reaction, which yields N-sulfofurfuryl chitosan sodium salt without polymer degradation and O-substitution and introduces a spacer between the sulfate group and the chitosan backbone, the sulfonic acid function was also added to chitosan. These chitosan sulfates have shown anticoagulant and hemagglutination properties as their structure is similar to heparin. Some of the amino groups in chitosan are changed into anionic centers during the sulfation process, improving the polymer's polyelectrolyte qualities. These improved capabilities can be exploited to create possible drug carriers in the form of micelles or microcapsules (Jain et al. 2013).

Chitosan is designed to produce composites that enhance specific properties including adsorption, mucoadhesive retention, inclusion complexation (Logigan et al. 2022), bacteriostaticity, biocompatibility, and biodegradability (D'Ayala et al. 2008). As expected in drug carrier systems and wound dressings, chitosan grafting with oligo-l-lactide improves hydrophilicity and regulates breakdown rate because the hydrophobic core of the micelles traps and regulates the release of hydrophobic medicines (Logigan et al. 2022). In recent decades, chitosan has been grafted with vinyl monomers copolymers, hydroxyethyl-methacrylate, and methyl methacrylate to control wound healing, tissue engineering, and cardiovascular medication release (Wijesekara and Xu 2024).

Chitosan cross-linking produces hydrogel with good mechanical qualities and a high drug-loading capacity, which may be used in controlled drug delivery systems (Logigan et al. 2022). Glutaraldehyde, genipin, ethylene glycol, diglycidyl ether, and diisocyanate cross-linking at chitosan –NH2 creates specialties such as nonionic/ionic drug interactions and pH sensitivity helps with gastric swelling, which is expected in site-specific drug release (Logigan et al. 2022). Chitosan cross-link microspheres are oral pharmacological agents that are biodegradable and non-toxic (Varshosaz 2007; Sinha et al. 2004) with no possibility for harm. Even after heparin incubation, tripolyphosphate-chitosan ionic gels exhibit notable physical stability without DNA release, encapsulating plasmid DNA/dsDNA for in vitro transfection, cellular absorption, and in vivo gene expression via intratracheal injection. In vivo intratracheal high β-galactosidase expression was mediated by endocytotic cellular nanoparticle uptake, which was followed by quick releases of cytoplasm, according to confocal investigations. A nonviral gene delivery method that can cause steric stabilization and targeting is chitosan-tripolyphosphate nanogel. (Csaba et al. 2009; Yammine et al. 2025). In bone regenerating procedures, calcium sulfate-encapsulated alginate-N-succinyl chitosan hydrogel pastes maintained their structural integrity and were found to reduce the resorption rate that causes bone defect healing (Mitra and Dey 2011).

2.3 *Biomedical Applications of Chitosan*

Chitosan can be developed and fabricated into different forms, enhancing its biomedical versatility:

Scaffolds based on nanomaterials have a lot of potential for further research because of their capacity to control infections and encourage wound healing (Blebea et al. 2025). Because of their specific qualities, which include increased surface area, size flexibility, and the capacity to include therapeutic substances, nanomaterials have become a potential alternative for wound treatment (Muzzarelli et al. 2015). The purpose of gauze, a conventional wound dressing, is to offer passive defense against the environment. Gauze with chitosan and antibacterial nanoparticles transforms into an interactive dressing. Compared to alternative coverings for superficial wounds, this is more affordable. By adding chitosan, Ag, and ZnO to cotton gauze, Abbasipour et al. created a nanocompound that has antibacterial properties against *S. aureus* and *E. coli*. Compared to chitosan/silver or chitosan/zinc nanoparticles, the dressing exhibited better qualities (Martins et al. 2014).

A chitosan-hyaluronic acid nanocomposite sponge was created by Anisha et al. and demonstrated the high porosity needed for wound treatment. The outcome demonstrates that fibroblast motility, adhesion, and proliferation were all improved by chondroitin sulfate nanoform. Mohanty et al. looked into the therapeutic effectiveness of chitosan-alginate sponge loaded with curcumin in rats. Curcumin was slowly and steadily released from the sponge, which also held onto the molecule for a considerable amount of time (Dongre 2017).

By ionic cross-linking and complexation, chitosan nanoparticles containing therapeutic compounds were created. Because medicines have a limited absorption in the stomach, treating stomach ulcers caused by *H. pylori* can be challenging. The majority of the medications are broken down before they reach the goal. Lin and colleagues developed pH-responsive chitosan that is loaded with nanoheparin and amoxicillin in order to solve the issue.

In response to acidic pH, this system releases the contents into the stomach. Studies conducted in vivo demonstrated that the chitosan nanoparticles directly interacted with the pathogen by penetrating cell-cell junctions. Various techniques were used to create chitosan nanospheres that included biomolecules and antibiotics. Chitosan nanoparticles dramatically boost nitric oxide generation and lymphocyte proliferation during wound healing (Bhattacharya et al. 2019). Chung assessed the impact of chitosan nanoparticles loaded with fibrinogen and ATP. A 60% decrease in acute lesions on the stomach mucosa was seen when chitosan/sodium tripolyphosphate loaded with *Arrabidaea chica* extract was applied (Abbasipour et al. 2014). Zhou investigated the impact of chitosan nanoparticles loaded with recombinant EGF (Anisha et al. 2013). The effectiveness of gold nanoparticles with chitosan/PVA nanocomposite was investigated by Hsu et al. It demonstrated enhanced fibroblast proliferation and hemostatic potential (Dai et al. 2009).

Different hydrophilic polymeric chains are cross-linked to generate hydrogel, a three-dimensional structural system (Cui et al. 2019).

Hydrogels have similarities with extracellular matrices, including fluidity and viscoelasticity. Superior hydrophilicity, which allows hydrogels to adsorb exudate (Khorasani et al. 2018), wound moisturization (Zhang et al. 2020), the ability to create a physical barrier against microbial contamination of the wound (Khorasani et al. 2018; Qu et al. 2018), and low adhesion force, which avoids repeated damage from dressing changes, are some of the benefits of hydrogels over other types of wound dressings. For the majority of research, chitosan is the favored native hydrogel among those composed of alginate, collagen, and chitosan.

The tensile strength of chitosan hydrogels can be highly enhanced by cross-linking with agents such as glutaraldehyde and genipin-N. Furthermore, substances like polyvinyl alcohol and carbon nanotubes help to create a strong interpenetrating network inside the hydrogels, improving their overall functionality (Bashir et al. 2020).

The incorporation of functional substances like β-glycerophosphate and photosensitizers has led to the creation of smart hydrogels that are thermosensitive, pH-sensitive, or photosensitive. These hydrogels are particularly useful in drug release control and tissue regeneration, indicating a promising area for future research (Rahmanian-Devin et al. 2021).

Hydrogels can be developed with self-healing property by adding substances like konjac glucomannan and vanillin. These hydrogels can reform their shape after rupture, which is beneficial for treating irregularly shaped wounds, thus providing continuous and effective treatment (Bashir et al. 2020). Hydrogels loaded with silver-like metal nanoparticles have antibacterial properties. Gram-positive *S. aureus* and Gram-negative *E. coli* are two frequent infections that these hydrogels have demonstrated efficacy against, enhancing their suitability for wound care applications. Drug incorporation in hydrogels enhances healing: incorporating therapeutic molecules with antimicrobial, free radical scavenging, and re-epithelializing efficiency into chitosan hydrogels can further expand their applications. These hydrogels' three-dimensional network structure facilitates the controlled release and storage of these medications while encouraging the migration and proliferation of vital cells involved in wound healing (Rahmanian-Devin et al. 2021). Chitosan-cetyltrimethylammonium bromide hydrogels loaded with mupirocin shows antibacterial property against bacteria like *S. aureus* and *S. pyogenes* (Mao et al. 2017). Burns to the skin frequently cause generation of free radicals, which raises reactive oxygen species (ROS) and causes oxidative stress. By shielding tissues from oxidative damage, antioxidants including vitamins A, D, and E can hasten the healing process.

Vitamin E's hydrolyzate, α-Tocopherol, protects collagen and glycosaminoglycans from oxidative stress. Vitamins D and A contribute to tissue repair by regulating inflammation, immune responses, and cell functions. Hydrogel carriers combining poloxamer, chitosan, and hyaluronic acid, loaded with vitamins A, D, and E, have shown promising results in treating skin burns without causing adverse skin reactions (Zhu et al. 2024).

2.3.1 Degradation and Biocompatibility

The biodegradation of chitosan in vivo occurs via enzymatic cleavage primarily by lysozyme. The degradation rate is influenced by DD, MW, and formulation structure. Enzymatic degradation produces non-toxic, resorbable products such as glucosamine, which can be further utilized by the body (Zhou et al. 2024). Biocompatible scaffold shows minimal foreign body reaction, well-tolerated in subcutaneous, dermal, and mucosal tissues. Immunogenicity is generally low, though high-MW or low-DD chitosan may elicit mild immune responses. Biodegradable and biocompatible nature positions chitosan as an ideal candidate for temporary wound coverings that support healing and then safely degrade (Mohamady Hussein et al. 2021).

2.3.2 Regulatory and Safety Considerations

Chitosan is generally approved by the US FDA for certain applications. However, safety and regulatory considerations depend on source, processing method, and final application. The chitosan products should meet these: Residual proteins and endotoxins must be removed during processing. Formulations should meet regulatory standards for sterilization and storage. Although derived from shellfish, chitosan is typically non-allergenic as proteins are removed. Several chitosan-based products have received CE mark and FDA approval for wound care (e.g., HemCon®) (Ho et al. 2022).

2.4 *Wound Healing Accelerated by Chitosan*

Wound healing is a highly dynamic, multistep biological process comprising four overlapping stages: hemostasis, inflammation, proliferation, and remodelling. Chitosan, a biopolymer derived primarily through the deacetylation of chitin, exhibits multifaceted biological activity that can positively modulate each of these healing stages. The mechanisms through which chitosan promotes wound healing are rooted in its molecular structure, physicochemical properties, and its interaction with cellular and extracellular components of skin tissue (Feng et al. 2021b).

2.4.1 Hemostasis: Blood Clot Formation

One of the earliest and most significant roles of chitosan in wound management is its ability to promote hemostasis. Upon injury, vascular constriction and platelet aggregation form the primary defense against blood loss. Chitosan's cationic nature, due to its abundant amine groups, plays a crucial role in initiating clot formation. The positive charges on chitosan attract negatively charged erythrocytes and platelets, enhancing aggregation and accelerating the formation of a hemostatic plug (Golmohammadi et al. 2020).

Moreover, chitosan has been shown to stimulate the release of thromboxane A2 and serotonin from activated platelets, further promoting vasoconstriction and platelet recruitment. This makes chitosan-based materials especially useful in trauma care, battlefield medicine, and surgical applications (Sekhon 2021).

Advanced chitosan formulations such as oxidized chitosan and carboxymethyl chitosan have demonstrated improved hemostatic efficiency and biocompatibility in preclinical studies. Commercial products like Celox™ and HemCon® exemplify successful clinical translations of this property (Araneda Cisternas and Varaprasad 2024).

2.4.2 Antimicrobial and Anti-inflammatory Activity of Chitosan

The inflammatory phase of wound healing involves the recruitment of immune cells such as neutrophils and macrophages to the wound site. These cells release pro-inflammatory cytokines and reactive oxygen species (ROS) to combat pathogens and initiate tissue repair. However, prolonged or excessive inflammation may result in delayed healing and chronic wound formation (Ellis et al. 2018).

Chitosan shows antimicrobial activity against a wide range of Gram-positive and Gram-negative bacteria, fungi, and yeasts. Its antimicrobial action is primarily attributed to the disruption of microbial cell membranes. Chitosan's polycationic nature allows it to bind to negatively charged microbial surfaces, increasing membrane permeability and leading to cell lysis. Additionally, it chelates essential nutrients and metals required for microbial metabolism, further suppressing microbial growth (Shoaib and Wang 2020). Chitosan also modulates the immune response. It has been shown to reduce the levels of pro-inflammatory cytokines such as IL-6, TNF-α, and IL-1β, while simultaneously promoting anti-inflammatory cytokines like IL-10. These immunomodulatory effects contribute to a shortened inflammatory phase and create an optimal environment for tissue regeneration (Ghattas et al. 2025).

In vivo studies on infected wounds treated with chitosan-based dressings have demonstrated reduced bacterial burden, decreased neutrophilic infiltration, and enhanced macrophage polarization toward the anti-inflammatory M2 phenotype (Lewicki et al. 2023).

2.4.3 Cell Proliferation and Migration

During the proliferative phase, fibroblasts, keratinocytes, and endothelial cells play key roles in forming granulation tissue, initiating angiogenesis, and promoting epithelialization. Chitosan facilitates cellular proliferation and migration by mimicking the native extracellular matrix (ECM), providing structural support and biochemical cues (Mawazi et al. 2024).

Chitosan's high affinity for ECM proteins like fibronectin and laminin encourages fibroblast adhesion and spreading. It also promotes the synthesis of collagen types I and III, glycosaminoglycans, and other matrix components, essential for the structural integrity of newly formed tissue (Singh et al. 2017).

Furthermore, chitosan scaffold enhances the activity of growth factors such as basic fibroblast growth factor (bFGF), vascular endothelial growth factor (VEGF), and epidermal growth factor (EGF). It can also serve as a delivery vehicle for these molecules, protecting them from enzymatic degradation and enabling their sustained release (Vijayan and Kumar 2019). Keratinocyte proliferation and migration are significantly enhanced by chitosan, as it supports epidermal stratification and restoration of the skin barrier. In vitro scratch assays and ex vivo skin explant models confirm chitosan's capability to accelerate wound closure (Feng et al. 2021b).

2.4.4 Angiogenesis Stimulation

The formation of new blood vessels, angiogenesis, is critical for supplying nutrients and oxygen to regenerating tissue. Chitosan contributes to angiogenesis through both direct and indirect mechanisms (Zahid et al. 2021). In vitro studies have shown that chitosan stimulates endothelial cell proliferation, migration, and tube formation. The direct effects of chitosan on endothelial cells are complemented by its ability to serve as a delivery vehicle for angiogenic factors, further boosting its angiogenic potential. Chitosan directly promotes the proliferation of human umbilical vein endothelial cells (HUVECs) by inhibiting apoptosis through the downregulation of Bax protein expression, thereby enhancing cell survival and proliferation (Farhadihosseinabadi et al. 2019). In vitro studies demonstrate that chitosan enhances tube formation, a critical step in angiogenesis, by supporting the structural development of endothelial cells into capillary-like networks (Dev et al. 2025).

Chitosan-based systems, such as chitosan-albumin microspheres, provide controlled release of endothelial cell growth factors (ECGF), leading to sustained angiogenic responses. This controlled release system ensures a prolonged and localized effect, enhancing neovascularization in vivo (Sinha et al. 2004). Chitosan-coated scaffolds, such as 2-N,6-O-sulfated chitosan (26SCS) on PLGA, improve the delivery and bioactivity of vascular endothelial growth factor (VEGF), further promoting angiogenesis through enhanced endothelial cell viability and tube formation (Wang et al. 2019b). The incorporation of nanocurcumin into chitosan-fibrin hydrogels has been shown to improve angiogenic responses, as evidenced by increased nitric oxide release and tube formation in vitro, as well as enhanced aortic sprouting ex vivo (Mohandas and Rangasamy 2021).

In in vivo, chitosan enhances the expression of pro-angiogenic factors such as VEGF and angiopoietin-1 while suppressing anti-angiogenic mediators. Chitosan hydrogels and scaffolds loaded with VEGF or PRP have been shown to significantly increase capillary density and vascularization in wound beds. Chitosan by-products, glucosamine and N-acetylglucosamine, also participate in biosynthetic pathways that influence endothelial function and vascular remodelling. Additionally, chitosan scaffolds' porosity and hydrophilicity allow for efficient nutrient and oxygen transport (Veith et al. 2019; Pal et al. 2024).

2.4.5 Epithelialization and Remodelling

The final stage of wound healing involves tissue remodelling and the re-establishment of a functional epithelium. Chitosan plays a pivotal role in these processes by regulating the matrix metalloproteinase (MMP) activity and supporting the organization of collagen fibers (Yadav and Palei 2024).

Chitosan enhances re-epithelialization by promoting keratinocyte migration and restoring dermal-epidermal junctions. It also reduces excessive scar formation by controlling fibroblast proliferation and preventing hypertrophic responses. Importantly, chitosan scaffolds serve as temporary matrices that degrade at a controlled rate, allowing for natural tissue replacement without provoking chronic inflammation. In animal models, in wound tissue chitosan-based membranes have resulted in improved tensile strength, better collagen alignment, and reduced scar formation compared to conventional dressings. These outcomes are critical for achieving both aesthetic and functional restoration of the skin (Ferreira et al. 2022).

3 Bioactive Molecule Delivery

Chitosan's ability to form hydrogels, nanoparticles, and scaffolds enables it to serve as a highly efficient delivery vehicle for a range of bioactive agents. Its mucoadhesive nature and controlled degradation profile allow for localized, sustained, and stimuli-responsive drug release (Ferreira et al. 2022).

Chitosan-based systems have been employed to deliver antibiotics, anti-inflammatory agents, growth factors, stem cells, and nucleic acids directly to the wound site. For instance, chitosan nanoparticles encapsulating plasmid DNA encoding VEGF have demonstrated accelerated angiogenesis and improved wound healing in diabetic models (Sinha et al. 2004). Functionalized chitosan materials with ligands or antibodies can further enhance targeted delivery, minimizing off-target effects and systemic toxicity. This targeted approach is particularly beneficial in chronic wounds, where impaired perfusion and persistent infection hinder therapeutic efficacy (Iacob et al. 2021).

3.1 *Immunomodulation and Stem Cell Interaction*

Chitosan is increasingly recognized for its immunomodulatory effects and its compatibility with stem cell-based therapies. It creates a favorable microenvironment for stem cell survival, proliferation, and differentiation (Yadav and Palei 2024).

Mesenchymal stem cells (MSCs) seeded on chitosan scaffolds exhibit enhanced viability and paracrine signalling, contributing to anti-inflammatory effects and tissue regeneration. Chitosan also modulates toll-like receptor (TLR) pathways, shifting immune responses from pro-inflammatory to regenerative phenotypes (Barbosa et al. 2019).

In chronic wounds where immune dysregulation is prominent, chitosan-based materials help recalibrate the inflammatory milieu, thereby supporting sustained healing. The incorporation of immunosuppressive drugs or gene therapy vectors into chitosan matrices further expands their therapeutic potential (Shi et al. 2006).

3.2 *Mechano-transduction and Cellular Signalling*

Chitosan can influence cellular behavior not only through biochemical interactions but also via mechano-transduction, the conversion of mechanical cues into cellular responses. Biomolecule loaded chitosan such as insulin loaded affects focal adhesion formation, cytoskeletal organization, and downstream signalling pathways like PI3K/Akt, MAPK, and Wnt/β-catenin (Dixit et al. 2023; Rahaman and Mukherjee 2025). These signalling cascades are crucial in regulating cell proliferation, migration, differentiation, and matrix synthesis. By tailoring the mechanical properties of chitosan scaffolds, researchers can guide cellular fate decisions and optimize tissue regeneration outcomes.

Additionally, chitosan scaffolds with conjugation to biomolecules have been shown to inhibit oxidative stress by scavenging free radicals and upregulating endogenous antioxidant enzymes such as SOD and catalase. These effects help maintain redox homeostasis in the wound bed and protect cells from oxidative damage (Zhang et al. 2018; Marrazzo and O'Leary 2020).

4 Formulations and Applications in Wound Care

Chitosan's versatility enables its application in a wide variety of wound dressing formats. These formulations are specifically designed to provide optimal healing conditions, protect against infection, manage wound exudate, and facilitate the delivery of bioactive agents to the wound site (Rajinikanth et al. 2024). The most commonly explored and clinically relevant formulations of chitosan are as follows:

4.1 Films and Membranes

Chitosan-based films and membranes have been widely studied and used due to their ease of application, conformability to wound surfaces, and their ability to maintain a moist wound environment, a critical factor in optimal wound healing. These films are typically fabricated via solvent casting, where chitosan is dissolved in dilute acids and then cast into thin layers (Rajinikanth et al. 2024; Moe et al. 2008). These films serve as protective barriers that can prevent microbial invasion and reduce wound contamination while allowing gaseous exchange. Additionally, their transparency allows for visual monitoring of wound progression without removal, thus minimizing patient discomfort and the risk of infection (Moe et al. 2008; Moreira et al. 2023).

Incorporation of therapeutic agents such as antibiotics (e.g., ciprofloxacin, gentamicin), anti-inflammatory compounds, and growth factors into chitosan films has been shown to enhance their efficacy (Ngadaonye et al. 2014). Recent innovations include multilayered chitosan films integrated with nanocarriers or herbal materials such as curcumin, *Aloe vera*, and *Centella asiatica* extracts. These hybrid films exhibit superior antioxidant, antimicrobial, and regenerative capacities (Jangra et al. 2025).

Biophysical properties like tensile strength, elasticity, and hydration rate can be tailored by blending chitosan with other biopolymers such as gelatin, collagen, alginate, or synthetic polymers like polyvinyl alcohol (PVA). These modifications ensure that the films can withstand mechanical stress while remaining flexible, making them suitable for jointed or mobile anatomical sites (El-Husseiny et al. 2022).

4.2 *Hydrogels*

Chitosan-based hydrogels are three-dimensional, hydrophilic polymer networks capable of retaining substantial amounts of water, thereby creating a moist and breathable environment conducive to tissue regeneration. These hydrogels are synthesized via physical (ionic) or chemical (covalent) cross-linking of chitosan chains (El-Husseiny et al. 2022; Gounden and Singh 2024).

Hydrogels have found utility in the management of dry or necrotic wounds, as they can rehydrate eschar, promote autolytic debridement, and reduce pain by cooling the wound site. Their viscoelastic nature ensures intimate contact with irregular wound beds, enhancing their functional integration (Gounden and Singh 2024). Functional hydrogels incorporating silver nanoparticles, nitric oxide donors, and platelet-rich plasma (PRP) have been reported to significantly enhance healing outcomes in infected wounds, diabetic ulcers, and burns. Additionally, injectable chitosan hydrogels are being explored for minimally invasive wound treatment and as fillers for tissue defects (Brumberg et al. 2021; Edwards 2010).

4.3 *Sponges and Foams*

Chitosan sponges and foams are prepared by freeze-drying or lyophilization techniques, resulting in highly porous and absorbent structures. These spongy matrices are suitable for wounds with high levels of exudate, as they can absorb fluids while maintaining a moist healing environment (Rajinikanth et al. 2024).

Their porous architecture supports cell migration and proliferation, angiogenesis, and ECM remodelling. Chitosan sponges are often utilized in emergency medicine and battlefield scenarios due to their hemostatic property. For instance, HemCon® dressings, derived from chitosan, have been widely adopted in military settings to manage hemorrhagic wounds (Dev et al. 2025; Brown et al. 2009).

A study showed that chitosan modified with amino acid proline promotes collagen deposition from fibroblast cells. These findings show the scaffold cues remodel the wound microenvironment (Linju and Rekha 2023). Additionally, the mechanical properties and degradation rates of chitosan sponges can be modulated by cross-linking or blending with other biopolymers like alginate, hyaluronic acid, or silk fibroin, making them suitable for chronic wound care and post-surgical applications (Kołodziejska et al. 2021).

4.4 *Nanoparticles and Nanofibers*

Nanotechnology has significantly enhanced the therapeutic potential of chitosan in wound healing. Chitosan nanoparticles, typically ranging from 50 to 300 nm in size, serve as efficient carriers for bioactive molecules. These nanoparticles enhance drug solubility, stability, and bioavailability while ensuring localized delivery at the wound site (Jafernik et al. 2023; Placha and Jampilek 2021). Nanoparticles can be synthesized through ionic gelation, emulsification, or spray-drying methods and can be loaded with a range of agents, including antimicrobial drugs (e.g., silver sulfadiazine), anti-inflammatory molecules, and nucleic acids (Alehosseini et al. 2022; Bashir et al. 2022).

Chitosan nanofibers, produced through electrospinning, mimic the extracellular matrix (ECM) and provide a biomimetic scaffold that encourages cell adhesion, migration, and differentiation. An example of nanofibrous mats which showed accelerated wound closure and skin regeneration in animal models are chitosan/silk fibroin mats and chitosan/PLLA nanofibrous membrane loaded with graphene oxide (Sethuram and Thomas 2023). Further innovation has led to the development of core-shell nanofibers, where chitosan encapsulates a drug-loaded core, allowing for sequential or dual-drug delivery such as chitosan/PCL membrane loaded with ciprofloxacin. Additionally, the surface of these nanofibers can be functionalized with peptides or antibodies to enhance targeted healing responses (Taokaew and Chuenkaek 2024).

4.5 Composite and Hybrid Dressings

To further enhance the functionality of chitosan-based wound dressings, composites incorporating other natural or synthetic polymers, nanomaterials, and therapeutic agents have been extensively explored. Such formulations leverage the strengths of individual components to provide synergistic healing effects.

Chitosan-alginate composites, for example, offer superior gelling behavior and ion exchange capabilities, which contribute to enhanced moisture retention and ionic homeostasis in the wound bed. They also help in granulation tissue development. These properties are crucial for supporting cell function and promoting angiogenesis (Rezaei and Ehtesabi 2022).

Similarly, chitosan-collagen and chitosan-gelatin composites mimic ECM and help cell adhesion. These hybrid systems are especially effective in enhancing granulation tissue formation and epithelialization. The incorporation of antimicrobial agents such as silver, zinc oxide, or essential oils into these composites has further improved their infection-resistance profile (Sethuram and Thomas 2023).

Recently, electrospun nanofiber mats and multilayered hydrogels composed of chitosan blended with hyaluronic acid or polyvinyl alcohol have demonstrated outstanding biocompatibility and wound closure rates. These smart materials with sensors monitor the wound in real time, releasing therapeutic agents in response to infection or inflammation (Valachová et al. 2022; Naseri et al. 2014).

Commercially available examples of chitosan composite dressings include Chitopack®, which combines chitosan with gauze fabric to manage bleeding and reduce microbial contamination. Other marketed products use bioadhesive chitosan gels with integrated lidocaine or anti-inflammatory drugs for postoperative wound management (Singh et al. 2017).

5 Clinical Applications

Chitosan-based wound healing products have transitioned from lab research to clinical use. Clinical applications of chitosan include acute and chronic wound management, surgical hemostasis, burn treatment, diabetic ulcers, and trauma care. Chitosan's rise in clinical settings is driven by its excellent biocompatibility, low immunogenicity, broad-spectrum antimicrobial action, and intrinsic hemostatic ability. Clinicians have reported high patient tolerance and favorable healing outcomes with chitosan-based dressings. Chitosan dressings are categorized into several forms based on their composition and function such as hemostatic agents which are designed to control bleeding and initiate the clotting process in surgical or emergency trauma settings. Chitosan moist wound dressings like gels, sponges, and films maintain a moist wound environment and enhance epithelial regeneration. Chitosan scaffolds also serve as a matrix for controlled release of growth factors, antimicrobials, or stem cells (Rajinikanth et al. 2024; Iacob et al. 2021). The widespread application across various wound types demonstrates chitosan's flexibility and adaptability.

Chitosan-based products have been approved for clinical use. These products vary in formulation, indication, and mechanism of action:

Product	Form	Application
HemCon® (HemCon Medical Technologies, USA)	Sponge	Hemorrhage control. It enhances clot formation and prevents microbial infection
ChitoGauze®	Gauze	Hemostatic material
Celox™ (Medtrade Products, UK)	Gauze, granule form	Rapidly forms a gel-like clot on contact with blood, making it valuable in emergency bleeding control
Chitopack® (Woorhi Mechatronics, South Korea)	Sponge, film	Used in postoperative wound care, particularly in dental and ENT surgery
KytoCel® (Aspen Medical Europe)	Sponge	Used in chronic wounds like diabetic foot ulcers and pressure ulcers. High absorbency and anti-infection properties

These products demonstrate the clinical trust and regulatory confidence in chitosan-based wound care (Cheung et al. 2015).

6 Conclusion

A wound is skin damage brought on by a chemical or physical trauma. Complete wound healing requires the use of an appropriate wound management strategy. Cotton gauze and other synthetic materials used in commercial wound dressings have issues with wound healing pace, moist environment near the site, and patient discomfort.

Alginate is a polyanionic copolymer, extracted from brown sea algae. Viscosity is one of its beneficial qualities; thermostable qualities, sol-gel transition, hydrophilicity, swelling capacity, and drug release behavior lead to numerous applications in biomedical field, including wound care, tissue engineering, and therapeutic delivery.

A cationic polymer produced by deacetylating chitin, chitosan provides a flexible and efficient platform for wound healing applications due to their multifunctional biological activities and adaptability to various formulations.

Alginate and chitosan have successfully shown their reliability as wound dressing material, and they are still the preferred biopolymers for basic scaffold in the field of tissue engineering and wound healing. Future research in this field may focus on creating novel biopolymers with altered properties that differ from the other polymers now on the market by altering the synthesis process and technology.

References

Rajinikanth B, S., Rajkumar, D. S. R., K, K., & Vijayaragavan, V. (2024). Chitosan-Based Biomaterial in Wound Healing: A Review. Cureus, 16(2), e55193. https://doi.org/10.7759/cureus.55193

Hay, I. D., Rehman, Z. U., Moradali, M. F., Wang, Y., & Rehm, B. H. (2013). Microbial alginate production, modification and its applications. Microbial biotechnology, 6(6), 637–650.

Abourehab, M. A. S., Pramanik, S., Abdelgawad, M. A., Abualsoud, B. M., Kadi, A., Ansari, M. J., & Deepak, A. (2022a). Recent Advances of Chitosan Formulations in Biomedical Applications. *International Journal of Molecular Sciences, 23*(18), 10975. https://doi.org/10.3390/ijms231810975

Lee, K. Y., & Mooney, D. J. (2012). Alginate: properties and biomedical applications. Progress in polymer science, 37(1), 106–126.

Tomić, S. L., Babić Radić, M. M., Vuković, J. S., Filipović, V. V., Nikodinovic-Runic, J., & Vukomanović, M. (2023). Alginate-based hydrogels and scaffolds for biomedical applications. Marine Drugs, 21(3), 177.

Remminghorst, U., & Rehm, B. H. (2006). Bacterial alginates: from biosynthesis to applications. Biotechnology letters, 28(21), 1701–1712.

Barbu, A., Neamtu, B., Zăhan, M., Iancu, G. M., Bacila, C., & Mireşan, V. (2021). Current trends in advanced alginate-based wound dressings for chronic wounds. Journal of personalized medicine, 11(9), 890.

Yang, J. S., Xie, Y. J., & He, W. (2011). Research progress on chemical modification of alginate: A review. Carbohydrate polymers, 84(1), 33–39.

Barbu, A., Neamţu, M. B., Zăhan, M. A. R. I. U. S., & Mireşan, V. I. O. A. R. A. (2020). Trends in alginate-based films and membranes for wound healing. Romanian. Biotechnological Letters, 25, 1683–1689.

Szekalska, M., Puciłowska, A., Szymańska, E., Ciosek, P., & Winnicka, K. (2016). Alginate: current use and future perspectives in pharmaceutical and biomedical applications. International journal of polymer science, 2016(1), 7697031.

Abourehab, M. A., Rajendran, R. R., Singh, A., Pramanik, S., Shrivastav, P., Ansari, M. J. & Deepak, A. (2022b). Alginate as a promising biopolymer in drug delivery and wound healing: A review of the state-of-the-art. International Journal of Molecular Sciences, 23(16), 9035.

Tønnesen, H. H., & Karlsen, J. (2002). Alginate in drug delivery systems. Drug development and industrial pharmacy, 28(6), 621–630.

Tavakoli, J., Laisak, E., Gao, M., & Tang, Y. (2019). AIEgen quantitatively monitoring the release of Ca2+ during swelling and degradation process in alginate hydrogels. Materials Science and Engineering: C, 104, 109951.

Zhou, R., Shi, X., Gao, Y., Cai, N., Jiang, Z., & Xu, X. (2015). Anti-inflammatory activity of guluronate oligosaccharides obtained by oxidative degradation from alginate in lipopolysaccharide-activated murine macrophage RAW 264.7 cells. Journal of agricultural and food chemistry, 63(1), 160–168.

Sahoo, D. R., & Biswal, T. (2021). Alginate and its application to tissue engineering. SN Applied Sciences, 3(1), 30.

Aderibigbe, B. A., & Buyana, B. (2018). Alginate in wound dressings. Pharmaceutics, 10(2), 42.

Trucillo, P., & Di Maio, E. (2021). Classification and production of polymeric foams among the systems for wound treatment. Polymers, 13(10), 1608.

Rezvani Ghomi, E., Khalili, S., Nouri Khorasani, S., Esmaeely Neisiany, R., & Ramakrishna, S. (2019). Wound dressings: Current advances and future directions. Journal of Applied Polymer Science, 136(27), 47738.

Gheorghita Puscaselu, R., Lobiuc, A., Dimian, M., & Covasa, M. (2020). Alginate: From food industry to biomedical applications and management of metabolic disorders. Polymers, 12(10), 2417.

Varaprasad, K., Jayaramudu, T., Kanikireddy, V., Toro, C., & Sadiku, E. R. (2020). Alginate-based composite materials for wound dressing application: A mini review. Carbohydrate polymers, 236, 116025.

Dhivya, S., Padma, V. V., & Santhini, E. (2015). Wound dressings–a review. BioMedicine, 5(4), 22.

Nayak, A. K., Mohanta, B. C., Hasnain, M. S., Hoda, M. N., & Tripathi, G. (2020a). Alginate-based scaffolds for drug delivery in tissue engineering. Alginates in drug delivery, 359–386.

Xie, F., Zou, L., Xu, Z., Ou, X., Guo, W., Gao, Y., & Gao, G. (2022). Alginate foam gel modified by graphene oxide for wound dressing. International Journal of Biological Macromolecules, 223, 391–403.

Oh, G. W., Nam, S. Y., Heo, S. J., Kang, D. H., & Jung, W. K. (2020). Characterization of ionic cross-linked composite foams with different blend ratios of alginate/pectin on the synergistic effects for wound dressing application. International journal of biological macromolecules, 156, 1565–1573.

Hegge, A. B., Andersen, T., Melvik, J. E., Bruzell, E., Kristensen, S., & Tønnesen, H. H. (2011). Formulation and bacterial phototoxicity of curcumin loaded alginate foams for wound treatment applications: studies on curcumin and curcuminoides XLII. Journal of pharmaceutical sciences, 100(1), 174–185.

Valerón Bergh, V. J., Johannessen, E., Andersen, T., & Tønnesen, H. H. (2018). Evaluation of porphyrin loaded dry alginate foams containing poloxamer 407 and β-cyclodextrin-derivatives intended for wound treatment. Pharmaceutical Development and Technology, 23(8), 761–770.

Namviriyachote, N., Lipipun, V., Akkhawattanangkul, Y., Charoonrut, P., & Ritthidej, G. C. (2019). Development of polyurethane foam dressing containing silver and asiaticoside for healing of dermal wound. Asian Journal of Pharmaceutical Sciences, 14(1), 63–77.

Wang, Y., Wang, C., Qiao, L., Feng, J., Zheng, Y., Chao, Y. & Li, M. (2018). Shape-adaptive composite foams with high expansion and absorption used for massive hemorrhage control and irregular wound treatment. Applied Materials Today, 13, 228–241.

Saraiva, M. M., Campelo, M. D. S., Camara Neto, J. F., Lima, A. B. N., Silva, G. D. A., Dias, A. T. D. F. F. & Ribeiro, M. E. N. P. (2023). Alginate/polyvinyl alcohol films for wound healing: Advantages and challenges. Journal of Biomedical Materials Research Part B: Applied Biomaterials, 111(1), 220–233.

George, M., Joseph, L., & Francis, L. T. (2017). Development and evaluation of silver sulphadiazine loaded sodium alginate gelatin film for wound dressing applications. Eur. J. Pharm. Med. Res, 4, 420–423.

Shao, W., Liu, H., Liu, X., Wang, S., Wu, J., Zhang, R. & Huang, M. (2015). Development of silver sulfadiazine loaded bacterial cellulose/sodium alginate composite films with enhanced antibacterial property. Carbohydrate polymers, 132, 351–358.

Rezvanian, M., Amin, M. C. I. M., & Ng, S. F. (2016). Development and physicochemical characterization of alginate composite film loaded with simvastatin as a potential wound dressing. Carbohydrate polymers, 137, 295–304.

Han, F., Dong, Y., Song, A., Yin, R., & Li, S. (2014). Alginate/chitosan based bi-layer composite membrane as potential sustained-release wound dressing containing ciprofloxacin hydrochloride. Applied surface science, 311, 626–634.

Li, S., Li, L., Guo, C., Qin, H., & Yu, X. (2017). A promising wound dressing material with excellent cytocompatibility and proangiogenesis action for wound healing: Strontium loaded Silk fibroin/Sodium alginate (SF/SA) blend films. International journal of biological macromolecules, 104, 969–978.

Dantas, M. D. M., Cavalcante, D. R. R., Araújo, F. E. N., Barretto, S. R., Aciole, G. T. S., Pinheiro, A. L. B. & Júnior, R. A. (2011). Improvement of dermal burn healing by combining sodium alginate/chitosan-based films and low level laser therapy. Journal of Photochemistry and Photobiology B: Biology, 105(1), 51–59.

Sharma, S., Sanpui, P., Chattopadhyay, A., & Ghosh, S. S. (2012). Fabrication of antibacterial silver nanoparticle—sodium alginate–chitosan composite films. Rsc Advances, 2(13), 5837–5843.

Guadarrama-Acevedo, M. C., Mendoza-Flores, R. A., Del Prado-Audelo, M. L., Urbán-Morlán, Z., Giraldo-Gomez, D. M., Magaña, J. J. & Leyva-Gómez, G. (2019). Development and evaluation of alginate membranes with curcumin-loaded nanoparticles for potential wound-healing applications. Pharmaceutics, 11(8), 389.

Oliveira, D. M. L., Rezende, P. S., Barbosa, T. C., Andrade, L. N., Bani, C., Tavares, D. S. & Severino, P. (2020). Double membrane based on lidocaine-coated polymyxin-alginate nanoparticles for wound healing: In vitro characterization and in vivo tissue repair. International Journal of Pharmaceutics, 591, 120001.

Tarusha, L., Paoletti, S., Travan, A., & Marsich, E. (2018). Alginate membranes loaded with hyaluronic acid and silver nanoparticles to foster tissue healing and to control bacterial contamination of non-healing wounds. Journal of Materials Science: Materials in Medicine, 29, 1–14.

Moreira Filho, R. N. F., Vasconcelos, N. F., Andrade, F. K., de Freitas Rosa, M., & Vieira, R. S. (2020). Papain immobilized on alginate membrane for wound dressing application. Colloids and Surfaces B: Biointerfaces, 194, 111222.

Shefa, A. A., Park, M., Gwon, J. G., & Lee, B. T. (2022). Alpha tocopherol-nanocellulose loaded alginate membranes and pluronic hydrogels for diabetic wound healing. Materials & Design, 224, 111404.

Ndlovu, S. P., Motaung, K. S., Razwinani, M., Alven, S., Adeyemi, S. A., Ubanako, P. N. & Aderibigbe, B. A. (2024). Capparis sepiaria-Loaded Sodium Alginate Single-and Double-Layer Membrane Composites for Wound Healing. Pharmaceutics, 16(10), 1313.

Pacheco, M. S., Kano, G. E., de Almeida Paulo, L., Lopes, P. S., & de Moraes, M. A. (2020). Silk fibroin/chitosan/alginate multilayer membranes as a system for controlled drug release in wound healing. International Journal of Biological Macromolecules, 152, 803–811.

Wang, L., Khor, E., Wee, A., & Lim, L. Y. (2002). Chitosan-alginate PEC membrane as a wound dressing: Assessment of incisional wound healing. Journal of Biomedical Materials Research: An Official Journal of The Society for Biomaterials, The Japanese Society for Biomaterials, and

The Australian Society for Biomaterials and the Korean Society for Biomaterials, 63(5), 610–618.

Nayak, A. K., Hasnain, M. S., Pal, K., Banerjee, I., & Pal, D. (2020b). Gum-based hydrogels in drug delivery. In Biopolymer-based formulations (pp. 605–645).

Hoare, T. R., & Kohane, D. S. (2008). Hydrogels in drug delivery: Progress and challenges. polymer, 49(8), 1993–2007.

Markovic, M. D., Spasojevic, P. M., Pantic, O. J., Savic, S. I., Savkovic, M. M. S., & Panic, V. V. (2024). Status and future scope of hydrogels in wound healing. Journal of Drug Delivery Science and Technology, 105903.

Barnett, S. E., & Varley, S. J. (1987). The effects of calcium alginate on wound healing. Annals of the Royal College of Surgeons of England, 69(4), 153.

Pereira, R., Carvalho, A., Vaz, D. C., Gil, M. H., Mendes, A., & Bártolo, P. (2013a). Development of novel alginate based hydrogel films for wound healing applications. International journal of biological macromolecules, 52, 221–230.

Pereira, R., Mendes, A., & Bártolo, P. (2013b). Alginate/Aloe vera hydrogel films for biomedical applications. Procedia CIRP, 5, 210–215.

Sezer, A. D., & Cevher, E. (2011). Biopolymers as wound healing materials: challenges and new strategies. Biomaterials applications for nanomedicine, 383–414.

Leise, B. S. (2018). Topical wound medications. Veterinary Clinics: Equine Practice, 34(3), 485–498.

Straccia, M. C., Gomez d'Ayala, G., Romano, I., Oliva, A., & Laurienzo, P. (2015). Alginate hydrogels coated with chitosan for wound dressing. Marine drugs, 13(5), 2890–2908.

Bagher, Z., Ehterami, A., Safdel, M. H., Khastar, H., Semiari, H., Asefnejad, A. & Salehi, M. (2020). Wound healing with alginate/chitosan hydrogel containing hesperidin in rat model. Journal of Drug Delivery Science and Technology, 55, 101379.

Ehterami, A., Salehi, M., Farzamfar, S., Samadian, H., Vaez, A., Ghorbani, S. & Sahrapeyma, H. (2019). Chitosan/alginate hydrogels containing Alpha-tocopherol for wound healing in rat model. Journal of Drug Delivery Science and Technology, 51, 204–213.

Kim, J. O., Choi, J. Y., Park, J. K., Kim, J. H., Jin, S. G., Chang, S. W., & Choi, H. G. (2008). Development of clindamycin-loaded wound dressing with polyvinyl alcohol and sodium alginate. Biological and Pharmaceutical Bulletin, 31(12), 2277–2282.

Balakrishnan, B., Mohanty, M., Fernandez, A. C., Mohanan, P. V., & Jayakrishnan, A. (2006). Evaluation of the effect of incorporation of dibutyryl cyclic adenosine monophosphate in an in situ-forming hydrogel wound dressing based on oxidized alginate and gelatin. Biomaterials, 27(8), 1355–1361.

Kamoun, E. A., Kenawy, E. R. S., Tamer, T. M., El-Meligy, M. A., & Eldin, M. S. M. (2015). Poly (vinyl alcohol)-alginate physically crosslinked hydrogel membranes for wound dressing applications: characterization and bio-evaluation. Arabian Journal of Chemistry, 8(1), 38–47.

Rajalekshmy, G. P., & Rekha, M. R. (2021a). Synthesis and evaluation of an alginate-methacrylate xerogel for insulin delivery towards wound healing applications. Therapeutic Delivery, 12(3), 215–234.

Wang, T., Wang, J., Wang, R., Yuan, P., Fan, Z., & Yang, S. (2019a). Preparation and properties of ZnO/sodium alginate bi-layered hydrogel films as novel wound dressings. New Journal of Chemistry, 43(22), 8684–8693.

Li, X., Chen, S., Zhang, B., Li, M., Diao, K., Zhang, Z., … & Chen, H. (2012). In situ injectable nano-composite hydrogel composed of curcumin, N, O-carboxymethyl chitosan and oxidized alginate for wound healing application. International journal of pharmaceutics, 437(1–2), 110–119.

Khampieng, T., Wongkittithavorn, S., Chaiarwut, S., Ekabutr, P., Pavasant, P., & Supaphol, P. (2018). Silver nanoparticles-based hydrogel: Characterization of material parameters for pressure ulcer dressing applications. Journal of Drug Delivery Science and Technology, 44, 91–100.

Liang, M., Chen, Z., Wang, F., Liu, L., Wei, R., & Zhang, M. (2019). Preparation of self-regulating/anti-adhesive hydrogels and their ability to promote healing in burn wounds. Journal of Biomedical Materials Research Part B: Applied Biomaterials, 107(5), 1471–1482.

Chen, T., Chen, Y., Rehman, H. U., Chen, Z., Yang, Z., Wang, M. & Liu, H. (2018). Ultratough, self-healing, and tissue-adhesive hydrogel for wound dressing. ACS applied materials & interfaces, 10(39), 33523–33531.

Golafshan, N., Rezahasani, R., Esfahani, M. T., Kharaziha, M., & Khorasani, S. N. (2017). Nanohybrid hydrogels of laponite: PVA-Alginate as a potential wound healing material. Carbohydrate polymers, 176, 392–401.

Stubbe, B., Mignon, A., Declercq, H., Van Vlierberghe, S., & Dubruel, P. (2019). Development of gelatin-alginate hydrogels for burn wound treatment. Macromolecular bioscience, 19(8), 1900123.

Mostafalu, P., Tamayol, A., Rahimi, R., Ochoa, M., Khalilpour, A., Kiaee, G. & Khademhosseini, A. (2018). Smart bandage for monitoring and treatment of chronic wounds. Small, 14(33), 1703509.

Shalumon, K. T., Anulekha, K. H., Nair, S. V., Nair, S. V., Chennazhi, K. P., & Jayakumar, R. (2011). Sodium alginate/poly (vinyl alcohol)/nano ZnO composite nanofibers for antibacterial wound dressings. International journal of biological macromolecules, 49(3), 247–254.

Hajiali, H., Summa, M., Russo, D., Armirotti, A., Brunetti, V., Bertorelli, R. & Mele, E. (2016). Alginate–lavender nanofibers with antibacterial and anti-inflammatory activity to effectively promote burn healing. Journal of Materials Chemistry B, 4(9), 1686–1695.

Üstündağ, G. C., Karaca, E., Özbek, S., & Çavuşoğlu, İ. (2010). In vivo evaluation of electrospun poly (vinyl alcohol)/sodium alginate nanofibrous mat as wound dressing. Textile and Apparel, 20(4), 290–298.

Fu, R., Li, C., Yu, C., Xie, H., Shi, S., Li, Z. & Lu, L. (2016). A novel electrospun membrane based on moxifloxacin hydrochloride/poly (vinyl alcohol)/sodium alginate for antibacterial wound dressings in practical application. Drug delivery, 23(3), 818–829.

Donaghue, V. M., Chrzan, J. S., Rosenblum, B. I., Giurini, J. M., Habershaw, G. M., & Veves, A. (1998). Evaluation of a Collagen-Alginate Wound Dressing in the Management. Adv. Wound Care, 11, 114–118.

Rashaan, Z. M., Krijnen, P., van den Akker-van Marle, M. E., van Baar, M. E., Vloemans, A. F., Dokter, J.,& Breederveld, R. S. (2016). Clinical effectiveness, quality of life and cost-effectiveness of Flaminal® versus Flamazine® in the treatment of partial thickness burns: study protocol for a randomized controlled trial. Trials, 17, 1–9.

Das, S., & Baker, A. B. (2016). Biomaterials and nanotherapeutics for enhancing skin wound healing. Frontiers in bioengineering and biotechnology, 4, 82.

Feng, P., Luo, Y., Ke, C., Qiu, H., Wang, W., Zhu, Y., Hou, R., Xu, L., & Wu, S. (2021a). Chitosan-Based Functional Materials for Skin Wound Repair: Mechanisms and Applications. *Frontiers in bioengineering and biotechnology*, *9*, 650598. https://doi.org/10.3389/fbioe.2021.650598

Kozma, M., Acharya, B., & Bissessur, R. (2022). Chitin, Chitosan, and Nanochitin: Extraction, Synthesis, and Applications. *Polymers*, *14*(19), 3989. https://doi.org/10.3390/polym14193989

Wang, C., Yuan, F., Jin, L., Du, X., & Cai, H. (2016). Evaluation of the Deacetylation Degree of Chitosan with Two-Abrupt-Change Coulometric Titration. *Electroanalysis*, *28*(2), 401–406. https://doi.org/10.1002/ELAN.201500387

Kołodziejska, M., Jankowska, K., Klak, M., & Wszoła, M. (2021). Chitosan as an Underrated Polymer in Modern Tissue Engineering. *Nanomaterials (Basel, Switzerland)*, *11*(11), 3019. https://doi.org/10.3390/nano11113019

Alemu, D., & Mondal, A. K. (2023). Study on the Physicochemical Properties of Chitosan and their Applications in the Biomedical Sector. *International Journal of Polymer Science*, *2023*, 1–13. https://doi.org/10.1155/2023/5025341

Roy, J. C., Salaün, F., Giraud, S., Ferri, A., Chen, G., & Guan, J. (2017). Solubility of Chitin: Solvents, Solution Behaviors and. *Solubility of polysaccharides*, 109.

Matica, A., Menghiu, G., & Ostafe, V. (2017). Biodegradability of chitosan based products. *New Frontiers in Chemistry*, *26*(1).

Dash, M., Chiellini, F., Ottenbrite, R. M., & Chiellini, E. (2011). Chitosan—A versatile semi-synthetic polymer in biomedical applications. Progress in polymer science, 36(8), 981–1014.

Dong, X., Cheng, Q., Long, Y., Xu, C., Fang, H., Chen, Y., & Dai, H. (2020). A chitosan based scaffold with enhanced mechanical and biocompatible performance for biomedical applications. *Polymer Degradation and Stability*, *181*, 109322.

Singh, R., Shitiz, K., & Singh, A. (2017). Chitin and chitosan: biopolymers for wound management. *International wound journal*, *14*(6), 1276–1289.

Aduba, D. C., & Yang, H. (2017). Polysaccharide Fabrication Platforms and Biocompatibility Assessment as Candidate Wound Dressing Materials. *Bioengineering*, *4*(1), 1. https://doi.org/10.3390/BIOENGINEERING4010001

Liu, Z., Xu, Y., Su, H., Jing, X., Wang, D., Li, S., … & Meng, L. (2023). Chitosan-based hemostatic sponges as new generation hemostatic materials for uncontrolled bleeding emergency: modification, composition, and applications. *Carbohydrate Polymers*, *311*, 120780.

Biranje, S., Madiwale, P. V., & Adivarekar, R. V. (2020). *Nanoscale Chitosan-Based Hemostasis Membrane*. *1*(3). https://doi.org/10.33696/HAEMATOLOGY.1.013

Confederat, L. G., Tuchilus, C. G., Dragan, M., Sha'at, M., & Dragostin, O. M. (2021). Preparation and Antimicrobial Activity of Chitosan and Its Derivatives: A Concise Review. *Molecules*, *26*(12), 3694. https://doi.org/10.3390/molecules26123694

Liu, H., Wang, C., Li, C., Qin, Y., Wang, Z., Yang, F., … & Wang, J. (2018). A functional chitosan-based hydrogel as a wound dressing and drug delivery system in the treatment of wound healing. *RSC advances*, *8*(14), 7533–7549.

Chen, Q., Qi, Y., Jiang, Y., Quan, W., Luo, H., Wu, K., Li, S., & Ouyang, Q. (2022). Progress in Research of Chitosan Chemical Modification Technologies and Their Applications. Marine Drugs, 20(8), 536. https://doi.org/10.3390/md20080536

Baharlouei, P., & Rahman, A. (2022). Chitin and Chitosan: Prospective Biomedical Applications in Drug Delivery, Cancer Treatment, and Wound Healing. *Marine Drugs*, *20*(7), 460. https://doi.org/10.3390/md20070460

Wang, W., Meng, Q., Li, Q., Liu, J., Zhou, M., Jin, Z., & Zhao, K. (2020). Chitosan Derivatives and Their Application in Biomedicine. *International Journal of Molecular Sciences*, *21*(2), 487. https://doi.org/10.3390/IJMS21020487

Cai, Z., Chen, P., Jin, H. J., & Kim, J. (2009). The effect of chitosan content on the crystallinity, thermal stability, and mechanical properties of bacterial cellulose—chitosan composites. *Proceedings of the Institution of Mechanical Engineers, Part C: Journal of Mechanical Engineering Science*, *223*(10), 2225–2230.

Abreu, F. R. de, & Campana-Filho, S. P. (2005). Preparation and characterization of carboxymethylchitosan. *Polimeros-Ciencia E Tecnologia*, *15*(2), 79–83. https://doi.org/10.1590/S0104-14282005000200004

Wijesekara, T., & Xu, B. (2024). New insights into sources, bioavailability, health-promoting effects, and applications of chitin and chitosan. *Journal of Agricultural and Food Chemistry*, *72*(31), 17138–17152.

Cao, J., He, G., Ning, X., Wang, C., Fan, L., Yin, Y., & Cai, W. (2021). Hydroxypropyl chitosan-based dual self-healing hydrogel for adsorption of chromium ions. *International journal of biological macromolecules*, *174*, 89–100.

Selvan, M. (2017). Characterization of bioactive chitosan and sulfated chitosan from Doryteuthis singhalensis (Ortmann, 1891). International Journal of Biological Macromolecules.

D'Ayala, G. G., Malinconico, M., & Laurienzo, P. (2008). Marine Derived Polysaccharides for Biomedical Applications: Chemical Modification Approaches. *Molecules*, *13*(9), 2069–2106. https://doi.org/10.3390/molecules13092069

Mourya, V. K., & Inamdar, N. N. (2008). Chitosan-modifications and applications: Opportunities galore. Reactive and Functional polymers, 68(6), 1013–1051

Jain, A., Gulbake, A., Shilpi, S., Jain, A., Hurkat, P., & Jain, S. K. (2013). A new horizon in modifications of chitosan: syntheses and applications. Critical Reviews™ in Therapeutic Drug Carrier Systems, 30(2).

Logigan, C.-L., Delaite, C., Tiron, C.-E., Peptu, C., Popa, M., & Peptu, C. A. (2022). Chitosan Grafted Poly (Ethylene Glycol) Methyl Ether Acrylate Particulate Hydrogels for Drug Delivery Applications. Gels, 8(8), 494. https://doi.org/10.3390/gels8080494

Varshosaz, J. (2007). The promise of chitosan microspheres in drug delivery systems. Expert opinion on drug delivery, 4(3), 263–273.

Sinha, V. R., Singla, A. K., Wadhawan, S., Kaushik, R., Kumria, R., Bansal, K., & Dhawan, S. (2004). Chitosan microspheres as a potential carrier for drugs. International journal of pharmaceutics, 274(1–2), 1–33.

Csaba, N., Köping-Höggård, M., & Alonso, M. J. (2009). Ionically crosslinked chitosan/ tripolyphosphate nanoparticles for oligonucleotide and plasmid DNA delivery. International journal of pharmaceutics, 382(1–2), 205–214. https://doi.org/10.1016/j.ijpharm.2009.07.028

Yammine, P., El Safadi, A., Kassab, R., El-Nakat, H., Obeid, P. J., Nasr, Z., Tannous, T., Sari-Chmayssem, N., Mansour, A., & Chmayssem, A. (2025). Types of Crosslinkers and Their Applications in Biomaterials and Biomembranes. *Chemistry*, *7*(2), 61. https://doi.org/10.3390/ chemistry7020061

Mitra, A., & Dey, B. (2011). Chitosan microspheres in novel drug delivery systems. *Indian journal of pharmaceutical sciences*, *73*(4), 355–366. https://doi.org/10.4103/0250-474X.95607

Muzzarelli, R. A., El Mehtedi, M., Bottegoni, C., Aquili, A., & Gigante, A. (2015). Genipin-Crosslinked Chitosan Gels and Scaffolds for Tissue Engineering and Regeneration of Cartilage and Bone. *Marine drugs*, *13*(12), 7314–7338. https://doi.org/10.3390/md13127068

Blebea, N.-M., Puşcaşu, C., Vlad, R.-A., & Hancu, G. (2025). Chitosan-Based Gel Development: Extraction, Gelation Mechanisms, and Biomedical Applications. Gels, 11(4), 275. https://doi. org/10.3390/gels11040275

Martins, A., Vieira, H., Gaspar, H., & Santos, S. (2014). Marketed marine natural products in the pharmaceutical and cosmeceutical industries: Tips for success. *Marine drugs*, *12*(2), 1066–1101.

Dongre, R. S. (2017). Marine polysaccharides in medicine. *Biological activities and application of marine polysaccharides. IntechOpen, London*, 181–206.

Bhattacharya, D., Ghosh, B., & Mukhopadhyay, M. (2019). Development of nanotechnology for advancement and application in wound healing: a review. *IET nanobiotechnology*, *13*(8), 778–785. https://doi.org/10.1049/iet-nbt.2018.5312

Abbasipour, M., Mirjalili, M., Khajavi, R., & Majidi, M. M. (2014). Coated cotton gauze with Ag/ZnO/chitosan nanocomposite as a modern wound dressing. *Journal of Engineered Fibers and Fabrics*, *9*(1), 155892501400900114.

Anisha, B. S., Sankar, D., Mohandas, A., Chennazhi, K. P., Nair, S. V., & Jayakumar, R. (2013). Chitosan-hyaluronan/nano chondroitin sulfate ternary composite sponges for medical use. *Carbohydrate Polymers*, 92(2), 1470–1476.

Dai, M., Zheng, X., Xu, X., Kong, X., Li, X., Guo, G., … & Qian, Z. (2009). Chitosan-alginate sponge: preparation and application in curcumin delivery for dermal wound healing in rat. BioMed Research International, 2009(1), 595126.

Cui, Z. K., Kim, S., Baljon, J. J., Wu, B. M., Aghaloo, T., & Lee, M. (2019). Microporous methacrylated glycol chitosan-montmorillonite nanocomposite hydrogel for bone tissue engineering. Nature communications, 10(1), 3523.

Khorasani, M. T., Joorabloo, A., Moghaddam, A., Shamsi, H., & MansooriMoghadam, Z. (2018). Incorporation of ZnO nanoparticles into heparinised polyvinyl alcohol/chitosan hydrogels for wound dressing application. International journal of biological macromolecules, 114, 1203–1215.

Zhang, B., He, J., Shi, M., Liang, Y., & Guo, B. (2020). Injectable self-healing supramolecular hydrogels with conductivity and photo-thermal antibacterial activity to enhance complete skin regeneration. Chemical Engineering Journal, 400, 125994.

Qu, J., Zhao, X., Liang, Y., Zhang, T., Ma, P. X., & Guo, B. (2018). Antibacterial adhesive injectable hydrogels with rapid self-healing, extensibility and compressibility as wound dressing for joints skin wound healing. Biomaterials, 183, 185–199.

Bashir, S., Hina, M., Iqbal, J., Rajpar, A. H., Mujtaba, M. A., Alghamdi, N. A., Wageh, S., Ramesh, K., & Ramesh, S. (2020). Fundamental Concepts of Hydrogels: Synthesis, Properties, and Their Applications. Polymers, 12(11), 2702. https://doi.org/10.3390/polym12112702

Rahmanian-Devin, P., Baradaran Rahimi, V., & Askari, V. R. (2021). Thermosensitive chitosan-β-glycerophosphate hydrogels as targeted drug delivery systems: an overview on preparation and their applications. Advances in pharmacological and pharmaceutical sciences, 2021(1), 6640893.

Mao, C., Xiang, Y., Liu, X., Cui, Z., Yang, X., Yeung, K. W. K., Pan, H., Wang, X., Chu, P. K., & Wu, S. (2017). Photo-Inspired Antibacterial Activity and Wound Healing Acceleration by Hydrogel Embedded with Ag/Ag@AgCl/ZnO Nanostructures. ACS nano, 11(9), 9010–9021. https://doi.org/10.1021/acsnano.7b03513

Zhu, J., Cheng, H., Zhang, Z., Chen, K., Zhang, Q., Zhang, C., Gao, W., & Zheng, Y. (2024). Antibacterial Hydrogels for Wound Dressing Applications: Current Status, Progress, Challenges, and Trends. Gels (Basel, Switzerland), 10(8), 495. https://doi.org/10.3390/gels10080495

Zhou, X., Yu, X., You, T., Zhao, B., Dong, L., Huang, C., Zhou, X., Xing, M., Qian, W., & Luo, G. (2024). 3D Printing-Based Hydrogel Dressings for Wound Healing. Advanced science (Weinheim, Baden-Wurttemberg, Germany), 11(47), e2404580. https://doi.org/10.1002/advs.202404580

Mohamady Hussein, M. A., Ulag, S., Abo Dena, A. S., Sahin, A., Grinholc, M., Gunduz, O., … Megahed, M. (2021). Chitosan/Gold Hybrid Nanoparticles Enriched Electrospun PVA Nanofibrous Mats for the Topical Delivery of *Punica granatum* L. Extract: Synthesis, Characterization, Biocompatibility and Antibacterial Properties. *International Journal of Nanomedicine*, *16*, 5133–5151. https://doi.org/10.2147/IJN.S306526

Ho, T. C., Chang, C. C., Chan, H. P., Chung, T. W., Shu, C. W., Chuang, K. P., Duh, T. H., Yang, M. H., & Tyan, Y. C. (2022). Hydrogels: Properties and Applications in Biomedicine. *Molecules (Basel, Switzerland)*, *27*(9), 2902. https://doi.org/10.3390/molecules27092902

Feng, P., Luo, Y., Ke, C., Qiu, H., Wang, W., Zhu, Y., … & Wu, S. (2021b). Chitosan-based functional materials for skin wound repair: Mechanisms and applications. Frontiers in Bioengineering and Biotechnology, 9, 650598.

Golmohammadi, R., Najar-Peerayeh, S., Tohidi Moghadam, T., & Hosseini, S. M. J. (2020). Synergistic Antibacterial Activity and Wound Healing Properties of Selenium-Chitosan-Mupirocin Nanohybrid System: An in Vivo Study on Rat Diabetic Staphylococcus aureus Wound Infection Model. *Scientific reports*, *10*(1), 2854. https://doi.org/10.1038/s41598-020-59510-5

Sekhon, U. D. S. (2021). Bio-Inspired Enzyme Responsive Nanotechnologies for the Treatment of Bleeding Dysfunctions. Case Western Reserve University.

Araneda Cisternas, M., & Varaprasad, K. (2024). Chitosan-Based Biomaterials for Hemostasis and Wound Healing.

Ellis, S., Lin, E. J., & Tartar, D. M. (2018). Immunology of Wound Healing. *Current Dermatology Reports*, *7*(4), 350–358. https://doi.org/10.1007/S13671-018-0234-9

Shoaib, M., & Wang, Z. (2020). Application of Chitosan as an Antimicrobial Agent. *Journal of Food and Nutritional Health*, *1*(1). https://doi.org/10.47275/2692-5222-106

Ghattas, M., Dwivedi, G., Chevrier, A., Horn-Bourque, D., Alameh, M. G., & Lavertu, M. (2025). Chitosan immunomodulation: insights into mechanisms of action on immune cells and signaling pathways. *RSC advances*, *15*(2), 896–909. https://doi.org/10.1039/d4ra08406c

Lewicki, S., Zwoliński, M., Hovagimyan, A., Stelmasiak, M., Szarpak, Ł., Lewicka, A., Pojda, Z., & Szymański, Ł. (2023). Chitosan-Based Dressing as a Sustained Delivery System for Bioactive Cytokines. *International journal of molecular sciences*, *25*(1), 30. https://doi.org/10.3390/ijms25010030

Mawazi, S. M., Kumar, M., Ahmad, N., & Mahmood, S. (2024). Recent Applications of Chitosan and Its Derivatives in Antibacterial, Anticancer, Wound Healing, and Tissue Engineering Fields. *Polymers*. https://doi.org/10.3390/polym16101351

Vijayan, A., A, S., & Kumar, G. S. V. (2019). PEG grafted chitosan scaffold for dual growth factor delivery for enhanced wound healing. *Scientific reports*, *9*(1), 19165. https://doi.org/10.1038/s41598-019-55214-7

Zahid, M., Lodhi, M., Rehan, Z. A., Tayyab, H., Javed, T., Javed, T., Shabbir, R., Mukhtar, A., Sabagh, A. E., Sabagh, A. E., Adamski, R., Sakran, M. I., Sakran, M. I., & Siuta, D. (2021). Sustainable Development of Chitosan/Calotropis procera-Based Hydrogels to Stimulate Formation of Granulation Tissue and Angiogenesis in Wound Healing Applications. *Molecules*, *26*(11), 3284. https://doi.org/10.3390/MOLECULES26113284

Farhadihosseinabadi, B., Zarebkohan, A., Eftekhary, M., Heiat, M., Moosazadeh Moghaddam, M., & Gholipourmalekabadi, M. (2019). Crosstalk between chitosan and cell signaling pathways. *Cellular and molecular life sciences: CMLS*, *76*(14), 2697–2718. https://doi.org/10.1007/s00018-019-03107-3

Dev, A. S., Mohan, N., & Mohan, R. (2025). Chitosan-based composite scaffolds for accelerated epidermal-dermal wound healing. *Exploration of BioMat-X*, *2*, 101336.

Wang, C., Yu, Y., Chen, H., Zhang, S., Wang, J., & Liu, C. (2019b). Construction of cytokine reservoirs based on sulfated chitosan hydrogels for the capturing of VEGF in situ. *Journal of Materials Chemistry B*, *7*(11), 1882–1892.

Mohandas, A., & Rangasamy, J. (2021). Nanocurcumin and arginine entrapped injectable chitosan hydrogel for restoration of hypoxia induced endothelial dysfunction. International Journal of Biological Macromolecules, 166, 471–482.

Veith, A. P., Henderson, K., Spencer, A., Sligar, A. D., & Baker, A. B. (2019). Therapeutic strategies for enhancing angiogenesis in wound healing. *Advanced drug delivery reviews*, *146*, 97–125. https://doi.org/10.1016/j.addr.2018.09.010

Pal, D., Das, P., Mukherjee, P., Roy, S., Chaudhuri, S., Kesh, S. S., ... & Nandi, S. K. (2024). Biomaterials-based strategies to enhance angiogenesis in diabetic wound healing. *ACS Biomaterials Science & Engineering*, *10*(5), 2725–2741.

Yadav, S., & Palei, N. N. (2024). Chitosan as Biomaterial for Wound healing: Mechanisms and Various applications. *Research Journal of Pharmacy and Technology*, *17*(10), 5102–5112.

Ferreira, P. G., Ferreira, V. F., da Silva, F. d. C., Freitas, C. S., Pereira, P. R., & Paschoalin, V. M. F. (2022). Chitosans and Nanochitosans: Recent Advances in Skin Protection, Regeneration, and Repair. *Pharmaceutics*, *14*(6), 1307. https://doi.org/10.3390/pharmaceutics14061307

Iacob, A. T., Lupascu, F. G., Apotrosoaei, M., Vasincu, I. M., Tauser, R. G., Lupascu, D., Giusca, S. E., Caruntu, I.-D., & Profire, L. (2021). Recent Biomedical Approaches for Chitosan Based Materials as Drug Delivery Nanocarriers. Pharmaceutics, 13(4), 587. https://doi.org/10.3390/pharmaceutics13040587

Barbosa, A. I., Coutinho, A. J., Costa Lima, S. A., & Reis, S. (2019). Marine Polysaccharides in Pharmaceutical Applications: Fucoidan and Chitosan as Key Players in the Drug Delivery Match Field. *Marine Drugs*, *17*(12), 654. https://doi.org/10.3390/md17120654

Shi, C., Zhu, Y., Ran, X., Wang, M., Su, Y., & Cheng, T. (2006). Therapeutic potential of chitosan and its derivatives in regenerative medicine. *Journal of Surgical research*, *133*(2), 185–192.

Dixit, K., Bora, H., Lakshmi Parimi, J., Mukherjee, G., & Dhara, S. (2023). Biomaterial mediated immunomodulation: An interplay of material environment interaction for ameliorating wound regeneration. *Journal of Biomaterials Applications*, *37*(9), 1509–1528.

Rahaman, J., & Mukherjee, D. (2025). Insulin for oral bone tissue engineering: a review on innovations in targeted insulin-loaded nanocarrier scaffold. *Journal of Drug Targeting*, *33*(5), 648–665. https://doi.org/10.1080/1061186X.2024.2445737

Zhang, L., Ma, Y., Pan, X., Chen, S., Zhuang, H., & Wang, S. (2018). A composite hydrogel of chitosan/heparin/poly (γ-glutamic acid) loaded with superoxide dismutase for wound healing. *Carbohydrate polymers*, *180*, 168–174.

Marrazzo, P., & O'Leary, C. (2020). Repositioning Natural Antioxidants for Therapeutic Applications in Tissue Engineering. Bioengineering, 7(3), 104. https://doi.org/10.3390/bioengineering7030104

Moe, S., Khaing, T. A., Zin Han, T., & Myat Mon, H. (2008). Effects of Chitosan Films on Wound Healing and Evaluation of Their Properties. In *International Conference on Sustainable Development: Issues and Prospects for the GMS*.

Moreira, V. M., Leite, J. M. D. S., Medeiros, K. D. A., Assis, K. M. A. D., Borges, J. C., Santana, L. M. B., ... & Damasceno, B. P. G. D. L. (2023). Pentoxifylline/chitosan films on wound healing: In vitro/in vivo evaluation. *Pharmaceutics*, *15*(4), 1122.

Ngadaonye, J. I., Geever, L. M., McEvoy, K. E., Killion, J., Brady, D. B., & Higginbotham, C. L. (2014). Evaluation of novel antibiotic-eluting thermoresponsive chitosan-PDEAAm based wound dressings. *International Journal of Polymeric Materials and Polymeric Biomaterials*, *63*(17), 873–883.

Jangra, N., Singla, A., Puri, V., Dheer, D., Chopra, H., Malik, T., & Sharma, A. (2025). Herbal bioactive-loaded biopolymeric formulations for wound healing applications. *RSC advances*, *15*(16), 12402–12442.

El-Husseiny, H. M., Mady, E. A., Hamabe, L., Abugomaa, A., Shimada, K., Yoshida, T., ... & Tanaka, R. (2022). Smart/stimuli-responsive hydrogels: Cutting-edge platforms for tissue engineering and other biomedical applications. *Materials Today Bio*, *13*, 100186.

Gounden, V., & Singh, M. (2024). Hydrogels and Wound Healing: Current and Future Prospects. *Gels*, *10*(1), 43. https://doi.org/10.3390/gels10010043

Brumberg, V., Astrelina, T., Malivanova, T., & Samoilov, A. (2021). Modern Wound Dressings: Hydrogel Dressings. *Biomedicines*, *9*(9), 1235. https://doi.org/10.3390/biomedicines9091235

Edwards J. (2010). Hydrogels and their potential uses in burn wound management. *British journal of nursing (Mark Allen Publishing)*, *19*(11), S12–S16. https://doi.org/10.12968/bjon.2010.19.Sup4.48419

Brown, M. A., Daya, M. R., & Worley, J. A. (2009). Experience with chitosan dressings in a civilian EMS system. *The Journal of emergency medicine*, *37*(1), 1–7.

Linju, M. C., & Rekha, M. R. (2023). Proline conjugated chitosan as wound healing material: In vitro studies on the influence of the scaffold on collagen production and wound healing. *International journal of biological macromolecules*, *242*(Pt 1), 124688. https://doi.org/10.1016/j.ijbiomac.2023.124688

Jafernik, K., Ładniak, A., Blicharska, E., Czarnek, K., Ekiert, H., Wiącek, A. E., & Szopa, A. (2023). Chitosan-Based Nanoparticles as Effective Drug Delivery Systems—A review. *Molecules*, *28*(4), 1963. https://doi.org/10.3390/molecules28041963

Placha, D., & Jampilek, J. (2021). Chronic Inflammatory Diseases, Anti-Inflammatory Agents and Their Delivery Nanosystems. *Pharmaceutics*, *13*(1), 64. https://doi.org/10.3390/pharmaceutics13010064

Alehosseini, E., Shahiri Tabarestani, H., Kharazmi, M. S., & Jafari, S. M. (2022). Physicochemical, Thermal, and Morphological Properties of Chitosan Nanoparticles Produced by Ionic Gelation. Foods, 11(23), 3841. https://doi.org/10.3390/foods11233841

Bashir, S. M., Ahmed Rather, G., Patrício, A., Haq, Z., Sheikh, A. A., Shah, M. Z. U. H., ... & Fonte, P. (2022). Chitosan nanoparticles: a versatile platform for biomedical applications. *Materials*, *15*(19), 6521.

Sethuram, L., & Thomas, J. (2023). Therapeutic applications of electrospun nanofibers impregnated with various biological macromolecules for effective wound healing strategy–a review. *Biomedicine & Pharmacotherapy*, *157*, 113996.

Taokaew, S., & Chuenkaek, T. (2024). Developments of Core/Shell Chitosan-Based Nanofibers by Electrospinning Techniques: A Review. *Fibers*, *12*(3), 26. https://doi.org/10.3390/fib12030026

Rezaei, A., & Ehtesabi, H. (2022). Fabrication of alginate/chitosan nanocomposite sponges using green synthesized carbon dots as potential wound dressing. *Materials Today Chemistry*, *24*, 100910.

Valachová, K., El Meligy, M. A., & Šoltés, L. (2022). Hyaluronic acid and chitosan-based electrospun wound dressings: Problems and solutions. *International Journal of Biological Macromolecules*, *206*, 74–91.

Naseri, N., Algan, C., Jacobs, V., John, M., Oksman, K., & Mathew, A. P. (2014). Electrospun chitosan-based nanocomposite mats reinforced with chitin nanocrystals for wound dressing. *Carbohydrate polymers*, *109*, 7–15.

Cheung, R. C. F., Ng, T. B., Wong, J. H., & Chan, W..Y. (2015). Chitosan: An Update on Potential Biomedical and Pharmaceutical Applications. Marine Drugs, 13(8), 5156–5186. https://doi.org/10.3390/md13085156

Marine Seaweed Polysaccharide-Based Scaffolds in Tissue Regeneration

Deepa Thomas and M. S. Latha

Abstract Marine seaweed polysaccharides have emerged as a potential biomaterial for tissue regeneration due to their unique properties, such as biocompatibility, biodegradability, and capability to mimic the extracellular matrix. This chapter reviews the current state of marine seaweed polysaccharide-based scaffolds in tissue regeneration, highlighting their potential applications in various tissues, including the bone, cartilage, skin, and nerve. We discuss the advantages and challenges of using marine seaweed polysaccharides as scaffold materials, as well as the future directions for research and advances in this field.

Keywords Marine seaweed polysaccharide · Tissue regeneration · Biodegradable · Scaffold

1 Introduction

Tissue engineering has emerged as a promising solution for repairing or replacing damaged or diseased tissues, as the human body's natural regenerative capabilities are often limited. Restoring tissue function through tissue regeneration is a complex process that requires the coordinated action of several cell types, growth hormones, and extracellular matrix constituents. Inflammation, cell proliferation, cell differentiation, tissue organisation, and tissue maturation are some of the discrete stages that make up this process, and they all cooperate to help replace or repair injured tissue.

D. Thomas
Research and Post Graduate Department of Chemistry, Bishop Moore College, Mavelikara, Kerala, India

M. S. Latha (✉)
Department of Chemistry, Sree Narayana College, Kollam, Kerala, India

Sree Narayana Guru College of Advanced Studies, Nangiarkulangara, Kerala, India

S. Jana et al. (eds.), *Multifunctional Marine Polysaccharides*,
https://doi.org/10.1007/978-981-95-4126-3_12

By understanding and harnessing the complexities of tissue regeneration, researchers aim to formulate innovative tissue engineering constructs that can effectively restore tissue function and promote healing (Wang et al. 2024).

Biomaterials are essential for tissue regeneration because they offer a structural framework that promotes tissue development and cell proliferation. The generation of functional tissue is eventually aided by them as they promote the regeneration process in a number of ways, including tissue organisation, growth factor and signalling molecule supply, cell adhesion and proliferation, and mechanical support. Biomaterials can also promote vascularization, which is an essential part of tissue regeneration, by offering a scaffold for cells to proliferate and interact (Farag 2023).

The three primary categories of biomaterials utilised in tissue regeneration are natural, synthetic, and hybrid biomaterials. Natural biomaterials, such as collagen, alginate, chitosan, hyaluronic acid, and fibrin, come from natural sources. These biomaterials are appropriate for tissue engineering applications since they are frequently biocompatible and biodegradable (Krishani et al. 2023). Conversely, synthetic biomaterials are materials that are created by humans, such as poly (ethylene glycol) (PEG), poly (glycolic acid) (PGA), poly (lactic acid) (PLA), poly (lactic-co-glycolic acid) (PLGA), and poly(caprolactone) (PCL). These biomaterials can be customised for certain uses and have a variety of qualities (Pérez et al. 2013). Collagen-PLA, alginate-PEG, and chitosan-PLGA are examples of hybrid biomaterials, which blend natural and synthetic ingredients to produce biomaterials with special qualities and benefits. These hybrid biomaterials are appropriate for numerous tissue engineering applications as they can provide enhanced mechanical, biocompatibility, and biodegradability (Lewandowska-Łańcucka et al. 2015).

Over the past two decades, research has extensively explored the potential of seaweed-derived polysaccharides in various biomedical applications, including tissue engineering, wound healing, drug delivery, and biosensors. These marine polysaccharides have become a crucial component of the rapidly growing marine bioindustry globally. Derived from diverse species of seaweed, such as red, brown, and green algae, marine seaweed polysaccharides are complex carbohydrates that have garnered substantial attention for their unique properties and potential uses in various fields, particularly tissue regeneration. Due to their exceptional biocompatibility, biodegradability, and bioactivity, these polysaccharides, including alginate, carrageenan, ulvan, and fucoidan, are considered ideal for creating scaffolds in tissue engineering and regenerative medicine applications. Their ability to support tissue and organ growth makes them a valuable resource in the development of innovative biomedical solutions (Chandika et al. 2015; Wang et al. 2023).

This chapter covers an extensive overview of scaffolds for tissue regeneration based on polysaccharides found in marine seaweed. It begins with an exploration of the inherent characteristics of these polysaccharides, followed by a detailed discussion of their application in regenerating specific tissues. The chapter additionally looks into the advantages and challenges of using them and concludes by suggesting possible directions for further research.

2 Properties of Marine Seaweed Polysaccharides

2.1 *Structural Composition*

Brown (Phaeophyceae), red (Rhodophyceae), and green (Chlorophyceae) seaweeds are the three main types of marine algae. Different polysaccharides with distinctive structural characteristics define each of these groupings. Green algae mostly generate ulvan, red algae produce agar and carrageenan, while brown algae are rich in alginate and fucoidan.

Alginate, derived from brown seaweed, is a linear anionic polysaccharide consisting of (1 $\rightarrow$ 4)-linked β-D-mannuronic acid (M) and α-L-guluronic acid (G) units. The ratio and sequential arrangement of these residues affect the gelation capacity and mechanical characteristics of alginate-based scaffolds. Carrageenan, obtained from red seaweed, comprises sulphated galactose units and exists in many forms (κ-, ι-, and λ-carrageenan) determined by the degree and position of sulphation. Ulvan, derived from green seaweed, is a sulphated heteropolysaccharide predominantly consisting of rhamnose, xylose, glucuronic acid, and iduronic acid. These structural differences yield distinct physicochemical and biological properties, facilitating customised scaffold designs for certain tissue regeneration applications (Narasimhan et al. 2023).

2.2 *Biocompatibility*

The remarkable biocompatibility of marine polysaccharides, including alginate, carrageenan, chitosan, and fucoidan, is primarily due to their structural similarity to glycosaminoglycans (GAGs) and other extracellular matrix (ECM) constituents. They are appropriate for biomedical applications, such as tissue engineering and regenerative medicine, because of their resemblance, which enables them to blend in perfectly with biological systems, simulating the normal cellular environment and supporting important physiological processes. Tissue regeneration depends on these biomaterials' support for vital cellular processes as adhesion, proliferation, migration, and differentiation. Their ability to create gels and their hydrophilic nature further improve nutrient diffusion and cell encapsulation, resulting in the perfect microenvironment for tissue formation and even boosting the viability of a variety of cell types (Carvalho et al. 2021).

Several in vitro and in vivo investigations have shown that hydrogels based on alginate and carrageenan are non-toxic and have the ability to preserve and even improve the survival of a variety of cell types. Furthermore, when cultivated in these marine-derived matrices, keratinocytes and neurones have demonstrated both healthy morphology and functional activity, highlighting their adaptability to a variety of tissue types (Iravani and Jamalipour Soufi 2021). Marine polysaccharides are a useful resource in the creation of novel biomedical solutions because their biocompatibility may be adjusted to fit particular applications by changes such as sulphation, acetylation, or combining with other polymers,

2.3 Biodegradability

The dynamic processes of tissue regeneration are ideally suited to the advantageous biodegradability profiles of marine polysaccharides, such as alginate, carrageenan, and fucoidan. The reason for their biodegradability is their polysaccharide structure, which enzymes like glycosidases may readily hydrolyse and then be metabolised by the body. During the healing process, the scaffold can be gradually replaced with newly produced tissue thanks to this regulated breakdown, facilitating a smooth transition. By altering variables including molecular weight, degree of crosslinking, and chemical composition, the rate of biodegradation can be adjusted, giving tissue engineers the freedom to customise the degradation profile to meet their unique requirements (Reddy et al. 2023).

In contrast to more substantially modified or blended systems, which provide longer structural stability, minimally crosslinked alginate hydrogels breakdown more quickly and are best suited for applications needing short-term support (Iqbal et al. 2024). Crucially, the breakdown products of marine polysaccharides are often non-toxic and easily absorbed or eliminated by the body, reducing the possibility of chronic buildup or inflammation. Because marine polysaccharides are biodegradable and biocompatible, they are a desirable option for biomedical applications where removing foreign substances is essential to preserve tissue health and function.

2.4 Gelation and Rheological Properties

Marine seaweed polysaccharides, including agar, carrageenan, and alginate, have special rheological and gelation characteristics that make them appropriate for a range of industrial and biological uses. Several processes, such as ionic gelation, thermal gelation, and pH-dependent gelation, can cause these polysaccharides to gel, producing hydrogels with specific characteristics. Its rheological characteristics—such as their viscoelasticity, thixotropy, and non-Newtonian behaviour—allow them to adapt to a variety of environmental factors, which makes them perfect for tissue engineering applications (Akter et al. 2024).

The shear-thinning behaviour of these marine polysaccharide gels makes them appropriate for 3D bioprinting and injectable formulations where recovery at rest and flow under stress are crucial. It is possible to accurately control their viscoelastic nature by varying variables including temperature, ionic conditions, molecular weight, and polymer concentration. The mechanical characteristics of biological tissues, such as stiffer cartilage and soft brain tissue, can thus be replicated by researchers. Furthermore, regulating the mechanical stiffness and gelation kinetics permits regulated cell behaviour, such as tissue organisation, migration, and differentiation inside the scaffold (Wang and Zhou 2024).

2.5 Mechanical Properties

As marine seaweed-derived polysaccharides must replicate the target tissue's natural ECM while offering sufficient structural support, their mechanical characteristics are essential in establishing their appropriateness for tissue engineering applications. Extracted from brown and red seaweeds, polysaccharides including alginate, carrageenan, and agar have mechanical properties that can be adjusted by crosslinking, chemical modification, or combining with other biomaterials. Depending on their concentration, molecular weight, and the presence of ions or co-polymers, these polymers naturally produce hydrogels with different levels of stiffness and elasticity.

Alginate hydrogels have demonstrated exceptional mechanical qualities, with tensile strengths between 10 and 100 kPa, which qualifies them for use in tissue engineering (Sahoo and Biswal 2021). Similarly, hydrogels based on carrageenan have been shown to have high compressive strengths, which makes them perfect for use in drug administration and wound dressing applications.

Even though marine polysaccharide hydrogels frequently have lower mechanical strengths than synthetic polymers, they can be strengthened by adding reinforcing agents like graphene oxide, nanocellulose, or bioactive ceramics to create composite materials with better durability, compressive modulus, and tensile strength (Yosri et al. 2024). Moreover, it is possible to tailor their mechanical behaviour to display viscoelasticity and stress relaxation, both of which are critical for sustaining dynamic cell-matrix interactions throughout tissue formation.

2.6 Bioactivity and Cell Interaction

Polysaccharides derived from marine seaweed, including carrageenan, alginate, and fucoidan, have been shown to have exceptional cell interaction and bioactivity qualities, which makes them appealing candidates for a range of biomedical uses. Numerous cellular processes, such as cell migration, differentiation, and proliferation, have been demonstrated to be modulated by these polysaccharides through their interactions with cells. These polymers, especially sulphated types like ulvan, carrageenan, and fucoidan, have been shown to have anti-inflammatory, anti-coagulant, antiviral, antioxidant, and anticancer properties (Xie et al. 2024). Structural characteristics that affect their interaction with cellular receptors and extracellular matrix components, such as molecular weight, degree of sulphation, and monosaccharide composition, are major determinants of their bioactivity.

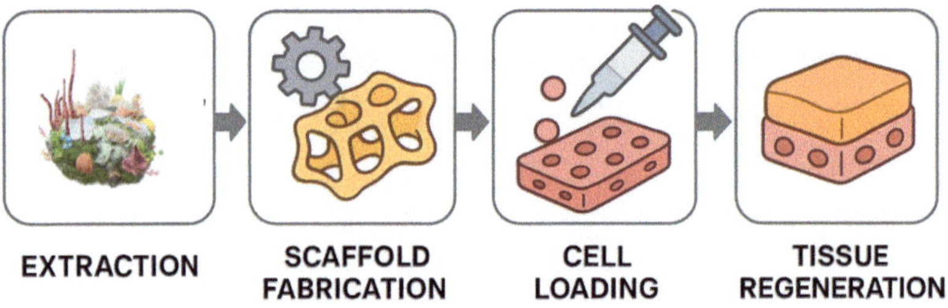

Fig. 1 Schematic overview of tissue engineering using marine polysaccharides

Additionally, alginate has demonstrated the ability to stimulate fibroblast proliferation and extracellular matrix remodelling, hence promoting tissue regeneration. The distinct chemical structures of marine seaweed-derived polysaccharides are responsible for their bioactivity and cell interaction characteristics. These structures can be altered using a variety of methods to enhance the bioactivity and specificity of the polysaccharides.

Thus, marine polysaccharides are pivotal in tissue engineering due to their exceptional biocompatibility, biodegradability, and inherent bioactivity. These biomaterials are engineered into 3D scaffolds, such as hydrogels, fibres, or sponges, which mimic the extracellular matrix, giving structural support for cell attachment, proliferation, and differentiation. The tissue engineering process involves scaffold fabrication, cell seeding, and cultivation under controlled conditions to promote tissue maturation. Marine polysaccharides not only provide structural support but also actively modulate cellular behaviour through their molecular architecture, promoting angiogenesis, immune modulation, and wound healing. Upon implantation, the scaffold degrades gradually, promoting native tissue regeneration driven by both structural and biochemical cues from the marine polysaccharide matrix. Figure 1 illustrates the schematic overview of tissue engineering using marine polysaccharides.

3 Biological Functions in Tissue Regeneration

3.1 Cell Adhesion, Proliferation, and Differentiation

The capacity of biomaterials to improve cell adhesion, proliferation, and lineage-specific differentiation is a crucial aspect of tissue regeneration. These cellular processes are facilitated by the biomimetic milieu provided by marine seaweed polysaccharides, specifically alginate, fucoidan, and carrageenan. When crosslinked into hydrogel matrices, alginate provides a porous scaffold structure that sustains cell viability and encourages cellular adhesion. Because fucoidan is sulphated, it has been demonstrated to improve stem cell and progenitor cell proliferation and neural development via modifying signalling pathways linked to growth factors like VEGF and FGF. Through their intricate carbohydrate backbones, carrageenan and ulvan also facilitate matrix interactions and cellular colonisation while offering vital biochemical cues.

3.2 *Angiogenesis and Extracellular Matrix Remodelling*

Angiogenesis, the formation of new blood vessels, is a critical process in wound healing, as it ensures the delivery of essential nutrients and oxygen to regenerating tissues. Marine polysaccharides have been found to play a significant role in promoting angiogenesis by stimulating the migration and proliferation of endothelial cells. By affecting matrix metalloproteinases' activity and the deposition of ECM proteins like collagen and fibronectin, these polysaccharides also contribute to ECM remodelling. ECM remodelling controls tissue morphogenesis and cell migration during regeneration in addition to restoring the structural integrity of tissues.

3.3 *Inflammation Modulation and Antimicrobial Activity*

Effective management of inflammation is critical for preventing chronic wound conditions and promoting a conducive healing environment. Marine seaweed polysaccharides have been shown to exhibit significant anti-inflammatory benefits through two key mechanisms: the polarization of M2 macrophages, which is associated with tissue repair, and the downregulation of pro-inflammatory cytokines. Furthermore, certain seaweed-derived polysaccharides possess inherent antibacterial properties, which reduce the risk of infection in wounds and implanted scaffolds. This dual functionality of marine polysaccharides, modulating immune response and inhibiting microbial colonization, enhances their therapeutic potential in tissue engineering applications. By regulating the immune response and preventing infection, these polysaccharides facilitate a more controlled and efficient regenerative process, ultimately promoting successful tissue repair and regeneration. Table 1 illustrates an overview of role of marine polysaccharide scaffolds in tissue regeneration.

4 Fabrication Strategies for Polysaccharide-Based Scaffolds

The fabrication of scaffolds based on marine seaweed polysaccharides is essential to evaluate their bioactivity, durability, and compatibility for specific tissue engineering application. These polysaccharides, which include alginate, fucoidan,

Table 1 Marine polysaccharide scaffolds in tissue regeneration

Polysaccharide	Structure	Scaffold form	Applications	Key benefits	References
Alginate	Linear polysaccharide composed of α-L-guluronic acid (G) and β-D-mannuronic acid (M) residues	Hydrogel, composite, foam	Bone, cartilage, wound healing	Biocompatibility, gelation under mild conditions, supports cell encapsulation, adhesion, proliferation, and differentiation	Lee and Mooney (2012)
Ulvan	Sulphated polyelectrolyte composed of recurrent disaccharides units (xylose and rhamnose) and glucuronic acid	Film, Hydrogel	Skin, nerve, cardiovascular	Sulphated structure promotes antioxidant and anti-inflammatory properties, enhances cell growth and differentiation	Flórez-Fernández et al. (2023)
Fucoidan	Sulphated polysaccharide composed of L-fucose and sulphate ester groups	Sponge, nanofiber, hydrogel	Wound healing, bone, angiogenesis	Anti-inflammatory, promotes angiogenesis, cell signalling modulation, and tissue repair	
Carrageenan	Sulphated polysaccharide composed of alternating β-D-galactose and α-D-galactose or 3,6-anhydro-α-D-galactose residues	Hydrogel, film	Cartilage, skin, soft tissue	ECM mimicry, mechanical strength, enhances chondrogenesis. Supports cell adhesion and proliferation	

carrageenan, and ulvan, can be transformed into three-dimensional structures that resemble the ECM using a variety of techniques. This creates an environment that is favourable for tissue regeneration and cell proliferation.

4.1 3D Bioprinting

Customised, cell-filled structures can be precisely fabricated in terms of both space and architecture through 3D bioprinting. Alginate, a marine-derived polysaccharide, has emerged as a leading bioink candidate, owing to its exceptional properties, including rapid gelation and excellent biocompatibility with living cells, making it an ideal material for 3D bioprinting applications. 3D printed scaffolds have demonstrated remarkable potential in various regenerative medicine applications, spanning from bone reconstruction to skin regeneration, exhibiting promising outcomes in facilitating tissue repair and regeneration.

4.2 Electrospinning

Electrospinning is employed to fabricate fibrous scaffolds that mimic the extracellular matrix, providing a favourable environment for tissue regeneration. To overcome the poor spinnability of marine polysaccharides and enhance their mechanical properties, blending them with synthetic polymers, such as polycaprolactone or polyethylene oxide, is a common strategy. Electrospun nanofibers loaded with seaweed-derived polysaccharides have demonstrated improved cell adhesion and proliferation, rendering them suitable for applications in skin and nerve regeneration. Moreover, surface functionalization with ulvan or fucoidan provides additional biological cues that guide tissue repair, further enhancing the regenerative potential of these scaffolds.

4.3 Hydrogel Formation

Hydrogels have emerged as a versatile scaffold structure in regenerative medicine, characterized by their high water content and tissue-like consistency. To encapsulate cells or therapeutic agents, hydrogels are often fabricated through ionic crosslinking, with calcium ions being particularly effective in the case of alginate. These hydrogels, which can be pre-formed or injectable, enable the sustained release of medications and growth factors at the wound site, promoting tissue repair and regeneration. Furthermore, the incorporation of carrageenan and fucoidan into hydrogel networks has been shown to enhance their biological functionality, particularly due to the interactions between their sulphate groups and growth factors, which facilitates the creation of a favourable environment for tissue regeneration.

4.4 Freeze-drying and Cryogelation

Freeze-drying, or lyophilization, is a widely employed technique for fabricating porous scaffolds with high surface areas and interconnected pore structures, which facilitate vascularization and nutrient transfer. This method is particularly effective when polysaccharides are combined with cellulose for skin tissue engineering applications or with bioactive ceramics for bone regeneration. The resulting scaffolds exhibit suitable compressive strength and biodegradation rates, which are consistent with the natural dynamics of tissue healing, thereby providing a supportive environment for tissue regeneration and repair (Madub et al. 2021).

5 Applications of Marine Seaweed Polysaccharide-Based Scaffolds in Tissue Regeneration

Figure 2 illustrates the applications of marine seaweed polysaccharide-based scaffolds in tissue regeneration.

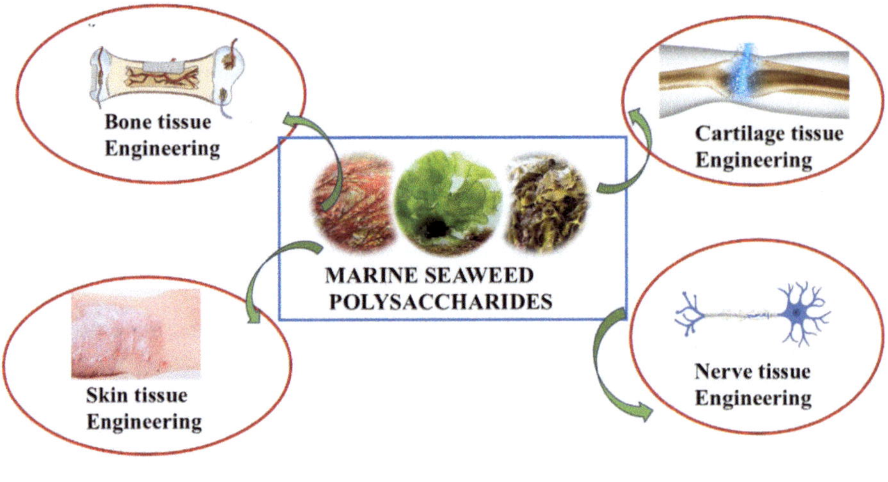

Fig. 2 Applications of marine seaweed polysaccharide-based scaffolds in tissue regeneration

5.1 Bone Tissue Regeneration

Traumatic, infectious, or surgically curable bone abnormalities present a major clinical issue. In order to enable bone regeneration, scaffolds need to encourage osteogenic differentiation, facilitate the integration of new bone tissue, and offer mechanical support. In these applications, marine seaweed polysaccharides have shown a great deal of promise.

Alginate, carrageenan, fucoidan, and ulvan polysaccharides derived from brown, red, and green algae are being investigated more and more for use in the creation of scaffolds in bone tissue regeneration. The goal of bone tissue engineering is to create biomaterials that can replicate the composition and capabilities of natural bone in order to support tissue repair and regeneration. Scaffolds made of marine seaweed polysaccharides have shown promise because of their special qualities, which include biocompatibility, biodegradability, and bioactivity.

The use of alginate as a scaffold material in bone tissue engineering has been thoroughly investigated. However, because of its limited mechanical strength, it is frequently combined with bioactive compounds or other polymers to improve its biological and physicochemical characteristics. The mechanical characteristics, bioactivity, and cell growth and differentiation of alginate scaffolds have all been demonstrated to be enhanced by alginate-based composites, which blend alginate with additional biomaterials. Alginate-based composites have a wide range of potential uses in bone tissue engineering. These composites can be utilised as a substitute to conventional bone grafts, lowering the risk of immunological rejection and disease transmission, and to repair bone abnormalities brought on by accident, illness, or surgery. Moreover, tissue-engineered bone replacements that can be utilised to replace or repair injured bone tissue can be made using alginate-based composite.

Alginate scaffolds' osteoconductivity and mechanical strength are enhanced by adding hydroxyapatite (HA). Comparing porous alginate-HA scaffolds to pure alginate scaffolds, Lin and Yeh showed that the former showed better in vitro cell adhesion and mineralisation (Lin and Yen 2004). The use of doped bioglass (such as Zn or Mg) or mesoporous bioactive glass improves scaffold bioactivity, promoting antibacterial and bone repair. The release of bioactive ions from these materials promotes angiogenesis and osteoblast development (Zamani et al. 2019). The mechanical characteristics and cell adhesion of alginate scaffolds are also enhanced when alginate is combined with collagen, a significant extracellular matrix component. Numerous bone tissue engineering applications, including as bone grafting, tissue engineering, and bone defect repair, have been investigated for these composites (Su et al. 2020). Alginate can be blended with natural polymers such as silk fibroin or chitosan to enhance its mechanical qualities and promote improved cell adhesion. For instance, regulated drug release and increased cell proliferation were demonstrated by composite microspheres made of hydroxyapatite, chitosan, and alginate (Guang et al. 2019).

The sulphated polysaccharide fucoidan is well-known for its angiogenic, osteoinductive, and anti-inflammatory qualities. Applications involving bone tissue engineering can benefit from its anticoagulant, biocompatible, and bioactive qualities. Fucoidan has been found to increase osteoblast proliferation and mineralisation by inducing the expression of bone morphogenetic proteins.

Composites based on fucoidan have been investigated for a number of bone tissue engineering applications, providing encouraging options for bone regeneration and repair. In particular, these composites offer a practical substitute for conventional bone transplants and lower the danger of immunological rejection and disease transmission when used to restore bone abnormalities brought on by accident, illness, or surgery. Furthermore, tissue engineering can use fucoidan-based composites to produce customised bone replacements that can replace or repair damaged bone tissue, encouraging bone development and regeneration.

These composites have been developed to improve its qualities by mixing it with biomaterials like collagen, hydroxyapatite, and nanoparticles. These composites have demonstrated enhanced cell adhesion, bioactivity, and mechanical characteristics, which makes them attractive for use in bone tissue engineering. Fucoidan-hydroxyapatite composites, for example, have been demonstrated to stimulate bone mineralisation and osteogenic differentiation.

Fucoidan is frequently used with synthetic polymers like PCL in composite scaffolds to enhance their mechanical strength and biological activity. Fucoidan-PCL scaffolds made with 3D printing have shown improved structural support and increased bone matrix deposition. When compared to PCL alone, these have demonstrated improved osteogenic differentiation and increased mineral deposition.

Blends containing hydroxyapatite increase the rigidity of the scaffold and offer reservoirs for calcium and phosphate to promote osteoconduction. The bioactivity and mechanical characteristics of fucoidan scaffolds are improved by the addition of HA (Jeong et al. 2013). Collagen-fucoidan composites enhance the mechanical characteristics and cell adherence of fucoidan scaffolds (Shanmugapriya and Kang 2021). The bioactivity of fucoidan is combined with the structural advantages of alginate or chitosan in fucoidan-alginate/chitosan hydrogels. For less invasive bone restoration, they function as 3D-printed scaffolds or injectable devices (Murugan et al. 2022). Nanoparticles like titanium dioxide or silica can be added to fucoidan scaffolds to enhance their mechanical characteristics and bioactivity (Amorim et al. 2023).

The potential of carrageenan-based scaffolds to support bone growth and regeneration has been shown in prior investigations, which explored them in great detail for bone tissue regeneration. Carrageenan-based scaffolds have been demonstrated in studies are able to replicate the extracellular matrix, creating an environment that is favourable for cell growth and differentiation. Osteoblast-seeded scaffolds based on carrageenan facilitated the mineralisation and development of bone tissue.

Prior research has shown that carrageenan-based scaffolds have improved mechanical integrity and osteoconductive characteristics, especially when combined with hydroxyapatite (HA), chitosan, or gelatine. κ-carrageenan/HA composites have demonstrated promising results for improving mineral deposition, osteoblast adhesion, and proliferation all of which are essential processes in bone regeneration. In vitro studies demonstrate these scaffolds' capacity to promote osteogenic development and cell survival utilising osteoblast-like cell lines like MG-63 and MC3T3-E1. Carrageenan-based structures may also aid in early-stage bone formation and vascularization, which is crucial for successful scaffold integration and long-term regeneration outcomes (González Ocampo et al. 2019).

Scaffolds made of carrageenan and bioactive glass particles improved bone healing in lesions of crucial size (Qamar et al. 2024). Additionally, growth factor-modified carrageenan-based scaffolds enhanced osteogenic differentiation and bone tissue production. Peptide-modified carrageenan-based scaffolds enhanced bone mineralisation, higher expression of osteogenic markers, and osteogenic differentiation and bone tissue development (Batool et al. 2021).

Ulvan is a sulphated polysaccharide derived from *Ulva* species. Due to its bioactivity, biocompatibility, structural resemblance to glycosaminoglycans, and potential for customisation, it has become an attractive biomaterial for bone tissue engineering. Recent research has demonstrated that ulvan can be successfully blended into composite scaffolds which promote osteogenesis. Ulvan- PCL hybrid scaffolds facilitated bone mineralisation and tissue development while exhibiting strong osteoinductive properties (Kikionis et al. 2021). For bone scaffold design, ulvan-loaded PDLLA scaffolds were appropriate as they maintained mechanical integrity and cell compatibility (Alves et al. 2012). Polymeric scaffolds functionalised with ulvan have also been demonstrated to affect mineral formation, resulting in enhanced biomineralisation appropriate for bone repair applications (Dash et al. 2014). Its function in regulating scaffold construction and improving osteogenic results was further validated by hybrid sponge-like scaffolds composed of gelatin and ulvan (Tziveleka et al. 2020). According to recent evaluations, ulvan exhibits pro-osteogenic, immunomodulatory, and antioxidant properties that recommend its use in regenerative medicine.

Scaffolds made of marine seaweed polysaccharides have enormous potential for bone tissue regeneration because they combine therapeutic utility with ecological sustainability. These natural biomaterials could be widely used in next-generation regenerative therapeutics with further multidisciplinary study.

5.2 Cartilage Tissue Regeneration

Alginate-based scaffolds have been shown strong potential in cartilage tissue engineering due to their biocompatibility and ability to support chondrocyte viability. These scaffolds enhance chondrocyte growth and differentiation, which facilitates the deposition of vital extracellular matrix elements for cartilage, including glycosaminoglycans and type II collagen (Yang et al. 2018). Additionally, they showed great promise for improving the mechanical integrity of cartilage tissue that has been created, especially with regard to compressive and tensile strength. These scaffolds are renowned for having biomechanical characteristics that can be adjusted to replicate cartilage's natural mechanical environment. Researchers assessed the printability and structural integrity of alginate-based bioinks through unconfined compression tests, revealing optimal rheological and compressive properties crucial for successful 3D cartilage bioprinting (Yang et al. 2018). The incorporation of collagen into alginate scaffolds enhanced their tensile and compressive properties, thereby improving the structural stability and durability of the bioprinted cartilage constructs (Jahani et al. 2024).

Fucoidan has garnered significant interest in regenerative medicine owing to its versatile bioactive properties, particularly its robust anti-inflammatory and antioxidant capacities, which play a vital role in counteracting cartilage degeneration and fostering repair in inflamed environments. Within the realm of cartilage tissue regeneration, fucoidan-based scaffolds have shown promise in facilitating chondrocyte growth and specialization, which in turn augments the production of critical extracellular matrix constituents, including type II collagen and glycosaminoglycans, essential for healthy cartilage formation. Fucoidan is a good choice for biodegradable scaffold formulations in biomedical applications because of its exceptional biosafety profile and minimal immunogenicity. Furthermore, as it originates from nature, it can be easily combined with other ECM mimetic substances like collagen, gelatine, or hyaluronic acid to form composite scaffolds that more closely resemble the natural cartilage microenvironment. The intricate biomechanical and biological needs of regenerating hyaline cartilage may be better supported by these hybrid scaffolds, which could ultimately result in more successful tissue engineering techniques.

The biological efficacy of fucoidan is attributed to its capacity to regulate cellular redox balance and modulate inflammatory signalling pathways, thereby creating a conducive microenvironment that fosters cartilage repair. Fucoidan-based hydrogels have been leveraged as a vehicle for intra-articular delivery of platelet-rich plasma, yielding notable anti-inflammatory effects through the suppression of inflammatory mediators, concurrently facilitating cartilage repair and regeneration. Nanomaterials loaded with fucoidan demonstrated significant anti-inflammatory properties, notably reducing pro-inflammatory cytokines while maintaining cell viability and mammalian cell compatibility. Fucoidan can be used as a delivery system for chemicals that support cartilage healing because its sulphate groups allow it to interact electrostatically with growth factors. Moreover, hydrogels based on fucoidan can be engineered to have both micro and macro porous structures, which makes them appropriate for cartilage tissue engineering, nutrition exchange, and 3D chondrocyte encapsulation. Injectable fucoidan-composite hydrogels have demonstrated translational potential in the treatment of osteochondral defects through intra-articular administration. Collectively, these findings position fucoidan-based biomaterials as promising tools for cartilage tissue engineering, owing to their dual capacity to promote tissue regeneration while suppressing degenerative inflammatory responses.

The structural analogy between carrageenan and the native glycosaminoglycans present in articular cartilage has generated significant interest in its potential applications for cartilage tissue engineering. By mimicking the natural extracellular matrix environment, carrageenan-based scaffolds can facilitate chondrogenesis, promoting the development and differentiation of chondrocytes. Research has shown that carrageenan-based hydrogels can foster the synthesis of cartilage-specific extracellular matrix components while also enhancing the bioactivity of growth factors through interactions with its sulphated groups, ultimately encouraging cartilage repair and regeneration.

Research has demonstrated that carrageenan-based scaffolds can enhance cartilage tissue regeneration, exhibiting superior mechanical properties and histological scores compared to control groups. By incorporating carrageenan into hydrogel matrices or composite scaffolds, chondrocyte adhesion and proliferation are significantly promoted. The polyanionic sulphate groups of carrageenan interact positively with cellular receptors, facilitating improved cell-matrix interactions that are essential for matrix deposition and cartilage-specific gene expression. Moreover, carrageenan's physicochemical compatibility with bioinks makes it an ideal candidate for 3D bioprinting of cartilage structures, enabling the maintenance of structural integrity and nutrient transport within engineered tissues. Notably, carrageenan-based scaffolds have also been shown to control the immune response, reducing inflammation and fostering a regenerative microenvironment that promotes tissue repair.

The cartilage regenerative potential of carrageenan is significantly enhanced when combined with other biomaterials, such as collagen and hyaluronic acid. Composite scaffolds comprising collagen and carrageenan have been shown to augment cartilage tissue formation by promoting the differentiation of mesenchymal stem cells into chondrocytes. Similarly, the combination of carrageenan with hyaluronic acid in composite scaffolds has been demonstrated to enhance chondrocyte proliferation and differentiation, leading to increased production of cartilage matrix components. These synergistic effects highlight the potential of carrageenan-based composite scaffolds for enhanced cartilage tissue engineering.

Ulvan has developed as a promising biomaterial in cartilage tissue engineering due to its structural similarity to glycosaminoglycans, key components of the cartilage extracellular matrix. Comprised of rhamnose, xylose, and uronic acids, ulvan's unique chemical composition imparts biological properties that facilitate cell adhesion, proliferation, and differentiation, all of which are essential for cartilage regeneration. Research on marine biopolymers as extracellular matrix analogues in cartilage scaffolds has demonstrated that the sulphated groups present in ulvan facilitate interactions with growth factors, thereby augmenting their bioactivity and ultimately promoting the regeneration of cartilage tissue. Furthermore, studies have shown that ulvan-based hydrogels can support chondrocyte growth and differentiation by enhancing the production of cartilage-specific extracellular matrix components (Morelli et al. 2016).

It has been demonstrated that ulvan-based scaffolds promote cartilage tissue regeneration, as evidenced by improved mechanical characteristics and histology scores as compared to control groups. Furthermore, it has been shown that these scaffolds alter the immune response, reducing inflammation and creating an environment that is favourable for regeneration. Ulvan-based hydrogels' hydrophilic nature promotes chondrocyte survivability, while their adjustable viscoelastic qualities make them appropriate for the load-bearing roles of cartilage. Ulvan-collagen and ulvan-alginate composite biomaterials have been created recently; these materials not only have increased compressive strength but also, in vitro, increase the expression of chondrogenic genes like SOX9 and aggrecan. These biomaterials are also interesting prospects for clinical translation in cartilage tissue engineering applications due to their favourable biodegradability and low immunogenicity (Cui et al. 2024).

5.3 Skin Tissue Regeneration

Marine seaweed polysaccharides possess distinct structural and biological characteristics which made them powerful scaffolds in the field of skin tissue regeneration. These natural polymers have been investigated more and more for use in regenerative skin therapies, drug delivery, and wound healing. They increase the suppleness of the skin and promote the creation of collagen. These polysaccharides have also been demonstrated to improve wound healing by encouraging the migration, differentiation, and proliferation of cells. Additionally, their antibacterial and anti-inflammatory properties lower the risk of infection and foster an environment that is favourable for tissue regeneration. Many studies have emphasised the use of marine polysaccharides as "engineered cues" for biomedical applications, pointing out that their characteristics including gel-forming ability, biocompatibility, and biodegradability make them useful in tissue engineering and wound healing. Research has highlighted the potential of marine seaweed polysaccharides in anti-aging skin therapies, demonstrating their ability to stimulate collagen production and safeguard skin structure. Moreover, these biomolecules have shown promising applications in the development of antimicrobial surfaces and scaffolds for tissue regeneration, underscoring their broad therapeutic potential.

The potential of alginate to promote skin tissue regeneration has been thoroughly investigated. Its ability to keep wounds moist due to its hydrophilic properties is essential for encouraging epithelialisation and reducing the formation of scars throughout the healing process. It has been demonstrated that hydrogels based on alginate offer a favourable environment for cell division and development, accelerating the regeneration of skin tissue. It has been shown that using alginate to regenerate skin tissue improves the efficacy of wound healing. Alginate-based dressings have been demonstrated to reduce scar formation, enhance tissue strength, and speed up wound closure. Its potential as a therapeutic agent is highlighted by the fact that it has been demonstrated to enhance skin regeneration rates when added to scaffolds and wound dressings (Cui et al. 2024).

Although unmodified alginate lacks cell-adhesive properties, its combination with other biomaterials, such as collagen, hyaluronic acid, gelatine, or bioactive nanoparticles, has been shown to significantly enhance its potential for skin regeneration. Composite scaffolds composed of alginate and collagen, for instance, have been demonstrated to promote the differentiation of fibroblasts into myofibroblasts, resulting in improved wound closure and tissue strength. These composite hydrogels exhibit enhanced cellular interactions and mechanical properties, facilitating more effective integration with host tissue. Moreover, alginate-based dressings have been engineered to deliver growth factors or antimicrobial agents directly to the wound site, thereby accelerating the regenerative process while preventing infection. Clinically, alginate-based wound dressings, including hydrogels and films, have been approved and widely used for the treatment of chronic wounds, burns, and surgical incisions (Peng et al. 2022).

Fucoidan has been demonstrated to expedite wound healing by upregulating the expression of growth factors and cytokines, thereby facilitating the skin regeneration process. Its multifaceted bioactive features, including anti-inflammatory, antioxidant, and pro-angiogenic effects, contribute to its potential in promoting wound healing. Fucoidan has been shown to modulate pivotal cellular behaviours, such as fibroblast proliferation, keratinocyte migration, and extracellular matrix remodelling, which are essential for effective wound healing. Moreover, fucoidan enhances skin hydration and elasticity by stimulating the production of hyaluronic acid and collagen, respectively. Furthermore, fucoidan provides a scaffold for cell growth and differentiation, supporting the creation of a favourable microenvironment for skin tissue engineering.

By upregulating the expression of growth factors which in turn promote angiogenesis and fibroblast activity, it aids in the regeneration of skin tissue. Because of its strong affinity for heparin-like growth factors, fucoidan can carry these molecules to the wound site over time, creating an environment that is beneficial to tissue repair. Additionally, it has been demonstrated that fucoidan inhibits the activity of matrix metalloproteinases which can break down vital ECM components and are frequently overexpressed in chronic wounds. Fucoidan creates an environment that is favourable for skin tissue regeneration by finding a balance between maintaining the extracellular matrix and triggering cellular functions (Ghahtan et al. 2024).

The combination of fucoidan with other biomaterials, such as collagen and hyaluronic acid, has been shown to enhance its skin regenerative potential. Composite scaffolds composed of fucoidan and collagen have been demonstrated to promote the differentiation of fibroblasts into myofibroblasts, leading to improved wound closure and tissue strength (Perumal et al. 2018).

Carrageenan is a great option for accelerating wound healing and skin regeneration due to its biological qualities, which include immunomodulatory, antioxidant, and anti-inflammatory characteristics. The migration and proliferation of skin cells, such as fibroblasts and keratinocytes, which are critical for tissue regeneration and wound closure, have been demonstrated to be enhanced by it. Due to its structural resemblance to the extracellular matrix's glycosaminoglycans, carrageenan promotes cell adhesion and proliferation. According to studies, scaffolds based on carrageenan improve neovascularisation and dermal cell migration, two essential steps for efficient skin healing. It has been demonstrated that hydrogels based on carrageenan can decrease scarring, increase tissue strength, and speed up wound closure. Carrageenan has the potential to be a therapeutic agent because it has been demonstrated to enhance skin regeneration results when added to scaffolds and wound dressings.

The synergistic combination of carrageenan with other biomaterials, such as collagen and hyaluronic acid, has been shown to enhance its skin regenerative potential. Composite scaffolds composed of collagen and carrageenan have been demonstrated to promote the differentiation of fibroblasts into myofibroblasts, resulting in improved tissue strength and wound closure. Furthermore, the combination of carrageenan and hyaluronic acid has been shown to augment the skin's regenerative capacity. Hybrid hydrogel systems composed of carrageenan, gelatine, and locust bean gum have been developed, exhibiting enhanced biological and mechanical performance. These systems have been shown to facilitate the regeneration of full-thickness skin wounds by serving as vehicles for therapeutic agents or stem cells. Notably, the combination of carrageenan and ulvan has been found to significantly improve the healing outcomes of second-degree burn treatments.

Ulvan is structurally comparable to the extracellular matrix glycosaminoglycans of mammals since it is made up of rhamnose, glucuronic acid, iduronic acid, and xylose. Its biocompatibility and potential to enhance cell adhesion, elasticity, and proliferation are supported by this structural mimicry. Its antioxidant and immunomodulatory qualities, which are essential for controlling inflammation during the wound healing process a critical component in promoting healthy skin regeneration, are also influenced by its sulphate level. Hydrogels based on ulvan have been demonstrated to decrease scar formation, increase tissue strength, and speed up wound closure. It has been demonstrated that adding ulvan to scaffolds and wound dressings enhances the results of skin regeneration, underscoring its potential as a pharmaceutical agent (Flórez-Fernández et al. 2023).

Ulvan has being investigated more and more in the creation of hydrogels, films, and nanocomposites for use as scaffold materials in skin tissue engineering and as wound dressings. These substances can be designed to distribute bioactive substances, such as growth factors and antibiotics, and they produce a moist healing environment. Additionally, to improve its mechanical stability and biological importance, ulvan can be crosslinked with other biopolymers like chitosan or carrageenan due to its physicochemical characteristics. In both in vitro and in vivo scenarios, these hybrid systems have shown enhanced wound closure rates and higher dermal fibroblast activity. It has been demonstrated that ulvan and hyaluronic acid increase the skin's capacity for regeneration (Hwang et al. 2023).

5.4 Nerve Tissue Regeneration

Nerve tissue regeneration is an intricate process that necessitates the coordinated effort of multiple cell types, growth factors, and ECM components. Despite significant advances in regenerative medicine, the regeneration of damaged nerve tissues remains a formidable challenge due to the complex structure and limited intrinsic repair capacity of the nervous system. Conventional strategies, such as nerve autografts, are hindered by donor site morbidity and limited availability.

Marine seaweed polysaccharides, including alginate, fucoidan, carrageenan, and ulvan, have emerged as promising candidates for nerve tissue regeneration due to their neuroprotective and neuroregenerative properties. Recent studies have established the capacity of these polysaccharides to promote nerve cell growth, differentiation, and survival. Alginate has been extensively used to fabricate injectable hydrogels and conduits for nerve guidance due to its gelation capability and porous structure, which mimics the ECM of neural tissues.

Fucoidan has been reported to enhance the proliferation and neuronal differentiation of neural stem cells, while carrageenan has shown efficacy in promoting axonal regeneration and improving post-injury motor function. Additionally, both carrageenan and ulvan demonstrate anti-inflammatory and antioxidant effects, essential for establishing a neuroprotective milieu. The sulphated groups within these polysaccharides help attenuate oxidative stress and neuroinflammatory responses, thereby enhancing neuronal survival and regeneration outcomes.

Alginate and fucoidan hydrogels have demonstrated efficacy as three-dimensional matrices for encasing Schwann cells and neural progenitors, providing a conducive environment for axonal elongation and guidance. To improve therapeutic results, these systems can be further functionalised using conductive additives or bioactive substances. In vivo studies have demonstrated that freeze-dried sponge scaffolds derived from alginate-ulvan-cellulose blends provide advantageous topographical and mechanical characteristics for peripheral nerve healing. Moreover, the development of scaffolds that are both structurally accurate and physiologically active is made possible by the incorporation of marine polysaccharides into 3D-printable bioinks. Their natural biofunctions, which include immune cell behaviour modulation and neovascularisation stimulation, make them more suitable for use in brain injury treatments and improved neural prostheses. Therefore, scaffolds based on seaweed polysaccharides offer a viable platform for the creation of cutting-edge neural tissue engineering solutions.

6 Advantages and Challenges of Marine Seaweed Polysaccharide-Based Scaffolds

The natural availability, biocompatibility, and bioactivity of marine seaweed polysaccharides—such as alginate, fucoidan, carrageenan, and ulvan—make them particularly advantageous for tissue regeneration. In order to enhance cell adhesion, proliferation, and differentiation, these polysaccharides can be combined to create hydrogels and other scaffold formats that closely mimic the extracellular matrix.

Their sulphated structures facilitate interactions with growth factors, which improve wound healing and angiogenesis. Moreover, a favourable milieu for tissue regeneration is produced by their natural anti-inflammatory, antioxidant, and antibacterial qualities. These polysaccharides' processability makes them suitable for use in bone, nerve, and skin tissue engineering.

Despite their encouraging promise, a number of obstacles prevent marine polysaccharide-based scaffolds from being widely used. Variability in chemical composition, which can result from variations in seaweed species and extraction techniques, is a significant barrier that eventually compromises uniformity and reproducibility.

Furthermore, many of these polysaccharides—alginate in particular—have low mechanical strength and no natural cell-binding sites; thus in order to improve their activity, they must be chemically modified or blended with other substances.

Clinical translation is also severely hampered by regulatory worries about long-term safety, scalability, and purity. Thorough research and development are necessary to address these issues and make it easier for marine polysaccharide-based scaffolds to go from laboratory studies to clinical applications.

7 Future Directions and Research Opportunities

The potential of marine seaweed polysaccharide-based scaffolds in tissue regeneration is vast, yet several avenues remain underexplored. With advancements in biomaterials science, biofabrication techniques, and cellular biology, the future holds promising opportunities for enhancing the performance and applicability of these scaffolds.

7.1 Advanced Scaffold Engineering and 3D Bioprinting

The integration of marine polysaccharides with 3D bioprinting technologies represents a transformative opportunity for tissue engineering. The tuneable gelation properties of materials like alginate and carrageenan make them excellent candidates for use as bioinks. 3D bioprinting permits for precise spatial control of scaffold architecture, enabling the fabrication of complex tissue constructs that closely mimic native tissues. Future research should focus on optimizing the rheological and mechanical properties of marine polysaccharide-based bioinks, improving cell viability during printing, and enhancing post-printing scaffold performance.

7.2 Composite and Hybrid Materials

Combining marine polysaccharides with other natural and synthetic biomaterials can overcome existing limitations such as mechanical weakness and limited bioactivity. Hybrid scaffolds that incorporate marine polysaccharides with materials like collagen, chitosan, polylactic acid, or polycaprolactone can offer synergistic benefits. Such composites can be tailored for specific tissue types, providing the necessary mechanical support while maintaining bioactivity. Further exploration of these combinations, including the use of nano- and microparticles for reinforcement, could open new frontiers in scaffold design.

7.3 Functionalization and Bioactive Molecule Incorporation

Chemical modification and functionalization of marine polysaccharides can significantly enhance their biological interactions. Strategies such as sulphation, oxidation, or grafting with peptides and growth factors can improve cell adhesion, proliferation, and differentiation. For instance, functionalizing alginate with RGD peptides or incorporating BMPs can direct osteogenic differentiation. Future studies should investigate the optimal methods for stable and targeted incorporation of bioactive molecules into marine polysaccharide matrices, as well as the controlled release mechanisms for sustained therapeutic effects.

7.4 Stem Cell and Immunomodulatory Interactions

The interaction between marine polysaccharide scaffolds and stem cells offers significant promise for regenerative medicine. Investigating how these materials influence stem cell behaviour—including differentiation pathways, proliferation rates, and immunomodulatory profiles—can guide the development of next-generation scaffolds. Moreover, recent research has highlighted the role of biomaterials in modulating the immune response. Marine polysaccharides with inherent anti-inflammatory properties, such as ulvan and fucoidan, could be engineered to promote a pro-regenerative immune environment, thereby enhancing tissue repair outcomes.

7.5 In Vivo Evaluation and Clinical Translation

Despite encouraging in vitro results, the in vivo performance of marine polysaccharide-based scaffolds must be thoroughly evaluated to ensure safety, efficacy, and reproducibility. Animal studies are essential to understand the biodegradation profile, immune response, integration with host tissue, and functional recovery in various tissue types. Long-term studies should focus on both the regenerative capacity and potential adverse effects of these materials. Furthermore, the path to clinical translation requires addressing regulatory requirements, scalability, and cost-effectiveness. Developing standardized protocols for extraction, purification, modification, and sterilization is vital to ensuring batch-to-batch consistency and regulatory approval.

7.6 *Sustainability and Environmental Impact*

Given the rising interest in marine-derived biomaterials, ensuring the sustainability of raw material sources is critical. Overharvesting of wild seaweed populations can lead to ecological imbalance and depletion of marine biodiversity. Thus, future efforts must include the development of sustainable aquaculture practices and the use of biotechnological approaches for large-scale production of specific polysaccharides. Additionally, the environmental impact of scaffold production and disposal should be minimized by developing green extraction methods and biodegradable formulations. It will be necessary to solve present constraints and investigate novel biomedical approaches in order to advance the use of marine seaweed polysaccharides in tissue regeneration. To improve their bioactivity, mechanical strength, and cell adhesiveness, polysaccharides like alginate, fucoidan, carrageenan, and ulvan can be chemically modified and functionalised. This is one important avenue for future research. For example, adding peptide motifs or mixing with nanomaterials might enhance the endurance of scaffolds and cell-material interactions, increasing their application in load-bearing tissues like tendon or bone. The incorporation of stimuli-responsive components, which allow scaffolds to release bioactive molecules in response to physiological cues like pH, temperature, or enzyme activity, is another potential approach that could enhance control over the healing process.

8 Conclusion

Scaffolds based on polysaccharides found in marine seaweeds have enormous potential for tissue regeneration because they provide an unmatched blend of biocompatibility, biodegradability, and physiological activity. Polysaccharides such as alginate, fucoidan, carrageenan, and ulvan, which are derived from sustainable marine sources, support vital regenerative processes like cell adhesion, proliferation, differentiation, angiogenesis, and immune modulation in a way that closely resembles the extracellular matrix in both structure and function.

The capability to generate different scaffold designs, such as hydrogels, sponges, and 3D-printed structures, increases their suitability for use in various tissue types, such as bone, nerve, and skin. Unlocking their full therapeutic potential requires continued interdisciplinary research focused on chemical modification, scaffold functionalisation, and scalable production methods, even though issues with mechanical strength, cell-binding affinity, and standardisation still exist.

Marine seaweed polysaccharide-based scaffolds have the potential to completely change the next wave of regenerative medicines by providing a revolutionary approach to tissue regeneration and repair as bioprinting, biomaterial engineering, and personalised medicine technologies progress.

References

Wang H, Li X, Xuan M, et al (2024) Marine biomaterials for sustainable bone regeneration. Giant 19:100298. https://doi.org/10.1016/J.GIANT.2024.100298

Farag MM (2023) Recent trends on biomaterials for tissue regeneration applications: review. Journal of Materials Science 2022 58:2 58:527–558. https://doi.org/10.1007/S10853-022-08102-X

Krishani M, Shin WY, Suhaimi H, Sambudi NS (2023) Development of Scaffolds from Bio-Based Natural Materials for Tissue Regeneration Applications: A Review. Gels 2023, Vol 9, Page 100 9:100. https://doi.org/10.3390/GELS9020100

Pérez RA, Won JE, Knowles JC, Kim HW (2013) Naturally and synthetic smart composite biomaterials for tissue regeneration. Adv Drug Deliv Rev 65:471–496. https://doi.org/10.1016/J.ADDR.2012.03.009

Lewandowska-Łańcucka J, Fiejdasz S, Rodzik Ł, et al (2015) Novel hybrid materials for preparation of bone tissue engineering scaffolds. J Mater Sci Mater Med 26:1–15. https://doi.org/10.1007/S10856-015-5564-6/METRICS

Chandika P, Ko SC, Jung WK (2015) Marine-derived biological macromolecule-based biomaterials for wound healing and skin tissue regeneration. Int J Biol Macromol 77:24–35. https://doi.org/10.1016/J.IJBIOMAC.2015.02.050

Wang Z, Xu Z, Yang X, et al (2023) Current application and modification strategy of marine polysaccharides in tissue regeneration: A review. Biomaterials Advances 154:213580. https://doi.org/10.1016/J.BIOADV.2023.213580

Kuznetsova TA, Andryukov BG, Besednova NN, Khotimchenko YS (2021) Polysaccharides from Marine Algae in Modern Technologies of Regenerative Medicine. Russian Journal of Marine Biology 2021 47:1 47:1–9. https://doi.org/10.1134/S1063074021010065

Narasimhan AM, Ravikumar A, Nambiar S, et al (2023) Marine seaweed polysaccharides in tissue engineering. Functional Ingredients from Algae for Foods and Nutraceuticals, Second Edition 519–551. https://doi.org/10.1016/B978-0-323-98819-3.00007-9

Carvalho DN, Reis RL, Silva TH (2021) Marine origin materials on biomaterials and advanced therapies to cartilage tissue engineering and regenerative medicine. Biomater Sci 9:6718–6736. https://doi.org/10.1039/D1BM00809A

Iravani S, Jamalipour Soufi G (2021) Algae-derived materials for tissue engineering and regenerative medicine applications: current trends and future perspectives. Emergent Materials 2021 5:3 5:631–652. https://doi.org/10.1007/S42247-021-00283-6

Reddy PN, Kolla HB, Berde CV, et al (2023) Biomedical Applications of Marine Biopolymers in Tissue Engineering and Regenerative Medicine. Marine Bioactive Molecules for Biomedical and Pharmacotherapeutic Applications 39–59. https://doi.org/10.1007/978-981-99-6770-4_3

Iqbal Y, Amin F, Usman Y, Farrukh Sarfraz M (2024) Alginate-Based hydrogels with inorganic Nanomaterials: A promising approach for wound healing and bone tissue regeneration. Eur Polym J 212:113057. https://doi.org/10.1016/J.EURPOLYMJ.2024.113057

Akter A, Sobuj MKA, Islam MS, et al (2024) Seaweed polysaccharides: Sources, structure and biomedical applications with special emphasis on antiviral potentials. Future Foods 10:100440. https://doi.org/10.1016/J.FUFO.2024.100440

Wang C, Zhou Y (2024) Sacrificial biomaterials in 3D fabrication of scaffolds for tissue engineering applications. J Biomed Mater Res B Appl Biomater 112:e35312. https://doi.org/10.1002/JBM.B.35312;PAGEGROUP:STRING:PUBLICATION

Venkatesan J, Lowe B, Anil S, et al (2015) Seaweed polysaccharides and their potential biomedical applications. Starch/Staerke 67:381–390. https://doi.org/10.1002/STAR.201400127;WGROUP:STRING:PUBLICATION

Sahoo DR, Biswal T (2021) Alginate and its application to tissue engineering. SN Appl Sci 3:1–19. https://doi.org/10.1007/S42452-020-04096-W/METRICS

Jafari A, Farahani M, Sedighi M, et al (2022) Carrageenans for tissue engineering and regenerative medicine applications: A review. Carbohydr Polym 281:119045. https://doi.org/10.1016/J.CARBPOL.2021.119045

Yosri N, Khalifa SAM, Attia NF, et al (2024) Sustainability in the green engineering of nanocomposites based on marine-derived polysaccharides and collagens: A review. Int J Biol Macromol 274:133249. https://doi.org/10.1016/J.IJBIOMAC.2024.133249

Xie C, Lee ZJ, Ye S, et al (2024) A Review on Seaweeds and Seaweed-Derived Polysaccharides: Nutrition, Chemistry, Bioactivities, and Applications. Food Reviews International 40:1312–1347. https://doi.org/10.1080/87559129.2023.2212055;WGROUP:STRING:PUBLICATION

Lee KY, Mooney DJ (2012) Alginate: Properties and biomedical applications. Prog Polym Sci 37:106–126. https://doi.org/10.1016/J.PROGPOLYMSCI.2011.06.003

Flórez-Fernández N, Rodríguez-Coello A, Latire T, et al (2023) Anti-inflammatory potential of ulvan. Int J Biol Macromol 253:126936. https://doi.org/10.1016/J.IJBIOMAC.2023.126936

Anupama AD, Udduttula A, Jaiswal AK (2023) Unveiling the secrets of marine—derived fucoidan for bone tissue engineering—A review. Front Bioeng Biotechnol 10:1100164. https://doi.org/10.3389/FBIOE.2022.1100164

Jin Y, Yu Q, Li S, et al (2023) Application of seaweed polysaccharide in bone tissue regeneration. Front Mar Sci 10:. https://doi.org/10.3389/FMARS.2023.1202422/PDF

Bilal M, Iqbal HMN (2020) Marine seaweed polysaccharides-based engineered cues for the modern biomedical sector. Mar Drugs 18:. https://doi.org/10.3390/MD18010007

Madub K, Goonoo N, Gimié F, et al (2021) Green seaweeds ulvan-cellulose scaffolds enhance in vitro cell growth and in vivo angiogenesis for skin tissue engineering. Carbohydr Polym 251:117025. https://doi.org/10.1016/J.CARBPOL.2020.117025

Lin HR, Yen YJ (2004) Porous alginate/hydroxyapatite composite scaffolds for bone tissue engineering: Preparation, characterization, and in vitro studies. J Biomed Mater Res B Appl Biomater 71:52–65. https://doi.org/10.1002/JBM.B.30065

Zamani D, Moztarzadeh F, Bizari D (2019) Alginate-bioactive glass containing Zn and Mg composite scaffolds for bone tissue engineering. Int J Biol Macromol 137:1256–1267. https://doi.org/10.1016/J.IJBIOMAC.2019.06.182

Su W, Ma L, Ran Y, et al (2020) Alginate-Assisted Mineralization of Collagen by Collagen Reconstitution and Calcium Phosphate Formation. ACS Biomater Sci Eng 6:3275–3286. https://doi.org/10.1021/ACSBIOMATERIALS.9B01841/SUPPL_FILE/AB9B01841_SI_001.PDF

Bi Y Guang, Lin Z Ting, Deng S Ting (2019) Fabrication and characterization of hydroxyapatite/sodium alginate/chitosan composite microspheres for drug delivery and bone tissue engineering. Materials Science and Engineering: C 100:576–583. https://doi.org/10.1016/J.MSEC.2019.03.040

Reys LL, Silva SS, Oliveira C, et al (2020) Marine-origin polysaccharides for tissue engineering and regenerative medicine: Chitosan and fucoidan as illustrative examples. Encyclopedia of Marine Biotechnology 2619–2650. https://doi.org/10.1002/9781119143802.CH118

Jeong HS, Venkatesan J, Kim SK (2013) Hydroxyapatite-fucoidan nanocomposites for bone tissue engineering. Int J Biol Macromol 57:138–141. https://doi.org/10.1016/J.IJBIOMAC.2013.03.011

Shanmugapriya K, Kang HW (2021) Synthesis of nanohydroxyapatite/collagen-loaded fucoidan-based composite hydrogel for drug delivery to gastrointestinal cancer cells. Colloids Surf B Biointerfaces 203:111769. https://doi.org/10.1016/J.COLSURFB.2021.111769

Murugan SS, Anil S, Venkatesan J (2022) Polysaccharides-based nanoparticles for bone tissue engineering. Polysaccharide Nanoparticles: Preparation and Biomedical Applications 603–614. https://doi.org/10.1016/B978-0-12-822351-2.00001-2

Amorim S, Dudik O, Soares da Costa D, et al (2023) Fucoidan-Coated Silica Nanoparticles Promote the Differentiation of Human Mesenchymal Stem Cells into the Osteogenic Lineage. ACS Biomater Sci Eng 9:4907–4915. https://doi.org/10.1021/ACSBIOMATERIALS.3C00265/SUPPL_FILE/AB3C00265_SI_001.PDF

González Ocampo JI, Machado de Paula MM, Bassous NJ, et al (2019) Osteoblast responses to injectable bone substitutes of kappa-carrageenan and nano hydroxyapatite. Acta Biomater 83: 425–434. https://doi.org/10.1016/J.ACTBIO.2018.10.023

Qamar SA, Junaid M, Riasat A, et al (2024) Carrageenan-Based Hybrids with Biopolymers and Nano-Structured Materials for Biomimetic Applications. Starch/Staerke 76:2200018. https://doi.org/10.1002/STAR.202200018;CSUBTYPE:STRING:SPECIAL;PAGE:STRING:ARTICLE/CHAPTER

Batool F, Özçelik H, Stutz C, et al (2021) Modulation of immune-inflammatory responses through surface modifications of biomaterials to promote bone healing and regeneration. J Tissue Eng 12:. https://doi.org/10.1177/20417314211041428

Kikionis S, Ioannou E, Aggelidou E, et al (2021) The marine polysaccharide ulvan confers potent osteoinductive capacity to pcl-based scaffolds for bone tissue engineering applications. Int J Mol Sci 22:1–20. https://doi.org/10.3390/IJMS22063086

Alves A, Duarte ARC, Mano JF, et al (2012) PDLLA enriched with ulvan particles as a novel 3D porous scaffold targeted for bone engineering. J Supercrit Fluids 65:32–38. https://doi.org/10.1016/J.SUPFLU.2012.02.023

Dash M, Samal SK, Bartoli C, et al (2014) Biofunctionalization of ulvan scaffolds for bone tissue engineering. ACS Appl Mater Interfaces 6:3211–3218. https://doi.org/10.1021/AM404912C

Tziveleka LA, Sapalidis A, Kikionis S, et al (2020) Hybrid sponge-like scaffolds based on ulvan and gelatin: Design, characterization and evaluation of their potential use in bone tissue engineering. Materials 13:. https://doi.org/10.3390/MA13071763

Yang X, Lu Z, Wu H, et al (2018) Collagen-alginate as bioink for three-dimensional (3D) cell printing based cartilage tissue engineering. Materials Science and Engineering: C 83:195–201. https://doi.org/10.1016/J.MSEC.2017.09.002

Jahani A, Nourbakhsh MS, Ebrahimzadeh MH, et al (2024) Biomolecules-Loading of 3D-Printed Alginate-Based Scaffolds for Cartilage Tissue Engineering Applications: A Review on Current Status and Future Prospective. Archives of Bone and Joint Surgery 12:92. https://doi.org/10.22038/ABJS.2023.73275.3396

Morelli A, Betti M, Puppi D, Chiellini F (2016) Design, preparation and characterization of ulvan based thermosensitive hydrogels. Carbohydr Polym 136:1108–1117. https://doi.org/10.1016/J.CARBPOL.2015.09.068

Cui Z, Jiang F, Li L, et al (2024) Advances in Biomedical Applications of Hydrogels from Seaweed-Derived Sulfated Polysaccharides: Carrageenan, Fucoidan, and Ulvan. Journal of Ocean University of China 23:1329–1346. https://doi.org/10.1007/S11802-024-5988-Z/METRICS

Peng W, Li D, Dai K, et al (2022) Recent progress of collagen, chitosan, alginate and other hydrogels in skin repair and wound dressing applications. Int J Biol Macromol 208:400–408. https://doi.org/10.1016/J.IJBIOMAC.2022.03.002

Ghahtan N, Dehghan N, Ullah M, et al (2024) From seaweed to healing: the potential of fucoidan in wound therapy. Nat Prod Res. https://doi.org/10.1080/14786419.2024.2358387;WGROUP:STRING:PUBLICATION

Perumal RK, Perumal S, Thangam R, et al (2018) Collagen-fucoidan blend film with the potential to induce fibroblast proliferation for regenerative applications. Int J Biol Macromol 106:1032–1040. https://doi.org/10.1016/J.IJBIOMAC.2017.08.111

Hwang PA, Chen HY, Chang JS, Hsu FY (2023) Electrospun nanofiber composite mat based on ulvan for wound dressing applications. Int J Biol Macromol 253:126646. https://doi.org/10.1016/J.IJBIOMAC.2023.126646

Marine Animal Polysaccharide Scaffolds in Tissue Engineering Applications

Krishnameera Sajayan and Kausik Kapat

Abstract Tissue engineering is the foothill of regenerative medicine owing to the development of artificial tissues and organs. This discipline involves engineering scaffolds that support cell growth and regeneration. Various materials, including polysaccharides derived from marine fauna, have been used to fabricate scaffolds. Seafaring animals, such as crustaceans, jellyfish, sponges, squids, and fish, have contributed significantly to the development of scaffold biomaterials as sources of polysaccharides. Most of them facilitate cell growth, adhesion, migration, and responses to molecular and physical environments. They have the advantages of low antigenicity, efficient extraction, and compatibility with other biomaterials, resulting in a biomimetic architecture. This chapter provides an overview of the recent advances in the development and application of marine animal polysaccharide-based scaffolds, focusing on their potential to treat various clinical conditions. This discussion also highlights emerging trends and future directions, emphasizing the role of sustainable marine biomaterials in advancing tissue engineering and regenerative medicine.

Keywords Marine animal · Polysaccharide · Scaffolds · Tissue engineering · Regenerative medicine

1 Introduction

Tissue engineering (TE) emerged as an interdisciplinary field in response to the limitations of allografts and autografts, which were often inadequate, difficult to obtain, or ineffective in fully restoring damaged tissues. The global TE market was valued at approximately USD 19.36 billion in 2024 and is expected to grow at a compound annual growth rate of 14.3% between 2025 and 2030 (Grand View Research 2025). Scaffolds are the fundamental building blocks of TE; they aid in

K. Sajayan · K. Kapat (✉)
Department of Medical Devices, National Institute of Pharmaceutical Education and Research Kolkata, Kolkata, West Bengal, India
e-mail: kausik.kapat@niperkolkata.ac.in

S. Jana et al. (eds.), *Multifunctional Marine Polysaccharides*,
https://doi.org/10.1007/978-981-95-4126-3_13

providing support for the tissues to grow, sustain, and develop for the required period of time (Suamte et al. 2023). An ideal scaffold mimics the extracellular matrix (ECM), supporting cell adhesion, proliferation, and differentiation. Hence, the materials used for scaffold fabrication must possess appropriate mechanical strength, porosity, biocompatibility, and tunable biodegradability based on specific applications (Kumar and Jacob 2022a).

Polysaccharides are among the most commonly used biomaterials in scaffold design due to their bioactivity and structural versatility. Notably, the marine ecosystem, characterized by its remarkable phylogenetic diversity, offers a vast source of such polysaccharides. It harbors an abundance of unique bioactive compounds with significant pharmaceutical potential (Ward et al. 2022). Over the last five decades, nearly 20,000 biologically active compounds have been isolated from marine flora, fauna, and microorganisms, many of which display antimicrobial and therapeutic properties (Srinivasan et al. 2021).

Marine-derived polysaccharides offer greater biodiversity and often require simpler extraction processes compared to terrestrial sources. They have various pharmacological activities, including anti-viral, anti-cardiovascular, antitumor, and immune-regulatory effects. For instance, hyaluronic acid can selectively target cancer cells by binding to overexpressed CD44 receptors. These biomolecules contain chemically active groups such as carboxyl, amine, and hydroxyl, which can be modified to enhance their properties and broaden their range of applications (Sun et al. 2021). These advantages have fueled the increasing use of marine-derived polysaccharides in scaffold fabrication for TE. In this chapter, we explore marine animal-derived polysaccharides and their direct applications in TE scaffolds.

2 Potential Sources of Marine Animal Polysaccharides

In a 2012 global study on marine species diversity, Appeltans et al. estimated the existence of approximately 201,587 marine species under the kingdom Animalia (Appeltans et al. 2012). Among the marine organisms, crustaceans (subphylum), along with mollusks and vertebrates (phyla), have emerged as significant sources of polysaccharides for scaffold fabrication. Notable marine animal-derived polysaccharides include chitin, chitosan (CT), fucoidan, and glycosaminoglycans (GAGs) such as chondroitin sulfate (CS) and hyaluronic acid (HA).

Crustaceans form a subphylum under the phylum Arthropoda. They are distinguished by their segmented body structure known as tagmata, compound eyes, a prominent exoskeleton, jointed appendages, and a ventral nerve cord (VanHook and Patel 2008). Exoskeletons from marine crustaceans like crabs, barnacles, lobsters, krill, crayfish, and shrimp are often regarded as marine waste. Globally, an estimated 6–8 million tons of this exoskeletal waste is generated each year (Vidal et al. 2022). Notably, these structures contain around 13–42% chitin, making them a significant and widely exploited source for the extraction of chitin and its derivative, CT (Xu et al. 2008).

Mollusca is another major phylum within the animal kingdom, comprising around 51,689 reported marine species (Appeltans et al. 2012). The members of this phylum, such as squid pen, crayfish, cuttlefish, snails, and mussels, often serve as sources for chitin and CT. The Echinodermata phylum includes invertebrates with pentameric radial symmetry, such as sea stars, sea urchins, sea cucumbers, and sea lilies (Arnone et al. 2015). Notably, sea cucumbers and sea urchins are an extraction source for fucoidan (Jayawardena et al. 2022).

Marine vertebrates are the primary sources for the extraction of CS and HA, owing to their abundance of cartilaginous and connective tissues. CS, in particular, is obtained from marine species with a high cartilage content, such as sharks, yellowfin tuna, skate, mackerel, tilapia, salmon, and black scraper. HA is typically extracted from fish eyeballs, the liver of stingrays, and processing by-products like the head, bones, and cartilage of sharks, zebrafish, and swordfish. Additionally, mollusks, bivalves, and other shellfish also serve as valuable sources of HA (Abdallah et al. 2020a). Some of the sources of marine animal-derived polysaccharides are listed in Table 1.

2.1 *Glycosaminoglycans (GAGs)*

2.1.1 Hyaluronic Acid

HA is a GAG without sulfation or protein conjugation. This polysaccharide is made up of glucuronic acid and N-acetylglucosamine with 100–20,000 repeating units (Fig. 1a). In comparison to other GAGs, HA has a larger size and is abundantly found in the human body, particularly in connective tissues, the umbilical cord, synovial fluid, and vitreous humor (Abdel-Rahman Rasha and Abdel-Mohsen 2023a). HA is widely utilized in the treatment of osteoarthritis and for skin regeneration, particularly in cases of severe burn injuries. In the cosmetic industry, it is commonly incorporated into anti-aging formulations, used as a dermal filler, and applied in various aesthetic and plastic surgical procedures (Abdel-Rahman Rasha and Abdel-Mohsen 2023a).

2.2 *Sulfated GAGs and Polysaccharides*

2.2.1 Chondroitin Sulfate

As shown in Fig. 1b, CS is a linear GAGs composed of repeating disaccharide units made of glucuronic acid (GlcA) and N-acetylgalactosamine (GalNAc), linked by β-(1 → 3) and β-(1 → 4) glycosidic bonds, forming a linear polymer of 40–70 units and 10–80 kDa. Each unit can be sulfated at GlcA C-2 and GalNAc C-4 or C-6 positions (Wang et al. 2022a). This anionic heteropolysaccharide forms the major

Table 1 Potential sources of marine animal-derived polysaccharides

Polysaccharide	Marine animal sources	References
Chitin/chitosan	*Penaeus kerathurus* (shrimp)	Hamdi et al. (2017)
	Macrobrachium rosenbergii (shrimp)	Iber et al. (2023)
	Litopenaeus vannamei (whiteleg shrimp)	Remesh et al. (2025a)
	Parapenaeus longirostris (deep water rose shrimp)	Remesh et al. (2025a)
	Portunus segnis (blue crab)	Hamdi et al. (2017)
	Portunus trituberculatus (swimming crab)	Hao et al. (2021)
	Allopetrolisthes punctatus (porcelain crab)	Castro et al. (2018)
	Scylla serrata (mud crab)	Carbohydrate Research (2023)
	Lithodes santolla (southern king crab)	Forero et al. (2023)
	Pontastacus leptodactylus (narrow-clawed crayfish)	Nuc et al. (2023)
	Faxonius limosus (spiny-cheek crayfish)	Nuc et al. (2023)
	Parastacus pugnax (Chilean crayfish)	Burgos-Díaz et al. (2021)
	Astacus leptodactylus (Turkish crayfish)	Kadak et al. (2023)
	Sepiella inermis (cuttlefish)	Mater Int (2022)
	Dosidicus gigas (squid pen)	Cabrera-Barjas et al. (2021)
	Uroteuthis duvaucelii (Indian squid)	Balitaan et al. (2020)
	Illex argentinus (squid pen)	Vázquez et al. (2017)
	Loligo formosana (squid pen)	Chandumpai et al. (2004)
	Telescopium telescopium (telescope snail)	Rajathy et al. (2021)
	Perna viridis (Asian green mussel)	Kaewprachu and Jaisan (2023)
	Ianthella labyrinthus (sea sponge)	Romano et al. (2022)
	Ianthella flabelliformis (sea sponge)	Romano et al. (2022)
	Pseudoceratina purpurea (sea sponge)	Romano et al. (2022)
	Ianthella basta (sea sponge)	Romano et al. (2022)
	Aplysina aerophoba (sea sponge)	Romano et al. (2022)
Chondroitin sulfate	*Squatina oculata* (shark)	Sim et al. (2007)
	Dipturus flavirostris (skate)	Lin et al. (2017)
	Katsuwonus pelamis (skipjack tuna)	Lin et al. (2017)
	Lophius litulon (monk fish)	Lin et al. (2017)
	Oncorhynchus keta (salmon)	Zhang et al. (2014)
	Thunnus albacares (yellowfin tuna)	Thomas and Mathew (2021)
	Oreochromis niloticus (Nile tilapia)	Yang et al. (2023)
	Raja porosa (skate)	Zhou et al. (2020)
	Salmo salar (aquatic salmon)	Lin et al. (2017)
	Scophthalmus maximus (flat fish)	Ren et al. (2018)
	Scomberomorus niphonius (mackerel)	Wang et al. (2022a)
	Thamnaconus modestus (black scraper)	Wang et al. (2022a)

(continued)

Table 1 (continued)

Polysaccharide	Marine animal sources	References
Hyaluronic acid	*Cyclopterus lumpus* (Lumpsucker fish)	Panagos et al. (2014)
	Thunnus thynnus (bluefin tuna)	Elhiss et al. (2024)
	Scyliorhinus canicula (cat shark)	Vázquez et al. (2015)
	Aetobatus narinari (sting ray)	Sadhasivam et al. (2013)
Fucoidan	*Paracentrotus lividus (*sea urchin*)*	Salem et al. (2017a)
	Holothuria fuscopunctata (elephant trunkfish)	Gao et al. (2020)
	Holothuria poli (spot cucumber)	Mansour et al. (2019a)
	Apostichopus japonicus (sea cucumber)	Yu et al. (2015)
	Acaudina molpadioides (sea cucumber)	Hu et al. (2019)
	Stichopus horrens (Selenka's sea cucumber)	Ustyuzhanina et al. (2018)
	Paracentrotus lividus (purple sea urchin)	Salem et al. (2017b)

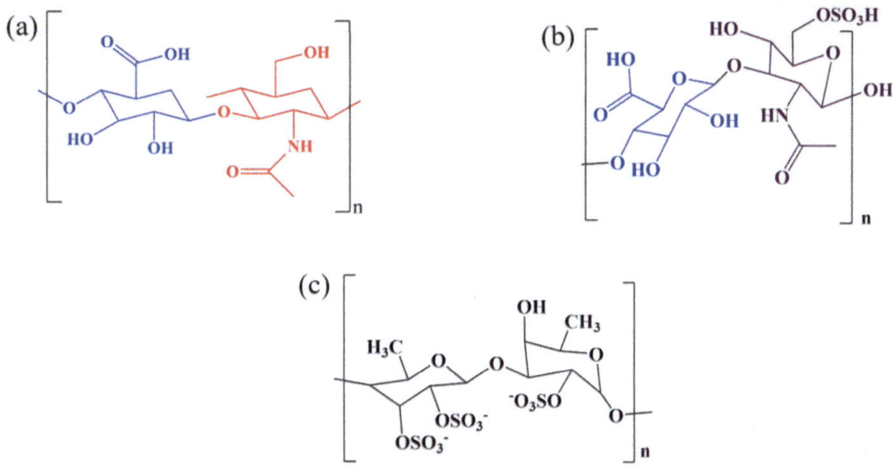

Fig. 1 Chemical structures of (**a**) hyaluronic acid, (**b**) chondroitin sulfate, and (**c**) fucoidan

component of cells and the ECM of vertebrates, bacteria, and invertebrates. In the body tissues, CS is found as a proteoglycan, i.e., a combination of polysaccharide and protein linked through a covalent bond (Konovalova et al. 2020). On a commercial scale, they are sourced from pigs' ears, nasal septa, and skin. Chicken cartilage and bovine trachea are also the major extraction sources of CS (Sharma et al. 2022a). Marine by-products such as fish fins, bones, cartilage, and scales are an alternative source for CS procurement. They serve as an abundant and cost-effective source for CS extraction, offering advantages in terms of availability and ease of processing. In the year 2021, CS had a US market value of 1211 million dollars, with projections indicating a 41% growth by 2030 (Urbi et al. 2022). The demand for this biopolymer is due to its wide range of applications in the medical field. CS is one of the major building blocks of cartilage. It supports joint health by stimulating *type II collagen production* and enhancing the *biosynthesis of proteoglycans*. It is usually taken as a dietary supplement and slow-acting medication for osteoarthritis, supplying glucosamine or other GAG components that support the development and repair of cartilage. Additionally, it also displays antioxidant, anti-viral, anti-infective, anti-inflammatory, and anti-apoptotic properties. In TE, it helps in regeneration, especially in epithelialization and neovascularization (Sharma et al. 2022a).

2.2.2 Fucoidan

Fucoidan, also referred to as sulfated fucan, is derived from both algae and marine invertebrates. When sourced from marine animals, fucoidan tends to have a homogeneous structure and lacks complex architecture, often observed in algal-derived variants. It is primarily made of L-fucose monomer units, with a sulfate group attached (Fig. 1c), which classifies it as a sulfated polysaccharide, similar to CS (Senni et al. 2011). The primary marine animal sources for fucoidan extraction are sea cucumbers and sea urchin eggs. In sea cucumbers, fucoidan is one of the key constituents of the body wall, where it accounts for approximately 3–8% of the dry weight (Chen et al. 2024). In drug delivery and biomedical applications, low MW and structurally homogeneous fucoidan is generally preferred due to its reduced antigenicity, enhanced bioavailability, and favorable functional properties (Liu et al. 2023).

2.3 *GAGs-Mimetic Polysaccharides*

2.3.1 Chitin

Chitin is a naturally occurring, linear biopolymer composed of N-acetyl-D-glucosamine units (Fig. 2a) and is among the most abundant biopolymers on Earth, with an estimated annual biosynthesis of nearly ten billion tons. Chitin is predominantly found in the phylum Arthropoda, where it constitutes the primary component of the exoskeleton. It is also present in other arthropods (insects), fungi, certain algae, and yeasts. In the context of marine organisms, chitin is abundantly available in members of the Crustacea and Mollusca subphyla (Kou et al. 2022). Chitin exists in three

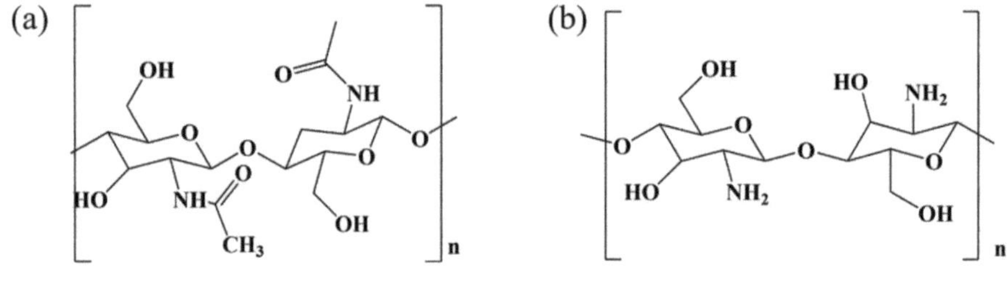

Fig. 2 Chemical structures of (**a**) chitin and (**b**) chitosan

polymorphic forms: alpha, beta, and gamma. Typically, chitin extracted from crustaceans is in the alpha form, while molluscan sources predominantly yield the beta form. Although chitin is an abundantly available polymer, its poor solubility and biodegradability hinder its use in biomedical research. This limitation arises from the presence of numerous hydroxyl, carbonyl, and acetyl amino groups, which establish strong intra- and intermolecular hydrogen bonds. This issue was overcome by developing chitosan, the deacetylated derivative of chitin (Tang et al. 2023).

2.3.2 Chitosan

CT is a widely used biomaterial for scaffold fabrication, produced by the deacetylation of chitin, wherein approximately 60% of acetyl groups are removed. This modification enhances its solubility and biodegradability. Structurally, CT is a linear polymer predominantly composed of β-1,4-linked D-glucosamine units and is characterized by a high density of free amino groups (Fig. 2b). These amino groups impart a positive charge and confer a basic nature to the polymer, making CT the only naturally occurring basic polysaccharide (Tang et al. 2023). CT has gained significant attention in TE due to its multiple advantageous properties, including non-toxicity, biodegradability, biological activity, and antibacterial effects. Its physical and mechanical properties can be tailored by adjusting factors such as molecular weight (MW), degree of deacetylation, and concentration. CT-based scaffolds are not only suitable for tissue regeneration but also serve as carriers for drug incorporation and sustained release, thereby enabling simultaneous treatment of associated diseases (Gholap et al. 2024).

2.4 Miscellaneous Polysaccharides

Several polysaccharides from marine animals like the sea cucumber (*Pattalus mollis*), including fucansulfate, fucosylated GAGs, and neutral glycans, exhibit strong anticoagulant properties but remain largely unexplored for TE applications, as research on these promising biomaterials is still in its early stages (Zheng et al. 2019).

3 Processing of Marine Animal Polysaccharides

Over the years, researchers have investigated numerous extraction techniques to enhance the yield, physicochemical characteristics, and biological activities of these polymers, aiming to tailor them for scaffold-based biomedical applications (Fig. 3) (Kang et al. 2023).

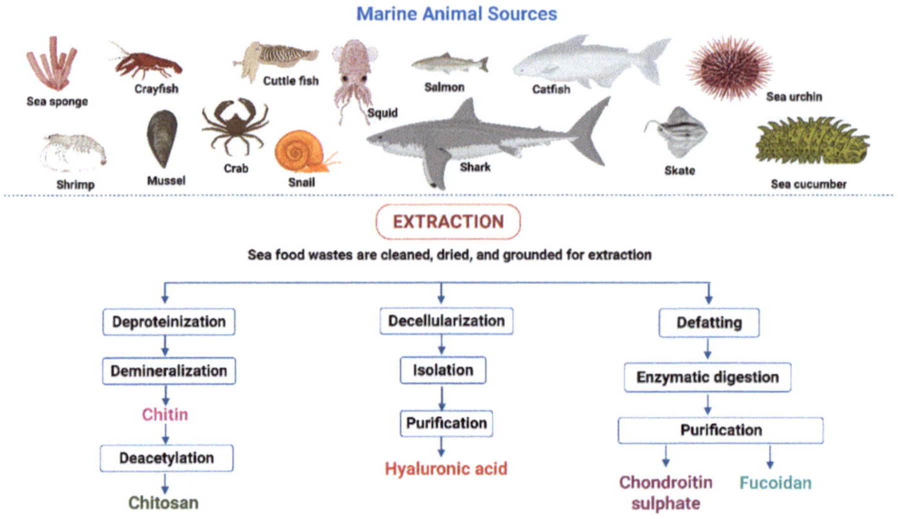

Fig. 3 Extraction process of marine polysaccharides

Chitin/Chitosan The extraction of chitin from crustaceans can be performed using biological or chemical treatments, both of which include deproteinization with alkali and demineralization using acid. The chemical approach typically involves the use of strong and concentrated chemicals under high-temperature conditions for extended periods. Common acids used for demineralization include sulfuric acid, nitric acid, hydrochloric acid, acetic acid, and methanoic acid, followed by alkaline treatment with sodium hydroxide to remove proteins. The extracted chitin often appears pink in color, which is then decolorized using agents such as potassium permanganate, oxalic acid, or hydrogen peroxide. Chitin is then converted into CT through deacetylation using 40–50% sodium or potassium hydroxide. In contrast, the biological leverages enzymes like alkaline proteases, pancreatin, devolvase, papain, pepsin, and trypsin, often derived from bacterial sources, for deproteinization. *Lactobacillus* species are commonly employed in this process, with crabs and shrimp serving as the primary sources of chitin. This chitin is then enzymatically converted into CT through bacterial or fungal deacetylase enzymes (Muthu et al. 2021).

Researchers have also investigated various alternative methods to extract chitin from squid pens with the objectives of increasing yield, enhancing antioxidant activity and physicochemical properties, and reducing processing time. In most of these approaches, the initial step involves drying the squid pens at 60 °C, followed by blending and sieving to obtain a fine powder. Among the alternative techniques explored are ultrasonic-assisted extraction and high hydrostatic pressure (HHP), which serve as more sustainable options compared to conventional chemical methods. In the HHP method, dried squid pen samples are vacuum heat-sealed in polyethylene bags containing 1% acetic acid and placed in a high-pressure chamber, where water acts as the pressure-transmitting medium. The system operates with a ramp-up rate of 300 MPa/min. Following treatment, the samples are dried at 50 °C to yield powder suitable for further chitin processing (Huang and Tsai 2020). In the ultrasonic-assisted extraction method, the ground squid pen is mixed with 1 M NaOH, and the mixture is subjected to ultrasonic waves at a frequency of 20 kHz and a high power of 750 W, while maintaining the temperature below 40 °C. After sonication, the resulting chitin is washed to neutral pH and vacuum filtered (Singh et al. 2019).

Hyaluronic Acid The extraction of HA from the marine sources is carried out using chemical, enzymatic, or detergent processes. However, the selection of the extraction technique depends on factors such as the type of marine organism, the intended application, and the desired properties of the final product. The process begins with the *disruption of the tissue's cellular matrix*, typically through physical techniques such as grinding or homogenization. This is followed by the extraction of HA using organic solvents, detergents, or enzymes.

Chemical extraction of HA is the most commonly used method, which involves several purification steps. The two main chemical extraction processes involve either acetone or a complexing agent, cetylpyridinium chloride (CPC). The CPC-based extraction process is more efficient and faster. This complexing agent selectively forms a complex with HA, separating it from other components of the tissue. Finally, the complex is purified using a charge-based anionic exchanger. For a milder and more selective alternative to harsh chemical treatments, enzymatic extraction is employed. In this method, specific enzymes such as chondroitinase, hyaluronidase, papain, and protease are utilized to degrade cellular components, followed by chemical purification procedures. In detergent-based extraction, the process starts with homogenization, followed by treatment with detergents like sodium deoxycholate or Triton X-100 to release HA. This is complemented by enzymatic digestion using DNase, RNase, and protease to remove residual nucleic acids and proteins. The final steps involve alcohol precipitation and purification through either chromatography or dialysis (Abdel-Rahman Rasha and Abdel-Mohsen 2023b).

Chondroitin Sulfate The best source for isolating CS would be materials that contain cartilage tissue, which is abundantly seen in marine fish waste. The process of extraction of CS contains multiple steps, initiated by defatting of the marine source. This is followed by enzymatic or alkaline hydrolysis to precipitate protein. The CS is then sedimented out from the solution, purified, and dried (Konovalova et al. 2020). The enzymes usually employed in hydrolysis are alcalase, papain, neutrase, bromelain, trypsin, and actinase (Abdallah et al. 2020b).

Isolation of CS from by-products of marine sources such as yellow goosefish, skate, and flat fish was studied by Im et al. The by-products (cartilage, bone, and head) were cleaned, dried, and ground. The grounded material was subjected to depolymerization of protein by alcalase and sodium carbonate buffer. The proteins were removed by precipitating them with trichloroacetic acid. The solution was further complexed with CPC. The final product was precipitated out by ethanol and lyophilized (Im et al. 2017). In a different study, crude CS was extracted from six different marine tissues by a rapid method by Wang et al. The author used enzymatic hydrolysis by the enzyme papin. This was followed by precipitating it with hexadecylpyridinium chloride. The final product was purified using a fast-flow anionic exchange column (Wang et al. 2022b).

Fucoidan The extraction of fucoidan generally involves processes like defatting, enzymatic digestion, and isolation of crude polysaccharide. This is followed by a purification process using anion-exchange chromatography or any other suitable techniques (Mansour et al. 2019b). The extraction of fucoidan from sea cucumber (*Holothuria poli*) was initiated by grinding its body wall into powder, followed by acetone treatment to remove lipid content. The homogenate was then digested using the papain enzyme and centrifuged. The supernatant was treated with CPC to precipitate the sulfated fucans. Later, it was purified using anion-exchange chromatography (Hou et al. 2025).

4 Properties

(a) *Physicochemical Properties*

Chitin is largely resistant to degradation, primarily due to its complete insolubility in both water and common organic solvents. Its rigid crystalline structure makes it difficult to dissolve under normal conditions. Only specific agents, such as concentrated thiocyanate solutions, mineral acids, calcium halides, and certain ionic liquids, have the ability to solubilize chitin. The solubility issue had restricted its use as a biomaterial in several areas of applications, including TE (Lee et al. 2023).

The degree of deacetylation and MW predominantly influence the functional and physicochemical properties of CT (Kadak et al. 2023). Among these, MW plays a critical role in its solubility, which in turn impacts its overall applications. Additionally, CT has strong inter- and intra-molecular H-bonds, which make it highly insoluble in many of the inorganic and organic solvents. A study showed that the mussel-derived CT had higher solubility (81–90%) than the crab, shrimp, and fish-derived CT (Kaewprachu and Jaisan 2023). Each monomer unit of CT contains amine as well as primary and secondary hydroxyl groups, enabling surface modifications through protonation. These chemical modifications can significantly influence its mechanical and biological behavior by altering key physicochemical properties such as crystallinity, solubility, and hydrophilicity. Hao et al. developed a low MW CT from swimming crabs. They used subcritical water treatment instead of traditional alkaline treatment. The extracted CT had improved thermal stability and compaction, which could be suitable for the fabrication of scaffolds through methods that involve high temperatures (Hao et al. 2021). Krishnan et al. demonstrated that cuttlebone-derived CT, when fabricated into a scaffold, holds uniform pores with a pore size of 30–40 μm. The scaffold exhibited porous microstructure and interconnectivity, which are essential features for cell proliferation and permeation. The cuttlebone CT possesses better physicochemical properties, such as higher solubility and fat and water binding capacities. These characteristics contribute to its effectiveness in scaffold fabrication (Krishnan et al. 2021).

On the other hand, HA lacks sulfate groups on its structure, and as a result, it does not carry a strong negative charge. Instead, HA is highly hydrophilic in nature and is available in various MW ranges, such as high, medium, and low, each offering distinct biological and physicochemical properties suitable for different biomedical applications (Abdel-Rahman Rasha and Abdel-Mohsen 2023b). Marine-derived HA possesses distinct physicochemical properties such as viscoelasticity, hydrophilicity, and excellent moisture retention. Its viscoelastic nature closely resembles that of native tissues, offering cushioning and shock absorption, particularly beneficial in joint-related TE applications where mechanical support is vital. Additionally, its strong hydrophilic character allows it to absorb and retain a large amount of water, making it an ideal hydrating agent for maintaining tissue lubrication and hydration. This capacity for moisture retention significantly contributes to its therapeutic value in regenerative and wound care treatments (Abdel-Rahman Rasha and Abdel-Mohsen 2023b). Furthermore, HA demonstrates extrusion and shear-thinning properties, making it highly suitable for 3D bioprinting applications in scaffold fabrication (Bui et al. 2023).

Marine-derived CS exhibits several physicochemical properties. It is an anionic heteropolysaccharide, which contributes to its unique interactions with other biomolecules. The MW of CS varies depending on its source. For example, CS isolated from black shark has a MW of approximately 55 kDa, while that from northern skate is around 47 kDa, and from salmon, about 64 kDa (Konovalova et al. 2020). A distinguishing characteristic of CS extracted from marine fish sources is the presence of disulfated disaccharides. The overall disaccharide content in the CS backbone can range from 1.3% to 10%, setting it apart from CS derived from terrestrial sources (Maccari et al. 2015). Its structure allows for the formation of complexes with metal ions, enhancing its functionality in TE. CS can form complexes with various ions (e.g., Sr, Ca, Mg), which can improve its bioactivity and effectiveness in treating bone-related disorders. These complexes can enhance the mechanical properties and biological activity of scaffolds used in TE (Sharma et al. 2022b).

Fucoidan is a hygroscopic, negatively charged polysaccharide, which is slightly soluble in acidic solutions and highly soluble in water (Luthuli et al. 2019). The hygroscopic nature of this polymer enhances its suitability for biomedical applications that require water retention, including the development of hydrogels for wound healing (Abbas et al. 2025). The MW and structural properties of fucoidan highly vary depending on its source (Zayed et al. 2020). For instance, the MW of fucoidan isolated from sea cucumber (*Holothuria poli*) was 1376.3 kDa and had 34.6% of sulfate content. Its structure had a repeating unit of tetrafucose and glucuronic acid branching (Mansour et al. 2019a). On the other hand, the fucoidan derived from sea urchin (*Paracentrotus lividus*) has a MW greater than 22,000 kD and is primarily made of arabinose along with glucose, fucose, and galactose. However, its sulfate content is relatively lesser at 22.4% (Salem et al. 2017a). In a different study conducted on fucoidan obtained from sea cucumber, cooking oil had a MW of

6.75 kDa and possessed 31.69% of sulfate moieties and 65.94 % of fucose. SEM analysis confirmed that this fucoidan has a porous sheet structure which is ideal for TE. It also has outstanding thermal stability and can withstand temperature from 30 to 200 °C (Cao et al. 2025). Fucoidan strongly binds to various compounds and macromolecules, mainly due to its negative charge, sulfation level, and molecular weight. Besides, fucoidan is highly stable in both acidic and alkaline conditions (Haggag et al. 2023).

(b) *Mechanical Properties*

Mechanical properties of the polysaccharide play a key role in the fabrication process as well as in maintaining scaffold integrity. Chitin exhibits remarkable mechanical properties primarily due to its abundant hydroxyl groups, which promote crystalline organization. Within this crystalline structure, a single crystal of chitin can consist of 18 to 28 polymer chains. The resulting chitin fibrils are stiff, strong, and lightweight and possess a high surface area. Notably, chitin also demonstrates a lower thermal expansion coefficient compared to materials such as aluminum, glass, steel, and copper. These characteristics make chitin a promising biomaterial for TE applications where enhanced mechanical strength is essential (Mushi 2021).

In contrary, CT does not possess the same mechanical strength as that of chitin. To improve its mechanical strength for scaffold fabrication, CT is often blended with other polymers. A study suggested that blending mussel-derived CT with conventional CT enhances the tensile strength, thereby improving the overall mechanical properties of the composite material (Kaewprachu and Jaisan 2023). Li et al. reported that CT derived from squid exhibited superior biochemical properties compared to crab-derived CT. This enhanced performance is attributed to the beta form of squid CT, which is known for its favorable characteristics in biomedical applications (Li et al. 2021). CT inherently possesses poor mechanical strength, which limits its standalone application in load-bearing tissues. Therefore, it is commonly combined with other polymers to enhance its mechanical properties, particularly for applications in bone TE, where structural integrity is crucial (Sukpaita et al. 2021).

The mechanical strength of HA is highly dependent on its molecular mass. High MW HA is generally preferred for applications requiring enhanced mechanical integrity and pronounced viscoelastic properties, such as in wound dressings and joint supplements (Iaconisi et al. 2023). In addition to rapid degradation limiting its long-term therapeutic efficacy, HA's naturally low mechanical strength may hinder its use in load-bearing applications. Chemical modification and crosslinking of HA through its hydroxyl and carboxyl groups or with polymers like methyl cellulose, collagen, polyacrylic acid, and poly(lactic-co-glycolic acid) (PLGA) can improve its mechanical strength and enzymatic degradation resistance (Iaconisi et al. 2023).

CS structure plays a vital role in retaining water and absorbing shock in cartilage, while its viscosity and mechanical properties depend on molecular weight and sulfation levels. Marine CS differs from terrestrial CS by having higher disulfation, longer GAG chains, and unique disaccharide units like GlcA(3S)-GalNAc(4S) (CS-K) (Wang et al. 2022b). Unlike synthetic single-polymer hydrogels, biopolymer hydrogels are generally very soft, with tensile moduli ranging from 10 to 10^4 Pa—much lower than that of load-bearing tissues like cartilage (0.1–1.0 MPa). However, the strength of CS hydrogels can be greatly enhanced through chemical modifications and by physically or chemically crosslinking with other polymers. For example, methacrylated CS crosslinked with poly(N,N-dimethylacrylamide) can form tough double network hydrogels with significantly improved mechanical properties (Zhu et al. 2025a).

Fucoidan has low apparent viscosity and exhibits pseudoplastic flow, limiting its use as a gelling or thickening agent. However, it can form gels, matrices, and films when mixed with oppositely charged polymers (Haggag et al. 2023). Mechanically stable 3D bioprinted fucoidan scaffolds (~700 kPa) were prepared from methacrylated, hydrothermally degraded fucoidan solution as light-curable bioink (Qureshi et al. 2025). Similarly, imine-crosslinked oxidized fucoidan-gelatin hydrogel provided controlled gelation and stable mechanical properties for over 28 days (Hsu et al. 2021). Conversely, photo-crosslinked methacrylate-hyaluronan and methacrylate-fucoidan hydrogels maintained hardness but exhibited a reduced elastic modulus with methacrylate-fucoidan addition (Sabu et al. 2022).

(c) *Biological Properties*

CT derived from marine animal sources exhibits a range of biological activities, including antibacterial, anti-inflammatory, anti-obesity, antifungal, and antioxidant properties (Remesh et al. 2025b). The crustacean-derived CT, especially from deep-water rose shrimp and whiteleg shrimp, was found to have antimicrobial activity against *Salmonella*, *Listeria*, and *Staphylococcus* species of bacteria. They were found to have more than 50% inhibition against these bacteria (Conde et al. 2024). Similarly, CT derived from telescope snail was found to have biofilm inhibiting and bactericidal activity against *Vibrio cholerae* and *Bacillus subtilis* (Rajathy et al. 2021). Crayfish-derived CT was also found to have antibacterial activity against *Staphylococcus aureus*, *Candida albicans*, and *Escherichia coli.* It was solvent-cast into films and evaluated for vaginal infections, demonstrating promising potential for therapeutic application in such conditions (Fourie et al. 2022). Beyond its antimicrobial efficacy, marine-derived CT exhibits excellent cytocompatibility and is known to stimulate anti-inflammatory cytokine production through macrophage activation. Due to its low toxicity, inert nature, and osteoconductive potential, CT is widely utilized in scaffold fabrication, especially in bone TE, where it is often combined with other biomaterials to enhance its performance (Islam et al. 2020). Abundance, biodegradability, biocompatibility, and antimicrobial traits of CT make it ideal for wound healing and TE of cartilage, intervertebral discs, vessels, cornea, skin, and gums (Guan et al. 2024).

The biological properties of HA involve anti-inflammatory effect, wound healing, immune-modulation, and cell signalling. It plays a vital role in tissue repair by promoting cell migration to injury sites, thereby accelerating the healing process. HA is extensively applied in bone and cartilage TE due to its anti-inflammatory nature and ability to provide joint lubrication. As a major component of synovial fluid, HA reduces friction between cartilage surfaces, which is crucial for smooth joint movement. These attributes make HA an ideal candidate for scaffold development in the treatment of conditions such as osteoarthritis (Yu et al. 2018).

CS, as naturally occurring component of tissue, exhibits several biological properties. It is well-known for its anticoagulant properties and is often considered a potential alternative to heparin. CS plays a significant role in bone and cartilage TE due to its ability to support cartilage structure and function, making it beneficial in managing osteoarthritis and enhancing joint mobility. Studies have shown that CS promotes the synthesis of cartilage matrix components, aiding in cartilage repair and regeneration (Cahyadi et al. 2025). Additionally, CS demonstrates anti-inflammatory and anti-adipogenic effects. Specifically, CS extracted from marine sources such as blue shark, mako shark, sharpspine skate, and stingray was found to inhibit lipid droplet accumulation in differentiating 3T3-L1 cells in a concentration-dependent manner (Li et al. 2019).

Fucoidan is a highly viscous, chondroitin sulfate-like polysaccharide with strong anti-inflammatory, antioxidant, antitumor, antithrombotic, antimicrobial, immunomodulatory, and cartilage-rejuvenating properties. The antioxidant and antimicrobial properties of fucoidan are mainly attributed to its negatively charged sulfate groups, which contribute to reactive oxygen species (ROS) scavenging and support an anionic antimicrobial mechanism (Qureshi et al. 2025). Fucoidan oligosaccharides derived from sea cucumbers have demonstrated significant anti-inflammatory and anti-obesity effects, along with the ability to inhibit hyperlipidemia in mice subjected to a high-fat diet. Additionally, their capacity to restore gut microbial balance suggests potential as a beneficial dietary supplement (Li et al. 2020). The presence of disulfated fucose content in fucoidan derived from sea cucumber has resulted in higher anticoagulant activity (Mansour et al. 2019a). Another study revealed that the fucoidan isolated from the sea cucumber cooking oil had higher antioxidant properties than its algal counterpart. It also has bacteriostatic and biofilm inhibition properties against *Helicobacter pylori* strains (Cao et al. 2025). The novel fucoidan from the sea cucumber (*Stichopus chloronotus*) was found to have lipid peroxidase inhibiting activity. It also promoted in vitro proliferation of RAW 246.7 cells and produced TNF-α and nitric oxide (Lu et al. 2019). Fucoidan supports stem cell proliferation, making it advantageous for cell culture studies in regenerative medicine. It has been widely explored in bone TE applications (Maccari et al. 2015).

5 Techniques for Fabrication of TE Scaffolds

Scaffolds for TE and regenerative medicine applications act as temporary ECM-like templates, guiding cells into two-dimensional (2D) and/or three-dimensional (3D) hierarchical structures. Scaffold parameters such as surface area, porosity, and pore interconnectivity—critical for cell attachment, migration, proliferation, and differentiation—can vary based on the fabrication technique used. Both conventional methods (e.g., lyophilization, solvent casting, electrospinning) and advanced techniques (e.g., 3D printing, stereolithography, bioplotting) have been used to fabricate biopolymer scaffolds, including those from marine sources (Setiawati et al. 2024). Due to its susceptibility to acid and enzymatic degradation (e.g., by lysozymes), chitosan is often combined with other polymers like hyaluronic acid or collagen or bioceramics such as β-tricalcium phosphate (β-TCP), hydroxyapatite, or biphasic calcium phosphate to fabricate scaffolds.

Satiawati et al. developed a crab-derived CT/collagen/hydroxyapatite scaffold by homogenizing hydroxyapatite and CT in solvents, blending with collagen in acetic acid, and freeze-drying the final suspension (Aydogdu et al. 2019). Polylactic acid (PLA)/β-TCP composite scaffolds with shrimp shell-derived chitosan were fabricated via 3D printing and coated with amoxicillin to achieve enhanced tissue regeneration with antimicrobial effects (Zhu et al. 2025b). Methacrylated fucoidan scaffolds were prepared by 3D bioprinting exhibited high mechanical strength (Fan et al. 2014). Electrospinning is widely used to produce hyaluronan-based scaffolds with high porosity and surface area. Electrospun marine HA/silk fibroin mats were made by blending different HA/silk fibroin ratios in water, and the scaffold morphology changed with the MW of HA (Mutsenko et al. 2017).

6 Applications in Tissue Engineering

Marine animal-derived polysaccharides have emerged as a promising focus in TE, with growing interest in their application for scaffold development in the bone, cartilage, cardiac, skin, and corneal TE. CT, in particular, has been extensively investigated for bone TE due to its excellent osteoconductive properties that support osteocyte proliferation. Additionally, the chitinous exoskeletons of sea sponges, with their naturally occurring microporous architecture, have garnered attention for scaffold fabrication. CS and HA are also key candidates in TE, owing to their ECM-mimicking characteristics that support cell culture. Despite their biological relevance, the direct use of CS and HA extracted from marine animal sources remains limited. Nonetheless, given their potential, future research should further explore these marine-derived biopolymers for advanced TE applications. A few of the polysaccharides derived from marine animal sources along with their application in TE scaffolds are mentioned in Table 2.

Bone TE CT is extensively utilized in scaffold development within the biomedical field, especially in bone TE, due to its excellent osteoconductive properties (Shaz et al. 2024). A key requirement for bone regeneration scaffolds is to exhibit porosity and mechanical properties that closely resemble natural bone. To mimic the ECM of the bone, a team of researchers developed scaffolds using CT extracted from mud crab (*Scylla serrata*) through a chemical process involving partial deacetylation under alkaline conditions. The extracted CT was then combined with collagen type I and hydroxyapatite to fabricate the scaffold. This composite system exhibited efficient nutrient transport and improved osteoconductivity. The resulting scaffold featured an average pore size of approximately 100 μm, which falls within the

Table 2 Marine animal polysaccharides used in TE scaffolds

Applications	Polysaccharides	Other scaffold components	Outcome	References
Bone TE	Chitosan	Collagen type I, hydroxyapatite	Osteoconductive Biocompatible with osteoblast, fibroblast, MG-63	Aydogdu et al. (2019)
	Chitin	–	Twofold increase in hMSCs within 7 days hMSC differentiation into adipogenic, chondrogenic, and osteogenic lineages	Guo et al. (2023)
	Chondroitin sulfate	Gelatin, nano hydroxyapatite	Osteogenic differentiation Enhanced osteoblast migration Repaired skull defects in mouse	Hong et al. (2021)
	Hyaluronic acid	Calcium phosphate	Supported viability and proliferation of osteoblast cells (MC3T3-E1)	Zheng et al. (2022)
	Hyaluronic acid	–	Supported osteoblast adhesion, growth, and differentiation	Chonanant et al. (2024)
Cartilage TE	Chitosan	Gelatin, collagen	Biocompatibility with TC28a2human chondrocytes Supported aggrecan gene expression	Carvalho et al. (2023)
	Chitosan, fucoidan, chondroitin sulfate	Collagen	Proliferation and viability of hASCs	Carvalho et al. (2020a)
	Methacrylated fucoidan	–	In vivo cartilage repair through antimicrobial and antioxidant activity	Fan et al. (2014)
	Chitosan, fucoidan	Collagen	Suitable for both acellular scaffolds and cell-laden systems	Jung et al. (2018)
Skin TE	Beta-chitin	Polyethylene oxide	Epithelial cell regeneration on SD rats	Reys et al. (2013)
	Chitosan	–	Cytocompatibility with L929 fibroblast-like cells	Zhou et al. (2024)
	Chitosan	Collagen	95.75% wound reduction in rats than control (22.25%) Facilitated skin regeneration formation	Puigmal et al. (2023)
	Hyaluronic acid	Decellularized Korean fish (*Seriola dumerili*) skin	Improved infiltration of cells into dermis and stimulated collagen synthesis	Bui et al. (2023)
	Hyaluronic acid	Silk	Improved biocompatibility	Mutsenko et al. (2017)

(continued)

Table 2 (continued)

Applications	Polysaccharides	Other scaffold components	Outcome	References
	Fucoidan, chitosan	Polyvinyl alcohol	Antibacterial efficacy against *E. coli* and *S. aureus* Biocompatibility with fibroblast cell lines	Sadeghi et al. (2022)
	Chondroitin sulfate	Polyvinyl alcohol, gelatin	Enhanced vascular and cellular infiltration Complete dermal regeneration	Schubert et al. (2019)
Cardiac TE	Chitin	–	iPSCs differentiated into cardiomyocytes within 20 days	Yan et al. (2024)
	Chondroitin sulfate	Decellularized heart valve	Enhanced resistance to enzymatic degradation, hemo- and biocompatibility, endothelialization, reduced proinflammatory responses	Lei et al. (2021)
	Hyaluronic acid	Fibrin	Reduced leaflet (heart valve) retraction	Wang et al. (2024)
Functional coating for magnesium stents	Fucoidan	Acrylamide, sulfobetaine methacrylate	Enhanced anti-corrosion performance, re-endothelialization, hemocompatibility, neovascularization	Garzón et al. (2024)
Corneal TE	Chitin, chitosan	Amino-polysaccharides	Corneal cells adhered, proliferated, and maintained their elongated morphology No hemorrhage, necrosis, or tumor formation	da Silva et al. (2025)
	Hyaluronic acid	Gelatin	Delivery of corneal MSC into deep corneal wounds Promoted wound closure within 48 h	Lai et al. (2012)
	Chondroitin sulfate	Gelatin	Good biocompatibility with rabbit corneal keratocytes	Kudiyarasu et al. (2024)

TE tissue engineering, *hMSC* human mesenchymal stromal cells, *hASC* human adipose-derived stem cells, *iPSC* induced pluripotent stem cells

optimal range for cell adhesion and proliferation. Biocompatibility assessments revealed favorable interactions with osteoblast-like cells, fibroblasts, and osteosarcoma cells (MG-63), confirming its cytocompatibility. Due to its relatively low compressive strength (2–12 MPa), the scaffold was proposed for use in treating fibrous cortical defects in non-load-bearing bone regions (Aydogdu et al. 2019).

Aplysina aerophoba, a marine sponge from the class Demospongiae, possesses a chitin-based 3D microporous skeleton. Mutsenko et al. explored its suitability for tissue TE applications through a series of in vitro assessments, including cytocompatibility, cell viability, proliferation, and cell attachment studies. Human mesenchymal stromal cells (hMSCs) cultured on the scaffold exhibited a twofold improvement in cell number over a period of 7 days. Furthermore, differentiation studies confirmed the scaffold's ability to support hMSC differentiation into adipogenic, chondrogenic, and osteogenic lineages. Based on these findings, the chitinous scaffold derived from *A. aerophoba* was proposed as a promising candidate for future TE research (Guo et al. 2023).

Traditional scaffolds used for bone repair often feature interconnected channel structures, which are not always ideal for the effective transport of cells and bioactive factors. To address this limitation, Guo et al. covalently incorporated CS/gelatin microspheres into a 3D-printed scaffold composed of modified gelatin and nanohydroxyapatite. These microspheres formed bridges within the scaffold framework, establishing channels that facilitated cell migration. Additionally, the controlled release of CS from the microspheres promoted osteogenesis and enhanced osteoblast migration. The scaffold successfully repaired skull defects in a mouse model and supported osteogenic differentiation. This study demonstrates the potential of CS-rich microspheres in creating a bridging effect to significantly enhance bone regeneration (Hong et al. 2021).

HA can serve as an injectable hydrogel for bone TE. In one study, thiolated HA hydrogels were crosslinked via disulfide bonds and incorporated with biphasic calcium phosphate nanoparticles. Various HA concentrations (1–5%) were evaluated, with the 3% formulation demonstrating optimal gelation time, degradation rate, and swelling behavior in vitro. This hydrogel supported the viability and proliferation of osteoblast cells (MC3T3-E1), confirming its biocompatibility. The findings suggest that this HA-based hydrogel is a promising candidate for applications in bone TE (Zheng et al. 2022).

Shaz et al. developed a porous composite scaffold by functionalizing nano-calcium sulfate and fucoidan with PLGA, aimed at promoting osteogenic differentiation of bone marrow stromal cells. The scaffold supported sustained cell proliferation and viability throughout the 28-day study period. It also enhanced the secretion of osteogenic markers such as alkaline phosphatase and osteocalcin. Furthermore, a significant upregulation of osteogenic gene expression was observed on days 14 and 28. The incorporation of fucoidan synergistically improved the scaffold's ability to stimulate osteogenic differentiation, indicating its strong potential as a candidate for bone TE applications (Carvalho et al. 2020b).

HA forms hydrogels that retain water, while HA scaffolds offer a 3D structure for cell growth and tissue formation. HA-based scaffolds supported osteoblast adhesion, growth, and differentiation, while releasing bone morphogenetic protein (BMP) to promote bone tissue regeneration (Chonanant et al. 2024).

Cartilage TE CT was extracted from *Macrobrachium rosenbergii* (shrimp) shell waste for the fabrication of scaffolds intended for cartilage TE. The extraction process involved thorough washing and grinding of the shell waste, followed by a standard chemical method as previously described. The resulting CT exhibited a degree of deacetylation of approximately 79%, which falls within the acceptable range compared to commercially available CT. Scaffold fabrication was carried out using the freeze-drying technique, combining the shrimp-derived CT with gelatin and collagen. The resulting scaffold displayed a pore size ranging from 88 to 278 μm, a water absorption capacity of 90%, and a degradation rate of 30% over a 21-day period. Cell viability, assessed via MTT assay, showed a progressive increase during the culture period, indicating good biocompatibility with human chondrocytes (TC28a2). Hematoxylin and eosin (H&E) staining after 21 days further confirmed cell infiltration and proliferation within the scaffold pores. Additionally, the scaffold supported the expression of the aggrecan gene, a key component of cartilage ECM (Carvalho et al. 2023).

High-strength 3D-printed scaffolds were fabricated using a natural bioink from degraded and methacrylated fucoidan, demonstrating effective in vivo cartilage repair through antimicrobial and antioxidant activity (Fan et al. 2014).

CT derived from *Dosidicus gigas* (squid pen) was evaluated for its potential biomedical applications by Reys et al. The extraction was carried out using conventional chemical methods. The extracted CT was fabricated into scaffolds through lyophilization and solvent casting techniques. These squid pen-derived CT scaffolds exhibited consistent morphology and structural stability. Furthermore, cytotoxicity studies using L929 fibroblast-like cells confirmed that the scaffolds were non-toxic (Zhou et al. 2024). Building on this work, the same research group developed cryogels incorporating the squid pen-derived CT, fucoidan extracted from brown algae, and jellyfish-derived collagen. For cryogel preparation, CT and collagen were dissolved in 1 M ammonium acetate, while fucoidan was solubilized in pure water. The mixed solutions were dispensed into 48-well plates and frozen at −80 °C, enabling a non-chemical crosslinking approach. The resulting cryogels were deemed suitable for both acellular scaffolds and cell-laden systems (Food and Agriculture Organization of the United Nations 2024). Further the researches included CS to the above formulation. To fabricate stable and cohesive cryogels, the authors employed cryoprocessed crosslinking at various subzero temperatures (−196 °C, −20 °C, and −80 °C). The resulting cryogels provided a favorable microenvironment that supported the proliferation and viability of human adipose-derived stem cells (hASCs). The authors suggested that this formulation holds promise for further investigation, particularly to evaluate its immunological response and chondrogenic differentiation potential (Carvalho et al. 2020a).

Skin TE Although chitin generally exhibits poor solubility, its beta form possesses notable wound healing properties. Recognizing this potential, Jung et al. developed electrospun nanofibers using beta-chitin derived from cuttlefish bone, an often discarded by-product of mollusks. The beta-chitin was dissolved in formic acid along with polyethylene oxide (PEO) to facilitate electrospinning. After fiber formation, the PEO was removed by washing with water, resulting in nanofibers with reduced diameter and enhanced hydrophilicity, as evidenced by water contact angle measurements. The authors attributed this increase in hydrophilicity to the smaller fiber diameter following PEO removal. When applied as a nanofiber web dressing on Sprague Dawley rats, the material effectively supported epithelial cell regeneration, an essential process in wound healing. These findings highlight the promising potential of beta-chitin nanofibers as scaffolding materials for future wound healing and tissue engineering applications (Reys et al. 2013).

Zou et al. developed a biofilm for wound healing applications using CT and acid-soluble collagen derived from the squid gladius (*Doryteuthis singhalensis*). The biopolymers were first dissolved in acetic acid and then mixed in a specific ratio of 8.5:1.5 (CT/collagen) to formulate the final biofilm under controlled laboratory conditions. In vivo studies revealed that rats treated with the developed biofilm exhibited a significant wound reduction of 95.75%, which was substantially higher than that of the control group (22.25%). The biofilm outperformed both collagen-only and CT-only films, which showed wound reductions of 63.25% and 52.67%, respectively. Furthermore, the biofilm demonstrated excellent biocompatibility and supported osteoblastic differentiation, indicating its potential use not only in wound healing but also in broader TE applications. The study emphasized that this CT-collagen hybrid film could effectively facilitate skin regeneration and stimulate granulation tissue formation, which are critical for accelerated and complete wound repair (Puigmal et al. 2023).

Decellularized ECMs are widely used as scaffolds in TE due to its ability to naturally improve the proliferation and migration of seeded cells. Bui et al. developed 3D printed scaffolds intended for human skin reconstruction. They decellularized Korean fish (*Seriola dumerili*) skin and incorporated it into HA hydrogel to develop bioink for 3D printing. The study revealed that introducing a higher concentration of decellularized ECM into HA hydrogel improved the injectability and printability. It also aided in increasing swelling and erosion of the scaffold, which are beneficial in nutrient movements and waste removal. This property of the scaffold is highly advantageous in wound healing. The presence of 30% decellularized ECM in HA hydrogel demonstrated higher cell viability in 7-day culture period. The same percentage improved infiltration of cells into the dermis and stimulated collagen synthesis, a crucial factor in skin regeneration. The authors successfully constructed bilayer skin model that can be used in wound healing and skin reconstruction (Bui et al. 2023).

Marine HA/silk fibroin scaffolds were electrospun from aqueous blends of varying compositions, showing improved biocompatibility and strong potential for skin tissue regeneration (Mutsenko et al. 2017). Piugmal et al. incorporated fucoidan into polyvinyl alcohol/CT nanofiber scaffolds to enhance their antibacterial properties for application in skin TE. The presence of fucoidan significantly improved the scaffold's antibacterial efficacy against *Escherichia coli* and *Staphylococcus aureus*. The electrospun nanofibers were uniform and bead-free, indicating successful fabrication. Additionally, fucoidan enhanced the scaffold's biocompatibility, as demonstrated by favorable results with fibroblast cell lines. The scaffold also exhibited good tensile strength, making it a promising candidate for skin TE (Sadeghi et al. 2022).

Electrospun mats typically suffer from limited thickness, resulting in poor load-bearing capacity, and their small pore size restricts cell infiltration—challenges that hinder their application in skin TE. To overcome these limitations, Sadeghi et al. developed a multilayered 3D nanofibrous scaffold composed of CS, gelatin, and polyvinyl alcohol. Layer-by-layer stacking was facilitated using ethanol, which brought adjacent fiber layers into close contact. The resulting scaffold enabled sustained release of CS, demonstrated improved mechanical strength, and supported enhanced vascular and cellular infiltration between the layers. When applied to full-thickness skin wounds on the dorsal region of rats, the scaffold promoted complete dermal regeneration, indicating its strong potential for treating deep skin injuries (Schubert et al. 2019).

Cardiac TE Schubert et al. introduced a chitin-based scaffold as a potential alternative to conventional absorbable hemostats. This bandage-like scaffold was derived from the chitinous skeleton of the marine sponge *Ianthella labyrinthus*. The fabrication process involved methanol extraction of bromotyrosines, followed by the removal of pigments, proteins, and cellular components. Subsequently, residual calcium carbonate was eliminated using sodium hydroxide. This entire procedure was repeated three times to obtain purified, colorless scaffolds. The resulting chitin scaffold demonstrated high thermal stability, making it suitable for sterilization through autoclaving. Induced pluripotent stem cells (iPSCs) were seeded onto the scaffold and successfully differentiated into cardiomyocytes, which were cultured for 20 days. The findings showed excellent cell adhesion and viability. Additionally, the scaffold exhibited strong capillary action, facilitating deep blood absorption into its microtubular structure. This platform was proposed as a promising model for investigating cardiac remodeling, tissue regeneration, and metabolic processes (Yan et al. 2024).

Tissue-engineered heart valves are receiving global attention for their potential to address the limitations of conventional valve replacements. Among these, decellularized heart valves stand out as a promising option due to their preserved natural 3D architecture and favorable biological characteristics. However, their clinical application is limited by inadequate mechanical strength, poor hemocompatibility, rapid degradation, and insufficient endothelialization. To address these limitations, Yan et al. employed oxidized CS to crosslink decellularized heart valves. This modification significantly enhanced the scaffold's resistance to collagenase- and elastase-mediated degradation, improved mechanical strength, and demonstrated superior hemocompatibility and biocompatibility in both in vitro and in vivo evaluations. Upon implantation into the rat aorta, the scaffold exhibited improved endothelialization, reduced proinflammatory responses, and maintained better patency. These findings suggest that this CS-based scaffolds hold promise as a next-generation valve prosthesis (Lei et al. 2021).

Leaflet retraction, characterized by the shrinkage, stiffening, or curling of valve leaflets, remains a significant challenge in the preclinical development of tissue-engineered heart valves. To address this, Lei et al. proposed that incorporating HA into a fibrin scaffold could enhance cell proliferation and minimize retraction. Utilizing a custom-designed high-throughput cell culture system, they observed that HA improved scaffold-cell interactions, triggering a cascade of morphological, mechanical, and cellular responses. These changes led to increased scaffold stiffness and compaction, effectively reducing leaflet retraction. The findings highlight the role of HA in modulating tissue remodeling and suggest its potential in mitigating retraction-related complications in engineered heart valves (Wang et al. 2024).

Magnesium alloys have been explored as biodegradable stents for the treatment of cardiovascular diseases; however, their clinical application is hindered by poor endothelialization and low corrosion resistance. To address these issues, Wang et al. developed a functional coating for magnesium stents aimed at enhancing both anti-corrosion performance and re-endothelialization. The coating involved the immobilization of fucoidan within a bioactive hydrogel synthesized through the copolymerization of acrylamide and sulfobetaine methacrylate. Fucoidan incorporation significantly improved hemocompatibility by reducing hemolysis, minimizing protein adsorption, and preventing clot formation. Additionally, the hydrogel coating enhanced the stent surface's wettability and corrosion resistance. The presence of immobilized fucoidan also facilitated endothelialization and neovascularization, underscoring its potential as an effective surface modification strategy for magnesium alloy stents (Garzón et al. 2024).

Corneal TE The gladius of squid is a flexible, internal structure located within the mantle that provides anchorage for muscle attachment. While its detailed architecture remains unclear, it is known to be primarily composed of chitin and serves as a viable source for chitin extraction. Rather than extracting CT from the gladius, Garzón et al. explored its direct use as a biomaterial for corneal tissue engineering. The study utilized the gladius of the *Illex coindetii* species and conducted histological analysis, revealing an acellular structure composed of densely packed parallel lamellae, devoid of blood vessels and glands. Given that the gladius primarily consists of chitin and CT aminopolysaccharides, it was evaluated for biocompatibility by implanting it subcutaneously in laboratory rats. After 30 days, the implants remained structurally intact, with no signs of hemorrhage, necrosis, or tumor formation in the surrounding tissues. Systemic evaluations also reported no abnormalities. Furthermore, the gladius was successfully cellularized using corneal cells, which adhered, proliferated, and maintained their elongated morphology. These findings suggest that the squid gladius holds significant potential as a scaffold material for corneal tissue engineering (da Silva et al. 2025).

Silva et al. utilized HA as a coating for gelatin nanofibers to fabricate electrospun scaffolds designed for the delivery of corneal mesenchymal stromal cells into deep corneal wounds. The scaffold effectively supported cell growth in vitro and promoted wound closure within 48 h. These results indicate the HA-based scaffold's potential as a therapeutic strategy for the treatment of deep corneal defects (Lai et al. 2012).

Lai et al. fabricated a 3D corneal keratocyte scaffold by crosslinking CS and gelatin using a carbodiimide-based method. The inclusion of CS enhanced both the light transmittance and water content of the scaffold. In terms of mechanical strength and hydrophilicity, the CS-based scaffold closely resembled native corneal tissue. It also demonstrated good biocompatibility with rabbit corneal keratocytes, promoting their proliferation and biosynthetic activity. These findings suggest that the CS-based scaffold holds significant promise for applications in corneal stromal TE (Kudiyarasu et al. 2024).

Future Prospect
According to a 2022 global survey, aquaculture production was estimated to be 223.2 million tonnes, comprising 185.4 million tonnes of marine fauna. Asia was regarded as the leading contributor of aquaculture, followed by Europe, Latin America, the Caribbean, Africa, North America, and Oceania (130). This data reflects the production of millions of seafood waste annually as a by-product of consumption. Such waste presents a valuable opportunity to be transformed into polysaccharides such as CS, CT, and HA. Hence, marine fauna serves as a sustainable resource for developing scaffolds that are bioactive, economical, and degradable.

However, there are challenges as well. Most extraction techniques currently rely on harsh chemical methods that can cause environmental risks. A shift toward eco-friendly extraction methods, such as biological or biotechnological approaches, is essential. Additionally, allergies caused by crustacean-derived CT need scientific attention. Furthermore, comprehensive long-term toxicity studies are needed, along with the establishment of strict regulatory frameworks for scaffolds intended for clinical use.

7 Conclusion

Marine animal-derived polysaccharides such as CT, HA, CS, and fucoidan have shown immense potential in TE due to their biocompatibility, biodegradability, and functional biological properties. These biopolymers support essential cellular functions and are suitable candidates for developing scaffolds in the bone, cartilage, skin, corneal, cardiac, and wound healing applications. However, their inherent limitations, such as poor mechanical strength (as seen with CT), necessitate blending with other biomaterials to enhance structural integrity for specific applications like bone TE. Additionally, variability in MW and sulfation patterns significantly influence their biological performance.

Marine animal-derived polysaccharides show a wide range of biological activities that support cell culture and differentiation, which are crucial factors for scaffold functioning. Nevertheless, challenges such as batch-to-batch variability, limited mechanical strength, and potential allergenicity, especially considering that shellfish is a known allergen, demand comprehensive preclinical evaluation. Overall, marine-derived polysaccharides offer a sustainable and functional platform for biomedical and TE innovations, provided their limitations are carefully addressed through scientific advancements and regulatory oversight.

References

Grand View Research [Internet]. [cited 2025 May 19]. Tissue Engineering Market Size And Share Report, 2030. Available from: https://www.grandviewresearch.com/industry-analysis/tissue-engineering-and-regeneration-industry

Suamte L, Tirkey A, Barman J, Jayasekhar Babu P. Various manufacturing methods and ideal properties of scaffolds for tissue engineering applications. Smart Materials in Manufacturing. 2023;1:100011.

Kumar A, Jacob A. Techniques in scaffold fabrication process for tissue engineering applications: A review. j app biol biotech. 2022a Apr 10;163–76.

Ward D, Melbourne-Thomas J, Pecl GT, Evans K, Green M, McCormack PC, et al. Safeguarding marine life: conservation of biodiversity and ecosystems. Rev Fish Biol Fisheries. 2022 Mar;32 (1):65–100.

Srinivasan R, Kannappan A, Shi C, Lin X. Marine Bacterial Secondary Metabolites: A Treasure House for Structurally Unique and Effective Antimicrobial Compounds. Marine Drugs. 2021 Sep 23;19(10):530.

Sun Y, Ma X, Hu H. Marine Polysaccharides as a Versatile Biomass for the Construction of Nano Drug Delivery Systems. Marine Drugs. 2021 Jun 16;19(6):345.

Appeltans W, Ahyong ST, Anderson G, Angel MV, Artois T, Bailly N, et al. The Magnitude of Global Marine Species Diversity. Current Biology. 2012 Dec;22(23):2189–202.

VanHook AM, Patel NH. Crustaceans. Current Biology. 2008 Jul 8;18(13):R547–50.

Vidal JL, Jin T, Lam E, Kerton F, Moores A. Blue is the new green: Valorization of crustacean waste. Current Research in Green and Sustainable Chemistry. 2022 Jan 1;5:100330.

Xu Y, Gallert C, Winter J. Chitin purification from shrimp wastes by microbial deproteination and decalcification. Appl MicrobiolBiotechnol. 2008 Jun 1;79(4):687–97.

Arnone MI, Byrne M, Martinez P. Echinodermata. In: Wanninger A, editor. Evolutionary Developmental Biology of Invertebrates 6: Deuterostomia [Internet]. Vienna: Springer; 2015 [cited 2025 May 20]. p. 1–58. Available from: https://doi.org/10.1007/978-3-7091-1856-6_1

Jayawardena TU, Nagahawatta DP, Fernando IPS, Kim YT, Kim JS, Kim WS, et al. A Review on Fucoidan Structure, Extraction Techniques, and Its Role as an Immunomodulatory Agent. Marine Drugs. 2022 Dec;20(12):755.

Abdallah MM, Fernández N, Matias AA, do Rosário Bronze M. Hyaluronic acid and Chondroitin sulfate from marine and terrestrial sources: Extraction and purification methods. Carbohydrate Polymers. 2020a;243:116441.

Hamdi M, Hammami A, Hajji S, Jridi M, Nasri M, Nasri R. Chitin extraction from blue crab (*Portunus segnis*) and shrimp (*Penaeus kerathurus*) shells using digestive alkaline proteases from *P. segnis* viscera. International Journal of Biological Macromolecules. 2017 Aug 1;101: 455–63.

Iber BT, Torsabo D, Chik CENCE, Wahab F, Abdullah SRS, Hasan HA, et al. Optimization of chitosan coagulant from dry legs of giant freshwater prawn, *Macrobrachium rosenbergii* in aquaculture wastewater treatment using response surface methodology (RSM). Journal of Environmental Chemical Engineering. 2023 Jun 1;11(3):109761.

Remesh SD, Sandrasaigaran P, Remesh S, Perumal V, Lip Vun JY, Gandhi S, et al. Antimicrobial and anti-biofilm activity of crustacean-derived chitosan against *Salmonella* typhimurium, *Staphylococcus aureus* and *Listeria monocytogenes*. Food Bioscience. 2025a Jun 1;68:106697.

Hao G, Hu Y, Shi L, Chen J, Cui A, Weng W, et al. Physicochemical characteristics of chitosan from swimming crab (Portunus trituberculatus) shells prepared by subcritical water pretreatment. Sci Rep [Internet]. 2021 Jan 18 [cited 2025 May 17];11(1). Available from: https://www.nature.com/articles/s41598-021-81318-0

Castro R, Guerrero-Legarreta I, Bórquez R. Chitin extraction from *Allopetrolisthes punctatus* crab using lactic fermentation. Biotechnology Reports. 2018 Dec 1;20:e00287.

Solid-state mechanochemical synthesis of chitosan from mud crab (Scylla serrata) chitin. Carbohydrate Research. 2023 Dec 1;534:108971.

Forero JC, Carvajal K, Guzmán F, Acevedo C, Osses N, Santana P. Use of Chitosan from Southern King Crab to Develop Films Functionalized with RGD Peptides for Potential Tissue Engineering Applications. Biomimetics. 2023 Jul;8(3):323.

Nuc Z, Brusotti G, Catenacci L, Grenha A, Pontes JF, Pinto da Silva J, et al. Pontastacus leptodactylus (Eschscholtz, 1823) and Faxonius limosus (Rafinesque, 1817) as New, Alternative Sources of Chitin and Chitosan. Water. 2023 Jan;15(17):3024.

Burgos-Díaz C, Opazo-Navarrete M, Palacios JL, Barahona T, Mosi-Roa Y, Anguita-Barrales F, et al. Synthesis of New Chitosan from an Endemic Chilean Crayfish Exoskeleton (Parastacus Pugnax): Physicochemical and Biological Properties. Polymers. 2021 Jan;13(14):2304.

Kadak AE, Küçükgülmez A, Çelik M. Preparation and Characterization of Crayfish (Astacus leptodactylus) Chitosan with Different Deacetylation Degrees. Iranian Journal of Biotechnology. 2023 Apr 1;21(2):e3253.

Extraction and Characterization of Chitosan from the Cuttlebone of Spineless Cuttlefish, Sepiella inermis. Mater Int. 2022 Dec 10;4(4):2.

Cabrera-Barjas G, González C, Nesic A, Marrugo KP, Gómez O, Delattre C, et al. Utilization of Marine Waste to Obtain β-Chitin Nanofibers and Films from Giant Humboldt Squid Dosidicus gigas. Marine Drugs. 2021 Apr;19(4):184.

Balitaan JNI, Yeh JM, Santiago KS. Marine waste to a functional biomaterial: Green facile synthesis of modified-β-chitin from *Uroteuthis duvaucelii* pens (gladius). International Journal of Biological Macromolecules. 2020 Jul 1;154:1565–75.

Vázquez JA, Noriega D, Ramos P, Valcarcel J, Novoa-Carballal R, Pastrana L, et al. Optimization of high purity chitin and chitosan production from *Illex argentinus* pens by a combination of enzymatic and chemical processes. Carbohydrate Polymers. 2017 Oct 15;174:262–72.

Chandumpai A, Singhpibulporn N, Faroongsarng D, Sornprasit P. Preparation and physicochemical characterization of chitin and chitosan from the pens of the squid species, *Loligo lessoniana* and *Loligo formosana*. Carbohydrate Polymers. 2004 Dec 7;58(4):467–74.

Rajathy T, Srinivasan M, Mohanraj T. Physicochemical and functional characterization of chitosan from horn snail gastropod Telescopium telescopium. Journal of Applied Pharmaceutical Science. 2021 Feb 5;11(2):052–8.

Kaewprachu P, Jaisan C. Physicochemical Properties of Chitosan from Green Mussel Shells (Perna viridis): A Comparative Study. Polymers. 2023 Jan;15(13):2816.

Romano G, Almeida M, Varela Coelho A, Cutignano A, Gonçalves LG, Hansen E, et al. Biomaterials and Bioactive Natural Products from Marine Invertebrates: From Basic Research to Innovative Applications. Marine Drugs. 2022 Apr;20(4):219.

Sim JS, Im AR, Cho SM, Jang HJ, Jo JH, Kim YS. Evaluation of chondroitin sulfate in shark cartilage powder as a dietary supplement: Raw materials and finished products. Food Chemistry. 2007 Jan 1;101(2):532–9.

Lin N, Mo X, Yang Y, Zhang H. Purification and sequence characterization of chondroitin sulfate and dermatan sulfate from fishes. Glycoconj J. 2017 Apr 1;34(2):241–53.

Zhang F, Xie J, Linhardt RJ. Isolation and structural characterization of glycosaminoglycans from heads of red salmon (Oncorhynchus nerka). Jacobs J BiotechnolBioeng. 2014;1(1):002.

Thomas DrL, KpDrM, Mathew DrS. Fish gills of Thunnus albacares: A novel source of chondroitin sulphate glycosaminoglycans. Int J Fish Aquat Stud. 2021 Jan 1;9(1):146–52.

Yang J, Shen M, Wu T, Chen X, Wen H, Xie J. Physicochemical, structural characterization, and antioxidant activities of chondroitin sulfate from *Oreochromis niloticus* bones. Food Science and Human Wellness. 2023 Jul 1;12(4):1102–8.

Zhou C, Mi S, Li J, Gao J, Wang X, Sang Y. Purification, characterisation and antioxidant activities of chondroitin sulphate extracted from *Raja porosa* cartilage. Carbohydrate Polymers. 2020 Aug 1;241:116306.

Ren Z, Ji Y, Wang Y, Dong L. Chondroitin sulfate from *Scophthalmus maximus* for treating osteoarthritis. International Journal of Biological Macromolecules. 2018 Mar 1;108:1158–64.

Wang Y, Ahmadi S, Yu C, Zhang L, Hu X, Ye X, et al. A rapid method for extraction, purification and structure analysis of chondroitin sulfate from six marine tissues. Food Quality and Safety. 2022a Jan 1;6:fyac057.

Panagos CG, Thomson D, Moss C, Bavington CD, Ólafsson HG, Uhrín D. Characterisation of hyaluronic acid and chondroitin/dermatan sulfate from the lumpsucker fish, *C. lumpus*. Carbohydrate Polymers. 2014 Jun 15;106:25–33.

Elhiss S, Hamdi A, Chahed L, Boisson-Vidal C, Majdoub H, Bouchemal N, et al. Hyaluronic acid from bluefin tuna by-product: Structural analysis and pharmacological activities. International Journal of Biological Macromolecules. 2024 Apr 1;264:130424.

Vázquez JA, Pastrana L, Piñeiro C, Teixeira JA, Pérez-Martín RI, Amado IR. Production of Hyaluronic Acid by Streptococcus zooepidemicus on Protein Substrates Obtained from Scyliorhinuscanicula Discards. Marine Drugs. 2015 Oct;13(10):6537–49.

Sadhasivam G, Muthuvel A, Pachaiyappan A, Thangavel B. Isolation and characterization of hyaluronic acid from the liver of marine stingray *Aetobatus narinari*. International Journal of Biological Macromolecules. 2013 Mar 1;54:84–9.

Salem YB, Amri S, Hammi KM, Abdelhamid A, Cerf DL, Bouraoui A, et al. Physico-chemical characterization and pharmacological activities of sulfated polysaccharide from sea urchin, *Paracentrotus lividus*. International Journal of Biological Macromolecules. 2017a Apr 1;97: 8–15.

Gao N, Chen R, Mou R, Xiang J, Zhou K, Li Z, et al. Purification, structural characterization and anticoagulant activities of four sulfated polysaccharides from sea cucumber *Holothuria fuscopunctata*. International Journal of Biological Macromolecules. 2020 Dec 1;164:3421–8.

Mansour MB, Balti R, Yacoubi L, Ollivier V, Chaubet F, Maaroufi RM. Primary structure and anticoagulant activity of fucoidan from the sea cucumber *Holothuria polii*. International Journal of Biological Macromolecules. 2019a Jan 1;121:1145–53.

Yu L, Xue C, Chang Y, Hu Y, Xu X, Ge L, et al. Structure and rheological characteristics of fucoidan from sea cucumber *Apostichopus japonicus*. Food Chemistry. 2015 Aug 1;180:71–6.

Hu S, Wang J, Wang J, Yang H, Yan X, Su L. Fucoidan from *Acaudinamolpadioides* improves insulin resistance by altering gut microbiota dysfunction. Journal of Functional Foods. 2019 Jun 1;57:59–67.

Ustyuzhanina NE, Bilan MI, Dmitrenok AS, Borodina EYu, Nifantiev NE, Usov AI. A highly regular fucansulfate from the sea cucumber *Stichopus horrens*. Carbohydrate Research. 2018 Feb 1;456:5–9.

Salem YB, Amri S, Hammi KM, Abdelhamid A, Cerf DL, Bouraoui A, et al. Physico-chemical characterization and pharmacological activities of sulfated polysaccharide from sea urchin, *Paracentrotus lividus*. International Journal of Biological Macromolecules. 2017b Apr 1;97: 8–15.

Abdel-Rahman Rasha M, Abdel-Mohsen AM. Marine Biomaterials: Hyaluronan. Marine Drugs. 2023a Jul 27;21(8):426.

Konovalova I, Novikov V, Kuchina Y, Dolgopiatova N. Technology and Properties of Chondroitin Sulfate from Marine Hydrobionts. KLS [Internet]. 2020 Jan 15 [cited 2025 May 18]; Available from: https://knepublishing.com/index.php/KnE-Life/article/view/6075

Sharma R, Kuche K, Thakor P, Bhavana V, Srivastava S, Mehra NK, et al. Chondroitin Sulfate: Emerging biomaterial for biopharmaceutical purpose and tissue engineering. Carbohydrate Polymers. 2022a Jun;286:119305.

Urbi Z, Azmi NS, Ming LC, Hossain MdS. A Concise Review of Extraction and Characterization of Chondroitin Sulphate from Fish and Fish Wastes for Pharmacological Application. CIMB. 2022 Aug 28;44(9):3905–22.

Senni K, Pereira J, Gueniche F, Delbarre-Ladrat C, Sinquin C, Ratiskol J, et al. Marine Polysaccharides: A Source of Bioactive Molecules for Cell Therapy and Tissue Engineering. Marine Drugs. 2011 Sep;9(9):1664–81.

Chen G, Yu L, Shi F, Shen J, Zhang Y, Liu G, et al. A comprehensive review of sulfatedfucan from sea cucumber: Antecedent and prospect. Carbohydrate Polymers. 2024 Oct 1;341:122345.

Liu S, Wang Q, Shao Z, Liu Q, He Y, Ren D, et al. Purification and Characterization of the Enzyme Fucoidanase from Cobetia amphilecti Utilizing Fucoidan from Undaria pinnatifida. Foods. 2023 Jan;12(7):1555.

Kou SG, Peters L, Mucalo M. Chitosan: A review of molecular structure, bioactivities and interactions with the human body and micro-organisms. CarbohydrPolym. 2022 Apr 15;282: 119132.

Tang W, Wang J, Hou H, Li Y, Wang J, Fu J, et al. Review: Application of chitosan and its derivatives in medical materials. International Journal of Biological Macromolecules. 2023 Jun 15;240:124398.

Gholap AD, Rojekar S, Kapare HS, Vishwakarma N, Raikwar S, Garkal A, et al. Chitosan scaffolds: Expanding horizons in biomedical applications. Carbohydrate Polymers. 2024 Jan 1;323: 121394.

Zheng W, Zhou L, Lin L, Cai Y, Sun H, Zhao L, et al. Physicochemical Characteristics and Anticoagulant Activities of the Polysaccharides from Sea Cucumber Pattalus mollis. Marine Drugs. 2019 Apr;17(4):198.

Kang MS, Jo HJ, Jang HJ, Kim B, Jung TG, Han DW. Recent Advances in Marine Biomaterials Tailored and Primed for the Treatment of Damaged Soft Tissues. Marine Drugs. 2023 Nov 25;21(12):611.

Muthu M, Gopal J, Chun S, Devadoss AJP, Hasan N, Sivanesan I. Crustacean Waste-Derived Chitosan: Antioxidant Properties and Future Perspective. Antioxidants. 2021 Feb 3;10(2):228.

Huang YL, Tsai YH. Extraction of chitosan from squid pen waste by high hydrostatic pressure: Effects on physicochemical properties and antioxidant activities of chitosan. International Journal of Biological Macromolecules. 2020 Oct 1;160:677–87.

Singh A, Benjakul S, Prodpran T. Ultrasound-Assisted Extraction of Chitosan from Squid Pen: Molecular Characterization and Fat Binding Capacity. Journal of Food Science. 2019 Feb 1;84 (2):224–34.

Abdel-Rahman Rasha M, Abdel-Mohsen AM. Marine Biomaterials: Hyaluronan. Marine Drugs. 2023b Jul 27;21(8):426.

Abdallah MM, Fernández N, Matias AA, Bronze M do R. Hyaluronic acid and Chondroitin sulfate from marine and terrestrial sources: Extraction and purification methods. Carbohydrate Polymers. 2020b Sep 1;243:116441.

Im AR, Sim JS, Park Y, Hahn BS, Toida T, Kim YS. Isolation and Characterization of Chondroitin Sulfates from the By- products of Marine Organisms. 2017.

Wang Y, Ahmadi S, Yu C, Zhang L, Hu X, Ye X, et al. A rapid method for extraction, purification and structure analysis of chondroitin sulfate from six marine tissues. Food Quality and Safety. 2022b Jan 1;6:fyac057.

Mansour MB, Balti R, Yacoubi L, Ollivier V, Chaubet F, Maaroufi RM. Primary structure and anticoagulant activity of fucoidan from the sea cucumber *Holothuria poli*. International Journal of Biological Macromolecules. 2019b Jan 1;121:1145–53.

Hou T, Liu X, Zhang S, Tang K, Liu S, Liu J, et al. Anti-inflammatory Effects of the Fucoidan from Sea Cucumber Apostichopus japonicus. Mar Biotechnol. 2025 Jan 20;27(1):32.

Lee S, Hao LT, Park J, Oh DX, Hwang DS. Nanochitin and Nanochitosan: Chitin Nanostructure Engineering with Multiscale Properties for Biomedical and Environmental Applications. Advanced Materials. 2023;35(4):2203325.

Krishnan S, Chakraborty K, Dhara S. Biomedical potential of β-chitosan from cuttlebone of cephalopods. Carbohydrate Polymers. 2021 Dec;273:118591.

Bui HTD, Cho W, Park JK, Lee MS, Kim HK, Yoo HS. Korean Amberjack Skin-Inspired Hyaluronic Acid Bioink for Reconstruction of Human Skin. ACS Omega. 2023 Jun 27;8(25): 22752–61.

Maccari F, Galeotti F, Volpi N. Isolation and structural characterization of chondroitin sulfate from bony fishes. Carbohydrate Polymers. 2015 Sep 20;129:143–7.

Sharma R, Kuche K, Thakor P, Bhavana V, Srivastava S, Mehra NK, et al. Chondroitin Sulfate: Emerging biomaterial for biopharmaceutical purpose and tissue engineering. Carbohydrate Polymers. 2022b Jun;286:119305.

Luthuli S, Wu S, Cheng Y, Zheng X, Wu M, Tong H. Therapeutic Effects of Fucoidan: A Review on Recent Studies. Marine Drugs. 2019 Sep;17(9):487.

Abbas MF, Karim DK, Kareem HR, Kamil MM, Al-Musawi MH, Asker MH, et al. Fucoidan and its derivatives: From extraction to cutting-edge biomedical applications. Carbohydrate Polymers. 2025 Jun 1;357:123468.

Zayed A, El-Aasr M, Ibrahim ARS, Ulber R. Fucoidan Characterization: Determination of Purity and Physicochemical and Chemical Properties. Marine Drugs. 2020 Nov;18(11):571.

Cao J, Qin L, Liu M, Yao M, Wang K, Lin H, et al. Fucoidan from sea cucumber cooking liquid: Structural analysis, physicochemical properties, and anti-*Helicobacter pylori* potential. International Journal of Biological Macromolecules. 2025 May 1;306:141593.

Haggag YA, Abd Elrahman AA, Ulber R, Zayed A. Fucoidan in Pharmaceutical Formulations: A Comprehensive Review for Smart Drug Delivery Systems. Marine Drugs. 2023 Feb;21(2):112.

Mushi NE. A review on native well-preserved chitin nanofibrils for materials of high mechanical performance. International Journal of Biological Macromolecules. 2021 May 1;178:591–606.

Li B, Wu X, Bao B, Guo R, Wu W. Evaluation of α-Chitosan from Crab Shell and β-Chitosan from Squid Gladius Based on Biochemistry Performance. Applied Sciences. 2021 Jan;11(7):3183.

Sukpaita T, Chirachanchai S, Pimkhaokham A, Ampornaramveth RS. Chitosan-Based Scaffold for Mineralized Tissues Regeneration. Marine Drugs. 2021 Oct;19(10):551.

Iaconisi GN, Lunetti P, Gallo N, Cappello AR, Fiermonte G, Dolce V, et al. Hyaluronic Acid: A Powerful Biomolecule with Wide-Ranging Applications—A Comprehensive Review. International Journal of Molecular Sciences. 2023 Jan;24(12):10296.

Zhu S, Zhou Z, Chen X, Zhu W, Yang M, Yu M, et al. High mechanical performance and multifunctional degraded fucoidan-derived bioink for 3D bioprinting. Carbohydrate Polymers. 2025a Jan 15;348:122805.

Qureshi AT, Afrin S, Asim S, Rizwan M. Imine Crosslinked, Injectable, and Self-Healing Fucoidan Hydrogel with Immunomodulatory Properties. Advanced Healthcare Materials. 2025. n/a (n/a):2405260.

Hsu FY, Chen JJ, Sung WC, Hwang PA. Preparation of a Fucoidan-Grafted Hyaluronan Composite Hydrogel for the Induction of Osteoblast Differentiation in Osteoblast-Like Cells. Materials. 2021 Jan;14(5):1168.

Sabu S, Sasidharan A, Venugopal V. Influence of Isolation Conditions on the Physicochemical and Biological Properties of Chitosan and Chitosan Oligosaccharides from Marine Crustacean Shell Wastes. In: Kim SK, editor. Chitooligosaccharides: Prevention and Control of Diseases [Internet]. Cham: Springer International Publishing; 2022 [cited 2025 May 23]. p. 333–52. Available from: https://doi.org/10.1007/978-3-030-92806-3_20

Remesh SD, Sandrasaigaran P, Remesh S, Perumal V, Lip Vun JY, Gandhi S, et al. Antimicrobial and anti-biofilm activity of crustacean-derived chitosan against Salmonella typhimurium, Staphylococcus aureus and Listeria monocytogenes. Food Bioscience. 2025b Jun;68:106697.

Conde A, Borges S, Baptista-Silva S, Veloso T, Pereira JL, Ventura SPM, et al. A crayfish chitosan-based bioactive film to treat vaginal infections: A sustainable approach. International Journal of Biological Macromolecules. 2024 Oct 1;277:134460.

Fourie J, Taute F, du Preez L, de Beer D. Chitosan Composite Biomaterials for Bone Tissue Engineering—a Review. Regen Eng Transl Med. 2022 Mar 1;8(1):1–21.

Islam MdM, Shahruzzaman Md, Biswas S, Nurus Sakib Md, Rashid TU. Chitosan based bioactive materials in tissue engineering applications-A review. Bioactive Materials. 2020 Mar 1;5(1): 164–83.

Guan X, Wang F, Zhou B, Sang X, Zhao Q. The nutritional function of active polysaccharides from marine animals: A review. Food Bioscience. 2024 Apr;58:103693.

Yu Y, Shen M, Song Q, Xie J. Biological activities and pharmaceutical applications of polysaccharide from natural resources: A review. Carbohydrate Polymers. 2018 Mar;183:91–101.

Cahyadi DD, Warita K, Takeda-Okuda N, Tamura J ichi, Hosaka YZ. Cartilaginous fishes-derived chondroitin sulfates potentially suppress lipid droplet accumulation in the differentiated 3T3-L1 adipocytes. Glycoconj J. 2025 Apr 1;42(2):77–86.

Li S, Li J, Mao G, Yan L, Hu Y, Ye X, et al. Effect of the sulfation pattern of sea cucumber-derived fucoidan oligosaccharides on modulating metabolic syndromes and gut microbiota dysbiosis caused by HFD in mice. Journal of Functional Foods. 2019 Apr 1;55:193–210.

Li Q, Jiang S, Shi W, Qi X, Song W, Mou J, et al. Structure characterization, antioxidant and immunoregulatory properties of a novel fucoidan from the sea cucumber *Stichopus chloronotus*. Carbohydrate Polymers. 2020 Mar 1;231:115767.

Lu SH, Hsia YJ, Shih KC, Chou TC. Fucoidan Prevents RANKL-Stimulated Osteoclastogenesis and LPS-Induced Inflammatory Bone Loss via Regulation of Akt/GSK3β/PTEN/NFATc1 Signaling Pathway and Calcineurin Activity. Marine Drugs. 2019 Jun;17(6):345.

Setiawati A, Tricahya K, Dika Octa Riswanto F, Dwiatmaka Y. Towards a sustainable chitosan-based composite scaffold derived from *Scylla serrata* crab chitosan for bone tissue engineering. Journal of Biomaterials Science, Polymer Edition. 2024 Jan 22;35(2):146–63.

Aydogdu MO, Oner ET, Ekren N, Erdemir G, Kuruca SE, Yuca E, et al. Comparative characterization of the hydrogel added PLA/β-TCP scaffolds produced by 3D bioprinting. Bioprinting. 2019 Mar 1;13:e00046.

Zhu S, Zhou Z, Chen X, Zhu W, Yang M, Yu M, et al. High mechanical performance and multifunctional degraded fucoidan-derived bioink for 3D bioprinting. Carbohydrate Polymers. 2025b Jan 15;348:122805.

Fan Z, Zhang F, Liu T, Zuo BQ. Effect of hyaluronan molecular weight on structure and biocompatibility of silk fibroin/hyaluronan scaffolds. International Journal of Biological Macromolecules. 2014 Apr 1;65:516–23.

Mutsenko VV, Bazhenov VV, Rogulska O, Tarusin DN, Schütz K, Brüggemeier S, et al. 3D chitinous scaffolds derived from cultivated marine demosponge *Aplysina aerophoba* for tissue engineering approaches based on human mesenchymal stromal cells. International Journal of Biological Macromolecules. 2017 Nov 1;104:1966–74.

Guo L, Chen H, Li Y, Zhou J, Chen J. Biocompatible scaffolds constructed by chondroitin sulfate microspheres conjugated 3D-printed frameworks for bone repair. Carbohydrate Polymers. 2023 Jan 1;299:120188.

Hong SY, Tran, Tuong Van Thi, Kang, Hoe Jin, Tripathi, Garima, Lee , ByongTaek, and Bae SH. Synthesis and characterization of biphasic calcium phosphate laden thiolated hyaluronic acid hydrogel based scaffold: physical and in-vitro biocompatibility evaluations. Journal of Biomaterials Science, Polymer Edition. 2021 Feb 11;32(3):337–54.

Zheng Z, Patel M, Patel R. Hyaluronic acid-based materials for bone regeneration: A review. Reactive and Functional Polymers. 2022 Feb 1;171:105151.

Chonanant C, Chancharoen P, Kiatkulanusorn S, Luangpon N, Klarod K, Surakul P, et al. Biocomposite Scaffolds Based on Chitosan Extraction from Shrimp Shell Waste for Cartilage Tissue Engineering Application. ACS Omega. 2024 Sep 10;acsomega.4c02910.

Carvalho DN, Gelinsky M, Williams DS, Mearns-Spragg A, Reis RL, Silva TH. Marine collagen-chitosan-fucoidan/chondroitin sulfate cryo-biomaterials loaded with primary human cells envisaging cartilage tissue engineering. International Journal of Biological Macromolecules. 2023 Jun 30;241:124510.

Carvalho DN, López-Cebral R, Sousa RO, Alves AL, Reys LL, Silva SS, et al. Marine collagen-chitosan-fucoidan cryogels as cell-laden biocomposites envisaging tissue engineering. Biomed Mater. 2020a Aug 28;15(5):055030.

Jung HS, Kim MH, Shin JY, Park SR, Jung JY, Park WH. Electrospinning and wound healing activity of β-chitin extracted from cuttlefish bone. Carbohydrate Polymers. 2018 Aug;193:205–11.

Reys LL, Silva SS, Oliveira JM, Caridade SG, Mano JF, Silva TH, et al. Revealing the potential of squid chitosan-based structures for biomedical applications. Biomed Mater. 2013 May 29;8(4):045002.

Zhou J, Li K, Ramasamy P. Chitosan-collagen biopolymer biofilm derived from cephalopod gladius; Evaluation of osteogenesis, angiogenesis and wound healing for tissue engineering application. International Journal of Biological Macromolecules. 2024 Nov;279:135078.

Puigmal AC, Ayran M, Ulag S, Altan E, Guncu MM, Aksu B, et al. Fucoidan-loaded electrospun Polyvinyl-alcohol/Chitosan nanofibers with enhanced antibacterial activity for skin tissue engineering. Journal of the Mechanical Behavior of Biomedical Materials. 2023 Dec 1;148:106163.

Sadeghi A, Fatemi MJ, Zandi M, Bagheri T, Ghadimi T, Tamimi M, et al. Multilayered 3-D nanofibrous scaffold with chondroitin sulfate sustained release as dermal substitute. International Journal of Biological Macromolecules. 2022 May 1;206:718–29.

Schubert M, Binnewerg B, Voronkina A, Muzychka L, Wysokowski M, Petrenko I, et al. Naturally Prefabricated Marine Biomaterials: Isolation and Applications of Flat Chitinous 3D Scaffolds from Ianthella labyrinthus (Demospongiae: Verongiida). International Journal of Molecular Sciences. 2019 Jan;20(20):5105.

Yan G, Fan M, Zhou Y, Xie M, Shi J, Dong N, et al. Chondroitin Sulfate Derivative Cross-Linking of Decellularized Heart Valve for the Improvement of Mechanical Properties, Hemocompatibility, and Endothelialization. ACS Appl Mater Interfaces. 2024 Jul 17;16(28): 35936–48.

Lei Y, Bortolin L, Benesch-Lee F, Oguntolu T, Dong Z, Bondah N, et al. Hyaluronic acid regulates heart valve interstitial cell contraction in fibrin-based scaffolds. Acta Biomaterialia. 2021 Dec 1;136:124–36.

Wang L, Xu R, Meng L, Zhang Q, Qian Z, Chen J, et al. A fucoidan-loaded hydrogel coating for enhancing corrosion resistance, hemocompatibility and endothelial cell growth of magnesium alloy for cardiovascular stents. Biomaterials Advances. 2024 Oct 1;163:213960.

Garzón I, Muñoz-Hurtado J, Pereira-Martínez J, Ionescu AM, Cardona JDLC, Tejada-Casado M, et al. Development of Novel Squid Gladius Biomaterials for Cornea Tissue Engineering. Marine Drugs. 2024 Nov 28;22(12):535.

da Silva GR, Song E, Chen KM, Chen F, Jiang L, Kim H, et al. Gelatin nanofibers coated with hyaluronic acid as a mesenchymal stromal cell scaffold for corneal regeneration. International Journal of Pharmaceutics. 2025 Jan 25;669:125009.

Lai JY, Li, Ya-Ting, Cho, Ching-Hsien, and Yu TC. Nanoscale modification of porous gelatin scaffolds with chondroitin sulfate for corneal stromal tissue engineering. International Journal of Nanomedicine. 2012 Feb 23;7:1101–14.

Kudiyarasu S, Karuppan Perumal MK, Rajan Renuka R, Manickam Natrajan P. Chitosan composite with mesenchymal stem cells: Properties, mechanism, and its application in bone regeneration. International Journal of Biological Macromolecules. 2024 Aug 1;275:133502.

Shaz N, Maran S, Genasan K, Choudhary R, Alias R, Swamiappan S, et al. Functionalization of poly (lactic-*co*-glycolic acid) nano-calcium sulphate and fucoidan 3D scaffold using human bone marrow mesenchymal stromal cells for bone tissue engineering application. International Journal of Biological Macromolecules. 2024 Jan 1;256:128059.

Carvalho DN, López-Cebral R, Sousa RO, Alves AL, Reys LL, Silva SS, et al. Marine collagen-chitosan-fucoidan cryogels as cell-laden biocomposites envisaging tissue engineering. Biomed Mater. 2020b Aug;15(5):055030.

Food and Agriculture Organization of the United Nations [Internet]. 2024 [cited 2025 May 17]. FAO Report: Global fisheries and aquaculture production reaches a new record high. Available from: https://www.fao.org/newsroom/detail/fao-report-global-fisheries-and-aquaculture-production-reaches-a-new-record-high/en

Multifunctional Marine Polysaccharides in Theranostic Applications

Kavipriya Murugaiyan, Sasvat Sayee Ram Ramesh, and Aravind Kumar Rengan

Abstract Marine polysaccharides have emerged as promising candidates in theranostic applications due to their unique physicochemical and biological properties. These biopolymers, derived from marine organisms such as algae, crustaceans, and microorganisms, offer biocompatibility, biodegradability, and bioactivity, making them suitable for a range of biomedical applications. Their ability to form hydrogels, films, and nanostructures enhances their utility in drug delivery systems, tissue engineering, and wound healing. The integration of marine polysaccharides in theranostic applications is driven by their multifunctional capabilities, including therapeutic efficacy and diagnostic potential. While marine polysaccharides hold significant promise in theranostic applications, challenges remain in optimising their properties for specific uses. The variability in polysaccharide characteristics based on their marine source and extraction methods can affect their performance. Additionally, further research is needed to fully understand their interactions with biological systems and to develop standardised protocols for their use in clinical settings. Despite these challenges, the potential of marine polysaccharides in theranostics continues to drive research and innovation in the field.

Keywords Marine polysaccharides · Theranostics · Carbon dots · Bioactive

1 Introduction

Polysaccharides are macromolecules comprising monosaccharide units linked by glycosidic bonds. These polysaccharides are commonly classified into four groups depending on their origin in occurrence, examples including storage or reserve, structural, gel forming, and based on their origin. Based on their composition, they could be further classified as homopolysaccharides and heteropolysaccharides (Delgado et al. 2019). Polysaccharides have hydrophobic groups that contribute to

K. Murugaiyan · S. S. R. Ramesh · A. K. Rengan (✉)
Department of Biomedical Engineering, Indian Institute of Technology-Hyderabad, Sangareddy, Telangana, India
e-mail: aravind@bme.iith.ac.in

S. Jana et al. (eds.), *Multifunctional Marine Polysaccharides*,
https://doi.org/10.1007/978-981-95-4126-3_14

their helical confirmation due to their stereoregularity. Their stability also depends on parameters like temperature and ionic concentration (Rinaudo 2008). Being water-soluble polymers, polysaccharides play a crucial role as thickening, gelling, and emulsifying agents (Li et al. 2024). According to the nature of monosaccharide components present, chain length, and the type of branching, they can be differentiated. Based on the charges present, they can be further classified as positively (e.g., chitosan) and negatively (e.g., alginate, heparin, hyaluronic acid, etc.) charged polysaccharides. Heteropolysaccharides such as GAGs (glycosaminoglycans) present on the cell surface and extracellular matrix have biological significance. They include heparin, heparan sulfate, hyaluronan, chondroitin sulfate, dermatan sulfate, and keratan sulfate (Mohammed et al. 2021; Sasisekharan et al. 2006; Boddohi and Kipper 2010). Marine polysaccharides primarily originate from macroalgae and phytoplankton, constituting a significant portion of organic matter in the ocean. They are complex carbohydrates that include various structural forms. These are sulfated polysaccharides such as fucoidans, carrageenans, and ulvans obtained from brown, red, and green algae, respectively. Additionally, marine bacteria, particularly those from the phylum *Bacteroidetes* and the *Flavobacteriales* order, contribute to polysaccharide production and degradation. These bacteria possess specialised enzymatic machinery to process polysaccharides, linking microbial activity to the cycling of these essential organic compounds in marine ecosystems. Marine bacteria also produce unique polysaccharides, such as exopolysaccharides, which exhibit diverse structural and functional properties (Arnosti et al. 2021; Jeewon et al. 2023; Sutapa et al. 2017). Generally, they can also be referred to as sources obtained from chitosan, microalgae and macroalgae, marine-based bacteria, fungi, and starfish (Yang et al. 2023). Polysaccharides obtained from macroalgae can be further classified into mucopolysaccharides, cell wall-structure polysaccharides, and storage polysaccharides (Tiwari et al. 2022). The increasing interest in these EPS is due to their biodegradability, biological activities, and biocompatibility, making them valuable for applications in food, cosmetics, biomedical industries, and environmental remediation (Qi et al. 2022). These polysaccharides exhibit diverse bioactive potential and functional characteristics, contributing to their application in pharmaceutical products aimed at disease control. Additionally, they are associated with lipopolysaccharides like dextran and hyaluronic acid, further enhancing their biocompatibility and utility in biomedical applications (Kamala et al. 2022) (Fig. 1).

2 Structural Diversity and Functional Properties

Polysaccharides are versatile biomolecules derived from various sources, including plants, fungi, and algae. Despite their natural benefits, their applications are restricted by limitations such as low solubility, inadequate biological activity, and unsuitable physicochemical properties. Chemical modifications, such as sulfation, acetylation, phosphorylation, and carboxymethylation, have been employed to overcome these limitations, enhancing their bioactivity and expanding their applications

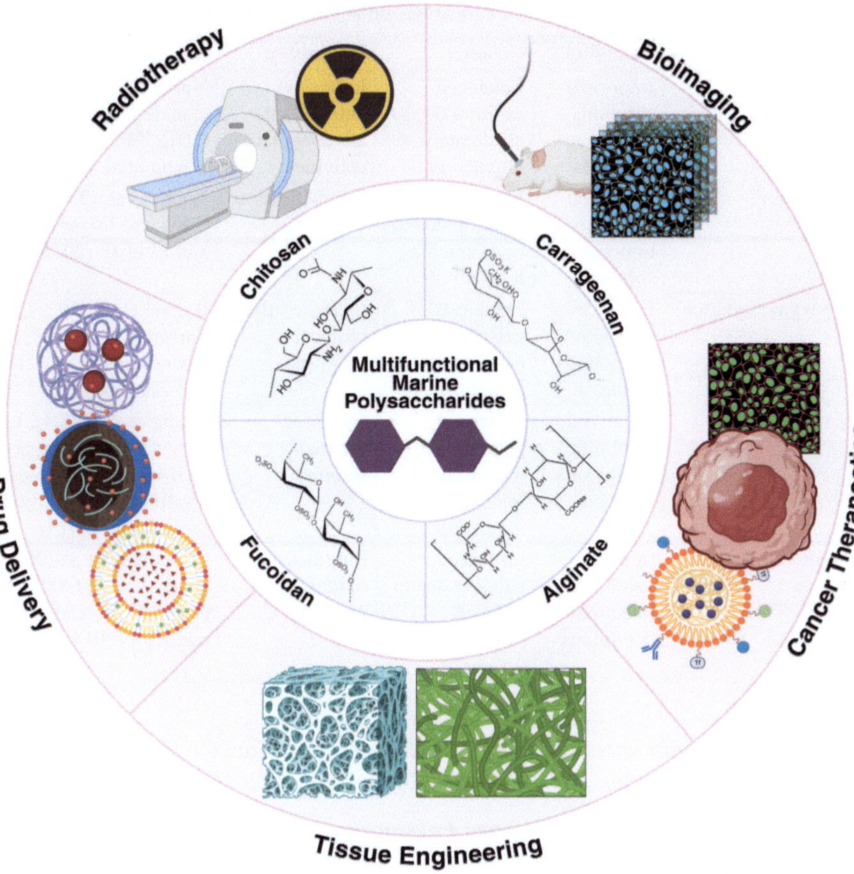

Fig. 1 Multifunctional marine polysaccharides in theranostic applications

(Wang et al. 2024a; Chemical Modification of Polysaccharides 2023; Li et al. 2022). They also help in improving solubility and gelation, which are critical for their performance in various systems. Chemical modifications of polysaccharides, such as etherification, esterification, and sulfation, enhance their amphiphilicity, solubility, and gelation properties (Zhou and Li 2024). Acetylation of polysaccharides introduces hydrophobic acetyl groups, increasing amphiphilicity and improving their crystallinity (Wang et al. 2024b). These chemical modifications depend on the polymer and the intended purpose of application. For example, chemical modifications of polysaccharides, such as galactomannans, include hydrolysis, esterification, and etherification which alter the structural characteristics and functional properties (Gómez-Rodríguez et al. 2023). Modifications such as sulfation and acetylation alter the molecular weight, substitution degree, and spatial architecture, influencing their biological activities. Understanding these relationships is essential for designing

Table 1 Impact of chitosan chemical modifications on solubility, gelation, and bioactivity

Modification	Solubility	Gelation	Bioactivity	References
Sulfonation/ sulfation	Improved solubility in aqueous solutions	Enhanced gelation due to electrostatic interaction	Enhanced antioxidant, anticoagulant activities	Niu et al. (2023), Singh et al. (2023), Wang et al. (2018, 2024a), and Zhang et al. (2024)
Acetylation	Improved solubility in organic solvents	Enhanced gelation due to hydrophobic interactions	Emulsification	Wang et al. (2024b), Chen and Edgar (2023), and Li et al. (2016)
Carboxymethylation	Improved solubility in aqueous solutions	Enhanced gelation due to negative charge	Increased rheological properties	Baghel et al. (2023), Zarrintaj et al. (2023), Nuerxiati et al. (2021), and Zhao et al. (2023)
Phosphorylation	Improved solubility in aqueous solutions	Enhanced gelation due to increased ionic interactions	Increased thermal stability	Zhang et al. (2024), Li et al. (2022), Wang et al. (2024a), and Chemical Modification of Polysaccharides (2023)
Hydrolysis	Improved solubility in aqueous conditions	Enhanced gelation due to reduced molecular weight	Provides antioxidant property	Choudhary et al. (2024), Aanisah et al. (2022), Qi et al. (2005), and Ngo and Kim (2014)

polysaccharides with specific functionalities as seen in Table 1 (Chemical Modification of Polysaccharides 2023; Shi et al. 2024; Li et al. 2016).

(A) *Solubility of Chemically Modified Polysaccharides*

Introduction to Solubility

Solubility is a key functional property of polysaccharides, influencing their applications in food, drug delivery, and biomedical engineering. Natural polysaccharides often exhibit limited solubility in water or organic solvents, which can hinder their utility. Chemical modifications, such as sulfonation, acetylation, and carboxymethylation, have been employed to improve solubility by altering the molecular structure and introducing functional groups (Zhou and Li 2024; Chen et al. 2024a; Li et al. 2022).

Sulfonation

Sulfonation involves the introduction of sulfate groups into the polysaccharide backbone, which enhances solubility by increasing the hydrophilicity of the molecule. Sulfated polysaccharides, such as sulfated fucoidan and sulfated galactomannans, have shown improved solubility in aqueous solutions. This modification also imparts additional biological activities, including antioxidant and anticoagulant properties (Niu et al. 2023; Singh et al. 2023).

Acetylation

Acetylation introduces acetyl groups to the hydroxyl groups of polysaccharides, reducing their hydrophilicity but improving their solubility in organic solvents. Acetylated polysaccharides, such as acetylated chitosan and acetylated cellulose, are widely used in food and pharmaceutical applications due to their enhanced stability and compatibility with organic systems (Wang et al. 2024b; Chen and Edgar 2023).

Carboxymethylation

Carboxymethylation is another widely used modification that enhances the solubility of polysaccharides in water. The introduction of carboxymethyl groups increases the negative charge on the polysaccharide chains, leading to improved hydration and solubility. Carboxymethylated polysaccharides, such as carboxymethyl starch and carboxymethyl chitosan, are commonly used in drug delivery systems and food applications due to their high solubility and stability (Baghel et al. 2023; Zarrintaj et al. 2023).

Other Modifications

Other modifications, such as phosphorylation and selenylation, also contribute to improved solubility. Phosphorylated polysaccharides exhibit enhanced solubility in aqueous solutions, while selenylated polysaccharides have shown improved solubility in both aqueous and organic solvents. These modifications also impart additional biological activities, such as antioxidant and immunomodulatory effects (Zhang et al. 2024; Li et al. 2022).

(B) *Gelation Properties of Chemically Modified Polysaccharides*

Introduction to Gelation

Gelation is another critical functional property of polysaccharides, influencing their applications in food, pharmaceuticals, and biomedicine. The gelation behaviour of polysaccharides is influenced by factors such as molecular weight, charge, and the presence of functional groups. Chemical modifications can significantly alter the gelation properties of polysaccharides, making them more suitable for specific applications (Chen et al. 2024b; Aggarwal et al. 2022).

Hydrolysis

Hydrolysis is a common modification method that reduces the molecular weight of polysaccharides, leading to improved gelation properties. Hydrolysed polysaccharides, such as hydrolysed guar gum and hydrolysed xanthan gum, exhibit enhanced gelation due to the formation of shorter polymer chains, which can form more stable networks (Chen et al. 2024a; Aanisah et al. 2022).

Sulfonation

Sulfonation not only improves solubility but also enhances the gelation properties of polysaccharides. Sulfated polysaccharides, such as sulfated alginate and sulfated carrageenan, form stronger gels due to the increased electrostatic interactions between the polymer chains. These gels are widely used in food and pharmaceutical applications due to their high stability and versatility (Niu et al. 2023; Singh et al. 2023).

Phosphorylation

Phosphorylation introduces phosphate groups to the polysaccharide backbone, which can enhance the gelation properties by increasing the ionic interactions between the chains. Phosphorylated polysaccharides, such as phosphorylated starch and phosphorylated cellulose, are commonly used in food and biomedical applications due to their improved gelation and stability (Zhang et al. 2024; Li et al. 2022).

Acetylation

Acetylation can also influence the gelation properties of polysaccharides. Acetylated polysaccharides, such as acetylated chitosan and acetylated cellulose, exhibit enhanced gelation due to the introduction of hydrophobic groups, which can promote the formation of more stable networks. These gels are widely used in drug delivery and tissue engineering applications (Wang et al. 2024b; Chen and Edgar 2023).

Carboxymethylation

Carboxymethylation enhances the gelation properties of polysaccharides by increasing the negative charge on the polymer chains, leading to stronger electrostatic interactions. Carboxymethylated polysaccharides, such as carboxymethyl starch and carboxymethyl chitosan, form highly stable gels that are commonly used in food, pharmaceutical, and biomedical applications (Baghel et al. 2023; Zarrintaj et al. 2023).

(C) *Bioactive Properties of Chemically Modified Polysaccharides*

Sulfation

Sulfation involves the introduction of sulfate groups into polysaccharides, significantly enhancing their biological activities. This modification is known to improve antioxidant, anticoagulant, and immunomodulatory properties. Sulfated polysaccharides have shown potential in drug delivery systems due to their ability to interact with drugs and improve bioavailability. In the food industry, sulfated polysaccharides can be used as stabilisers and thickeners, while in agriculture, they may serve as soil conditioners (Wang et al. 2018, 2024a; Nuerxiati et al. 2021).

Acetylation

Acetylation introduces acetyl groups, increasing the hydrophobicity of polysaccharides and enhancing their physicochemical properties. This modification improves water solubility and emulsification capabilities, making acetylated polysaccharides suitable for food applications as emulsifiers and texture modifiers. In drug delivery, acetylated polysaccharides can improve drug encapsulation efficiency and release profiles (Wang et al. 2024b; Li et al. 2016).

Phosphorylation

Phosphorylation enhances the solubility and thermal stability of polysaccharides, improving their antioxidant and immunomodulatory activities. This modification is particularly beneficial in the food industry for creating stable food formulations and in agriculture for improving soil fertility (Wang et al. 2024a; Li et al. 2022).

Carboxymethylation

Carboxymethylation increases the negative charge of polysaccharides, improving their water solubility and rheological properties. This modification is useful in drug delivery for controlled release systems and in the food industry as thickening agents (Nuerxiati et al. 2021; Zhao et al. 2023).

Other Properties of Polysaccharides

Biodegradability

Polysaccharides are inherently biodegradable, making them environmentally friendly. For instance, cellulose-based biocomposites degrade naturally in soil or seawater, with their biodegradability controlled by factors such as temperature and chemical modifications (Kitagawa et al. 1994). Similarly, alginate-based films exhibit complete biodegradation in aqueous environments, while chitosan-based films show faster initial degradation rates but may not degrade entirely (Vidmar et al. 2023). This property is crucial for reducing environmental impact in packaging and medical applications.

Mechanical Strength

The mechanical strength of polysaccharides can be enhanced through modifications and blending. For example, cellulose-chitosan composites demonstrate high tensile strength, particularly when chitosan content is optimised between 10% and 20% (Kitagawa et al. 1994). Alginate films, when crosslinked with calcium chloride, exhibit improved mechanical properties, making them suitable for packaging applications (Wardejn et al. 2024). Additionally, the incorporation of nanocellulose into chitosan and alginate films significantly enhances their tensile strength and barrier properties (Lavrič et al. 2021).

Barrier Properties

Polysaccharide-based films often exhibit excellent barrier properties against oxygen and water vapour. Chitosan films, when modified with nanofillers like nanocellulose, show reduced water absorption and improved hydrophobicity, making them ideal for food packaging (Lavrič et al. 2021). Alginate films, when blended with chitosan or starch, also demonstrate superior oxygen and carbon dioxide barrier properties compared to conventional materials like polylactic acid (Janik et al. 2022).

3 Theranostic Applications

3.1 Chitosan

Chitosan is composed of β(1-4)-linked D-glucosamine and N-acetyl-D-glucosamine units, which contribute to its unique physicochemical properties (Román-Doval et al. 2023; Mohan 2021). The presence of free amino groups in chitosan allows for chemical modifications, enhancing its functionality and solubility across different pH levels (Biswal and Swain 2023; Sayed et al. 2024). Chitosan exhibits excellent biocompatibility and biodegradability, making it suitable for biomedical applications such as tissue engineering and drug delivery systems (Kim et al. 2018; Mohan 2021). The following sections delve into the specific applications and advancements of chitosan in theranostics.

3.1.1 Cancer Therapy

Chitosan-based nanoparticles have been extensively studied for cancer theranostics due to their ability to deliver both therapeutic and imaging agents simultaneously. These nanoparticles can be functionalised with photosensitisers, photothermal agents, and quantum dots to enhance imaging and treatment efficacy (Soubhagya and Prabaharan 2021; Dar and Khan 2019). The cationic nature of chitosan facilitates the targeted delivery of antitumor agents, proteins, and genes, improving the specificity and effectiveness of cancer treatments (Yu et al. 2023; Dar and Khan 2019). Chitosan derivatives, such as those modified with N-aminophthalimide, have shown enhanced antitumor activity against cancer cells, indicating their potential as effective theranostic agents (Kandile et al. 2024).

3.1.2 Imaging

Magnetic nano-scale MOFs were designed using iron-oxide nanoparticles with O-carboxymethyl chitosan and then the growth of IRMOF-3 shells on the surface. Encapsulation of folic acid ensures targeting, and carbon dots serve as fluorescent probes in the (Fe_3O_4@OCMC2@IRMOF-3/FA@CDs) NMOFs. The NMOFs were further loaded with doxorubicin as an anticancer agent against HeLa cells. The nanoprobes showed increased drug loading capacity, pH-responsive drug release, superparamagnetic property, MRI, optical imaging, and selective targeting of cancer cells compared to normal cells. Chitosan/MOF composites are being explored frequently with different metal cores such as Cu, Co, Fe, Zr, Al, Ag, and various bimetallic combinations. The composites are studied for different applications such as energy conversion and storage, catalysis, sensing, and drug delivery (Chowdhuri et al. 2016). IR-820 was conjugated with chitosan using carboxyl-derivatised (IR linker) with a zero-length crosslinker. An amide bond was formed between

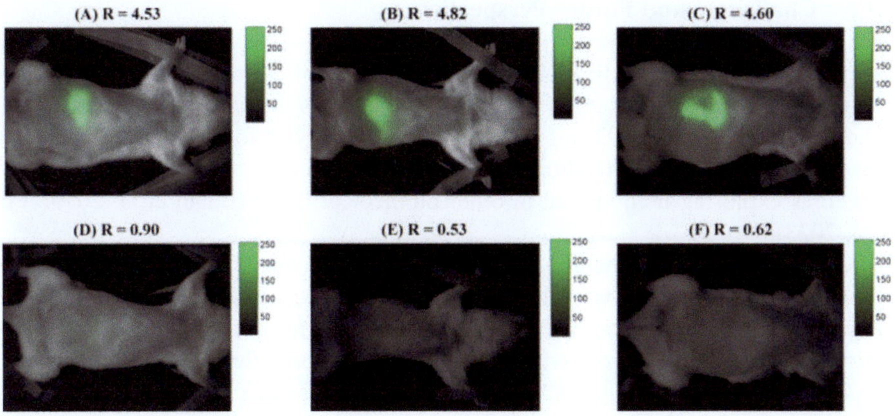

Fig. 2 IR820-chitosan conjugate imaging showed consistent abdominal signals at 45 minutes post-injection (R = 4.65 ± 0.15) that decreased to 14.6% of initial intensity by 24 h (R = 0.68 ± 0.19). Ex vivo analysis confirmed gastrointestinal retention and faecal elimination as the primary clearance route. (Srinivasan et al. 2013)

them, and their cytotoxicity was studied in MES-SA, Dx5, and SKOV-3. The developed IR820-chitosan conjugate was eliminated via the hepatobiliary system, sparing the other organs, unlike the free IR-820, which makes them suitable for optical imaging as seen in Fig. 2 (Srinivasan et al. 2013).

3.1.3 Radiotherapy

Chitosan-based nanospheres have been developed as carriers for radionuclides like 89Sr, which are used in radiopharmaceutical treatments for cancer therapy. These nanospheres exhibit second harmonic generation (SHG) properties, making them suitable for both therapeutic and diagnostic applications. The integration of fructose-based metal-organic frameworks with chitosan enhances the loading and delivery of radionuclides, providing a novel approach to radiotherapy theranostics (Cioci et al. 2024).

3.1.4 Wound Healing and Tissue Engineering

Chitosan's mucoadhesive and antimicrobial properties make it an excellent candidate for wound healing applications. It promotes cell proliferation and angiogenesis, which are crucial for tissue regeneration (Mawazi et al. 2024). In theranostic applications, chitosan-modified textiles have been developed for wound dressings, combining antimicrobial properties with the sustained release of therapeutic agents. These materials can visually indicate the presence of infections, providing a diagnostic function alongside treatment (Staneva et al. 2023).

3.1.5 Challenges and Future Perspectives

Despite the promising applications, the development of chitosan-based theranostic systems faces challenges such as regulatory hurdles and the need for further clinical validation (Yadav et al. 2024). Future research is likely to focus on optimising the functionalisation and modification of chitosan to enhance its theranostic capabilities, as well as exploring its potential in other biomedical fields (Balan et al. 2019; Yu et al. 2023).

While chitosan-based theranostic systems show great promise, it is important to consider the broader context of theranostics in biomedical research. The integration of diagnostic and therapeutic functions into a single platform is a growing trend, with various materials being explored for their potential in this field. Chitosan's unique properties make it a strong candidate, but ongoing research and development are essential to fully realise its potential and address existing challenges.

3.2 Carrageenan

Carrageenan is composed of linear, sulfated galactans, which are polysaccharides made up of alternating 3-linked β-d-galactopyranose (G-units) and 4-linked α-d-galactopyranose (D-units) or 4-linked 3,6-anhydro-α-d-galactopyranose (DA-units). The presence of sulfate groups and the 3,6-anhydro-bridge on the 4-linked galactose residue are key structural features that determine the type of carrageenan. Carrageenan is also characterised by its water-soluble potassium, sodium, magnesium, and calcium-sulfate esters of galactose and 3,6-anhydrogalactose copolymer. The primary sources of carrageenan are red seaweeds, particularly from the genera Eucheuma and Kappaphycus, which account for over 90% of global production. The three main types of carrageenan are kappa (κ), iota (ι), and lambda (λ), each with distinct structural and functional properties (van de Velde and Rollema 2006; Afoakwah et al. 2023a; Rupert et al. 2022; Rahmawati et al. 2023).

- *Kappa-carrageenan*: Known for its strong gelling properties, it is widely used in food products due to its abundance
- *Iota-carrageenan*: Forms soft gels and is often used in dairy products
- *Lambda-carrageenan*: Does not gel but is used for its thickening properties (van de Velde and Rollema 2006; Rahmawati et al. 2023)

Commercially available carrageenans often show structural variations and may contain hybrid forms, such as kappa-iota hybrids, which can affect their functionality (Hale et al. 2024). The following sections delve into the specific applications and advancements of carrageenan in theranostics.

3.2.1 Tissue Engineering and Wound Healing

Carrageenan is extensively used in tissue engineering due to its ability to mimic glycosaminoglycans, which are crucial for cell signalling and tissue repair. It is particularly effective in bone and cartilage tissue engineering and wound healing applications, where its gel-forming properties facilitate cell growth and tissue regeneration (Selvaprithiviraj et al. 2023; Das and Bal 2024).

3.2.2 Drug Delivery Systems

Carrageenan is utilised in various drug delivery systems, including hydrogels, nanoparticles, and emulsions, to enhance the delivery of bioactive compounds. Its high water solubility and ability to form stable gels makes it ideal for controlled and targeted drug release, improving the efficacy of therapeutic agents (Jayeoye et al. 2025; Gull et al. 2025).

3.2.3 Antitumor and Immunomodulatory Effects

Carrageenan exhibits antitumor properties by modulating the immune response and inhibiting tumour growth. It enhances the immune system's ability to target cancer cells, making it a promising adjuvant in cancer immunotherapy. Studies have shown that carrageenan can delay cell cycle progression in cancer cells, thereby inhibiting their proliferation (Luo et al. 2015; Prasedya et al. 2016; Kamala and Sivaperumal 2023).

3.2.4 Antiviral Activity

Carrageenan has demonstrated potent antiviral properties, particularly against human papillomavirus (HPV). It can prevent HPV infection and promote the clearance of existing infections, suggesting its potential as a complementary strategy to HPV vaccination (Laurie et al. 2021).

3.2.5 Immunomodulator

Carrageenan is used as an inflammatory agent in experimental models to study immune processes and the efficacy of anti-inflammatory drugs. It can activate innate immune pathways and alter gut microbiota, providing insights into inflammatory bowel diseases and allergic reactions. The ability of carrageenan to modulate immune responses and affect tumour microenvironments is being explored for diagnostic purposes. Its role in enhancing immune cell infiltration and cytokine production in tumours can aid in the development of diagnostic tools for cancer (Borsani et al. 2021; Luo et al. 2015).

3.2.6 Challenges and Future Perspectives

While carrageenan's therapeutic and diagnostic applications are promising, there are concerns regarding its safety, particularly in the context of inflammatory bowel diseases and allergic reactions. Some studies suggest that carrageenan can activate inflammatory pathways and alter gut microbiota, which may contribute to disease pathogenesis. Therefore, while carrageenan holds significant potential, further research is needed to fully understand its safety profile and optimise its applications in medicine.

3.3 *Alginate*

Alginate is extracted from brown seaweeds such as *Laminaria*, *Sargassum*, and *Macrocystis*. It is found in the cell walls and intercellular spaces of these algae as salts of sodium and calcium. The primary structure of alginate is a linear copolymer composed of mannuronic (M) and guluronic (G) acids, which can vary in proportion and sequence, affecting its properties (Afoakwah et al. 2023b). Alginate is known for its gelling, thickening, and film-forming abilities, which are utilised in various applications (Qin et al. 2018). It is an elastic, irreversible hydrocolloid, making it suitable for dental impressions due to its hydrophilicity and ability to record fine details (Vert et al. 2012). Alginate is also recognised for its antimicrobial properties, which are beneficial in pharmaceutical and biomedical applications (Kumar et al. 2023a). The following sections delve into the specific applications and advancements of chitosan in theranostics.

3.3.1 Drug Delivery

Alginate's ability to form hydrogels and encapsulate therapeutic agents makes it an excellent candidate for drug delivery systems. These systems can be engineered to provide controlled and targeted release of drugs, enhancing therapeutic efficacy while minimising side effects. Alginate-based nanosystems have been shown to effectively deliver therapeutic compounds, offering an eco-friendly alternative for controlled release (Lakkakula et al. 2022; Preman et al. 2022). pH-responsive zirconium-based MOFs were synthesised using UiO-66-NH_2 with 3,4-dihydroxybenzaldehyde(DHBD) to form DHBD@MOF. The developed MOF was further loaded along with the drug 5-FU(5-Fluorouracil) into a carboxymethyl cellulose and alginate hydrogel. In vitro release studies in simulated gastric and

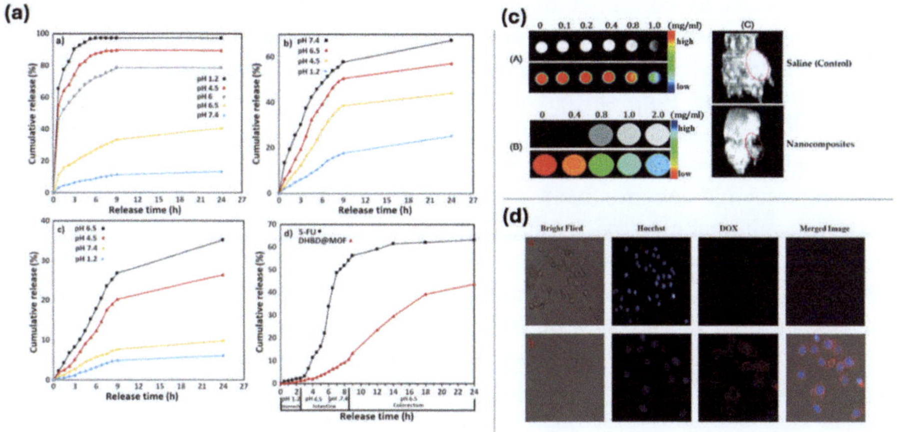

Fig. 3 (**a**) DHBD@MOF prodrug showed pH-dependent release with maximum delivery at acidic pH 1.2 (97.20%) versus physiological pH 7.4 (13.28%), enabling targeted drug release at acidic cancer sites (Binaeian and Rohani 2024). (**b**) M-MSN(Dox/Ce6)/PEM/P-gp shRNA nanocomposites demonstrated concentration-dependent MR (Fe-mediated darkening) and CT (Au-mediated brightening) contrast, enabling dual-modal imaging capability (Yang et al. 2017). (**c**) HepG2 cells were Hoechst-stained and incubated with DOX-COAL-g-PEG-FA/RhB theranostic prodrug nanogels (100 μg/mL) for 12 h, with cellular uptake assessed by fluorescence microscopy (Pei et al. 2018). (**b** is reproduced from an open-access article distributed under the terms of the Creative Commons Attribution 4.0 (CC BY-4.0) license)

intestinal fluids showed that the system provided protected burst release, ensuring controlled release at targeted sites (Fig. 3a; Binaeian and Rohani 2024).

3.3.2 Imaging Applications

Alginate's biocompatibility and ability to form stable nanocomposites make it suitable for molecular imaging applications. For instance, alginate/iron oxide nanocomposites have been used for theranostic molecular imaging in brain tumour models, demonstrating significant potential in both in vitro and in vivo settings (Su and Cheng 2015). NIR-responsive gold nanorods, along with superparamagnetic iron oxide particles, were loaded into alginate hydrogel beads. The formed beads were spherical with a diameter of 362.2 ± 22.7 μm. It was further loaded with doxorubicin, which was released in a sustained manner upon laser irradiation and allowed precise monitoring of the carrier beads using MRI imaging mode (Yoon et al. 2019). The core/shell structured magnetic mesoporous silica nanoparticles (M-MSNs) were synthesised using a modified sol-gel process. The Fe_3O_4-Au nanocrystals were incorporated to provide magnetic properties. The nanoparticles were coated with alginate/chitosan multilayers to create a pH-responsive drug delivery system. This coating also facilitated the adsorption of P-gp shRNA (P-glycoprotein small hairpin RNA) through electrostatic interactions. P-gp shRNA is used as part of a multifunctional nanocomposite system to reverse multidrug resistance in cancer therapy. The average size was found to be 280 nm, and they exhibited a positive surface charge, which is crucial for binding with negatively charged P-gp shRNA. The successful loading of Dox and Ce6 was confirmed by UV-vis spectroscopy. The release of these drugs was pH-dependent, with a higher release rate in acidic conditions, which is beneficial for targeting the acidic tumour microenvironment. The nanoparticles showed excellent biocompatibility with minimal cytotoxicity and haemolysis, making them suitable for in vivo applications. The combination of chemotherapy, photodynamic therapy (PDT), and gene therapy using these nanocomposites showed a synergistic effect in killing cancer cells both in vitro and in vivo. This was evidenced by significant tumour ablation in treated mice. The nanocomposites were effective as dual-modal imaging agents for MR and CT imaging (Fig. 3b), enhancing the visualisation of tumours in both in vitro and in vivo settings (Yang et al. 2017). A dual-responsive nanogel system was created using oxidised alginate, folic acid, and rhodamine-B terminated polyethylene glycols crosslinked with cysteamine. The formed nanogel exhibited strong fluorescence of rhodamine in an acidic environment and targeted cancer cells (Fig. 3c). The disulfide crosslinks, and acid-labile conjugation of doxorubicin increased the nanogel's sensitivity (Pei et al. 2018).

3.3.3 Tissue Engineering and Regenerative Medicine

Alginate's gel-forming ability allows it to be used as a scaffold in tissue engineering, replicating the extracellular matrix and supporting cell growth and tissue regeneration. This property is particularly useful in regenerative medicine, where alginate-based materials can aid in the healing of bone injuries, cartilage repair, and new bone regeneration (Preman et al. 2022; Sahoo and Biswal 2021).

3.3.4 Cell Delivery

Alginate's structural similarity to extracellular matrices and its ability to form hydrogels make it an ideal vehicle for cell delivery. This application is crucial in regenerative medicine, where alginate can support the transplantation and growth of cells in damaged tissues (Kesharwani et al. 2024; Xu and Lam 2018).

3.3.5 Multifunctionality

Alginate's ability to encapsulate both therapeutic and diagnostic agents allows for the development of theranostic systems that can simultaneously diagnose and treat diseases. This dual functionality is particularly beneficial in cancer treatment, where alginate-based systems can deliver chemotherapeutic agents while providing imaging capabilities to monitor treatment progress (Kothale et al. 2020; Su and Cheng

2015). The non-toxic and biodegradable nature of alginate ensures that it can be safely used in theranostic applications without adverse effects. This safety profile is critical for applications involving direct contact with biological tissues (Medha Gayatri and Vasanthi 2024; Hurtado et al. 2020).

3.3.6 Challenges and Future Perspectives

While alginate's properties make it highly suitable for theranostic applications, challenges remain in optimising its performance for specific uses. The development of alginate-based systems requires careful consideration of factors such as gelation conditions, crosslinking methods, and the incorporation of additional materials to enhance mechanical strength and functionality. Future research may focus on overcoming these challenges to fully realise the potential of alginate in theranostics.

3.4 Fucoidan

Fucoidan is a fucose-containing sulfated polysaccharide (FCSP) that constitutes 5–20% of the dry weight of brown seaweeds (Yang and Lim 2021). The simplest molecular structure of fucoidan, derived from *Fucus vesiculosus*, consists of 44.1% fucose, 26.3% sulfate, and 31.1% ash, with a small proportion of amino glucose (Tutuncu 2019). Its structure and composition can vary significantly depending on the species of algae from which it is extracted (Deghrigue et al. 2025; Jayawardena et al. 2022). Fucoidan exhibits a wide range of biological activities, including antioxidant, anticoagulant, antithrombotic, anti-inflammatory, antiviral, anti-lipidemic, anti-metastatic, anti-diabetic, and anticancer effects (Wang et al. 2022). It has been shown to reduce pro-inflammatory processes, suppress cancer cell proliferation, activate apoptosis signals in cancer cells, and inhibit vascular endothelial growth factor (VEGF) formation, thereby reducing angiogenesis and metastasis (Hees 2021). Fucoidan also has neuroprotective effects, potentially slowing neurodegenerative processes and providing therapeutic value for brain injuries and neurodegenerative diseases (Wang et al. 2021).

3.4.1 Cancer Theranostics

Fucoidan has been investigated for its anticancer properties, particularly in hepatocellular carcinoma. Functionalisation of iron oxide nanoparticles with fucoidan has shown promise in reducing cell invasion and migration, as well as decreasing reactive oxygen species production in cancer cells (Zhang et al. 2022). A fucoidan-based theranostic nanogel has been developed to enhance imaging and photodynamic therapy (PDT) of cancer. This nanogel targets P-selectin, overexpressed in tumour cells, allowing for selective imaging and treatment of

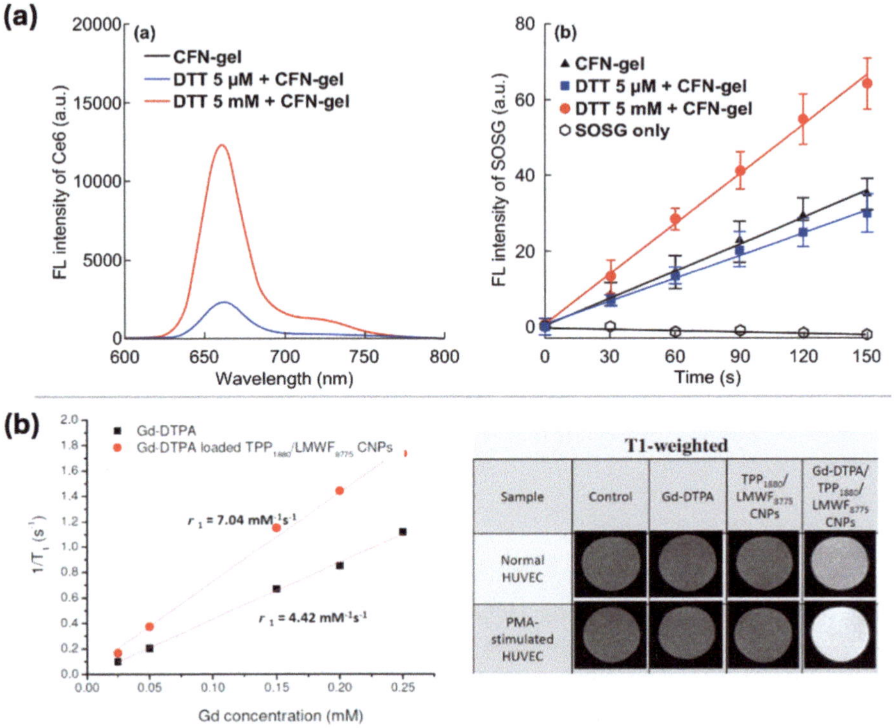

Fig. 4 (**a**) CFN-gel exhibited redox-responsive fluorescence activation and singlet oxygen generation upon DTT treatment, with concentration-dependent fluorescence enhancement and time-dependent SOSG signal increase during 670-nm laser irradiation (Cho et al. 2020). (**b**) T1 relaxation rates were plotted against Gd concentration for Gd-DTPA complex and Gd-DTPA loaded TPP1880/LMWF8775 CNPs, with T1-weighted MR imaging of inflammatory HUVECs at 0.5 mM Gd equivalent concentration (Cheng et al. 2020). (**a** is reproduced from an open-access article distributed under the terms of the Creative Commons Attribution 4.0 (CC BY-4.0) license)

tumours (Cho et al. 2020). Fucoidan-based theranostic nanogel (CFN-gel) was developed with a redox-responsive linker and photosensitiser. The developed gel showed no fluorescence or phototoxicity during systemic administration and acquired its photoactivity in response to intracellular redox potential (Fig. 4a), enabling increased PDT and selective imaging of tumours (Cho et al. 2020). Self-assembled complex nanoparticles (CNPs) were prepared by low-molecular-weight fucoidan and thermolysin hydrolysed protamine peptide (TPP_{18}). CNPs showed selective targeting of phorbol-12-myristate 13-acetate(PMA) stimulated and inflamed HUVEC cells, highly expressing P-selectin. They further loaded the nanoparticles with Gd-DTPA, which exhibited reduced cytotoxicity, selective accumulation in the activated HUVEC cells, and increased MRI intensity (Fig. 4b; Cheng et al. 2020).

3.4.2 Cardiovascular and Cerebrovascular Applications

Fucoidan exhibits lipid-lowering, anti-atherosclerosis, and anticoagulation effects, making it beneficial for cardiovascular and cerebrovascular diseases. It enhances cholesterol transport, inhibits lipid synthesis, and reduces lipid accumulation, contributing to its therapeutic potential in these conditions (Wang et al. 2022).

3.4.3 Neuroprotective Effects

Fucoidan's neuroprotective properties have been highlighted in studies focusing on brain disorders. It mitigates oxidative stress, supports mitochondrial function, and reduces neuroinflammation, suggesting its potential in treating neurodegenerative diseases (Batista et al. 2024).

3.4.4 Anti-inflammatory and Imaging Applications

Fucoidan has demonstrated significant anti-inflammatory effects, particularly in lung inflammation models. Additionally, radiolabelled fucoidan (99mTc-fucoidan) has been used for imaging inflammation sites, showcasing its dual role in therapy and diagnosis (Costa et al. 2022).

3.4.5 Autophagy Regulation

Fucoidan has been identified as a regulator of autophagy, a cellular process crucial for maintaining homeostasis. Its ability to modulate autophagy pathways presents opportunities for treating diseases such as cancer and liver disorders (Zhang et al. 2022).

3.4.6 Challenges and Future Perspectives

While fucoidan's potential in theranostic applications is promising, challenges remain in its clinical translation. The need for further clinical trials to validate its efficacy and safety is crucial, particularly in the context of neuroprotective and cancer therapies. Additionally, the development of efficient methods for its commercialisation and the determination of optimal dosages for therapeutic use are necessary steps to fully realise its potential in the pharmaceutical and nutraceutical industries.

4 Carbon Dots

CDs exhibit unique photoluminescence, which is beneficial for applications in bioimaging and biosensing, providing high sensitivity and precise identification. CDs are known for their low toxicity and high chemical stability, making them suitable for biomedical applications. Their ability to disperse in water enhances their applicability in biological environments (Wang et al. 2025; Ullah et al. 2025; Chen et al. 2025).

4.1 Synthesis Methods

- *Top-Down and Bottom-Up Approaches:* CDs can be synthesised using various techniques, including top-down methods like laser ablation and bottom-up methods such as pyrolysis (Ullah et al. 2025).
- *Biogenic Synthesis:* Utilising natural sources and waste materials offers an eco-friendly and sustainable alternative for CD production (Ullah et al. 2025). Polysaccharides like chitosan and fucoidan are subjected to hydrothermal processes, yielding CDs with distinct photoluminescent properties. Marine polysaccharides such as alginate and carrageenan serve as effective precursors, allowing for the natural doping of CDs with heteroatoms like nitrogen and sulfur (Gasilova et al. 2023; Torres et al. 2023).
- *Non-biomass Waste Conversion*: CDs can also be derived from non-biomass waste, contributing to waste management and environmental sustainability (Chen et al. 2024c).

4.2 Applications

- *Biomedical Applications:* CDs are used in diagnostics, therapy, and theranostics, including bioimaging, biosensing, and novel oncology treatments (Wang et al. 2025; Ullah et al. 2025).
- *Energy and Environmental Applications:* CDs have potential uses in energy regeneration, such as in LEDs and solar cells, and in promoting plant growth (Chen et al. 2024c).

4.3 Marine Polysaccharide-Derived Carbon Dots

Marine polysaccharide-derived CQDs are used for both therapy (like drug delivery) and diagnosis (like imaging), which is why they are referred to as theranostic agents.

They can be tagged with fluorescent markers that help doctors visualise diseases in real time. The high biocompatibility of CQDs makes them ideal carriers for drugs, ensuring that medications reach targeted areas without causing major side effects. Their strong and tunable fluorescent properties allow them to be used in various imaging techniques, from standard optical imaging to Raman imaging and even MRI when doped with certain elements. Nitrogen-doped chitosan-based carbon dots (N-CDs) were prepared by the hydrothermal carbonisation method. They had a high quantum yield (35%) and also exhibited excellent solubility, pH resistance, and increased ion strength. They enabled fluorescence imaging of *E. coli* and *B. subtilis* without causing cytotoxicity, highlighting its potential for imaging applications (Sun et al. 2021). CDs were prepared from chitin using deep eutectic solvents (ChCl/sulfonic acid). They showed high sensitivity towards Fe^{3+} ions, having a detection limit of 0.43 μM and a concentration range of 40–600 μM (Feng et al. 2022). Co-doped CDs were prepared with boron and sulfur using K-carrageenan. They exhibited increased blue-green fluorescence and photostability. It also showed high selectivity and sensitivity for glucose detection and also performed as a drug delivery vehicle for the anti-diabetic drug metformin (Das et al. 2019). Thus, carbon dots prepared from these renewable sources can help in developing sustainable theranostic agents (Torres et al. 2023).

4.4 Challenges and Future Prospects

Although promising, there are challenges like ensuring consistent quality during scale-up, enhancing the quantum yield (brightness), and understanding how these particles behave in the body over the long term. Future research is focused on overcoming these hurdles, which includes optimising the synthesis techniques and modifying the surface properties to improve functionality and safety (Torres et al. 2023; Maheshwari et al. 2025).

5 Toxicological and Regulatory Considerations of Marine Polysaccharides

Marine polysaccharides, derived from various marine organisms, have garnered significant attention due to their potential applications in pharmaceuticals, wound healing, and other biomedical fields. These polysaccharides, such as alginate, chitosan, and carrageenan, are valued for their biocompatibility, biodegradability, and low toxicity, making them suitable for diverse therapeutic applications. However, their toxicological and regulatory considerations are crucial for ensuring safe and effective use.

Toxicological Considerations

- *Non-toxic Nature*: Marine polysaccharides are generally considered non-toxic, as demonstrated in studies involving sulfated polysaccharides from marine algae like *Padina tetrastromatica* and *Ulva fasciata*. These studies showed no significant toxicological changes in vital organs, haematology, or serum toxicity parameters in animal models, even at specific doses.
- *Antioxidant and Anticoagulant Activities*: These polysaccharides have been shown to enhance antioxidant status and exhibit anticoagulant activities without adverse effects, further supporting their safety profile.
- *Biocompatibility and Biodegradability*: Marine polysaccharides are inherently biocompatible and biodegradable, which reduces the risk of adverse reactions when used in medical applications such as wound dressings and drug delivery systems (Lekshmi et al. 2019; Jing et al. 2021; Kumar et al. 2023b).

Regulatory Considerations

- *Regulatory Guidelines*: The development and use of marine polysaccharides in pharmaceuticals and other applications must adhere to regulatory guidelines to ensure safety and efficacy. This includes conducting comprehensive toxicological evaluations and adhering to test guidelines set by organisations such as the OECD (Organisation for Economic Co-operation and Development).
- *Approval for Clinical Use*: Some marine polysaccharides have been successfully converted into commercial products for clinical use, such as wound dressings, indicating that they have met regulatory requirements for safety and efficacy (Lekshmi et al. 2019; Jing et al. 2021).

6 Conclusion

Marine polysaccharides such as alginate, chitosan, and carrageenan have diverse applications in drug delivery, biomedicine, and food technology. Their unique properties, such as biocompatibility, biodegradability, and non-toxicity, make them ideal materials for these fields. As research continues to uncover their potential, these polysaccharides are expected to play an increasingly important role in advancing healthcare and food production technologies. While marine polysaccharides offer promising applications, it is essential to consider potential challenges such as variability in composition and bioactivity due to differences in source organisms and extraction methods. Additionally, the ecological impact of harvesting marine resources must be managed to ensure sustainability. These factors highlight the need for ongoing research and development to optimise the use of marine polysaccharides in various applications while adhering to regulatory standards.

References

Delgado LL, Masuelli M. Lismet Lazo Delgado and Martin Masuelli. Polysaccharides: Concepts and Classification. Evolution Poly Tech J 2019, 2(2): 180013.

Rinaudo M. Main properties and current applications of some polysaccharides as biomaterials. Polymer International. 2008 Mar;57(3):397–430.

Li K, Liu X, Jiang F, Zhang B, Qiao D, Xie F. In the process of polysaccharide gel formation: A review of the role of competitive relationship between water and alcohol molecules. International Journal of Biological Macromolecules. 2024 Nov;281:136398.

Mohammed ASA, Naveed M, Jost N. Polysaccharides; Classification, Chemical Properties, and Future Perspective Applications in Fields of Pharmacology and Biological Medicine (A Review of Current Applications and Upcoming Potentialities). J Polym Environ. 2021 Aug;29(8): 2359–71.

Sasisekharan R, Raman R, Prabhakar V. GLYCOMICS APPROACH TO STRUCTURE-FUNCTION RELATIONSHIPS OF GLYCOSAMINOGLYCANS. Annu Rev Biomed Eng. 2006 Aug 1;8(1):181–231.

Boddohi S, Kipper MJ. Engineering Nanoassemblies of Polysaccharides. Advanced Materials. 2010 Jul 27;22(28):2998–3016.

Arnosti C, Wietz M, Brinkhoff T, Hehemann JH, Probandt D, Zeugner L, et al. The Biogeochemistry of Marine Polysaccharides: Sources, Inventories, and Bacterial Drivers of the Carbohydrate Cycle. Annu Rev Mar Sci. 2021 Jan 3;13(1):81–108.

Jeewon R, Aullybux AA, Puchooa D, Nazurally N, Alrefaei AF, Zhang Y. Marine Microbial Polysaccharides: An Untapped Resource for Biotechnological Applications. Marine Drugs. 2023 Jul 24;21(7):420.

Sutapa BM, Dhruti A, Gopa RB. Pharmacological, pharmaceutical, cosmetic and diagnostic applications of sulfated polysaccharides from marine algae and bacteria. Afr J Pharm Pharmacol. 2017 Feb 8;11(5):68–77.

Yang S, Li D, Liu W, Chen X. Polysaccharides from marine biological resources and their anticancer activity on breast cancer. RSC Med Chem. 2023;14(6):1049–59.

Tiwari S, Amala Claret E, Chauhan VS. Algae as a Source of Polysaccharides and Potential Applications. In: Algal Biorefineries and the Circular Bioeconomy [Internet]. 1st ed. Boca Raton: CRC Press; 2022 [cited 2025 Jun 4]. p. 257–93. Available from: https://www.taylorfrancis.com/books/9781003195405/chapters/10.1201/9781003195405-9

Qi M, Zheng C, Wu W, Yu G, Wang P. Exopolysaccharides from Marine Microbes: Source, Structure and Application. Marine Drugs. 2022 Aug 12;20(8):512.

Kamala K, Sivaperumal P, Dharani G. Polysaccharides from Marine Micro- and Macro-Organisms. In: Marine Biochemistry [Internet]. 1st ed. Boca Raton: CRC Press; 2022 [cited 2025 Jun 4]. p. 271–84. Available from: https://www.taylorfrancis.com/books/9781003303916/chapters/10.1201/9781003303916-11

Wang Z, Zheng Y, Hu Y, Yang L, Liu X, Zhao R, et al. Improvement of antibacterial activity of polysaccharides via chemical modification: A review. International Journal of Biological Macromolecules. 2024a Jun;269:132163.

Chemical Modification of Polysaccharides: A Review of Synthetic Approaches, Biological Activity and the Structure–Activity Relationship. Molecules [Internet]. 2023 Aug 1 [cited 2025 Jun 6];28. Available from: https://scispace.com/papers/chemical-modification-of-polysaccharides-a-review-of-4k16t3xxg0

Li ZW, Du ZM, Wang YW, Feng YX, Zhang R, Yan XB. Chemical Modification, Characterization, and Activity Changes of Land Plant Polysaccharides: A Review. Polymers. 2022 Oct 4;14(19): 4161.

Zhou T, Li X. Chemically modified seaweed polysaccharides: Improved functional and biological properties and prospective in food applications. Comp Rev Food Sci Food Safe. 2024 Jul;23(4): e13396.

Wang X, Wang Z, Shen M, Yi C, Yu Q, Chen X, et al. Acetylated polysaccharides: Synthesis, physicochemical properties, bioactivities, and food applications. Critical Reviews in Food Science and Nutrition. 2024b Jun 10;64(15):4849–64.

Gómez-Rodríguez GH, Lizardi-Mendoza J, Argüelles-Monal W, Álvarez-Bajo O, López-Franco YL, Gómez-Rodríguez GH, et al. Chemical modifications of galactomannans: synthesis and structure-function analysis. Biotecnia. 2023 Aug;25(2):126–35.

Shi L, He Q, Li J, Liu Y, Cao Y, Liu Y, et al. Polysaccharides in fruits: Biological activities, structures, and structure-activity relationships and influencing factors-A review. Food Chemistry. 2024 Sep;451:139408.

Li S, Xiong Q, Lai X, Li X, Wan M, Zhang J, et al. Molecular Modification of Polysaccharides and Resulting Bioactivities. Comp Rev Food Sci Food Safe. 2016 Mar;15(2):237–50.

Chen X, Shen M, Yu Q, Chen Y, Xie J. Recent advance in chemistry modified methods of natural polysaccharides and their applications. Trends in Food Science & Technology. 2024a Feb;144: 104317.

Niu C, Liu Y, Yang Y, Wang R, Li T. Advances in sulfonated modification and bioactivity of polysaccharides. International Journal of Biological Macromolecules. 2023 Dec;253:126400.

Singh S, Sharma PK, Malviya R, Gupta A. Modified Polysaccharides and their Biomedical Applications: Advancement and Strategies. CMS. 2023 Sep;16(3):316–51.

Chen J, Edgar KJ. Synthetic Routes to Hydrogels and Polysaccharide-Based Block Copolymers. In: Cheng HN, Gross RA, editors. ACS Symposium Series [Internet]. Washington, DC: American Chemical Society; 2023 [cited 2025 Jun 6]. p. 163–85. Available from: https://pubs.acs.org/doi/abs/10.1021/bk-2023-1450.ch010

Baghel M, Sakure K, Giri TK, Maiti S, Nakhate KT, Ojha S, et al. Carboxymethylated Gums and Derivatization: Strategies and Significance in Drug Delivery and Tissue Engineering. Pharmaceuticals. 2023 May 22;16(5):776.

Zarrintaj P, Ganjali MR, Salmankhani A, Mashhadzadeh AH, Munir MT, Salehnia F, et al. Carboxymethylated polysaccharides in drug delivery. In: Tailor-Made Polysaccharides in Drug Delivery [Internet]. Elsevier; 2023 [cited 2025 Jun 6]. p. 63–81. Available from: https://linkinghub.elsevier.com/retrieve/pii/B9780128212868000124

Zhang XX, Zhang WW, Ni ZJ, Thakur K, Zhang JG, Khan MR, et al. Effects of different chemical modifications on physicochemical and antioxidation properties of Lycium barbarum seed dreg polysaccharides. Food Chemistry: X. 2024 Jun;22:101271.

Chen Y, Zhang N, Chen X. Structurally Modified Polysaccharides: Physicochemical Properties, Biological Activities, Structure–Activity Relationship, and Applications. J Agric Food Chem. 2024b Feb 21;72(7):3259–76.

Aggarwal S, Koser K, Chakravarty A, Ikram S. Understanding how the substituents of polysaccharides influence physical properties. In: Innovation in Nano-Polysaccharides for Eco-sustainability [Internet]. Elsevier; 2022 [cited 2025 Jun 6]. p. 119–32. Available from: https://linkinghub.elsevier.com/retrieve/pii/B978012823439600009X

Aanisah N, Wardhana YW, Chaerunisaa AY, Budiman A. Review on Modification of Glucomannan as an Excipient in Solid Dosage Forms. Polymers. 2022 Jun 23;14(13):2550.

Nuerxiati R, Mutailipu P, Abuduwaili A, Dou J, Aisa HA, Yili A. Effects of different chemical modifications on the structure and biological activities of polysaccharides from *Orchis chusua* D. Don. Journal of Food Science. 2021 Jun;86(6):2434–44.

Wang Z, Xie J, Shen M, Nie S, Xie M. Sulfated modification of polysaccharides: Synthesis, characterization and bioactivities. Trends in Food Science & Technology. 2018 Apr;74:147–57.

Zhao T, Yang M, Ma L, Liu X, Ding Q, Chai G, et al. Structural Modification and Biological Activity of Polysaccharides. Molecules. 2023 Jul 14;28(14):5416.

Choudhary A, Bains A, Sridhar K, Dhull SB, Goksen G, Sharma M, et al. Recent advances in modifications of exudate gums: Functional properties and applications. International Journal of Biological Macromolecules. 2024 Jun;271:132688.

Qi H, Zhao T, Zhang Q, Li Z, Zhao Z, Xing R. Antioxidant activity of different molecular weight sulfated polysaccharides from Ulva pertusa Kjellm (Chlorophyta). J Appl Phycol. 2005 Dec;17 (6):527–34.

Ngo DH, Kim SK. Antioxidant Effects of Chitin, Chitosan, and Their Derivatives. In: Advances in Food and Nutrition Research [Internet]. Elsevier; 2014 [cited 2025 Jun 7]. p. 15–31. Available from: https://linkinghub.elsevier.com/retrieve/pii/B9780128002681000020

Kitagawa R, Nishiyama M, Hosokawa J, Kubo T, Yoshihara K, Endo T, et al. New application of cellulose and chitosan for biodegradable polymer material. In: Studies in Polymer Science [Internet]. Elsevier; 1994 [cited 2025 Jun 6]. p. 451–8. Available from: https://linkinghub.elsevier.com/retrieve/pii/B9780444817082500506

Vidmar B, Oberlintner A, Stres B, Likozar B, Novak U. Biodegradation of polysaccharide-based biocomposites with acetylated cellulose nanocrystals, alginate and chitosan in aqueous environment. International Journal of Biological Macromolecules. 2023 Dec;252:126433.

Wardejn S, Wacławek S, Dudek G. Improving Antimicrobial Properties of Biopolymer-Based Films in Food Packaging: Key Factors and Their Impact. IJMS. 2024 Nov 22;25(23):12580.

Lavrič G, Oberlintner A, Filipova I, Novak U, Likozar B, Vrabič-Brodnjak U. Functional Nanocellulose, Alginate and Chitosan Nanocomposites Designed as Active Film Packaging Materials. Polymers. 2021 Jul 30;13(15):2523.

Janik W, Nowotarski M, Shyntum DY, Banaś A, Krukiewicz K, Kudła S, et al. Antibacterial and Biodegradable Polysaccharide-Based Films for Food Packaging Applications: Comparative Study. Materials. 2022 Apr 29;15(9):3236.

Román-Doval R, Torres-Arellanes SP, Tenorio-Barajas AY, Gómez-Sánchez A, Valencia-Lazcano AA. Chitosan: Properties and Its Application in Agriculture in Context of Molecular Weight. Polymers. 2023 Jan;15(13):2867.

P B, Mohan M. 8—Chitosan-based bionanocomposite in regenerative medicine. In: Ahmed S, Annu, editors. Bionanocomposites in Tissue Engineering and Regenerative Medicine [Internet]. Woodhead Publishing; 2021 [cited 2025 Jun 11]. p. 169–85. (Woodhead Publishing Series in Biomaterials). Available from: https://www.sciencedirect.com/science/article/pii/B9780128212806000349

Biswal A, Swain SK. Chitosan: A Smart Biomaterial. In: Swain SK, Biswal A, editors. Chitosan Nanocomposites: Bionanomechanical Applications [Internet]. Singapore: Springer Nature; 2023 [cited 2025 Jun 11]. p. 1–25. Available from: https://doi.org/10.1007/978-981-19-9646-7_1

Sayed AM, Hasnain SS, Abdelrady YA. Chapter 2—Introduction to chitosan and its nanocomposites. In: Ali N, Bilal M, Khan A, Nguyen TA, editors. Chitosan-Based Hybrid Nanomaterials [Internet]. Elsevier; 2024 [cited 2025 Jun 11]. p. 25–45. Available from: https://www.sciencedirect.com/science/article/pii/B9780443218910000020

Kim CH, Park SJ, Yang DH, Chun HJ. Chitosan for Tissue Engineering. In: Chun HJ, Park K, Kim CH, Khang G, editors. Novel Biomaterials for Regenerative Medicine [Internet]. Singapore: Springer; 2018 [cited 2025 Jun 11]. p. 475–85. Available from: https://doi.org/10.1007/978-981-13-0947-2_25

Soubhagya AS, Prabaharan M. Chitosan-Based Theranostics for Cancer Therapy. In: Jayakumar R, Prabaharan M, editors. Chitosan for Biomaterials IV [Internet]. Cham: Springer International Publishing; 2021 [cited 2025 Jun 9]. p. 271–92. (Advances in Polymer Science; vol. 288). Available from: https://link.springer.com/10.1007/12_2021_96

Dar MJ, Khan GM. Chitosan-based nanoparticles: promising biomedical applications in specific drug delivery and targeting. In: Materials for Biomedical Engineering [Internet]. Elsevier; 2019 [cited 2025 Jun 9]. p. 215–57. Available from: https://linkinghub.elsevier.com/retrieve/pii/B9780128169131000088

Yu F, Zhu Y, Shang X, Yuan H, Hu F. Rationally-designed Chitosan-based Polymeric Nanomaterials According to Intrinsic Characteristics for Cancer Therapy and Theranostics: A Review. Current Medicinal Chemistry. 2023. 30(12):1368–85.

Kandile NG, Ahmed MElS, Mohamed MI, Mohamed HM. Therapeutic applications of sustainable new chitosan derivatives and its nanocomposites: Fabrication and characterization. International Journal of Biological Macromolecules. 2024 Jan;254:127855.
Chowdhuri AR, Singh T, Ghosh SK, Sahu SK. Carbon Dots Embedded Magnetic Nanoparticles @Chitosan @Metal Organic Framework as a Nanoprobe for pH Sensitive Targeted Anticancer Drug Delivery. ACS Appl Mater Interfaces. 2016 Jul 6;8(26):16573–83.
Srinivasan S, Manchanda R, Fernandez-Fernandez A, Lei T, McGoron AJ. Near-infrared fluorescing IR820-chitosan conjugate for multifunctional cancer theranostic applications. Journal of Photochemistry and Photobiology B: Biology. 2013 Feb 5;119:52–9.
Cioci A, Benzi P, Canepa C, Mortati L, Alvarez de la Paz A, Garnica-Palafox IM, et al. Fructose-Based Metal–Organic Framework as a Means to Synthesize Sr-Loaded Chitosan Nanospheres with NLO Properties for Theranostic Applications in Radiotherapy. Inorganics. 2024 Sep;12(9): 231.
Mawazi SM, Kumar M, Ahmad N, Ge Y, Mahmood S. Recent Applications of Chitosan and Its Derivatives in Antibacterial, Anticancer, Wound Healing, and Tissue Engineering Fields. Polymers. 2024 Jan;16(10):1351.
Staneva D, Atanasova D, Grabchev I. Fluorescent Composite Cotton Fabric Modified with Crosslinked Chitosan for Theranostic Applications. Applied Sciences. 2023 Jan;13(23):12660.
Yadav S, Singh A, Palei NN, Pathak P, Verma A, Yadav JP. Chitosan-Based Nanoformulations: Preclinical Investigations, Theranostic Advancements, and Clinical Trial Prospects for Targeting Diverse Pathologies. AAPS PharmSciTech. 2024 Nov 5;25(8):263.
Balan V, Malihin S, Verestiuc L. Chitosan-Based Systems for Theranostic Applications. In: Jana S, Jana S, editors. Functional Chitosan: Drug Delivery and Biomedical Applications [Internet]. Singapore: Springer; 2019 [cited 2025 Jun 9]. p. 343–84. Available from: https://doi.org/10.1007/978-981-15-0263-7_12
van de Velde F, Rollema HS. High Resolution NMR of Carrageenans. In: Webb GA, editor. Modern Magnetic Resonance [Internet]. Dordrecht: Springer Netherlands; 2006 [cited 2025 Jun 11]. p. 1605–10. Available from: https://doi.org/10.1007/1-4020-3910-7_178
Afoakwah NA, Komla MG, Ali A, Ahmed S. 24—Extraction, structural properties, and applications of carrageenan gum. In: Ahmed S, Ali A, editors. Natural Gums [Internet]. Elsevier; 2023a [cited 2025 Jun 11]. p. 647–68. Available from: https://www.sciencedirect.com/science/article/pii/B9780323994682000243
Rupert R, Rodrigues KF, Thien VY, Yong WTL. Carrageenan From Kappaphycus alvarezii (Rhodophyta, Solieriaceae): Metabolism, Structure, Production, and Application. Front Plant Sci [Internet]. 2022 May 10 [cited 2025 Jun 11];13. Available from: https://www.frontiersin.org/journals/plant-science/articles/10.3389/fpls.2022.859635/full
Rahmawati I, Liviawaty E, Pratama RI, Junianto. Carrageenan in Seaweed (Eucheuma sp.) and Use of Carrageenan in Fishery Food Products: A Review. AJFAR. 2023 Jul 17;23(6):1–10.
Hale J, Gerhäuser J, Gaukel V, Wefers D. Commercially available carrageenans show broad variation in their structure, composition, and functionality [Internet]. ChemRxiv; 2024 [cited 2025 Jun 11]. Available from: https://chemrxiv.org/engage/chemrxiv/article-details/662ebc0a418a5379b0f93be1
Selvaprithiviraj V, Yegappan R, Muthuswamy S. 17—Carrageenan in tissue engineering and biomedical applications. In: Jayakumar R, Murali VP, editors. Natural Biopolymers in Drug Delivery and Tissue Engineering [Internet]. Woodhead Publishing; 2023 [cited 2025 Jun 9]. p. 449–80. (Woodhead Publishing Series in Biomaterials). Available from: https://www.sciencedirect.com/science/article/pii/B9780323988278000102
Das IJ, Bal T. Exploring carrageenan: From seaweed to biomedicine—A comprehensive review. International Journal of Biological Macromolecules. 2024 May 1;268:131822.
Jayeoye TJ, Eze FN, Muangsin N, Singh S. Carrageenan in Drug Delivery Therapeutics. In: Handbook of Research in Marine Pharmaceutics. Apple Academic Press; 2025.

Gull N, Jabeen S, Islam A, Khan SM, Khan RU. Carrageenan-based Carriers for Therapeutic Delivery. [cited 2025 Jun 9]; Available from: https://books.rsc.org/books/edited-volume/2012/chapter/4596375/Carrageenan-based-Carriers-for-Therapeutic

Luo M, Shao B, Nie W, Wei XW, Li YL, Wang BL, et al. Antitumor and Adjuvant Activity of λ-carrageenan by Stimulating Immune Response in Cancer Immunotherapy. Sci Rep. 2015 Jun 22;5(1):11062.

Prasedya ES, Miyake M, Kobayashi D, Hazama A. Carrageenan delays cell cycle progression in human cancer cells in vitro demonstrated by FUCCI imaging. BMC Complementary and Alternative Medicine. 2016 Aug 4;16(1):270.

Kamala K, Sivaperumal P. Seaweed-derived carrageenan: A potential adjuvant in the management of oral malignancies. Oral Oncology Reports. 2023 Sep 1;7:100063.

Laurie C, El-Zein M, Coutlée F, de Pokomandy A, Franco EL. Carrageenan as a Preventive Agent Against Human Papillomavirus Infection: A Narrative Review. Sexually Transmitted Diseases. 2021 Jul;48(7):458.

Borsani B, De Santis R, Perico V, Penagini F, Pendezza E, Dilillo D, et al. The Role of Carrageenan in Inflammatory Bowel Diseases and Allergic Reactions: Where Do We Stand? Nutrients. 2021 Oct;13(10):3402.

Afoakwah NA, Komla MG, Ali A, Ahmed S. 24—Extraction, structural properties, and applications of carrageenan gum. In: Ahmed S, Ali A, editors. Natural Gums [Internet]. Elsevier; 2023b [cited 2025 Jun 11]. p. 647–68. Available from: https://www.sciencedirect.com/science/article/pii/B9780323994682000243

Qin Y, Jiang J, Zhao L, Zhang J, Wang F. Chapter 13—Applications of Alginate as a Functional Food Ingredient. In: Grumezescu AM, Holban AM, editors. Biopolymers for Food Design [Internet]. Academic Press; 2018 [cited 2025 Jun 12]. p. 409–29. (Handbook of Food Bioengineering). Available from: https://www.sciencedirect.com/science/article/pii/B978012811449000013X

Vert M, Doi Y, Hellwich KH, Hess M, Hodge P, Kubisa P, et al. Terminology for biorelated polymers and applications (IUPAC Recommendations 2012). Pure and Applied Chemistry. 2012 Jan 11;84(2):377–410.

Kumar A, Kothari A, Kumar P, Singh A, Tripathi K, Gairolla J, et al. Introduction to Alginate: Biocompatible, Biodegradable, Antimicrobial Nature and Various Applications. In: Alginate—Applications and Future Perspectives [Internet]. IntechOpen; 2023a [cited 2025 Jun 12]. Available from: https://www.intechopen.com/chapters/86975

Lakkakula J, Roy A, Krishnamoorthy K, Alghamdi S, Almehmadi M, Gujarathi P, et al. Alginate-Based Nanosystems for Therapeutic Applications. Journal of Nanomaterials. 2022;2022(1): 6182815.

Preman NK, Jain S, Sanjeeva SG, Johnson RP. 10—Alginate derived nanoassemblies in drug delivery and tissue engineering. In: Venkatesan J, Kim SK, Anil S, P. d R, editors. Polysaccharide Nanoparticles [Internet]. Elsevier; 2022 [cited 2025 Jun 9]. p. 247–80. (Micro and Nano Technologies). Available from: https://www.sciencedirect.com/science/article/pii/B9780128223512000115

Binaeian E, Rohani S. pH-responsive prodrug containing Zr-based MOF and aldehyde-based drug; anionic hydrogel coating as a smart delivery system. Advanced Powder Technology. 2024 Jan;35(1):104316.

Su CH, Cheng FY. In vitro and in vivo applications of alginate/iron oxide nanocomposites for theranostic molecular imaging in a brain tumor model. RSC Adv. 2015 Oct 20;5(109):90061–4.

Yoon S, Chang J, Kwon N, Moon S, Park Y, Han KH, et al. Multifunctional Nanomaterial-alginate Drug Delivery and Imaging System for Cancer Therapy. BioChip J. 2019 Sep 1;13(3):236–42.

Yang H, Chen Y, Chen Z, Geng Y, Xie X, Shen X, et al. Chemo-photodynamic combined gene therapy and dual-modal cancer imaging achieved by pH-responsive alginate/chitosan multilayer-modified magnetic mesoporous silica nanocomposites. Biomater Sci. 2017;5(5): 1001–13.

Pei M, Jia X, Zhao X, Li J, Liu P. Alginate-based cancer-associated, stimuli-driven and turn-on theranostic prodrug nanogel for cancer detection and treatment. Carbohydrate Polymers. 2018 Mar;183:131–9.

Sahoo DR, Biswal T. Alginate and its application to tissue engineering. SN Appl Sci. 2021 Jan 8;3 (1):30.

Kesharwani P, Sharma S, Chaudhary V, Goyal R, Gautam RK. Biomedical Applications of Alginates. In: Biopolymers for Biomedical Applications [Internet]. John Wiley & Sons, Ltd; 2024 [cited 2025 Jun 9]. p. 53–86. Available from: https://onlinelibrary.wiley.com/doi/abs/10.1002/9781119865452.ch3

Xu Z, Lam MT. Alginate Application for Heart and Cardiovascular Diseases. In: Rehm BHA, Moradali MF, editors. Alginates and Their Biomedical Applications [Internet]. Singapore: Springer; 2018 [cited 2025 Jun 9]. p. 185–212. Available from: https://doi.org/10.1007/978-981-10-6910-9_7

Kothale D, Verma U, Dewangan N, Jana P, Jain A, Jain D. Alginate as Promising Natural Polymer for Pharmaceutical, Food, and Biomedical Applications. CDD. 2020 Oct 27;17(9):755–75.

B. Medha Gayatri, A. V. Vasanthi. Alginate Microbeads Technology for Pharmaceutical Applications. IJARSCT. 2024 Nov 27;492–505.

Hurtado A, Selgas R, Aroca ÁS. El alginato y sus inmensas aplicaciones industriales. Nereis Interdisciplinary Ibero-American Journal of Methods, Modelling and Simulation. 2020 Jun 26;(12):137–49.

Yang JY, Lim SY. Fucoidans and Bowel Health. Marine Drugs. 2021 Aug;19(8):436.

Tutuncu M. An Introduction to Bioactivity of Fucoidan. BJSTR [Internet]. 2019 Feb 4 [cited 2025 Jun 12];14(1). Available from: https://biomedres.us/fulltexts/BJSTR.MS.ID.002480.php

Deghrigue M, Cherif D, Lajili S, Mesmia H ben, Muller CD, Majdoub H, et al. Structural characterizations and bioactivities of fucoidans from *Dictyopteris membranacea* and *Padina pavonica* with in silico investigations. International Journal of Biological Macromolecules. 2025 May 1;307:142133.

Jayawardena TU, Nagahawatta DP, Fernando IPS, Kim YT, Kim JS, Kim WS, et al. A Review on Fucoidan Structure, Extraction Techniques, and Its Role as an Immunomodulatory Agent. Mar Drugs. 2022 Nov 30;20(12):755.

Wang K, Xu X, Wei Q, Yang Q, Zhao J, Wang Y, et al. Application of fucoidan as treatment for cardiovascular and cerebrovascular diseases. Therapeutic Advances in Chronic Disease. 2022 Jan 1;13:20406223221076891.

Hees B. Fucoidan aus Braunalgen. Deutsche Zeitschrift für Onkologie. 2021 Dec 8;53:148–56.

Wang Y, Wang Q, Han X, Ma Y, Zhang Z, Zhao L, et al. Fucoidan: a promising agent for brain injury and neurodegenerative disease intervention. Food Funct. 2021 May 11;12(9):3820–30.

Zhang N, Xue, Meilan, Sun, Ting, Yang, Jia, Pei, Zhongqian, and Qin K. Fucoidan as an Autophagy Regulator: Mechanisms and Therapeutic Potentials for Cancer and Other Diseases. Nutrition and Cancer. 2022 May 28;74(5):1568–79.

Cho MH, Li Y, Lo PC, Lee H, Choi Y. Fucoidan-Based Theranostic Nanogel for Enhancing Imaging and Photodynamic Therapy of Cancer. Nano-Micro Lett. 2020 Feb 4;12(1):47.

Cheng TM, Li R, Kao YCJ, Hsu CH, Chu HL, Lu KY, et al. Synthesis and characterization of Gd-DTPA/fucoidan/peptide complex nanoparticle and *in vitro* magnetic resonance imaging of inflamed endothelial cells. Materials Science and Engineering: C. 2020 Sep 1;114:111064.

Batista P, Cunha SA, Ribeiro T, Borges S, Baptista-Silva S, Oliveira-Silva P, et al. Fucoidans: Exploring its neuroprotective mechanisms and therapeutic applications in brain disorders. Trends in Food Science & Technology. 2024 Jan 1;143:104300.

Costa B, Corrêa LB, Silva PM e, Jannini de Sá YAP, Guimarães FV, Alencar LMR, et al. Using pure Fucoidan and radiolabeled Fucoidan (99mTc-Fucoidan) as a new agent for inflammation diagnosis and therapy. Food Hydrocolloids for Health. 2022 Dec 1;2:100049.

Wang J, Fu Y, Gu Z, Pan H, Zhou P, Gan Q, et al. Multifunctional Carbon Dots for Biomedical Applications: Diagnosis, Therapy, and Theranostic. [cited 2025 Jun 15]; Available from: https://onlinelibrary.wiley.com/doi/10.1002/smll.202303773

Ullah M, Awan UA, Ali H, Wahab A, Khan SU, Naeem M, et al. Carbon Dots: New Rising Stars in the Carbon Family for Diagnosis and Biomedical Applications. Journal of Nanotheranostics. 2025 Mar;6(1):1.

Chen BB, Liu QQ, Liu ML, Huang CZ. Introduction to Photoluminescent Carbon Dots. [cited 2025 Jun 15]; Available from: https://books.rsc.org/books/edited-volume/2140/chapter/7764157/Introduction-to-Photoluminescent-Carbon-Dots

Gasilova ER, Poshina D, Sitnikova AO, Skorik YA. Photoluminescence of Carbon Dots Obtained by Hydrothermal Treatment of Polysaccharide Solutions. In: 2023 International Conference on Electrical Engineering and Photonics (EExPolytech) [Internet]. 2023 [cited 2025 Jun 15]. p. 293–5. Available from: https://ieeexplore.ieee.org/document/10318796

Torres FG, Gonzales KN, Troncoso OP, Cañedo VS. Carbon Quantum Dots Based on Marine Polysaccharides: Types, Synthesis, and Applications. Marine Drugs. 2023 Jun;21(6):338.

Chen W, Yin H, Cole I, Houshyar S, Wang L. Carbon Dots Derived from Non-Biomass Waste: Methods, Applications, and Future Perspectives. Molecules. 2024c Jan;29(11):2441.

Sun L, Zhang H, Wang Y, Xiong Z, Zhao X, Xia Y. Chitosan-derived N-doped carbon dots for fluorescent determination of nitrite and bacteria imaging. Spectrochimica Acta Part A: Molecular and Biomolecular Spectroscopy. 2021 Apr 15;251:119468.

Feng M, Wang Y, He B, Chen X, Sun J. Chitin-Based Carbon Dots with Tunable Photoluminescence for Fe3+ Detection. ACS Appl Nano Mater. 2022 May 27;5(5):7502–11.

Das P, Maity PP, Ganguly S, Ghosh S, Baral J, Bose M, et al. Biocompatible carbon dots derived from κ-carrageenan and phenyl boronic acid for dual modality sensing platform of sugar and its anti-diabetic drug release behavior. International Journal of Biological Macromolecules. 2019 Jul 1;132:316–29.

Maheshwari S, Singh A, Verma A. Polysaccharide-Based Carbon Quantum Dots: Synthesis and Theranostic Applications—A Review. Biomedical Materials & Devices. 2025 May 12;1–24.

Lekshmi VS, Rauf, Arun A., and Muraleedhara Kurup G. Toxicological Evaluation of Bioactive Sulfated Polysaccharides from the Edible Marine Algae Padina tetrastromatica and Ulva fasciata in Sprague-Dawley Rats. Journal of Biologically Active Products from Nature. 2019 Mar 4;9 (2):79–96.

Jing X, Sun Y, Ma X, Hu H. Marine polysaccharides: green and recyclable resources as wound dressings. Mater Chem Front. 2021 Jul 26;5(15):5595–616.

Kumar M, Kumar D, Garg Y, Mahmood S, Chopra S, Bhatia A. Marine-derived polysaccharides and their therapeutic potential in wound healing application—A review. International Journal of Biological Macromolecules. 2023b Dec 31;253:127331.

3D Printed Marine Polysaccharides in Biological Applications

Sujata Das, Upadhyayula Suryanarayana Murty, and Subham Banerjee

Abstract Three-dimensional (3D) printing is an innovative computer-aided additive manufacturing technique for fabricating complex structures in three dimensions layer by layer. This approach is anticipated to have enormous potential in several areas, including the food, pharmaceutical, and biological sectors. In recent years, several bioprinting techniques and bio-ink materials have been introduced. Nevertheless, the development of affordable and environmental friendly bio-ink materials with exceptional properties (mechanical integrity, printability, viscoelasticity, biocompatibility, and biodegradability) remains a critical requirement. In recent years, natural polysaccharides derived from marine resources have received greater attention as effective and sustainable sources of bio-ink formulations because of their abundance and biological activity in comparison to polymers derived from other sources. Particular focus is given to the working principles, material requirements, and potential applications of popular 3D-printing technologies that employ marine-sourced polysaccharides. Marine polysaccharides (e.g., chitosan, alginate, hyaluronic acid, fucoidan, laminarin, gelatin, and carrageenan) frequently employed for 3D printing are also included. Owing to recent rapidly emerging technological advances, a variety of marine-derived polysaccharides possess significant biological applications, including drug delivery, tissue engineering (cartilage and bone tissue engineering), antimicrobial, and wound healing applications. The future opportunities and challenges of applying marine polysaccharides to 3D printing in the pharmaceutical and biomedical industries were also addressed.

Keywords Marine polysaccharides · 3D printing · Drug delivery · Tissue engineering · Biomaterials

---

S. Das · U. S. Murty · S. Banerjee (✉)
Department of Pharmaceutics, National Institute of Pharmaceutical Education and Research (NIPER), Guwahati, Changsari, Assam, India

S. Jana et al. (eds.), *Multifunctional Marine Polysaccharides*,
https://doi.org/10.1007/978-981-95-4126-3_15

1 Introduction

Three-dimensional (3D) printing is a type of additive manufacturing in which materials are extruded or bound in consecutive layers to create 3D objects within the desired framework (Prasad and Smyth 2016). Additive manufacturing (AM) allows individuals to print a series of materials layer by layer while modifying the properties and shape of each layer. Although AM is currently regarded as a scalable manufacturing process, it is still regarded as a subset of fast prototyping, which includes methods for rapidly developing models and prototypes (Günther et al. 2014). Over the past three decades, there has been a steady increase in the use of additive manufacturing techniques, such as 3D printing in biomedical engineering (Pham and Dimov 2012). These technologies have been explored for their use in drug delivery. More recently, the FDA approved the 3D printed orodispersible tablet Spritam® (levetiracetam), demonstrating the ability of 3D printing to produce intricate and unique dosage forms (Yu et al. 2008; Rowe et al. 2000; Moulton and Wallace 2014). The ability to precisely control the spatial distribution of an active pharmaceutical ingredient (API) within a dosage form, develop complex geometries, deposit very small amounts of API, minimize waste, and enable the quick fabrication of various compositions to support screening procedures or the development of customized dose strengths are some advantages of employing additive manufacturing techniques for dosage form design (Rowe et al. 2000; Moulton and Wallace 2014; Alomari et al. 2015; Katstra et al. 2000).

With the growing demand for personalized medicine and tailored tissues, the convergence of marine polysaccharides (PLS) with 3D bioprinting has opened new avenues for the development of functional and customizable biological constructs (such as organs, cartilage, skin, and neural tissue). In the pharmaceutical industry, 3D bioprinting also presents a plethora of options, such as in vitro/in vivo modelling, design of innovative drug discovery systems, and advancements in drug administration and screening systems (Vyas and Udyawar 2018; Peng et al. 2017). The American Society for Testing and Materials (ASTMs) International has classified 3D printing technologies into seven main categories based on feedstock materials and layer manufacturing techniques: direct energy deposition, binder jetting, vat photopolymerization, powder bed fusion, material extrusion, material jetting, and sheet lamination (Song et al. 2024; Trenfield et al. 2019). One of the earliest 3D printing techniques, jet-based bioprinting, is similar to the traditional 2D jet printing (Ng and Shkolnikov 2024; Zhang et al. 2021). Inkjet, microvalve, laser-assisted, and acoustic bioprinting methods are all included in jet-based bioprinting (Ng et al. 2020). The methods of extrusion-based bioprinting and fused deposition modelling are based on the fusion of materials, followed by extrusion and deposition (Yilmaz et al. 2021). Three types of extrusion-based bioprinting can be distinguished based on the bio-ink dispensing system: piston-, screw-, or pneumatic-driven (Ozbolat and

Hospodiuk 2016). Vat polymerization-based bioprinting, which encompasses two-photon polymerization, digital light processing, and stereolithography, depends on liquid resin polymerization after exposure to UV-visible light at a specific wavelength (Bagheri and Jin 2019). In 3D bioprinting, bio-inks, soft biomaterials comprised of live cells/tissues and/or physiologically active molecules, are crucial for the effective fabrication of 3D frameworks (Ji and Guvendiren 2017; Hospodiuk et al. 2017; Zhang et al. 2019). Bio-inks must have several essential characteristics, such as printability (i.e., viscoelastic properties), print fidelity, structural integrity, and biocompatibility, because the bioprinting process depends primarily on the deposition of bio-inks into designed geometries developed via computer-aided design (CAD) models (Hospodiuk et al. 2017; Zhang et al. 2019). In contrast, 3D printing is the process of developing intricate, noncellular networks (also known as scaffolds) that are then seeded with live cells and/or physiologically active substances after printing (Adepu et al. 2017).

The enhanced biocompatibility, biodegradability, and flexibility of marine biopolymers originating from marine sources have drawn considerable interest in the field of biomedicine. Through their interactions with biological systems, these polymers permit cell regeneration, control drug administration, and encourage tissue repair. They have several advantages over traditional synthetic polymers (e.g., PVA (polyvinyl alcohol), PLA (polylactic acid), PLGA (polylactide-co-glycolide), and PCL (polycaprolactone)) and are frequently employed in biological applications, including drug delivery systems, tissue engineering, wound healing, and bone regeneration. Unlike terrestrial animals, polysaccharides produced from shellfish, algae, fungi, crustacean shells, and corals have various structural and biological applications. Marine-derived biomaterials, including chitosan, hyaluronic acid, alginate, carrageenan, ulvan, laminarin, and fucoidan, have received considerable attention because of their great potential for biological applications.

The integration of these marine PLS with 3D bioprinting technology has revolutionized the fabrication of complex biological constructs. 3D bioprinting facilitates the accurate deposition of biomaterials and cells, thereby enabling the fabrication of structures that closely resemble native tissue architecture. This synergy enhanced cell adhesion, proliferation, and differentiation, thereby promoting the development of functional tissue constructs. The amalgamation of marine polysaccharides with 3D bioprinting offers a sustainable and versatile platform for developing personalized therapeutic solutions. By exploiting the unique properties of these natural polymers, researchers can fabricate scaffolds that not only replicate the structural and functional attributes of native tissues but also address the limitations associated with synthetic materials. This approach holds significant promise for advancing regenerative medicine and developing tailored treatments for a myriad of medical conditions.

2 Additive Manufacturing Applications of Marine Polysaccharides

In recent years, bioprinting has attracted considerable attention. Marine organisms contain an extensive library of biopolymers that exhibit various biological signals. Owing to the large diversity of marine polysaccharides and their ease of separation, marine biomaterials have been employed in 3D bioprinting. Marine-derived compounds possess chemical structures and functions that make them suitable for a variety of applications. In 3D bioprinting, marine-derived macromolecules such as hyaluronic acid, carrageenan, chitosan, and alginate are frequently employed in regenerative medicine applications. The biomaterials used in 3D bioprinting address the requirements of printability, mechanical integrity, and biocompatibility. Marine-derived bio-inks for 3D bioprinting possess the characteristics and benefits required for tissue engineering and regenerative medicine applications. Sulfated PLS, such as carrageenan, fucoidan, and sulfated polysaccharides from green algae, have several beneficial characteristics, including enhanced sheared cell differentiation and biomineralization, hydrogel formation, alkaline phosphatase activity, scaffolding, and extracellular matrix imitation (Chegu Krishnamurthi et al. 2024).

Research into the possible uses of marine biopolymers and related compounds in several fields, such as drug delivery, wound healing within healthcare research, tissue engineering in biotechnology, and nanotechnology, as well as their potential benefits as pharmaceutical compounds, is imperative given the potential advantages of marine biomaterials in technological and medical fields (Lim et al. 2019). Different 3D-printing applications of marine PLS for drug delivery, tissue engineering, and antimicrobial applications are presented in Fig. 1. Table 1 presented different types of 3D printing technologies whereas Table 2 represents 3D printing results for different marine polymers for biological applications.

2.1 *Drug Delivery*

Marine-derived polysaccharides (PLS) have attracted interest as drug delivery vehicles because of their potential to provide more customized and minimally intrusive therapeutic approaches. Polysaccharides obtained from marine organisms are frequently used as pharmaceutical delivery systems. These PLS are suitable for fabricating intricate prototypes that can be progressively released over a prolonged period owing to their biodegradability and stimulus responsiveness. These devices can be manufactured in a variety of forms, including hydrogels, capsules, and particles, and can be designed for protection. Numerous bio-polysaccharides reduce drug loading, which may substantially mitigate the adverse effects of drugs. These materials can be employed as diagnostic and signalling indicators to guide the delivery of carriers to targeted locations. Viral vector-related health hazards restrict the applications of such systems in gene therapy (Chegu Krishnamurthi et al. 2024; Senapati et al.

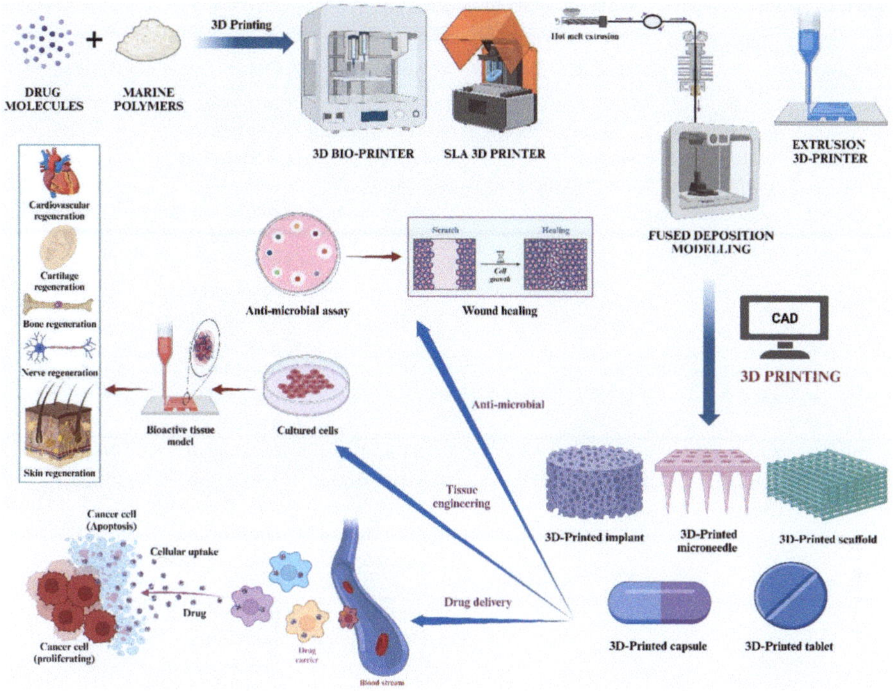

Fig. 1 3D-printing applications of marine polysaccharides in different biomedical approaches. (Created with Biorender.com)

2018). However, biomaterials provide several benefits for encapsulating genetic material and other target molecules, such as protection and stabilization, enhanced solubility that allows for longer release, biocompatibility, and biodegradability (Chegu Krishnamurthi et al. 2024). Marine polysaccharides are useful biomaterials for the development of 3D printed drug delivery systems (DDS) owing to their solubility, pH sensitivity, biodegradability, biocompatibility, and reduced toxicity.

In 2024, Su et al. developed a 3D printed scaffold composed of sodium alginate, caffeic-acid-grafted chitosan, and nanoclay for controlled local delivery in the management of postoperative breast cancer. The tumor suppression rate of the scaffolds on MCF-7 breast adenocarcinoma cells was demonstrated using a 14-day in vitro drug-release assay. Additionally, the scaffolds demonstrated strong antibacterial activity over prolonged periods. In vivo experiments have demonstrated that implantation of 3D scaffolds into postoperative deformities can suppress cancer cells that remain after surgery, reduce inflammation, encourage angiogenesis, restore tissue abnormalities resulting from surgery, and may be employed in breast cancer management (Su et al. 2024).

Another group developed a hydroxybutyl-methacrylated chitosan-based microneedle using a digital light processing (DLP) printer with dual temperature and photoresponsive properties. When exposed to temperature, the microneedles

Table 1 Different types of 3D printing technologies

3D Printing platform technology		Materials	Advantages	Disadvantages	References
Material extrusion	Fused deposition modelling (FDM)	Prefabricated filaments containing lower melting point polymers	Easy and inexpensive printing Quick processing Clean printing technique	Improper printing precision and accuracy Requirements for supporting structure Inadequate surface finish Very few polymeric materials available	Thurzo et al. (2022), Nahoum (1964), and Yassir et al. (2022)
	Semi-solid extrusion (SSE)	Semi-solid materials	Easy and inexpensive printing Room temperature printing Disposable syringe use for convenient material change	Fabricated semisolid materials with appropriate characteristics Post-processing is frequently necessary Poor printing accuracy	Wang et al. (2023)
Selective laser sintering (SLS)		Polymers with large melting point, ceramics	Prototypes with excellent physical and mechanical properties High accuracy Supporting materials not required	Expensive equipment Structure damage potential due to high-energy laser Poorly finished surface Shrinking and distortion of prototypes	Thurzo et al. (2022), Nahoum (1964), and Yassir et al. (2022)
Stereolithography (SLA)		Photopolymerized resins	Printing at room temperature Excellent printing speed High accuracy printing Capacity to print intricate geometric components Resistant to high temperature	Expensive equipment Unsuitable for large-scale manufacturing Time-consuming process Requirement for post-printing process Large material	Thurzo et al. (2022), Nahoum (1964), Yassir et al. (2022), Lin et al. (2020), Sehrawat et al. (2022), Dalaie et al. (2021), and Zinelis et al. (2022))

(continued)

Table 1 (continued)

3D Printing platform technology	Materials	Advantages	Disadvantages	References
		A smooth surface texture	consumption as supporting base is required Low precision than polyjet method Availability of very few polymeric resins	
Digital light processing (DLP)	Photopolymerized resins	Printing at room temperature Excellent printing speed Good printing accuracy and precision A smooth surface texture Develop intricate geometric structures Quick printing process Uniform layer thickness	Requirement for post-printing procedure Supporting base required	Thurzo et al. (2022), Yassir et al. (2022), Lin et al. (2020), Sehrawat et al. (2022), Dalaie et al. (2021), and Zinelis et al. (2022)
Binder jet 3D printer	Powder bed / polymeric ink	No supporting base required Variety of materials available High printing speed and cost effective	Requirement for complex post-printing procedure Low resolution and surface finish Insufficient flexibility in product Equipment cost is very high	Wang et al. (2023)
Polyjet 3D printer	Photopolymers	A smooth surface texture Develop intricate geometric structures Uniform layer thickness Excellent	Unsuitable for large-scale manufacturing Time-consuming printing process Large material consumption	Thurzo et al. (2022), Nahoum (1964), Yassir et al. (2022), Lin et al. (2020), Sehrawat

(continued)

Table 1 (continued)

3D Printing platform technology	Materials	Advantages	Disadvantages	References
		printing accuracy and precision Capacity to spray multiple materials simultaneously, to develop prototype with the appropriate mechanical and color characteristics	Equipment cost is very high	et al. (2022), and Dalaie et al. (2021)

displayed 4D characteristics, changing needle dimensions and improving mechanical strength, sharpness, and resolution. They discovered that these microneedles could penetrate soft tissues and load, transport, and release drug molecules over an extended period. Overall, chitosan-based microneedles exhibit promising potential as non-dermal drug delivery systems (Che et al. 2024). Interestingly, Zaer et al. developed a pH sensitive 3D printed alginate-gelatin scaffold encapsulated with doxorubicin-incorporated niosomes using a pneumatic piston extrusion 3D printer for the treatment of cancer (Fig. 2). The scaffolds demonstrated biodegradability, reduced cellular proliferation, enhanced cytotoxicity, decreased levels of metastasis-associated genes (Bcl-2, MMP-2, and MMP-9), and upregulation of apoptotic genes (CASP-3, CASP-8, and CASP-9) in mammary carcinoma (MCF-7) cells. The 3D printed scaffold significantly increased apoptosis and reduced necrosis, according to the flow cytometry data. This study demonstrated that the application of niosomal formulations and 3D printing could be a successful approach to the advancement of innovative nanoplatforms intended for drug delivery applications (Zaer et al. 2023).

3D printed two layered implantable scaffolds composed of chitosan and poly-ε-caprolactone were developed using a bioprinter for prolonged release of 5-fluorouracil. Continuous release of the drug resulted in an effective therapeutic concentration range throughout the administration period, whereas rapid release of the drug resulted in the prompt achievement of an effective therapeutic concentration. To improve the radiation, gold nanoparticles were placed in the second layer, which was composed of poly-ε-caprolactone, as a polymeric matrix. The implant demonstrated reduced cellular migration and higher cytotoxicity in human breast adenocarcinoma (MCF-7) cells (Di Luca et al. 2022). Fang et al. developed a sandwich composite composed of an encapsulated 3D printed scaffold and an electrospun fiber consisting of doxorubicin for tumor treatment (Fig. 3a). To stop bleeding and cancer metastasis, the lyophilized 3D printed porous scaffold quickly absorbed and aggregated the blood cells and scattered the tumor cells. Subsequently, the microtubules of the vascular endothelial cells were damaged by the selective

Table 2 3D printed marine polysaccharides for biological applications

Drug	Marine polysaccharide(s)	Delivery system	Additive manufacturing techniques	Disease target	Inference	References
Levofloxacin	Chitosan-MTAC, collagen, elastin	3D printed hydrogel	Pneumatic extrusion-based 3D bioprinter	Wound healing	The hydrogel demonstrated biocompatibility, antibacterial activity, and enhanced wound healing activity	Lazaridou et al. (2025)
Letrozole	Alginate, gelatin	3D printed scaffold	Pneumatic piston extrusion 3D printer	Breast cancer (MCF-7)	The scaffold displayed enhanced cytotoxicity, altered gene expression, greater apoptosis, reduced necrosis, increased ROS (reactive oxygen species) generation towards tumor cells	Mahdizadeh et al. (2024)
Curcumin-carbon dots	Chitosan, sodium alginate, nanoclay	3D printed hybrid scaffold	Extrusion-based 3D printer	Breast cancer (MCF-7)	The scaffold demonstrated postoperative tumor growth suppression, decreased inflammation, and promoted angiogenesis	Su et al. (2024)
–	Hydroxybutyl methacrylated chitosan	4D printed microneedle	DLP printer	Non-dermal drug delivery	The microneedle displayed extended-release pattern and penetrated soft tissue	Che et al. (2024)
Atorvastatin	Chitosan, PVA, HPMC	3D printed mucoadhesive film	Extrusion-based 3D printer	Oral candidiasis	The 3D printed film helped to mitigate microbial infection and related inflammation	Nour et al. (2023)
Doxorubicin	Alginate and gelatin	3D scaffold	Pneumatic piston extrusion 3D printer	Cancer (MCF-7)	The pH sensitive scaffold displayed enhanced cytotoxicity, apoptosis, and metastasis suppression	Zaer et al. (2023)
Paclitaxel	Alginate, gelatin	3D printed scaffold	Pneumatic piston extrusion-based 3D printer	Anticancer (MCF-7)	The scaffold demonstrated enhanced cytotoxicity, apoptosis, and suppression of metastasis	Hosseini et al. (2023)
Copper-doxorubicin	Sodium alginate, Pluronic F127	3D hydrogel scaffold	Extrusion-based 3D printer	Postoperative cancer therapy (H22)	The hydrogel showed increased apoptosis and ferroptosis, and tumor growth suppression	Dang et al. (2023)

(continued)

Table 2 (continued)

Drug	Marine polysaccharide(s)	Delivery system	Additive manufacturing techniques	Disease target	Inference	References
5-fluorouracil	Chitosan, PCL	3D printed implant	3D bioprinter	Breast cancer treatment	The insoluble implant demonstrated tailoring drug release pattern to meet the distinctive requirements of every patient	Di Luca et al. (2022)
Oxaliplatin	Sodium alginate (NPs), Eudragit L100-55	3D printed tablet	FDM printer with HME	Colon cancer (CT-26)	The printed tablet demonstrated excellent colon targeted drug release, tumor targeting ability, anticancer efficacy in CT-26 cells	Mirdamadian et al. (2022)
Combretastatin + Doxorubicin	Chitosan, gelatin, alginate, calcium chloride	3D printed scaffold	Extrusion-based 3D printer	Postoperative tumor therapy	The sandwich scaffold displayed disruption of microtubules, vascular disorders, and suppression of cell migration	Fang et al. (2022)
Methotrexate	Alginate, gelatin, TPGS	Oral 3D printed tablet	Extrusion-based 3D printer	Maintenance chemotherapy	The tablet exhibited prolonged release behavior, inhibition of P-gp efflux, and enhanced cellular uptake at gastrointestinal region	Kondiah et al. (2022)
Epirubicin	Alginate	3D printed hydrogel	Direct ink writing 3D printer (cryo-printng)	Breast cancer (MCF-7)	The hydrogel displayed increased cytotoxicity and cellular death towards tumor cells	Remaggi et al. (2022)
Doxorubicin	Alginate, gelatin, starch	3D printed capsules	FDM 3D printer	Controlled release	The capsules exhibited prolonged release pattern over 7 hours	Jingwen et al. (2021)
Levodopa	Chitosan, PLA	Scaffold	Extrusion-based 3D printer	Parkinson's disease	The scaffold showed excellent bio-compatibility, extended drug release pattern, uncompromised cell prolif-eration, and dose dependent cytotoxicity	Saylam et al. (2021)

Doxorubicin, O_2	Alginate	3D printed construct	3D bioprinter	Malignant melanoma (Colo 818)	The 3D scaffold displayed reduced cellular proliferation of cancerous cells	Motealleh et al. (2021)
Coumarin-6	Carboxy methyl chitosan, hyaluronic acid	3D hydrogel scaffold	3D bioprinter	Cancer and wound healing	The scaffold displayed prolonged release behavior and enhanced proliferation of fibroblast cells over 14 days	Puertas-Bartolomé et al. (2021)
Camptothecin	Chitosan, poly lactic acid, eudragit FS30D	Printfills (3D printed system)	Printfills (FDM and IVF technique)	Colon-specific delivery (Caco2)	The system displayed excellent intestinal permeability, targeted release at colonic pH, thereby preventing drug deterioration across the GIT	Almeida et al. (2021)
Doxorubicin	Alginate, gelatin, PCL	3D fiber scaffold	Extrusion-based 3D printer	Cancer therapy and wound healing	The scaffold displayed suppression of tumor cell progression and promote wound healing	Liu et al. (2021)
Doxorubicin, 5-fluorouracil	Alginate	3D scaffold	3D bioprinter	Breast carcinoma (MDA-MB-231and MCF-7)	Reduced cellular viability, downregulation of gene expression was demonstrated by the scaffold	Svanström et al. (2021)
Doxorubicin	Alginate, PDA	3D hydrogel scaffold	Co-axial 3D printer	Breast cancer	The scaffold displayed NIR responsive-customizable drug release by inducing photothermal effect and high anticancer activity	Wei et al. (2020)
Doxorubicin	Calcium alginate	Microfluidic chip	Projet 3500 HD MAX printer with Visjet	Breast cancer (MCF-7)	The chip demonstrated pH responsive drug release, increased cellular death towards human breast tumor cells	Cai et al. (2019)
Doxorubicin	Methacrylamide chitosan	3D printed microswimmers	Two photon direct laser writing technique	Light triggered drug delivery	The microswimmer biodegradability, biocompatibility, and displayed light triggered customizable drug delivery	Bozuyuk et al. (2018)

(continued)

Table 2 (continued)

Drug	Marine polysaccharide(s)	Delivery system	Additive manufacturing techniques	Disease target	Inference	References
Vancomycin, IGF-1	Chitosan, PEG, PLA	3D printed scaffold	Fused deposition modelling (FDM) 3D printer	Bone tissue engineering	The scaffold exhibited higher antibacterial activity and complete bone repair efficacy	Salehi et al. (2025)
–	Collagen, chitosan, and fucoidan	3D scaffold	Pneumatic driven extrusion plotter	Tissue engineering	The scaffold showed outstanding shape integrity and cellular migration	Carvalho et al. (2023)
Doxorubicin	Alginate	3D core shell fiber	Co-axial 3D printer	Tissue engineering	Stimuli responsive drug release	Wei et al. (2023)
Doxorubicin, BSA	Alginate	3D hollow fiber scaffold	Co-axial 3D printer	Tissue engineering	The scaffold displayed magnetically driven customizable drug delivery to the intended site	Wang et al. (2021)
Methotrexate	Alginate, Pluronic F127	Shape memory hydrogel	Extrusion-based 3D printer	Tissue engineering	The shape memory hydrogel displayed outstanding biocompatibility, immediate drug release, and unaffected cell proliferation of fibroblast cells	Wang et al. (2018)
–	Hyaluronic acid, methacrylated mucin	3D printed scaffold	Extrusion bioprinter	Lung tissue engineering	The scaffold displayed porous behavior, enhanced stability, biocompatibility, higher lung cell attachment and cell migration	Sasikumar et al. (2024)
—	Cysteamine grafted hyaluronic acid	3D printed hydrogel	Extrusion bioprinter	Tissue engineering	The hydrogel demonstrated self-healing, better cell support, enhanced osteoblast cell attachment and proliferation	Nagaraja et al. (2024)
Tyrosol	Thiolated hyaluronic acid, methacrylated HA	3D printed structure	SLA 3D printer	Nerve tissue engineering	The system exhibited excellent loading capacity, efficient Schwann cell proliferation and peripheral nerve regeneration	Buckley et al. (2024)

–	Methacrylated κ-carrageenan, bioactive silica nanoparticles	3D printed scaffold	DLP 3D printer	Bone tissue engineering	The scaffold showed no cytotoxicity, greater cell viability, biocompatibility, and higher osteogenic growth	Kumari et al. (2024)
–	PVA, gelatin, carrageenan	3D printed heart valve	BIO X6 bioprinter	Cardia tissue engineering	The system exhibited no persistent inflammation, can tolerate aortic environment	Jafari et al. (2024)
Clove extract	Sodium alginate, agar-agar	3D printed scaffold	Extrusion-based 3D printer	Antibacterial, wound healing and tissue engineering	The scaffold exhibited higher radical scavenging capacity, enhanced antibacterial activity, and skin regeneration	Gillani et al. (2024)
Vancomycin/ doxorubicin	Sodium alginate, gelatin	3D hydrogel	3D printer	Antibacterial/ Anti-tumor	The hydrogel was biocompatible, porous, and demonstrated bone graft characteristics and anti-tumor activity	Teterina et al. (2018)
Titanium	Chitosan, ZnO	3D printed implant	Selective laser melting / electrophoretic deposition	Antibacterial	The implant exhibited excellent antibacterial activity, hydroxyapatite precipitation, and increased bioactivity	Long et al. (2025)
Vancomycin	Chitosan, mesoporous bioactive glass	3D printed scaffold	Liquid deposition modelling 3D printer	Antibacterial	The scaffold demonstrated enhanced antibacterial efficacy against *S. aureus*, better cell attachment, and cell biocompatibility	Parvinnasab et al. (2025)
Vancomycin	Chitosan, cerium oxide, alginate	3D printed scaffold	Extrusion-based printer	Antibacterial and wound management	The scaffold displayed increased antibacterial activity, antioxidant activity, and ROS scavenging efficacy	Shahroudi et al. (2025)

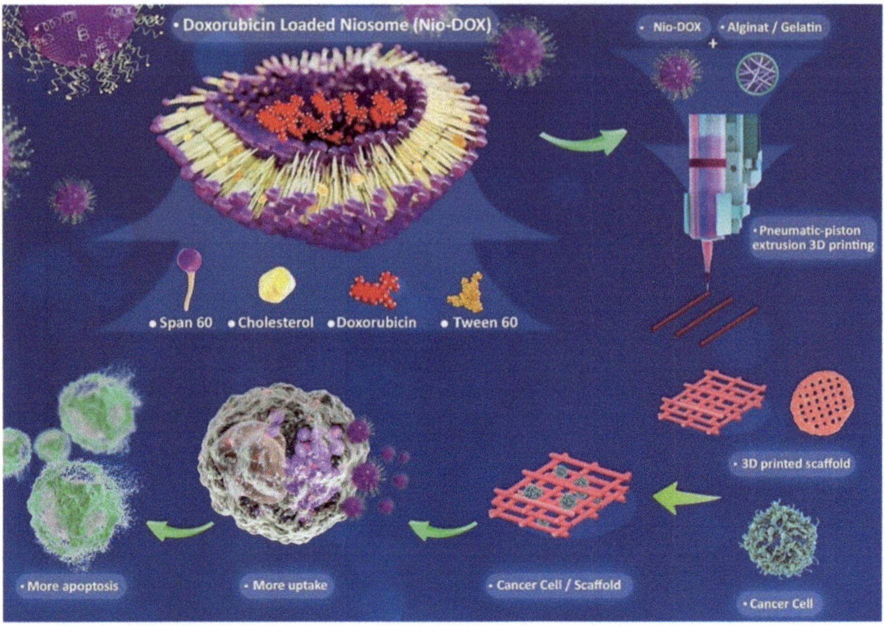

Fig. 2 Schematic illustration of pH-responsive drug delivery by 3D printed doxorubicin-loaded niosomes functionalized with gelatin and alginate. (Adapted with permission from Zaer et al. 2023)

release of combretastatin from the scaffold, leading to vascular distortion and inadequate delivery of nutrients to the solid tumor. The prolonged release of doxorubicin from the electrospun fiber sandwiched between the two layers significantly reduced the migration of peripheral tumor tissues and inhibited metastasis in RM-1 tumor-bearing mice. Combination of effective vascular disruption with chemotherapy, this integrated multifunctional implant technology offers a potential approach to postsurgical tumor therapy (Fang et al. 2022).

Kondiah and co-workers designed methotrexate-loaded nanoparticles integrated with an alginate-gelatin hydrogel to develop 3D printed tablet using an extrusion-based 3D printer for oral delivery. The findings also indicate a printing accuracy of 95%. A needle (25 G) having 25 mm of internal diameter, and an ideal printing pressure of 1400 kPa was employed to generate the 3D printed hydrogel/nanocomposite system. A regulated and extended release of methotrexate throughout a 24-hour period at pH 6.8 was seen in the in vitro release profile. P-gp ATPase efflux inhibition observed in the in silico model suggested improved gastrointestinal absorption of methotrexate. It is possible that chemotherapy difficulties associated with traditional medicines can be solved using a hydrogel-based tablet made using a 3D printer (Kondiah et al. 2022).

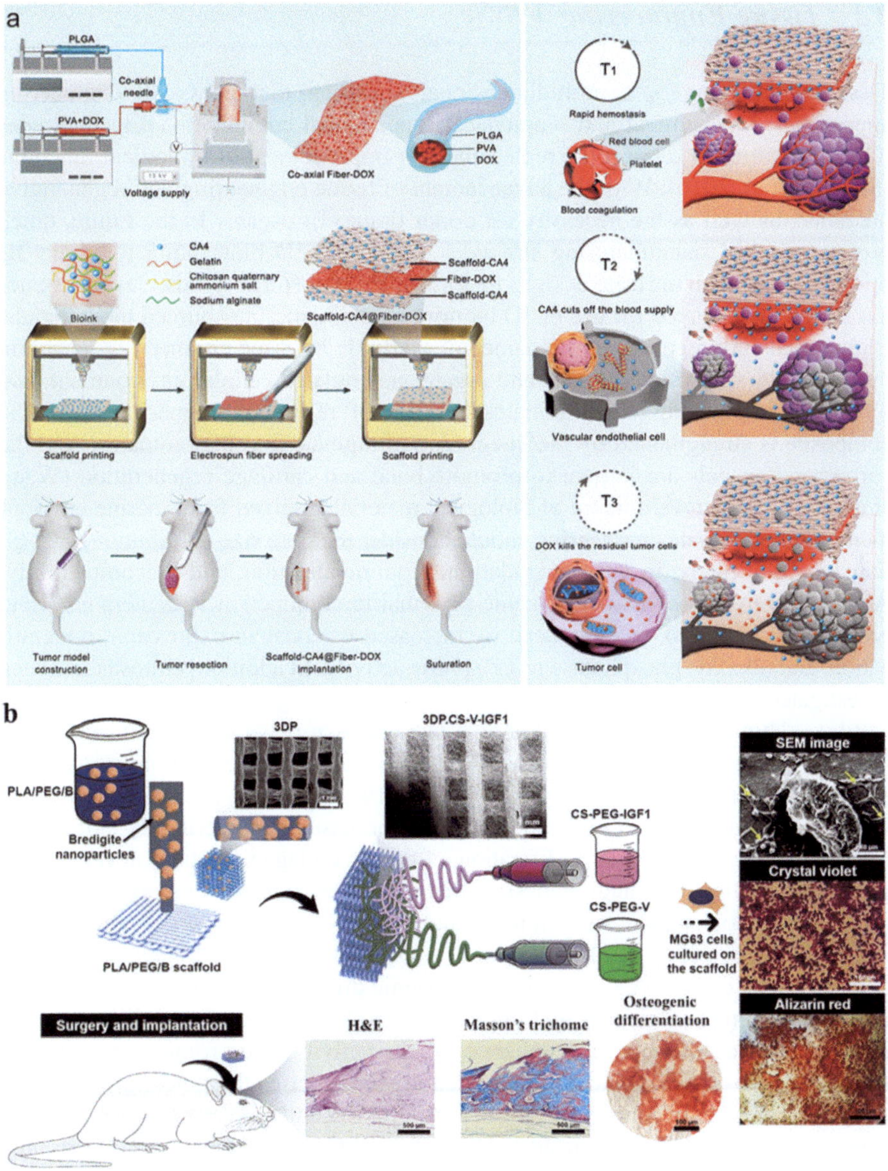

Fig. 3 (**a**) Schematic representation of combretastatin A4 and doxorubicin co-loaded 3D printed sandwich-like sponge/electrospun fiber composite for inhibiting bleeding and postoperative prostate tumor recurrence. Adapted with permission from Fang et al. (2022). (**b**) Schematic representation of antibacterial and osteogenic activity of vancomycin and IGF-1 encapsulated chitosan/PLA-PEG 3D printed scaffold. Adapted with permission from Salehi et al. (2025)

2.2 Tissue Engineering

Tissue engineering is a multidimensional approach that uses cell engineering approaches, biochemical and biophysical aspects, and computational technologies (CAD software) to support the replacement or improvement of biological functions (Mathew et al. 2016). With the advancement of tissue engineering and regenerative medicine, as well as the necessity for donor tissues or organs, In the future, quick prototyping and manufacturing strategies will allow 3D bioprinting to create 3D printed tissues with intricate designs for customized consumer goods. Several tissues have been investigated for use in 3D bioprinting using marine-sourced biomaterials. Biomaterials are regarded as fundamental scaffolds in tissue engineering, enabling the formation of artificial tissues and organs, a simulated cellular environment, and bio-signal impulsion, which initiates a series of regeneration mechanisms. The composite is strengthened by the integration of alginate into the biomatrix, and the corresponding gels are known to promote bone and cartilage regeneration (Wang et al. 2016). The development of biological materials derived from marine environments for bone tissue engineering should consider the pore size distribution, adsorption, swelling index, in vitro degradation, biomineralization, and biocompatibility. Alginate hydrogels exhibit osteogenic potential in conjunction with stem cells and growth factors (GFs), as evidenced by increased osteocalcin expression, mineralization, and alkaline phosphatase (ALP) phase activity. In addition, chitosan has been investigated for the repair of damaged tissues, including skin, muscles, bone, and cartilage. Numerous studies have shown that chitosan plays an integral role in cell attachment, increased mineralization, ALP activity, bone regeneration, and corneal endothelial tissue engineering (Cui et al. 2019; Tayebi et al. 2021). Fucoidan facilitates the development of bone cells in bone tissue engineering by stimulating GF activation, fibroblast proliferation, fibrous collagen matrix development, osteoconductivity, and angiogenesis when combined with other polysaccharides, such as low molecular weight chitosan and heparin-binding growth factors FGF-1 and FGF-2 (Chen et al. 2021; Venkatesan et al. 2014). Ulvan hydrogels increase the mineralization capacity by promoting osteogenic differentiation in conjunction with GFs and enzymes. Chitosan and chemically modified ulvan function together to mimic the extracellular matrix, enhance cellular activity, and promote tissue regeneration. Moreover, enzymatically modified ulvan increases the potential for mineralization and ATPase activity (Sudha et al. 2020). Recently, Salehi et al. developed a vancomycin and IGF-1 encapsulated chitosan-PEG nanofiber coated 3D printed scaffold using fused deposition modelling for bone tissue engineering applications (Fig. 3b). The scaffold demonstrated enhanced antimicrobial activity against *Staphylococcus aureus*. Furthermore, IGF-1 release was found to improve MG63 cell adhesion and migration, while counteracting the negative effects of vancomycin release on cell behavior. Preclinical in vivo investigations in a rat calvarial defect model confirmed that the group treated with 3D printed scaffold exhibited complete bone tissue healing in 8 weeks (Salehi et al. 2025).

In 2023, Carvalho et al. developed 3D printed construct consisting of fucoidan, chitosan, and collagen, using a pneumatic-driven extrusion plotter for tissue engineering. The 3D construct exhibited intriguing shear recovery capabilities at an 80% threshold and favorable shape integrity, delivering a stable structure free from deformation. The construct demonstrated excellent cell proliferation, suggesting flexibility, strong cell adherence to the scaffolds, and the provision of favorable environments for cells. The blending of fucoidan, chitosan, and collagen to produce biomaterial ink may offer strong structural support for printed items, as well as a proper environment for maintaining cell proliferation and migration, making the material suitable for printing in tissue engineering strategies (Carvalho et al. 2023).

Saylam et al. developed an encapsulated 3D printed tissue scaffold composed of chitosan and PLA for PD management. The scaffolds were 3D printed using a 30-gauge syringe needle. The incorporation of chitosan into PLA increased the weight loss and swelling behavior of the scaffolds. The scaffold demonstrated excellent biocompatibility, extended drug release behavior over a period of 14 days, and unaffected proliferation of mesenchymal stem cells (Saylam et al. 2021). Laminarin is a nontoxic, biodegradable marine polysaccharide. Interestingly, another group fabricated 3D printed constructs using bio-ink composed of laminarin-boronic acid and alginate double network hydrogel for tissue engineering applications. The 3D printed construct exhibited better mechanical integrity, resulting in a stable construct formation. The hydrogel construct demonstrated a uniform cell distribution after printing and remarkable cell viability for a prolonged time, which shows wide biological applications (Amaral et al. 2021).

Skin, skeletal muscle, neural, ophthalmic, hepatic, and dental tissue engineering have reported comparable outcomes to 3D bioprinting. Odontogenic stem cell proliferation and natural odontogenic potential have been demonstrated using alginate, dentin extracellular matrix, and stem cell bio-inks in regenerative dentistry (Athirasala et al. 2018). Similarly, human tooth pulp stem cells encapsulated in a 3D printed scaffold of gelatin and alginate enhanced the odontoblastic and osteogenic proliferation of these cells, leading to the greater development of bone-like structures (Alipour et al. 2021).

2.3 Antimicrobial Applications

Most plants and algae are structural storage units. Both sulfated and algal polysaccharides have found beneficial applications in medicine and nutrition (Santinon et al. 2022). It is believed that the glycoprotein receptors on the PLS (polysaccharides) cell surface, which bind to chemicals in bacterial DNA, cell walls, and cytoplasmic membranes, induce antibacterial action. Bacterial DNA binding is rendered possible by protein leakage, and the cytoplasmic membrane becomes more permeable (Lima et al. 2022). Several marine polysaccharides have been effectively used in drug delivery as oral antibiotics to prevent *Helicobacter pylori* biofilms from attaching to the stomach mucosa and inhibiting the growth of

Escherichia coli and *Staphylococcus aureus (*Venkatesan et al. 2022*)*. The cationic nature of chitosan contributes to its antibacterial properties against bacteria, yeast, fungi, and algae. Alginate and chitin films derived from marine environments are appropriate materials for wound dressings because of their adhesive properties, versatility, transparency, and cytocompatibility. Biomaterials can continuously modify their development, composition, and activity to dynamically alter their environments (Chegu Krishnamurthi et al. 2024). Recently, Li et al. developed a self-supporting 3D printed hydrogel composed of carboxymethyl chitosan and nanoclay, which exhibited high print fidelity and intricate 3D printability. The 3D printed hydrogel demonstrated biodegradability, enhanced antibacterial and proangiogenic activities, and efficient diabetic wound healing properties (Li et al. 2025). Ahmed et al. developed 3D printed film containing thyme and cinnamon oil-encapsulated γ-cyclodextrin and sodium alginate for antimicrobial applications. The core-shell patch was fabricated using a coaxial 3D printer, which displayed better mechanical and optical properties. The 3D printed patch exhibited enhanced inhibitory and bactericidal activities against pathogens and reduced biofilm formation (Ahmed et al. 2024).

In 2023, Nour et al. designed 3D printed mucoadhesive film composed of polyvinyl alcohol, chitosan, and hydroxypropyl methylcellulose loaded with atorvastatin-propylene glycol liposomes for the management of oral candidiasis. In human gingival fibroblasts, liposomes display sufficient colloidal stability and cytocompatibility in vitro. The created 3D printed films demonstrated mucoadhesion, appropriate swelling, controlled drug release pattern over 24 h, and growth suppression of *Candida albicans*. The 3D printed film reduced inflammation in vivo and promoted notable antifungal activity in a rabbit model of oral candidiasis. The findings of this study validated the use of medication repurposing as a potentially effective strategy to address antibiotic resistance (Nour et al. 2023). Yang and co-workers developed 3D printed scaffold composed of polylactide-co-glycolide (PLGA) and hydroxyapatite (HA) and then grafted quaternized chitosan (also known as hydroxypropyl trimethyl ammonium chloride chitosan) onto the printed scaffolds. In addition to its osteoconductive characteristics, the composite scaffold inhibited bacterial adhesion and biofilm development. Thus, there is a significant clinical application potential with the 3D printed scaffold (Yang et al. 2018).

2.4 Biological Imaging

Inflammation disrupts homeostasis at several levels and can be triggered by several factors including infection, damage, and pollution exposure. The demand for novel products that can potentially be used to treat inflammatory processes and selectively image inflammatory locations is a prevalent problem.

Costa et al. assessed the effectiveness of fucoidan as a medicinal and imaging agent by 2022. Researchers have examined fucoidan in two inflammatory models, lung (LPS) and arthritis, with the aim of achieving therapeutic aims. Radiolabelled fucoidan was evaluated as a radioligand (LPS) for inflamed lungs by using 99mTc. These findings demonstrated the anti-inflammatory and therapeutic activities of fucoidan, particularly in a lung model (LPS). Additionally, an imaging program confirmed the strong chemoattraction of radiolabelled fucoidan (99mTc-Fucoidan) to inflammatory locations with substantial bioaccumulation, thereby facilitating its conceptualization for imaging applications (Costa et al. 2022).

Jian-bo et al. synthesized a phase-transitional contrast agent (FPCA) modified with fucoidan and evaluated its efficacy in hepatoma cell targeting and in vitro ultrasound imaging. Perfluoropentane-containing nanoliposomes were developed using ultrasonic emulsification and thin-film hydration. FPCA nanoparticles were synthesized by chemically grafting fucoidan, and their chemical and physical properties were assessed. By applying ultrasonic diagnostic equipment, the imaging features of phase-transited FPCA were evaluated using both contrast-enhanced and two-dimensional ultrasounds. The effectiveness of FPCA in targeting hepatoma cells was assessed and confirmed using flow cytometry and fluorescence confocal imaging. When combining contrast-enhanced and two-dimensional ultrasound, FPCA showed significant improvement in imaging (Jian-bo et al. 2022).

Zapata et al. developed λ-carrageenan oligosaccharide-based (λ-COS)-based nanoparticles (NPs) encapsulating both divalent manganese (Mn^{2+}) releasable ions and ferrite cores to evaluate their efficacy in MRI and in vivo biodistribution applications. Depolymerized λ-CAR derivatives were assessed as possible NP scaffolds for investigating unique chemistries, particular functions, and in vivo biological interactions. In vitro experiments and cell-based models showed that λ-COS and λ-COS-NP were significantly more biocompatible than native λ-CAR, particularly in terms of suppressing proinflammatory activity. The resultant nanostructure was a λ-COS-based hybrid nanoparticle (NP) with microwave assistance. The λ-COS scaffold functioned as a macromolecular chelator for Mn^{2+} ions as well as a coating to enclose the ferrite cores. In vivo MRI studies demonstrated that λ-COS-NP is appropriate for the common use of Mn^{2+}-based intracellular contrast in MEMRI through the partial release of Mn^{2+} into the plasma for imaging of the myocardium and hepatobiliary system. MRI investigations revealed that the ferrite core coating of λ-COS-NPs achieved a favorable vascular lifespan compared to other polysaccharide-based NPs and was cleared by hepatic macrophages. Significant contrast enhancement may indicate accumulation at the target site, and the ferrite core, released Mn^{2+}, or λ-COS coating could trigger further bioactivity, which is promising for targeted therapy (Porta-Zapata et al. 2025).

3 Conclusion

Ocean is a rich source of biopolymers. As biopolymers can tolerate a wide range of environmental stresses and stimuli, they have been employed as raw materials in biological applications, and marine polysaccharides are particularly suitable. The important characteristics of marine PLS that allow their use in the production of DDS (drug delivery systems) include their nontoxic profile, biodegradability, biocompatibility, and responsiveness to stimuli. These characteristics make them suitable raw materials for the fabrication of intricate delivery systems, enabling the controlled release of target molecules. Over the past 20 years, marine biomimetic materials have been extensively employed in tissue-regeneration technologies. Marine biomaterials and their derivatives could potentially be advantageous for biomedical applications, owing to the distinct chemical and biological properties of each polymer.

The biomedical and pharmaceutical industries have been completely transformed by revolutionary technology known as 3D printing. However, despite tremendous progress and rapid development, there are still certain challenges in employing bio-ink derived from marine sources for 3D bioprinting that need to be resolved. Currently, it is necessary to address the lack of ability of bio-inks composed of marine-derived biopolymers to develop structurally stable prototypes (Khiari 2024). Certain physical characteristics, including stiffness, swelling ratio, poor mechanical strength, and degradation, limit the use of marine polysaccharides in 3D printing applications. As a result, tissue-specific material biomimicry can be achieved by the physical or chemical alteration of natural biomaterials, such as the methacrylation of natural polymers for biological applications. In light of this, future studies pertaining to the fabrication of bio-inks based on marine polysaccharides must concentrate on enhancing the biological and mechanical characteristics of the bio-ink (e.g., cell attachment and migration and stability). Second, a significant obstacle in 3D bioprinting is poor resolution. The development of marine polysaccharide-based bio-inks for 3D intricate structures is essential for the broad-spectrum use of the technology in the pharmaceutical and biomedical sectors. In conclusion, 3D printing with marine polysaccharides-based bio-inks presents a plethora of benefits for pharmaceutical and biological applications. However, in vivo testing remains crucial to establish combinations of different materials to enhance the performance of marine-derived polysaccharides. Currently, there are few clinical applications for marine-derived biomaterial-based regenerative medicine. More precisely, chitosan, alginate, fucoidan, and gelatin, which are found in significant amounts, have a promising future for the development of bio-inks.

Funding Acknowledgments This article framed under the joint funding support program for the project titled *"Establishment of Centre for Marine Therapeutics"* funded under Therapeutic Chemicals Program (TCP) sponsored by the Department of Science & Technology (DST), Ministry of Science & Technology, Govt. of India, New Delhi [Sanctioned File No. DST/TDT/TC/KSM/2022/05(G)], and the Department of Pharmaceuticals (DoP), Ministry of Chemicals and Fertilizers, Govt. of India, New Delhi [Sanctioned File No. DoP-50,020/41/2021-(NIPER)].

References

Prasad, L.K. and H. Smyth, *3D Printing technologies for drug delivery: a review.* Drug development and industrial pharmacy, 2016. **42**(7): p. 1019–1031.

Günther, D., et al., *Continuous 3D-printing for additive manufacturing.* Rapid Prototyping Journal, 2014. **20**(4): p. 320–327.

Pham, D. and S.S. Dimov, *Rapid manufacturing: the technologies and applications of rapid prototyping and rapid tooling*. 2012: Springer Science & Business Media.

Yu, D.G., et al., *Three-dimensional printing in pharmaceutics: promises and problems.* Journal of pharmaceutical sciences, 2008. **97**(9): p. 3666–3690.

Rowe, C., et al., *Multimechanism oral dosage forms fabricated by three dimensional printing™.* Journal of controlled release, 2000. **66**(1): p. 11–17.

Moulton, S.E. and G.G. Wallace, *3-dimensional (3D) fabricated polymer based drug delivery systems.* Journal of Controlled Release, 2014. **193**: p. 27–34.

Alomari, M., et al., *Personalised dosing: Printing a dose of one's own medicine.* International journal of pharmaceutics, 2015. **494**(2): p. 568–577.

Katstra, W., et al., *Oral dosage forms fabricated by Three Dimensional Printing™.* Journal of controlled release, 2000. **66**(1): p. 1–9.

Vyas, D. and D. Udyawar, *A review on current state of art of bioprinting.* 3D printing and additive manufacturing technologies, 2018: p. 195–201.

Peng, W., et al., *3D bioprinting for drug discovery and development in pharmaceutics.* Acta biomaterialia, 2017. **57**: p. 26–46.

Song, Y., et al., *An overview of selective laser sintering 3D printing technology for biomedical and sports device applications: Processes, materials, and applications.* Optics & Laser Technology, 2024. **171**: p. 110459.

Trenfield, S.J., et al., *Shaping the future: recent advances of 3D printing in drug delivery and healthcare.* Expert opinion on drug delivery, 2019. **16**(10): p. 1081–1094.

Ng, W.L. and V. Shkolnikov, *Optimizing cell deposition for inkjet-based bioprinting.* International Journal of Bioprinting, 2024.

Zhang, J., et al., *3D bioprinting of human tissues: biofabrication, bioinks, and bioreactors.* International journal of molecular sciences, 2021. **22**(8): p. 3971.

Ng, W.L., et al., *Vat polymerization-based bioprinting—process, materials, applications and regulatory challenges.* Biofabrication, 2020. **12**(2): p. 022001.

Yilmaz, B., et al., *Bioprinting: A review of processes, materials and applications.* Bioprinting, 2021. **23**: p. e00148.

Ozbolat, I.T. and M. Hospodiuk, *Current advances and future perspectives in extrusion-based bioprinting.* Biomaterials, 2016. **76**: p. 321–343.

Bagheri, A. and J. Jin, *Photopolymerization in 3D printing.* ACS Applied Polymer Materials, 2019. **1**(4): p. 593–611.

Ji, S. and M. Guvendiren, *Recent advances in bioink design for 3D bioprinting of tissues and organs.* Frontiers in bioengineering and biotechnology, 2017. **5**: p. 23.

Hospodiuk, M., et al., *The bioink: A comprehensive review on bioprintable materials.* Biotechnology advances, 2017. **35**(2): p. 217–239.

Zhang, Y., et al., *Biomaterials based on marine resources for 3D bioprinting applications.* Marine drugs, 2019. **17**(10): p. 555.

Adepu, S., et al., *Three-dimensional bioprinting for bone tissue regeneration.* Current Opinion in Biomedical Engineering, 2017. **2**: p. 22–28.

Chegu Krishnamurthi, M., et al., *Exploitation of Marine-Derived Multifunctional Biomaterials in Biomedical Engineering and Drug Delivery*, in *Marine Bioactive Molecules for Biomedical and Pharmacotherapeutic Applications*. 2024, Springer. p. 231–250.

Lim, Y.-S., et al., *Marine collagen as a promising biomaterial for biomedical applications.* Marine drugs, 2019. **17**(8): p. 467.

Senapati, S., et al., *Controlled drug delivery vehicles for cancer treatment and their performance.* Signal transduction and targeted therapy, 2018. **3**(1): p. 7.
Su, Y., et al., *Caffeic acid-grafted chitosan/sodium alginate/nanoclay-based multifunctional 3D-printed hybrid scaffolds for local drug release therapy after breast cancer surgery.* Carbohydrate Polymers, 2024. **324**: p. 121441.
Che, Q.T., et al., *4D-printed microneedles from dual-sensitive chitosan for non-transdermal drug delivery.* International Journal of Biological Macromolecules, 2024. **261**: p. 129638.
Zaer, M., et al., *Doxorubicin-loaded Niosomes functionalized with gelatine and alginate as pH-responsive drug delivery system: A 3D printing approach.* International Journal of Biological Macromolecules, 2023. **253**: p. 126808.
Di Luca, M., et al., *3D printed biodegradable multifunctional implants for effective breast cancer treatment.* International Journal of Pharmaceutics, 2022. **629**: p. 122363.
Fang, Y., et al., *Implantable sandwich-like scaffold/fiber composite spatiotemporally releasing combretastatin A4 and doxorubicin for efficient inhibition of postoperative tumor recurrence.* ACS Applied Materials & Interfaces, 2022. **14**(24): p. 27525–27537.
Kondiah, P.P., et al., *An Oral 3D Printed PLGA-Tocopherol PEG Succinate Nanocomposite Hydrogel for High-Dose Methotrexate Delivery in Maintenance Chemotherapy.* Biomedicines, 2022. **10**(7): p. 1470.
Salehi, S., et al., *Antibacterial and osteogenic properties of chitosan-polyethylene glycol nanofibre-coated 3D printed scaffold with vancomycin and insulin-like growth factor-1 release for bone repair.* International Journal of Biological Macromolecules, 2025. **298**: p. 139883.
Mathew, A.P., et al., *Tissue engineering: principles, recent trends and the future.* Nanomedicine and Tissue Engineering: State of the Art and Recent Trends, 2016: p. 31–82.
Wang, Y., et al., *A biomimetic silk fibroin/sodium alginate composite scaffold for soft tissue engineering.* Scientific Reports, 2016. **6**(1): p. 39477.
Cui, Z.-K., et al., *Microporous methacrylated glycol chitosan-montmorillonite nanocomposite hydrogel for bone tissue engineering.* Nature communications, 2019. **10**(1): p. 3523.
Tayebi, T., et al., *Biofabrication of chitosan/chitosan nanoparticles/polycaprolactone transparent membrane for corneal endothelial tissue engineering.* Scientific Reports, 2021. **11**(1): p. 7060.
Chen, Y., et al., *Preparation of fucoidan-based electrospun nanofibers and their interaction with endothelial cells.* Frontiers in Bioengineering and Biotechnology, 2021. **9**: p. 739209.
Venkatesan, J., I. Bhatnagar, and S.-K. Kim, *Chitosan-alginate biocomposite containing fucoidan for bone tissue engineering.* Marine drugs, 2014. **12**(1): p. 300–316.
Sudha, P., T. Gomathi, and S.K. Kim, *Ulvan in tissue engineering.* Encyclopedia of marine biotechnology, 2020. **2**: p. 1335–1350.
Carvalho, D.N., et al., *Assessing non-synthetic crosslinkers in biomaterial inks based on polymers of marine origin to increase the shape fidelity in 3D extrusion printing.* Biomedical Materials, 2023. **18**(5): p. 055017.
Saylam, E., et al., *Levodopa-loaded 3D-printed poly (lactic) acid/chitosan neural tissue scaffold as a promising drug delivery system for the treatment of Parkinson's disease.* Applied Sciences, 2021. **11**(22): p. 10727.
Amaral, A.J., et al., *Double network laminarin-boronic/alginate dynamic bioink for 3D bioprinting cell-laden constructs.* Biofabrication, 2021. **13**(3): p. 035045.
Athirasala, A., et al., *A dentin-derived hydrogel bioink for 3D bioprinting of cell laden scaffolds for regenerative dentistry.* Biofabrication, 2018. **10**(2): p. 024101.
Alipour, M., et al., *The osteogenic differentiation of human dental pulp stem cells in alginate-gelatin/Nano-hydroxyapatite microcapsules.* BMC biotechnology, 2021. **21**: p. 1–12.
Santinon, C., et al., *Chemical modifications in the structure of seaweed polysaccharides as a viable antimicrobial application: A current overview and future perspectives.* Algal Research, 2022. **66**: p. 102796.
Lima, R., C. Fernandes, and M.M. Pinto, *Molecular modifications, biological activities, and applications of chitosan and derivatives: A recent update.* Chirality, 2022. **34**(9): p. 1166–1190.

Venkatesan, J., S.S. Murugan, and G.H. Seong, *Fucoidan-based nanoparticles: Preparations and applications.* International Journal of Biological Macromolecules, 2022. **217**: p. 652–667.

Li, S., et al., *High Self-Supporting Chitosan-Based Hydrogel Ink for In Situ 3D Printed Diabetic Wound Dressing.* Advanced Functional Materials, 2025. **35**(5): p. 2414625.

Ahmed, J., Y. Zhang, and M. Maniruzzaman, *Fabrication of 3D-printed thyme and cinnamon essential oils in γ-cyclodextrin encapsulates/sodium alginate-methylcellulose antimicrobial films with a core-shell structure.* Food Packaging and Shelf Life, 2024. **46**: p. 101406.

Nour, E.M., et al., *Atorvastatin liposomes in a 3D-printed polymer film: a repurposing approach for local treatment of oral candidiasis.* Drug Delivery and Translational Research, 2023. **13**(11): p. 2847–2868.

Yang, Y., et al., *Dual-functional 3D-printed composite scaffold for inhibiting bacterial infection and promoting bone regeneration in infected bone defect models.* Acta biomaterialia, 2018. **79**: p. 265–275.

Costa, B., et al., *Using pure Fucoidan and radiolabeled Fucoidan (99mTc-Fucoidan) as a new agent for inflammation diagnosis and therapy.* Food Hydrocolloids for Health, 2022. **2**: p. 100049.

Jian-bo, H., et al., *Fucoidan-Modified Phase-Transitional Contrast Agent for Ultrasound Imaging and Targeting of Hepatoma Cells.* Journal of Sichuan University (Medical Science Edition), 2022. **53**(5).

Porta-Zapata, M., et al., *Synthesis and Characterization of λ-Carrageenan Oligosaccharide-Based Nanoparticles: Applications in MRI and In Vivo Biodistribution Studies.* Biomacromolecules, 2025.

Khiari, Z., *Recent developments in bio-ink formulations using marine-derived biomaterials for three-dimensional (3D) bioprinting.* Marine Drugs, 2024. **22**(3): p. 134.

Thurzo, A., et al., *Utilization of a 3D printed orthodontic distalizer for tooth-borne hybrid treatment in Class II unilateral malocclusions.* Materials, 2022. **15**(5): p. 1740.

Nahoum, H.I., *The vacuum formed dental contour appliance.* NY State Dent J, 1964. **9**: p. 385–390.

Yassir, Y.A., et al., *Clinical effectiveness of clear aligner treatment compared to fixed appliance treatment: an overview of systematic reviews.* Clinical oral investigations, 2022. **26**(3): p. 2353–2370.

Wang, S., et al., *A Review of 3D Printing Technology in Pharmaceutics: Technology and Applications, Now and Future.* Pharmaceutics, 2023. **15**(2): p. 416.

Lin, C.-H., et al., *Mechanical properties, accuracy, and cytotoxicity of UV-polymerized 3D printing resins composed of Bis-EMA, UDMA, and TEGDMA.* The Journal of prosthetic dentistry, 2020. **123**(2): p. 349–354.

Sehrawat, S., et al., *The expanding domains of 3D printing pertaining to the speciality of orthodontics.* Materials Today: Proceedings, 2022. **50**: p. 1611–1618.

Dalaie, K., S.M. Fatemi, and S. Ghaffari, *Dynamic mechanical and thermal properties of clear aligners after thermoforming and aging.* Progress in orthodontics, 2021. **22**: p. 1–11.

Zinelis, S., et al., *Comparative analysis of mechanical properties of orthodontic aligners produced by different contemporary 3D printers.* Orthodontics & craniofacial research, 2022. **25**(3): p. 336–341.

Lazaridou, M., et al., *3D-printed hydrogels based on amphiphilic chitosan derivative loaded with levofloxacin for wound healing applications.* International Journal of Polymeric Materials and Polymeric Biomaterials, 2025. **74**(2): p. 67–84.

Mahdizadeh, N., et al., *Delivery of letrozole-encapsulated niosomes via a 3D bioprinting gelatin–alginate scaffold for potential breast cancer treatment.* Cancer Nanotechnology, 2024. **15**(1): p. 33.

Hosseini, F., et al., *3D-printing-assisted synthesis of paclitaxel-loaded niosomes functionalized by cross-linked gelatin/alginate composite: Large-scale synthesis and in-vitro anti-cancer evaluation.* International Journal of Biological Macromolecules, 2023. **242**: p. 124697.

Dang, W., et al., *Implantable 3D printed hydrogel scaffolds loading copper-doxorubicin complexes for postoperative chemo/chemodynamic therapy.* ACS Applied Materials & Interfaces, 2023. **15**(4): p. 4911–4923.

Mirdamadian, S.Z., et al., *3D printed tablets containing oxaliplatin loaded alginate nanoparticles for colon cancer targeted delivery. An in vitro/in vivo study.* International Journal of Biological Macromolecules, 2022. **205**: p. 90–109.

Remaggi, G., et al., *Alginate self-crosslinking ink for 3D extrusion-based cryoprinting and application for epirubicin-HCl delivery on MCF-7 cells.* Molecules, 2022. **27**(3): p. 882.

Jingwen, L., et al., *3D printing of bioinspired compartmentalized capsular structure for controlled drug release.* Journal of Zhejiang University. Science. B, 2021. **22**(12): p. 1022.

Motealleh, A., et al., *3D-printed oxygen-carrying nanocomposite hydrogels for enhanced cell viability under hypoxic and normoxic conditions.* Biomacromolecules, 2021. **22**(11): p. 4758–4769.

Puertas-Bartolomé, M., et al., *Development of bioactive catechol functionalized nanoparticles applicable for 3D bioprinting.* Materials Science and Engineering: C, 2021. **131**: p. 112515.

Almeida, A., et al., *3D printed systems for colon-specific delivery of camptothecin-loaded chitosan micelles.* European Journal of Pharmaceutics and Biopharmaceutics, 2021. **167**: p. 48–56.

Liu, C., et al., *3D printed hydrogel/PCL core/shell fiber scaffolds with NIR-triggered drug release for cancer therapy and wound healing.* Acta Biomaterialia, 2021. **131**: p. 314–325.

Svanström, A., et al., *Optimized alginate-based 3D printed scaffolds as a model of patient derived breast cancer microenvironments in drug discovery.* Biomedical Materials, 2021. **16**(4): p. 045046.

Wei, X., et al., *3D printed core-shell hydrogel fiber scaffolds with NIR-triggered drug release for localized therapy of breast cancer.* International Journal of Pharmaceutics, 2020. **580**: p. 119219.

Cai, S., et al., *3D-printed concentration-controlled microfluidic chip with diffusion mixing pattern for the synthesis of alginate drug delivery microgels.* Nanomaterials, 2019. **9**(10): p. 1451.

Bozuyuk, U., et al., *Light-triggered drug release from 3D-printed magnetic chitosan microswimmers.* ACS nano, 2018. **12**(9): p. 9617–9625.

Wei, H., et al., *Three-Dimensional Printing Multi-Drug Delivery Core/Shell Fiber Systems with Designed Release Capability.* Pharmaceutics, 2023. **15**(9): p. 2336.

Wang, Z., et al., *Magnetically-driven drug and cell on demand release system using 3D printed alginate based hollow fiber scaffolds.* International Journal of Biological Macromolecules, 2021. **168**: p. 38–45.

Wang, Y., et al., *Three-dimensional printing of shape memory hydrogels with internal structure for drug delivery.* Materials Science and Engineering: C, 2018. **84**: p. 44–51.

Sasikumar, S.C., U. Goswami, and A.M. Raichur, *3D Bioprinting with Visible Light Cross-Linkable Mucin-Hyaluronic Acid Composite Bioink for Lung Tissue Engineering.* ACS Applied Bio Materials, 2024. **7**(8): p. 5411–5422.

Nagaraja, K., et al., *3D Bioprintable Self-Healing Hyaluronic Acid Hydrogel with Cysteamine Grafting for Tissue Engineering.* Gels, 2024. **10**(12): p. 780.

Buckley, C., et al., *Hyaluronic acid hybrid formulations optimised for 3D printing of nerve conduits and the delivery of the novel neurotrophic-like compound tyrosol to enhance peripheral nerve regeneration via Schwann cell proliferation.* International Journal of Pharmaceutics, 2024. **661**: p. 124477.

Kumari, S., et al., *Visible light-based 3D bioprinted composite scaffolds of κ-carrageenan for bone tissue engineering applications.* Journal of Materials Chemistry B, 2024. **12**(7): p. 1926–1936.

Jafari, A., et al., *Formulation and Evaluation of PVA/Gelatin/Carrageenan Inks for 3D Printing and Development of Tissue-Engineered Heart Valves.* Advanced Functional Materials, 2024. **34**(7): p. 2305188.

Gillani, S.M.H., et al., *Development of 3D printed sodium alginate/agar-agar/cloves scaffolds for potential wound healing applications.* Materials Letters, 2024. **377**: p. 137357.

Teterina, A.Y., et al. *Hydrogels based on polysaccharide-calcium phosphate with antibacterial/antitumor activity for 3D printing*. in *IOP Conference Series: Materials Science and Engineering*. 2018. IOP Publishing.

Long, S., et al., *Enhanced surface antimicrobial, biocompatible and mechanical properties of 3D printed titanium alloys by electrophoretic deposition of chitosan/ZnO*. Colloids and Surfaces B: Biointerfaces, 2025. **245**: p. 114274.

Parvinnasab, A., et al., *Balanced enhancement of antibacterial activity and biocompatibility in chitosan-vancomycin 3D-printed scaffolds through mesoporous bioactive glass addition*. Journal of Drug Delivery Science and Technology, 2025: p. 106637.

Shahroudi, S., et al., *Efficacy of 3D-printed chitosan-cerium oxide dressings coated with vancomycin-loaded alginate for chronic wounds management*. Carbohydrate Polymers, 2025. **349**: p. 123036.

Part III
Food Technology Applications

Marine Polysaccharides in Food Processing and Preservation

Vikramaditya Banerjee, Supriya Kumar Bose, Aparna Chaudhuri, Sabyasachi Ghosh, and Swarup Roy

Abstract Rising environmental concerns associated with the depletion of nonrenewable resources and the accumulation of persistent waste are fueling increased interest in biodegradable marine biopolymers as sustainable alternatives. Marine polysaccharides represent a diverse class of natural biopolymers derived from marine animals, seaweeds, and microorganisms, offering immense potential in food processing and preservation. This chapter presents a comprehensive overview of their sources and classification, highlighting key examples such as chitosan and chitin from crustaceans, alginate and carrageenan from seaweeds, and gellan and xanthan gum from marine microbes. The structural and chemical properties of these polysaccharides are discussed in detail, including their molecular architectures, glycosidic linkages, functional group modifications such as acetylation and sulfation, net charge, molecular weight, and conformational flexibility, all of which influence their behavior in food systems. The chapter also explores the wide-ranging applications of marine-derived polysaccharides in food processing. These include their roles in developing gluten-free products, encapsulating nutrients and flavors, modifying texture, and enabling the production of low-fat and low-calorie foods. Their contribution to food preservation is equally significant, particularly due to their antimicrobial and antioxidant properties, as well as their use in edible films and coatings that extend the shelf life of perishables. Finally, the chapter outlines emerging trends and future perspectives, emphasizing sustainable extraction technologies and novel formulation strategies that position marine

V. Banerjee
Department of Applied Biology, Maulana Abul Kalam Azad University of Technology, Haringhata Farm, West Bengal, India

S. K. Bose · A. Chaudhuri · S. Ghosh (✉)
Department of Biotechnology, School of Life Science, Swami Vivekananda University, Barrackpore, West Bengal, India

S. Roy (✉)
Department of Food Technology and Nutrition, School of Agriculture, Lovely Professional University, Phagwara, India

Department of Food and Nutrition, Kyung Hee University, Seoul, Republic of Korea

S. Jana et al. (eds.), *Multifunctional Marine Polysaccharides*,
https://doi.org/10.1007/978-981-95-4126-3_16

polysaccharides as key enablers in advancing health-focused and eco-friendly food innovations.

Keywords Marine polysaccharides · Marine biopolymers · Biodegradable materials · Food processing · Food preservation · Sustainable food packaging

1 Introduction

Marine ecosystems represent one of the planet's richest reservoirs of bioactive and functional compounds. Among these, marine polysaccharides stand out as an exceptionally diverse and versatile group of natural polymers that have found widespread applications in the food industry (Zhang et al. 2025a; Mardhekar et al. 2025). Extracted primarily from seaweeds, marine microbes, and marine invertebrates, these polysaccharides significantly contribute to food processing and preservation due to their unique physicochemical properties and biological activities. Their roles span from traditional functions such as gelling, thickening, and stabilizing to emerging applications as bioactive agents in functional and health-promoting foods (Ghosh et al. 2025a; Tukenmez Emre et al. 2025). Marine polysaccharides include a wide range of chemically distinct molecules such as alginate, agar, carrageenan, fucoidan, ulvan, chitin, chitosan, gellan gum, xanthan gum, and dextran. Each exhibits specific structural characteristics that determine its functional behavior in food systems (Tukenmez Emre et al. 2025; Jafarzadeh et al. 2024). For example, alginate, extracted from brown algae, is important for its ability to form heat-stable gels in the existence of divalent cations like calcium (Carrasqueira et al. 2025). This property is widely exploited in restructured foods, edible coatings, and encapsulation of sensitive ingredients such as probiotics and flavors. Similarly, agar, derived from red algae, forms strong, clear thermoreversible gels that are indispensable in confectionery, bakery fillings, and microbiological media (Subramanian et al. 2024).

Carrageenan, another red algal polysaccharide, is a key texturizing agent used extensively in dairy applications, such as chocolate milk and processed cheese, because of its unique ability to interact with milk proteins and stabilize emulsions (Jabeen et al. 2025). According to the International Market Analysis Research and Consulting Group (IMARC), the Indian food processing industry was worth US $336.4 billion in 2023 and is predictable to increase at a compound annual growth rate (CAGR) of 8.8%, reaching approximately US$735.5 billion by 2032 (IMARC 2025). Gellan gum and xanthan gum, produced by marine and terrestrial bacteria, have become essential hydrocolloids in modern food formulations. These microbial-derived gums provide excellent thickening and stabilizing effects, maintain product consistency across a wide pH and temperature range, and improve sensory qualities in sauces, dressings, and gluten-free baked goods (Zhang et al. 2020).

Beyond their technological functionalities, marine polysaccharides increasingly attract attention for their natural origin and health benefits, aligning with the growing consumer demand for clean-label, plant-based, and sustainable ingredients. For instance, chitosan obtained by deacetylating chitin from crustacean shells possesses potent antimicrobial activity against bacteria and fungi. This property makes chitosan an effective preservative and edible film component, extending shelf life and enhancing food safety without the use of synthetic additives (Guarnieri et al. 2022; Altaf et al. 2022). Likewise, fucoidan from brown seaweeds and ulvan from green algae exhibit antioxidant, anti-inflammatory, and immunomodulatory effects, offering opportunities to formulate functional foods that support health and well-being (Carvalho et al. 2025a). Marine polysaccharides also contribute to preservation strategies by acting as moisture regulators, oxygen barriers, and carriers for natural preservatives. The global food preservatives market was valued at USD 3.12 billion in 2024 and is probable to increase from USD 3.25 billion in 2025 to around USD 4.85 billion by 2034, registering a CAGR of 4.51% during the 2025–2034 period (Precedence Research 2025).

Edible coatings and films based on alginate, chitosan, and composite formulations have demonstrated effectiveness in preserving fresh fruits, vegetables, seafood, and meat products by reducing water loss, delaying oxidation, and inhibiting microbial growth (Orhotohwo et al. 2025). These applications are particularly relevant in addressing global challenges such as food spoilage, waste reduction, and the need for safer, more sustainable preservation solutions (Carvalho et al. 2025b). In addition to their technical and health-related advantages, marine polysaccharides are generally recognized as safe by food safety authorities and are biodegradable, making them environmentally responsible alternatives to synthetic additives and packaging materials (Carrasqueira et al. 2025). The utilization of marine biomass and microbial fermentation to produce these biopolymers supports the circular economy and valorizes underused marine resources, including by-products from the seafood industry (Venugopal 2022).

The objective of this chapter is to comprehensively explore the sources and classification of marine polysaccharides, including those derived from animals, plants (seaweeds), and marine microbes. Additionally, the chapter provides an overview of the structure and chemistry of marine polysaccharides, detailing their molecular architecture and linkages, functional chemical features such as acetylation, sulfation, and charge distribution, as well as their molecular weight and structural flexibility. The chapter systematically highlights the diverse applications of marine-derived polysaccharides in food processing, covering their roles in the development of gluten-free products, nutrient and flavor encapsulation, texture modification, and formulation of low-calorie and low-fat foods. Their significance in food preservation was also discussed, emphasizing their antimicrobial and antioxidant properties, utility in edible coatings and films, and contributions to extending the shelf life of perishable products. Finally, the chapter describes the emerging trends and future prospects for the use of marine polysaccharides in food processing and preservation.

2 Sources and Classification of Marine Polysaccharides

Marine ecosystems are an unparalleled reservoir of biologically active compounds, among which marine polysaccharides have gained exceptional attention due to their structural diversity, functional properties, and broad range of applications in the food industry. These polysaccharides are high-molecular-weight carbohydrate polymers produced by marine organisms as structural components, storage molecules, or protective agents. They can be systematically categorized based on their biological origin into three main groups: animal-derived, microbial-derived, and plant (seaweed)-derived (Bose et al. 2023) (Fig. 1).

2.1 *Animal-Derived Marine Polysaccharides*

Marine animals, particularly crustaceans, mollusks, and some marine invertebrates, produce polysaccharides that play important structural and bioactive roles. Chitin is a structural component forming the exoskeletons of crustaceans (e.g., shrimp, crabs, lobsters), mollusk shells, and the cell walls of some fungi and it is the most abundant polysaccharide in marine animals. Chitosan is produced by the partial deacetylation of chitin through chemical or enzymatic methods. Unlike chitin, chitosan is soluble in dilute acids due to its free amino groups. This cationic biopolymer possesses remarkable biological activities, including antimicrobial, antioxidant, and film-

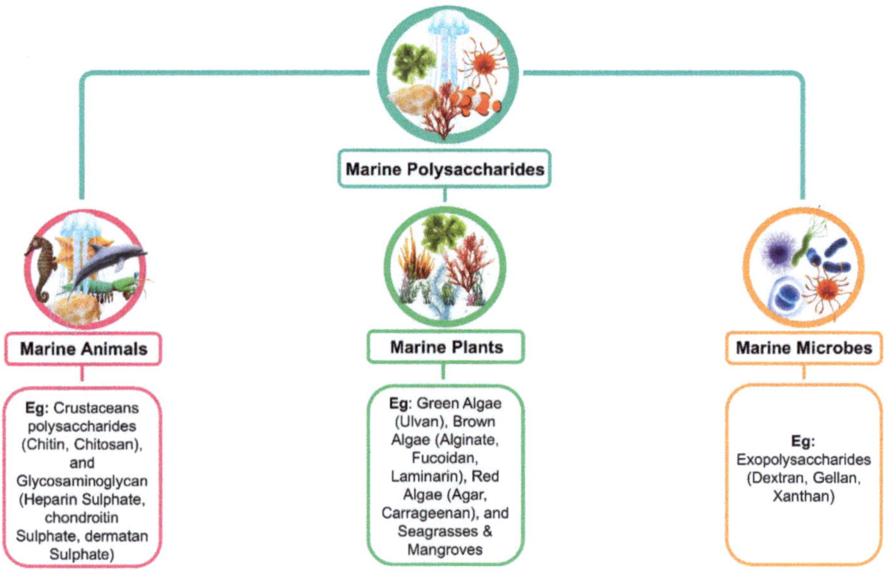

Fig. 1 Classification of marine polysaccharides based on their biological origin

forming properties, making it valuable in edible coatings, drug delivery systems, and water treatment. Although heparin and glycosaminoglycans are less abundant in marine species compared to mammals, some marine invertebrates like mollusks, sea cucumbers, and tunicates contain sulfated glycosaminoglycans such as heparin and heparan sulfate. These polysaccharides are composed of alternating uronic acids and glucosamine units with extensive sulfation, conferring potent anticoagulant and anti-inflammatory activities. Marine-derived heparin is increasingly explored as a safer alternative to mammalian sources due to reduced risk of contamination (Carvalho et al. 2025a).

2.2 *Plant (Seaweed)-Derived Marine Polysaccharides*

Marine plants, commonly known as seaweeds (algae), are prolific producers of structurally diverse polysaccharides with critical ecological, biological, and industrial roles. There are approximately 8000 known species of seaweeds found in marine environments worldwide (Bose et al. 2023). These polysaccharides account for a major fraction of seaweed biomass and serve as structural components, storage carbohydrates, and protective agents. Because of their unique composition and functionality, they have become indispensable in the food sector. They are traditionally classified into brown (Phaeophyceae), red (Rhodophyceae), and green (Chlorophyceae) algae. Each group produces distinctive polysaccharides with unique structural motifs and functional roles. The plant polysaccharides are better known as gelling and thickening agents. Animal-derived marine polysaccharides stand out for their structural support, biocompatibility, and unique biological activities such as anticoagulant and antimicrobial effects.

Alginate, fucoidan, and laminaran are some common examples of brown algae polysaccharides. Alginate is extracted mainly from Laminaria, Ascophyllum, and Macrocystis species, alginates. In food processing, alginates serve as gelling agents, stabilizers, and encapsulation materials due to their ability to form heat-stable gels in the presence of divalent cations like calcium (Kalita et al. 2025). Fucoidan occurs in significant amounts in brown algae such as *Fucus vesiculosus* and *Undaria pinnatifida*. Notably, fucoidan exhibits potent bioactivities, including anticoagulant, antiviral, and immunomodulatory effects. Laminaran, serving as a storage glucan, is soluble in water and contributes to the carbon reserves in brown algae.

A few important algae polysaccharides are carrageenan and agar (agarose and agaropectin). Carrageenans are sulfated galactans extracted primarily from Kappaphycusalvarezii and *Chondrus crispus*. Different types κ-, ι-, and λ-carrageenan have specific gelling and thickening properties. These polysaccharides are extensively used as food stabilizers, gelling agents, and emulsifiers. Agar, derived from Gelidium and Gracilaria species, is a mixture of agarose (the gelling fraction) and agaropectin (the charged fraction). Agar is renowned for forming strong thermoreversible gels, widely utilized in microbiological media, confectionery, and food texturization (Oun et al. 2024).

Green algae polysaccharides ulvan, sourced primarily from Ulva and Enteromorpha species, ulvan is a sulfated heteropolysaccharide rich in rhamnose, xylose, glucuronic acid, and iduronic acid. Ulvan has unique gelling and bioactive properties, supporting its emerging use as a functional food ingredient and hydrogel-forming agent.

2.3 *Microbe-Derived Marine Polysaccharides*

Marine microbes, including bacteria and fungi, produce a variety of extracellular polysaccharides (EPS). These microbial polysaccharides are typically secreted into the surrounding environment as a protective matrix, promoting cell adhesion, biofilm formation, nutrient trapping, and defense against desiccation and predation. Over the past decades, marine microbial EPS have attracted growing interest in the food industry due to their unique rheological properties, functional versatility, and bioactivities. Notably, some of these biopolymers are commercially produced and used as thickeners, stabilizers, and gelling agents.

Gellan gum, produced by marine bacteria *Sphingomonas elodea*, gellan gum is composed of a linear tetrasaccharide repeat of glucose, glucuronic acid, and rhamnose. In the presence of cations, it forms firm, transparent gels, making it valuable in plant-based beverages, desserts, and biomedical formulations. Although xanthan gum is primarily sourced from terrestrial strains, xanthan gum can also be produced by marine isolates of *Xanthomonas* species. Xanthan exhibits excellent thickening and stabilizing properties, maintaining viscosity across a wide pH and temperature range. Marine bacteria such as *Leuconostoc* strains synthesize dextran a homopolysaccharide of glucose. Dextran is utilized as a plasma expander, stabilizer, and food additive. Marine-derived fungi also produce β-glucans and other exopolysaccharides with promising antioxidant and immunomodulatory functions.

3 Structure and Chemistry of Marine Polysaccharides

Marine polysaccharides are formed from complex carbohydrates extracted from seaweeds and marine invertebrates that have structures suited to withstand high salt, stress from oxidation and high pressure (Carrasqueira et al. 2025). Most of these polymers consist of sugar units stuck together through glycosidic bonds, and a lot of them go through changes with sulfation, acetylation or uronic acid substitution. The way food system chemicals are built and made affects their performance in things like gelation, forming a film layer, emulsification, and bioactivity (Zhang et al. 2022).

3.1 Molecular Structure and Linkages of Marine Polysaccharides

Most marine polysaccharides are heteropolymers with varied monomeric building blocks (Table 1). Alginates are linear copolymers of β-D-mannuronic acid (M) and α-L-guluronic acid (G) together by (1 → 4) glycosidic bonds. The ratio and arrangement of M and G blocks determine gel strength and flexibility. These form homopolymeric M-M or G-G areas or regions of alternating M-G blocks. The way G blocks are laid down in sequence affects the stiffness and calcium-binding power of the gel through the "egg-box" mechanism, essential for cold-set gelation (Zhang et al. 2022). Carrageenans are sulfated galactans containing a series of repeating disaccharides from 3-linked β-D-galactopyranose to 4-linked α-D-galactopyranose (Jiao et al. 2011). Structurally, they consist of alternating 3-linked β-D-galactopyranose and 4-linked α-D-galactopyranose residues, with varying degrees of sulfation. Carrageenans are grouped by their sulfate groups into κ-type, ι-type, and λ-type. The gel-forming capacity of κ- and ι-carrageenan comes from their 3,6-anhydrogalactosyl link, which is not part of λ-carrageenan and makes it only suitable for thickening (Rupert et al. 2022).

Like carrageenan, agar is another red algal polysaccharide with much of the same structure but less sulfation. The main components of these chains are β-D-galactose and 3,6-anhydro-α-L-galactose (Rupert et al. 2022). Agarose is a linear polymer of repeating units of D-galactose and 3,6-anhydro-L-galactose linked via alternating β-(1 → 4) and α-(1 → 3) bonds (Padmesh and Singh 2021). The unique thermal abilities of agar are due to the formation of its double helix and subsequent aggregation upon cooling. Xanthan gum consists of a cellulose-like β-(1 → 4)-linked glucose backbone with trisaccharide side chains containing mannose and glucuronic acid (Kang et al. 2023). Fucoidan comes from brown algae and contains many branches, sulfate groups and L-fucose. Fucoidan is a complex sulfated polysaccharide composed primarily of α-(1 → 3)-linked L-fucose residues with sulfate substitutions and occasional branching. In addition, small components like galactose, xylose, and uronic acids might be found (Mensah et al. 2023).

Ulvan from green algae (Ulva, Enteromorpha) consists mostly of rhamnose, glucuronic acid, iduronic acid, and xylose. Ulvanobiuronic acid 3-sulfate types A and B are major repeating parts of the ulvan structure, giving it bioactivity and a high anionic charge density (Gao et al. 2025). Chemically, chitin is a linear homopolymer composed of β-(1 → 4)-linked N-acetyl-D-glucosamine units. Due to its crystalline and insoluble nature, it mainly serves as a mechanical barrier, providing rigidity and protection to marine invertebrates. A high degree of deacetylation makes chitosan water-soluble in acidic circumstances, improving its solubility, cationic charge, and interaction with many substances (Oladzadabbasabadi et al. 2024). Marine bacteria such as *Leuconostoc* strains synthesize dextran a homopolysaccharide of glucose linked mainly by α-(1 → 6) bonds with occasional α-(1 → 3) branches (Du et al. 2022).

Table 1 Major marine sources, structural details, and functions of the important polysaccharides present in the marine sources (Zhang et al. 2025a; Carrasqueira et al. 2025; Subramanian et al. 2024; Bose et al. 2023; De Jesus et al. 2015; Ghosh et al. 2025b; Ghosh et al. 2024)

Source type	Polysaccharide	Marine sources	Monomers unit	Linkage type	Functional role
Marine plant/algae/ seaweed	Alginate	Brown algae (Macrocystis, Laminaria)	Mannuronic, Guluronic acids	β-(1 $\rightarrow$ 4)	Gel formation, drug delivery
	Carrageenan	Red algae (Chondrus, Kappaphycus)	Galactose, 3,6-anhydro-D-galactose	β-(1 $\rightarrow$ 3), α-(1 $\rightarrow$ 4)	Thickening, food stabilizer, gelling
	Agar (agarose)	Red algae (Gelidium, Gracilaria)	D-galactose, 3,6-anhydro-L-galactose	β-(1 $\rightarrow$ 3), β-(1 $\rightarrow$ 4)	Thermoreversible gels, food additives, microbiological media
	Fucoidan	Brown algae (Fucus, Laminaria)	L-fucose (sulfated), galactose, uronic acids	α-(1 $\rightarrow$ 3) or α-(1 $\rightarrow$ 4)	Anticoagulant, antioxidant, antiviral
	Ulvan	Green algae (Ulva/sea lettuce)	Rhamnose, xylose, iduronic acid, glucuronic acid	Mixed α/β-linkages	Chelation, hydrogel formation, antioxidant films
Marine animal	Chitosan	Shrimp/crab shells	D-glucosamine (deacetylated N-acetylglucosamine)	β-(1 $\rightarrow$ 4)	Antimicrobial, pH-responsive films, good mechanical
	Chitin	Shrimp, crab exoskeleton	N-acetyl-D-glucosamine	β-(1 $\rightarrow$ 4)	Highly translucent, antibacterial properties, structural support, precursor for chitosan
	Heparin	Mast cells, marine invertebrates (e.g., mollusks)	D-glucosamine and uronic acid	α-(1 $\rightarrow$ 4)	Anticoagulant, anti-angiogenic, stabilizer
Marine microbe	Dextran	Marine bacteria (*Leuconostoc*, others)	D-glucose	Mainly α-(1 $\rightarrow$ 6) with α-(1 $\rightarrow$ 3) branches	Plasma expander, additive, stabilizer, improves softness
	Gellan	*Sphingomonas* spp.	Glucose, rhamnose, glucuronic acid	β-(1 $\rightarrow$ 4)	Gelling agent, food stabilizer, plant-based milks
	Xanthan	*Xanthomonas* spp. (marine isolates)	β-D-glucose backbone, D-mannose, glucuronic acid side chains	β-(1 $\rightarrow$ 4), β-(2 $\rightarrow$ 1), β- (4 $\rightarrow$ 1), α-(1 $\rightarrow$ 3),	Emulsifying, thickening, agents, rheology modifiers in food/pharma

3.2 Functional Chemistry: Charge, Acetylation, and Sulfation

Post-polymer modifications are central to the biofunctionality of marine polysaccharides. The compounds fucoidan, carrageenan, and ulvan usually feature sulfation. Sulfate groups give them anionic properties, make them soluble in water and allow them to bind with proteins, enzymes, and metal ions. One reason κ-carrageenan can form gels is due to how the sulfate groups are positioned with 3,6-anhydro bridges (Zhou et al. 2021). Acetylation found in chitin and ulvan influences how crystalline the molecule is, how many water molecules it binds, and its interactions with different bacteria. When chitin is processed into chitosan, it becomes more available, can combat microbes, and is better suited for use in foods (Oladzadabbasabadi et al. 2024). These anionic polysaccharides (alginate, carrageenan, and ulvan) maintain a negative charge that helps them form ionic and electrostatic bonds (Cunha and Grenha 2016). Due to the positively charged amino groups at acidic pH, chitosan can form polyelectrolyte complexes with anionic polysaccharides for use in film-coating and encapsulation technologies (Luo and Wang 2014).

3.3 Molecular Weight and Structural Flexibility of Marine Polysaccharides

The physicochemical and biological activities of marine polysaccharides are affected primarily by their molecular weight (mw) in food systems. It affects the texture and gelation process of their aqueous solutions and also their activity with biomolecules, as well as their use in antioxidant or antimicrobial products (De Jesus et al. 2015). Using techniques like ultrasonication, controlled depolymerization, acid hydrolysis or certain enzyme treatments can be done to control the molecular weight precisely. These fucoidan-based derivatives (~30–150 kDa) experience faster and increased uptake by cells (Flórez-Fernández et al. 2023). In addition, making ulvan with a reduced molecular weight enhances its ability to form emulsions and films, making it useful in nano-delivery or biodegradable packaging (Gao et al. 2025). Native fucoidan and carrageenan, which have high molecular weight (>500 kDa), tend to result in thick solutions that can strongly gel. When used in food, this means the gels are more solid, bond well and retain a larger amount of moisture. On the other hand, molecules with a high molecular mass might not function as well as antioxidants or agents against bacteria, since receptor binding is blocked by steric hindrance (Cunha and Grenha 2016). In addition, how the glycosidic links are built and how much the polymer is branched can affect the structure of polysaccharides in liquids. When a polymer has a flexible backbone with few rigid inhibitors, it can easily form a network that leads to film or emulsion development; however, linear polymers, with their strength from rigidity, typically produce gels (Lutsyk et al. 2024). Food products can be given their special properties by changing the molecular weight and molecular architecture.

4 Application of Marine-Derived Polysaccharides in Food Processing

Nowadays, forms of marine polysaccharides (MPs), including alginate, carrageenan, agar, fucoidan, ulvan, chitin, and chitosan, are widely used in modern food formulations. Fish canning, processing of lobsters, and waste materials landed from fisheries are some of the richest sources of biopolymers such as gelatin, collagen, chitin, and chitosan (Bose et al. 2023). Chitin, found in many products from mollusks and crustaceans, often comes from the shells of crabs and shrimp. Both chitin and collagen play important roles in building the body. It is common to make chitosan out of chitin since chitosan dissolves in water. Because of their colloidal nature, being produced from renewable sources, and meeting regulations, processors have the opportunity to alter the texture of products, maintain sensitive ingredients in place, and replace unhealthy items without harming their sales (Crini 2022). Isolating, studying, and using marine biomaterials play a major role in the growth of marine biotechnology industries. Recently, advancements in technology have made it possible to separate bioactive materials from marine samples better. Nowadays, marine biopolymers are gaining prominence in the market, which interests marine researchers and consumers (Carrasqueira et al. 2025). Some important marine polysaccharides used in food processing are tabulated in Table 2.

4.1 Development of Gluten-Free Product

The key problem with implementing gluten-free (GF) products is that gluten helps hold gas inside during fermentation and provides the structure in the dough during baking. This issue is being solved by using marine polysaccharides, as they recover some of the key properties of gluten. Adding hydrocolloids like alginate, carrageenan, and chitosan during bread baking improves the volume and texture of the crumbs and the overall lifespan of the bread (V et al. 2025). Combining hydroxypropyl methylcellulose (HPMC) and propylene glycol alginate (PGA) in the production of gluten-free bread (GFB) improves the shape, texture, and specific volume compared to making bread with HPMC alone (Zhao et al. 2021). An investigation compared carrageenan, carboxymethylcellulose, guar gum, and xanthan gum concerning bread makeup, demonstrating that they are crucial for increasing loaf volume and for helping bread keep moisture longer, owing to a process known as starch retrogradation, meaning starch hardens instantly (Das et al. 2014). Apart from bread, chitosan contributes significantly to GF noodles by promoting protein aggregation and providing a similar pliable feel to durum wheat semolina when combined with carboxymethylcellulose (Padalino et al. 2011). Its antimicrobial properties make it possible for products to remain good on shelves, so marine polysaccharides are useful in gluten-free foods that are becoming popular.

Table 2 Important roles of major polysaccharides in food processing

Polysaccharides	Inclusion level	Examples in the food matrix	Food processing function	References
Ulvan	0.5%	Nutraceuticals in chicken sausages	Encapsulation, UV protection	Alboofetileh et al.)2025)
Alginate	0.5–2%	Re-structured meats, probiotic juices	Cold-set gelation, encapsulation	Kim et al. (2018) and Tan et al. (2023)
Fucoidan	0.4–0.8%	Bread matrix, beverages	Bioactive carrier, antioxidant	Koh et al. (2020)
Agar	0.5% and 1.0%	Confectionery gels	Rapid-set, calorie-dilution	Tarahi et al. (2023)
κ/ι-carrageenan	0.1–0.5%	Dairy desserts, frankfurters	Thermoreversible gel, water-binding	Zarzycki et al. (2019)
Chitosan	0.0025–0.01%	Low-fat yoghurt, gluten-free noodles	Fat mimetic, viscosity booster	Kurchenko et al. (2024)
Dextran	0.5%	Bread	Better the hardness and improve the shelf life	Zannini et al. (2014)
Gellan	0.5%	Meat	Enhanced stability, texture, and water retention in modified meat batters	Totosaus and Pérez-Chabela (2009)
Xanthan	0.3% and 0.4%	Gluten-free cakes	Enhanced quality attributes, including softer texture, higher specific volume, and slower staling rate	Preichardt et al. (2011)

4.2 *Encapsulation of Nutrients and Flavors*

When formulating functional foods, using marine polysaccharides is important since they structure and help the nutrients. This is because naturally derived polymers interact well with water and ions, making them suitable for wrapping and protecting fragile molecules such as probiotics, vitamins, and essential oils from getting destroyed in food and digestion. For a long time, alginate has played an important part because it can easily form a gel due to interaction with divalent cations such as calcium. Ionic gelation using $CaCl_2$ is the best method for microencapsulating probiotics in alginate. Research conducted on ten studies from 2017 to 2022 showed that using alginate to encapsulate *Lactobacillus* made it last longer in the fridge and be more immune to gastric fluids (Pandey et al. 2024). Viable bacteria must be transferred to the intestine in abundance to help improve health. Combining compounds into one capsule is another breakthrough. When inulin prebiotic fibers are incorporated in alginate matrices, scientists have succeeded in building symbiotic microcapsules that look after probiotics and aid their growth inside the belly of the host (Pandey et al. 2024). Using encapsulation, the delivery of prebiotics like omega-3 fatty acids, phytochemicals, and fibers to the colon increased as a result of introducing symbiotic into alginate inulin cores (Kvakova et al. 2021). Meanwhile, chitosan, a derivative of chitin that holds opposite electrons to polysaccharides alginate and carrageenan, allows the creation of several protective layers inside them (Oladzadabbasabadi et al. 2024). As a result, these structures protect molecules carried inside capsules by making them less permeable to acid. Not only do marine polysaccharides defend against attacks, but they can also be used for delivering important molecules. Because it is an anionic sulfated substance, fucoidan can attract positively charged compounds like nisin (Gruškienė et al. 2024).

4.3 Texture Modification

At present, the food industry relies on polysaccharides from seaweeds (alginate, agar, carrageenan, and fucoidan), thanks to their special physiological properties (Senadheera et al. 2023). Carrageenans are useful because they gel easily; the ability of κ and ι carrageenans to gel even after mild temperature changes has made them essential in dairy and meat products over many years. Using low levels (0.2% w/w) of κ-carrageenan, the test frankfurters showed strong gels and improved togetherness, cutting down on the use of phosphates for clean label formulations (Cao et al. 2022). Combining κ-carrageenan and locust bean gum reduced the gelling and liquefying properties of the gel in sodium ham prototypes (Arda et al. 2009). Alginate is used mostly in restructured seafood and analogue meats, as the Ca^{2+} crosslinks it makes remain stable and sliceable after heat is applied. A previous study showed that an emulsion gel made from gelatin and sodium alginate replaced pork fat in luncheon meat (Lee et al. 2025). In the gel which contained 40% corn oil, the ratio of gelatin to sodium alginate was 1.9, and this seemed to make it healthier because the gel contained a higher percentage of polyunsaturated fatty acids than pork fat. They are part of an overall movement toward developing processed food that supports good health and the environment. Faced with high standards, marine polysaccharides respond effectively and benefit food by offering clean-label solutions and a range of functions needed in the future.

4.4 Use in Low-Calorie and Low-Fat Products

Due to concerns about obesity, heart disease and diabetes, the food industry must try to lower the fat in common products without losing their appeal to consumers. Fat is important for both flavor and fullness, as well as for texture, thickness and overall stability. In other words, to replace fat, new solutions are needed that can recreate its oiliness, emulsifying power and soft texture. The use of marine polysaccharides, mainly carrageenan, PGA, agar and chitosan, is preferred as a fat replacement since they help form creaminess, keep water in place and stabilize both air and oil droplets with very few calories (Wanniarachchi et al. 2025). Both carrageenan and PGA have significant value in making frozen desserts and dairy products. After water is added, these polysaccharides become larger and bond with the milk proteins to create a thick, creamy texture. According to a recent study, seaweeds were found to be superior to other types of functional fat replacers in low-fat ice creams (Akhtar et al. 2023). Products that used κ-carrageenan or PGA had better overrun, suffered lower melting rates, and seemed as creamy as regular full-fat options, without any visible signs of off-flavor or aftertaste. Therefore, these discoveries prove that marine polysaccharides are important in developing better food choices. These foods meet global health and sustainability targets since the use of plant proteins makes the product low in calories and fat, yet still tasty and healthy enough for consumers (Senadheera et al. 2023). The results suggest that small amounts (0.1–2%) of marine polysaccharides can improve many different and useful properties in various foods. Alginate is best for cold-set gelation and encapsulation in products such as restructured meats and probiotic beverages. κ/ι-Carrageenan adds the property of reversible gelation and moisture retention, which makes it ideal for meat and dairy applications. Agar is chosen in confectionery due to its swift setting time and low-calorie content. Chitosan imitates fat and helps thicken low-fat and gluten-free foods. With fucoidan and ulvan present, antioxidants and sun protection can be included in functional foods and beverages (Fig. 2).

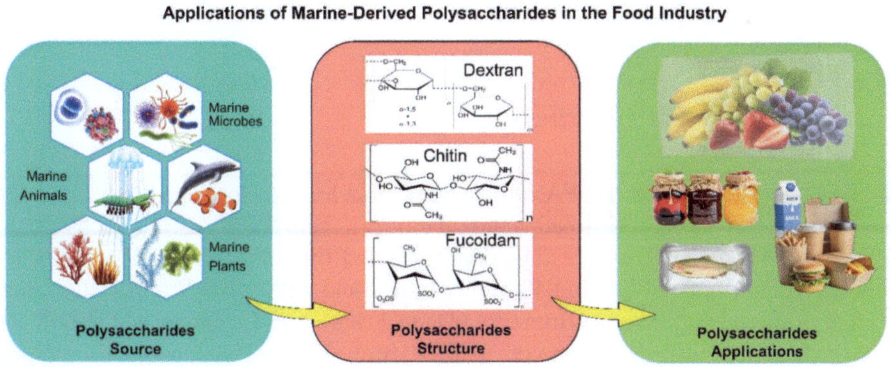

Fig. 2 Role of marine polysaccharides in enhancing food quality and shelf life

5 Application of Marine-Derived Polysaccharides in Food Preservation

They have gained significant interest in food preservation owing to their biodegradability, biocompatibility, non-toxicity, and multifunctional bioactivities. Here are the main applications: Besides their function in food processing, marine-derived polysaccharides have an important role in natural preservation.

5.1 Antimicrobial Activity

Chitosan is considered the best marine biopolymer when it comes to directly controlling pathogens. Giving chicken fillets a 2% chitosan dip significantly lowered *Salmonella typhimurium* and *E. coli* by 2.3–3.8 log CFU g^{-1} in just 48 h at 4 °C, which was much better than the results from chicken being rinsed with 1% lactic acid (El-Khawas et al. 2020). Introducing kaolinite clay and *Ficus carica* polyphenols into a chitosan film made it stronger and reduced the presence of mixed spoilage bacteria, suggesting that blending them synergistically into a matrix covers more microbes (El Mouzahim et al. 2023). Unlike highly cationic fucoidan, sulfated fucoidan still creates oxidative stress in bacteria. Applying the electrostatic connection of fucoidan micro-spray to the antibacterial bacteriocin nisin kept *Listeria monocytogenes* out of detectable numbers from 6.7 or 5 log CFU per ml or g in sliced turkey breast after ten days of refrigeration. The combination was more effective than nisin by itself at the same pH level (Sivarooban et al. 2007). In summary, these findings prove that marine polysaccharides are adaptable, suitable for labelling and can replace synthetic compounds used as preservatives.

5.2 Antioxidant Properties

While it's mostly the high-PUFA content in fish that leads to spoilage, some research has shown that adding seaweed antioxidants can help keep marine foods fresh longer. Low-molecular weight fucoidan generated by sonication mainly work to remove free radicals. Following 40 min of ultrasound with a 103 W cm^{-2} dose, the weight of fucoidan decreased from 950 kDa to 318 kDa and it enhanced the DPPH-scavenging free radicals (improved to 87% from 28%). The model oil-in-water emulsion also lasted 35% longer at 25 °C (Bagale et al. 2023). Several studies have shown that ulvan possesses specific properties, for example, it forms gels and offers good bioactivities, such as being able to fight bacteria and viruses. Such properties could help it become a suitable material for food wrappings and films (Wang et al. 2023). Moreover, mixing other natural polymers into ulvan-based films and coatings can give them improved mechanical features, better ability to preserve food, and make them more practical. In research, chitosan coating developed with bergamot juice powder controls enzyme activity, browning, and maintains the quality of stored fresh-cut fruit salads (Demircan and Velioglu 2024). It is predicted that using ulvan, a renewable material for food packaging, will experience rapid growth in the future. At the same time, more investigations are necessary to confirm the safety of ulvan in the meals and the effects that ulvan-based edible films might have on the appearance and quality of various products.

5.3 Edible Coatings and Films

Marine polysaccharide-based coatings for fresh produce now provide benefits beyond a shiny surface. First, the alginate–chitosan probiotic films act as a living shield. According to the MDPI study, strawberries with 3% sodium alginate, which were seeded with *Lacticaseibacillus casei* LC03 and overlayered with 0.5% fungal chitosan, kept their color and firmness for 12 days at 4 °C, while uncoated strawberries lasted only for six days in the same way. Further, noticeably less weight was lost, and the probiotic population still reached 8 log CFU g^{-1}, which further confirmed simultaneous oxygen shielding and competitive-exclusion benefits (Da Silva Simões et al. 2025). Secondly, nanostructuring helps increase the passive defense of the material. By using chitosan nanoparticles with propolis polyphenols, the respiration of strawberries was decreased by 30%, and around 92% of their initial antioxidant capacity was preserved for 8–12 days (Martínez-González et al. 2020). Third, layer-by-layer (LbL) engineering gives the structure the ability to respond to "on-demand" actions. Microcapsules containing thyme oil and made from shells of chitosan and alginate released their contents when external pH decreased, which often precedes microbial spoilage, producing inhibition zones against *E. coli* and *S. aureus* in vitro (Esteve-Redondo et al. 2024). This smart release approach prevents flavor contamination and also makes food safer. Overall, combining different biochemical properties (from probiotics, polyphenols and essential oils) with the versatile matrices created from alginate, chitosan, and ulvan allows researchers to transform simple edible coatings into packaging that meets both shelf life and sustainability objectives.

5.4 Shelf-Life Extension of Perishables

Marine polysaccharide films have progressed from laboratories to practical and scalable solutions that can be applied to food packaging for longer product shelf life. For example, chitosan-based coatings enriched with cinnamon oil make them very effective at preserving fresh-cut apples. Previously (Solís-Contreras et al. 2021) reported that apple wedges coated in chitosan–cinnamon oil film maintained excellent quality and faced much reduced browning plus microbial growth for 25 days at

4 °C, compared to uncoated samples kept in the same way. Chilled meat applications with κ-carrageenan–chitosan glazes have demonstrated a substantial delay in spoilage. The recent study (Montaño-Sánchez et al. 2020) found that coating pork loins with the glaze reduced TBARS (thiobarbituric acid reactive substances) values by half, and the meat remained completely safe for more than 25 days, just as nitrite-cured without chemical preservatives. According to a previous study (Zhang et al. 2025b), applying the water-soluble form of chitosan to meat during processing at conveyor-line speed decreases psychrotroph counts on refrigerated pork by about 50%. The studies indicate that using marine polysaccharide films lengthens the shelf life of products and also fits well into the commercial production of foods (Table 3).

Table 3 Several products made by polysaccharide-based preservatives

Product	Polysaccharide system	Mechanism	Shelf-life extension	References
Apple cubes	Alginate coating (often paired with lactic acid bacteria or other antimicrobials)	Barrier + carrier for probiotics/ antimicrobials	8 days	Bambace et al. (2025)
Watermelon, melon, strawberry	Chitosan + vanillin nanoparticle film	Antimicrobial + antibiofilm	Extended by ≥4 days	Rodriguez et al. (2024)
Fish and meat-based products	Ulvan/ZnO biodegradable film	Antimicrobial + O_2 barrier	Currently in research	Wang et al. (2023)
Fresh cheese	Alginate + bacteriocin-producing lactic acid bacteria	Barrier + antimicrobial peptides	10 days	Silva et al. (2022)
Pork meat	Alginate coating + hydroxyapatite complexes	Barrier + inhibition of odor/catabolic enzymes	Extended, up to end of storage	Montone et al. (2023)
Goat meat, burger, patties	κ-Carrageenan–chitosan glaze	Lipid-oxidation inhibition	14 days	Şengül and Şen (2025)
Rainbow trout (*Oncorhynchus mykiss*)	Nisin-fucoidan complex spray	Controlled bacteriocin release	12 to 16 days	Behnam et al. (2015)
Frankfurter sausage/meat	κ-Carrageenan + reduced animal fat	Texture improvement + water retention	Not specifically stated	Bao et al. (2025)
Strawberries	Alginate + lactic acid bacteria coating	Barrier + probiotic antagonism	15 days	González-Cuello et al. (2024)

6 Emerging Trends and Future Perspectives

The increasing focus on health, sustainability, and clean-label products is driving a surge of interest in marine polysaccharides as functional materials for food processing and preservation. One major trend is their incorporation into functional and personalized nutrition. Bioactive polysaccharides such as fucoidan, ulvan, and chitosan offer antioxidant, anti-inflammatory, immunomodulatory, and prebiotic benefits, supporting the development of foods that promote digestive health and disease prevention. Advances in encapsulation and controlled-release delivery systems using alginate and chitosan will help create next-generation nutraceuticals and fortified products. Hybrid formulations combining marine polysaccharides with plant proteins and other biopolymers are expected to improve textures and functionalities in plant-based meat and dairy alternatives. Alginate and gellan gum can improve gelation and water retention in vegan cheeses, while carrageenan stabilizes non-dairy beverages, catering to clean-label and allergen-free trends. Sustainable, biodegradable packaging is another important area of innovation. Edible films and coatings made from alginate, carrageenan, and chitosan are emerging as eco-friendly alternatives to synthetic plastics. These materials can be enhanced with natural antimicrobials and antioxidants to extend shelf life while supporting circular economy principles. Nanotechnology and biopolymer engineering will further enable customized film properties such as strength, transparency, and barrier performance. In production, digital and precision technologies will transform extraction and modification processes. Green methods like enzyme-assisted and subcritical water extraction will improve yields and reduce environmental impacts, while targeted molecular tailoring will deliver consistent quality and compliance with regulations. Finally, active and intelligent packaging using marine polysaccharides is poised to improve food safety by incorporating freshness sensors and antimicrobial systems. Valorizing underused marine biomass, such as crustacean shells and seaweed, aligns with the blue bioeconomy and adds value while reducing waste. Collectively, these innovations position marine polysaccharides as key enablers of a healthier, more sustainable food future.

7 Conclusion

This chapter has provided a comprehensive overview of marine polysaccharides, detailing their diverse origins from animal, plant (seaweed), and microbial sources. By reviewing their molecular structures, linkages, and functional chemical modifications such as acetylation and sulfation, also highlighted how these unique features determine their behavior and versatility in food applications. Marine polysaccharides play critical roles in food processing, where they contribute to the development of gluten-free formulations, enhance texture, encapsulate nutrients and flavors, and support the production of low-calorie and low-fat products. Their importance in food preservation has also been emphasized, particularly their antimicrobial and antioxidant activities, which help maintain product safety and quality. The use of edible coatings and films derived from marine polysaccharides presents sustainable solutions to extend shelf life and reduce reliance on synthetic preservatives and packaging materials. Finally, emerging trends including green extraction technologies, bioactive delivery systems, and biodegradable packaging innovations underscore their growing relevance in meeting consumer demands for healthier, more sustainable food products. So, these insights demonstrate that marine polysaccharides are poised to play an increasingly vital role in the future of food processing and preservation.

References

Zhang J, Tang J, Shi S, et al (2025a) Research progress on marine polysaccharide-based Pickering emulsions and their potential applications in the food industry. Food Research International 208: 116073. https://doi.org/10.1016/j.foodres.2025.116073

Mardhekar S, Luong P, Seeberger PH (2025) Exploring marine glycans: structure, function, and the frontier of chemical synthesis. RSC Chem Biol. https://doi.org/10.1039/d5cb00090d

Ghosh S, Mandal RK, Mukherjee A, Roy S (2025a) Nanotechnology in the manufacturing of sustainable food packaging: a review. Discover Nano 20:. https://doi.org/10.1186/s11671-025-04213-x

Tukenmez Emre U, Sirin S, Nigdelioglu Dolanbay S, Aslim B (2025) Harnessing polysaccharides for sustainable food packaging. Polym Bull 82:2779–2825. https://doi.org/10.1007/s00289-025-05659-w

Jafarzadeh S, Nooshkam M, Zargar M, et al (2024) Green synthesis of nanomaterials for smart biopolymer packaging: challenges and outlooks. J Nanostruct Chem 14:113–136. https://doi.org/10.1007/s40097-023-00527-3

Carrasqueira J, Bernardino S, Bernardino R, Afonso C (2025) Marine-Derived Polysaccharides and Their Potential Health Benefits in Nutraceutical Applications. Marine Drugs 23:60. https://doi.org/10.3390/md23020060

Subramanian S et al. (2024) Applications of marine polysaccharides in biomedical field and food industry. In: Advanced Biophysical Techniques for Polysaccharides Characterization. Elsevier, pp 61–80

Jabeen F, Zil-e-Aimen, Ahmad R, et al (2025) Carrageenan: structure, properties and applications with special emphasis on food science. RSC Adv 15:22035–22062. https://doi.org/10.1039/d5ra03296b

IMARC (2025) India Food Processing Market Report by Sector (Dairy, Fruits and Vegetables, Meat and Poultry Processing, Fisheries, Packaged Foods, Beverages, and Others), and Region 2025–2033

Zhang N, Li X, Ye J, et al (2020) Effect of Gellan Gum and Xanthan Gum Synergistic Interactions and Plasticizers on Physical Properties of Plant-Based Enteric Polymer Films. Polymers 12:121. https://doi.org/10.3390/polym12010121

Guarnieri A, Triunfo M, Scieuzo C, et al (2022) Antimicrobial properties of chitosan from different developmental stages of the bioconverter insect Hermetia illucens. Sci Rep 12:. https://doi.org/10.1038/s41598-022-12150-3

Altaf A, Usmani Z, Dar AH, Dash KK (2022) A comprehensive review of polysaccharide-based bionanocomposites for food packaging applications. Discov Food 2:. https://doi.org/10.1007/s44187-022-00011-x

Carvalho ACF et al. (2025a) Valorization of agrowaste derived materials for food packaging application. In: Sustainable Materials for Food Packaging and Preservation. Elsevier, pp 199–221

Precedence Research (2025) Food Preservatives Market Drives Innovation in Shelf Life and Clean-Label Trends. Precedence Research

Orhotohwo OL, Lucci P, Jaiswal AK, et al (2025) Enhancing the functional properties of chitosan-alginate edible films using spent coffee ground extract for fresh-cut fruit preservation. Current Research in Food Science 11:101124. https://doi.org/10.1016/j.crfs.2025.101124

Carvalho ACF, Ghosh S, Hoffmann TG, et al (2025b) Valuing agro-industrial waste in the development of sustainable food packaging based on the system of a circular bioeconomy: A review. Cleaner Waste Systems 11:100275. https://doi.org/10.1016/j.clwas.2025.100275

Venugopal V (2022) Green processing of seafood waste biomass towards blue economy. Current Research in Environmental Sustainability 4:100164. https://doi.org/10.1016/j.crsust.2022.100164

Bose I, Nousheen, Roy S, et al (2023) Unveiling the Potential of Marine Biopolymers: Sources, Classification, and Diverse Food Applications. Materials 16:4840. https://doi.org/10.3390/ma16134840

Kalita P, Roy PK, Bhattacharjee B, et al (2025) Alginate-based coating in post-harvest fruits preservation: A comprehensive review. International Journal of Biological Macromolecules 320:145799. https://doi.org/10.1016/j.ijbiomac.2025.145799

Oun AA, Roy S, Hong SJ, et al (2024) Development of smart colorimetric indicators for tracking kimchi freshness by loading aronia extract in agar, κ-carrageenan, and cellulose nanofiber films. International Journal of Biological Macromolecules 270:132343. https://doi.org/10.1016/j.ijbiomac.2024.132343

Zhang B, Lan W, Xie J (2022) Chemical modifications in the structure of marine polysaccharide as serviceable food processing and preservation assistant: A review. International Journal of Biological Macromolecules 223:1539–1555. https://doi.org/10.1016/j.ijbiomac.2022.11.034

Jiao G, Yu G, Zhang J, Ewart HS (2011) Chemical Structures and Bioactivities of Sulfated Polysaccharides from Marine Algae. Marine Drugs 9:196–223. https://doi.org/10.3390/md9020196

Rupert R, Rodrigues KF, Thien VY, Yong WTL (2022) Carrageenan From Kappaphycus alvarezii (Rhodophyta, Solieriaceae): Metabolism, Structure, Production, and Application. Front Plant Sci 13:. https://doi.org/10.3389/fpls.2022.859635

Padmesh S, Singh A (2021) Agars: Properties and Applications. In: Inamuddin, Ahamed MI, Boddula R, Altalhi T (eds) Polysaccharides, 1st ed. Wiley, pp 75–93

Kang J, Yue H, Li X, et al (2023) Structural, rheological and functional properties of ultrasonic treated xanthan gums. International Journal of Biological Macromolecules 246:125650. https://doi.org/10.1016/j.ijbiomac.2023.125650

Mensah EO, Kanwugu ON, Panda PK, Adadi P (2023) Marine fucoidans: Structural, extraction, biological activities and their applications in the food industry. Food Hydrocolloids 142:108784. https://doi.org/10.1016/j.foodhyd.2023.108784

Gao J, Chen Z, Kaewprachu P, et al (2025) Structural and rheological properties of ulvan polysaccharides and their potential for food packaging applications. Food Chemistry 488:144850. https://doi.org/10.1016/j.foodchem.2025.144850

Oladzadabbasabadi N et al. (2024) Polymer–nano-chitin and polymer–nano-chitosan composites for food packaging. In: Nanostructured Materials for Food Packaging Applications. Elsevier, pp 137–156

Du R, Pei F, Kang J, et al (2022) Analysis of the structure and properties of dextran produced by Weissella confusa. International Journal of Biological Macromolecules 204:677–684. https://doi.org/10.1016/j.ijbiomac.2022.02.038

Zhou Y, Chen F-Q, Chen S, et al (2021) Preparation and Characterization of κ-Carrageenan Modified with Maleic Anhydride and Its Application in Films. Marine Drugs 19:486. https://doi.org/10.3390/md19090486

Cunha L, Grenha A (2016) Sulfated Seaweed Polysaccharides as Multifunctional Materials in Drug Delivery Applications. Marine Drugs 14:42. https://doi.org/10.3390/md14030042

Luo Y, Wang Q (2014) Recent development of chitosan-based polyelectrolyte complexes with natural polysaccharides for drug delivery. International Journal of Biological Macromolecules 64:353–367. https://doi.org/10.1016/j.ijbiomac.2013.12.017

De Jesus Raposo M, De Morais A, De Morais R (2015) Marine Polysaccharides from Algae with Potential Biomedical Applications. Marine Drugs 13:2967–3028. https://doi.org/10.3390/md13052967

Flórez-Fernández N, Vaamonde-García C, Torres MD, et al (2023) Relevance of the Extraction Stage on the Anti-Inflammatory Action of Fucoidans. Pharmaceutics 15:808. https://doi.org/10.3390/pharmaceutics15030808

Lutsyk V, Wolski P, Plazinski W (2024) The Conformation of Glycosidic Linkages According to Various Force Fields: Monte Carlo Modeling of Polysaccharides Based on Extrapolation of Short-Chain Properties. J Chem Theory Comput 20:6350–6368. https://doi.org/10.1021/acs.jctc.4c00543

Ghosh S et al. (2025b) Nanotechnology in edible films and coatings. In: Advancements in Nanotechnology for Food and Packaging. Elsevier, pp 349–376

Ghosh S et al. (2024) Applications of types of polysaccharides for the food industry. In: Advanced Biophysical Techniques for Polysaccharides Characterization. Elsevier, pp 327–355

Crini G (2022) Chitin and Chitosan. Elsevier

V AS, Dubey PK, Roy S (2025) Development of gluten-free functional snack bar for gluten intolerant population by utilizing pseudocereals and dates. Food Chemistry Advances 7: 100999. https://doi.org/10.1016/j.focha.2025.100999

Zhao F, Li Y, Li C, et al (2021) Co-supported hydrocolloids improve the structure and texture quality of gluten-free bread. LWT 152:112248. https://doi.org/10.1016/j.lwt.2021.112248

Das L, Raychaudhuri U, Chakraborty R (2014) Effects of hydrocolloids as texture improver in coriander bread. J Food Sci Technol. https://doi.org/10.1007/s13197-014-1296-8

Padalino L, Mastromatteo M, Sepielli G, Nobile MAD (2011) Formulation Optimization of Gluten-Free Functional Spaghetti Based on Maize Flour and Oat Bran Enriched in b-Glucans. Materials 4:2119–2135. https://doi.org/10.3390/ma4122119

Pandey RP, Gunjan, Himanshu, et al (2024) Nanocarrier-mediated probiotic delivery: a systematic meta-analysis assessing the biological effects. Sci Rep 14:. https://doi.org/10.1038/s41598-023-50972-x

Kvakova M, Bertkova I, Stofilova J, Savidge TC (2021) Co-Encapsulated Synbiotics and Immobilized Probiotics in Human Health and Gut Microbiota Modulation. Foods 10:1297. https://doi.org/10.3390/foods10061297

Gruškienė R, Galinskaitė A, Kavleiskaja T, et al (2024) Fucoidan as a carrier of antimicrobial peptide: Preparation and characterization of nisin-loaded particles. LWT 191:115598. https://doi.org/10.1016/j.lwt.2023.115598

Senadheera TRL, Hossain A, Shahidi F (2023) Marine Bioactives and Their Application in the Food Industry: A Review. Applied Sciences 13:12088. https://doi.org/10.3390/app132112088

Cao C, Yuan D, Kong B, et al (2022) Effect of different κ-carrageenan incorporation forms on the gel properties and in vitro digestibility of frankfurters. Food Hydrocolloids 129:107637. https://doi.org/10.1016/j.foodhyd.2022.107637

Arda E, Kara S, Pekcan Ö (2009) Synergistic effect of the locust bean gum on the thermal phase transitions of κ-carrageenan gels. Food Hydrocolloids 23:451–459. https://doi.org/10.1016/j.foodhyd.2008.02.010

Lee S, Jo K, Kim S, et al (2025) Constructing stable emulsion gel from gelatin and sodium alginate as pork fat substitute: Emphasis on lipid digestion in vitro. Food Hydrocolloids 160:110739. https://doi.org/10.1016/j.foodhyd.2024.110739

Wanniarachchi PC, Paranagama IT, Idangodage PA, et al (2025) Natural polymer-based hydrogels: Types, functionality, food applications, environmental significance and future perspectives: An updated review. Food Biomacromolecules 2:84–105. https://doi.org/10.1002/fob2.70000

Akhtar A, Nasim I, Din MSU, et al (2023) Effects of different fat replacers on functional and rheological properties of low-fat mozzarella cheeses: A review. Trends in Food Science & Technology 139:104136. https://doi.org/10.1016/j.tifs.2023.104136

Alboofetileh M, Jeddi S, Subi TM, Vasanthi HR (2025) Sulfated polysaccharides from Ulva rigida as antioxidant and antibacterial enhancers in chicken sausages. Algal Research 86:103940. https://doi.org/10.1016/j.algal.2025.103940

Kim T-K, Shim J-Y, Hwang K-E, et al (2018) Effect of hydrocolloids on the quality of restructured hams with duck skin. Poultry Science 97:4442–4449. https://doi.org/10.3382/ps/pey309

Tan LL, Ang KL, Loo SCJ (2023) Alginate encapsulation improves probiotics survival in carbonated sodas and beers. PLoS ONE 18:e0283745. https://doi.org/10.1371/journal.pone.0283745

Koh HSA, Lim SEV, Lu J, Zhou W (2020) Bioactivity enhancement of fucoidan through complexing with bread matrix and baking. LWT 130:109646. https://doi.org/10.1016/j.lwt.2020.109646

Tarahi M, Mohamadzade Fakhr-davood M, Ghaedrahmati S, et al (2023) Physicochemical and Sensory Properties of Vegan Gummy Candies Enriched with High-Fiber Jaban Watermelon Exocarp Powder. Foods 12:1478. https://doi.org/10.3390/foods12071478

Zarzycki P, Ciołkowska AE, Jabłońska-Ryś E, Gustaw W (2019) Rheological properties of milk-based desserts with the addition of oat gum and κ-carrageenan. J Food Sci Technol 56:5107–5115. https://doi.org/10.1007/s13197-019-03983-4

Kurchenko V, Halavach T, Yantsevich A, et al (2024) Chitosan and its derivatives regulate lactic acid synthesis during milk fermentation. Front Nutr 11:. https://doi.org/10.3389/fnut.2024.1441355

Zannini E, Waters DM, Arendt EK (2014) The application of dextran compared to other hydrocolloids as a novel food ingredient to compensate for low protein in biscuit and wholemeal wheat flour. Eur Food Res Technol 238:763–771. https://doi.org/10.1007/s00217-014-2161-8

Totosaus A, Pérez-Chabela ML (2009) Textural properties and microstructure of low-fat and sodium-reduced meat batters formulated with gellan gum and dicationic salts. LWT - Food Science and Technology 42:563–569. https://doi.org/10.1016/j.lwt.2008.07.016

Preichardt LD, Vendruscolo CT, Gularte MA, Moreira ADS (2011) The role of xanthan gum in the quality of gluten free cakes: improved bakery products for coeliac patients. International Journal of Food Science & Technology 46:2591–2597. https://doi.org/10.1111/j.1365-2621.2011.02788.x

El-Khawas KM, Mashat BH, Attala OA, Kassem GMA (2020) Control of *Salmonella* and *Escherichia coli* in chilled chicken fillets using chitosan and lactic acid. CyTA - Journal of Food 18:445–450. https://doi.org/10.1080/19476337.2020.1772887

El Mouzahim M, Eddarai EM, Eladaoui S, et al (2023) Food packaging composite film based on chitosan, natural kaolinite clay, and Ficus. carica leaves extract for fresh-cut apple slices preservation. International Journal of Biological Macromolecules 233:123430. https://doi.org/10.1016/j.ijbiomac.2023.123430

Sivarooban T, Hettiarachchy NS, Johnson MG (2007) Inhibition of Listeria monocytogenes Using Nisin with Grape Seed Extract on Turkey Frankfurters Stored at 4 and 10°C. Journal of Food Protection 70:1017–1020. https://doi.org/10.4315/0362-028x-70.4.1017

Bagale U, Kadi A, Malinin A, et al (2023) Impact of a Sonochemical Approach to the Structural and Antioxidant Activity of Brown Algae (Fucoidan) Using the Box–Behnken Design Method. Processes 11:1884. https://doi.org/10.3390/pr11071884

Wang H, Cao Z, Yao L, et al (2023) Insights into the Edible and Biodegradable Ulvan-Based Films and Coatings for Food Packaging. Foods 12:1622. https://doi.org/10.3390/foods12081622

Demircan B, Velioglu YS (2024) Control of Browning, Enzyme Activity, and Quality in Stored Fresh-cut Fruit Salads through Chitosan Coating Enriched with Bergamot Juice Powder. Foods 13:147. https://doi.org/10.3390/foods13010147

Da Silva Simões CV, Stamford TCM, Berger LRR, et al (2025) Edible Alginate–Fungal Chitosan Coatings as Carriers for Lacticaseibacillus casei LC03 and Their Impact on Quality Parameters of Strawberries During Cold Storage. Foods 14:203. https://doi.org/10.3390/foods14020203

Martínez-González MDC, Bautista-Baños S, Correa-Pacheco ZN, et al (2020) Effect of Nanostructured Chitosan/Propolis Coatings on the Quality and Antioxidant Capacity of Strawberries During Storage. Coatings 10:90. https://doi.org/10.3390/coatings10020090

Esteve-Redondo P, Heras-Mozos R, Simó-Ramírez E, et al (2024) Innovative Systems for the Delivery of Naturally Occurring Antimicrobial Volatiles in Active Food-Packaging Technologies for Fresh and Minimally Processed Produce: Stimuli-Responsive Materials. Foods 13:856. https://doi.org/10.3390/foods13060856

Solís-Contreras GA, Rodríguez-Guillermo MC, De La Luz Reyes-Vega M, et al (2021) Extending Shelf-Life and Quality of Minimally Processed Golden Delicious Apples with Three Bioactive Coatings Combined with Cinnamon Essential Oil. Foods 10:597. https://doi.org/10.3390/foods10030597

Montaño-Sánchez E, Torres-Martínez BDM, Vargas-Sánchez RD, et al (2020) Effects of Chitosan Coating with Green Tea Aqueous Extract on Lipid Oxidation and Microbial Growth in Pork Chops during Chilled Storage. Foods 9:766. https://doi.org/10.3390/foods9060766

Zhang X, Na F, Zhang M, Yang W (2025b) Microbial Control in the Processing of Low-Temperature Meat Products: Non-Thermal Sterilization and Natural Antimicrobials. Foods 14:225. https://doi.org/10.3390/foods14020225

Bambace MF, Alvarez MV, Moreira MDR (2025) Alginate coatings applied on apple cubes as a vehicle for *Lacticaseibacillus casei*: probiotic viability and overall quality of a new functional product. J Sci Food Agric 105:74–83. https://doi.org/10.1002/jsfa.13805

Rodriguez OT, Valero MF, Gómez-Tejedor JA, Diaz L (2024) Performance of Biodegradable Active Packaging in the Preservation of Fresh-Cut Fruits: A Systematic Review. Polymers 16: 3518. https://doi.org/10.3390/polym16243518

Silva SPM, Ribeiro SC, Teixeira JA, Silva CCG (2022) Application of an alginate-based edible coating with bacteriocin-producing Lactococcus strains in fresh cheese preservation. LWT 153: 112486. https://doi.org/10.1016/j.lwt.2021.112486

Montone AMI, Malvano F, Taiano R, et al (2023) Alginate Coating Charged by Hydroxyapatite Complexes with Lactoferrin and Quercetin Enhances the Pork Meat Shelf Life. Foods 12:553. https://doi.org/10.3390/foods12030553

Şengül E, Şen DB (2025) Development and Characterization of κ-Carrageenan-Based Edible Films Enriched With Resveratrol or Quercetin for Shelf-Life Extension of Goat Meat Burger Patties. Journal of Food Science 90:. https://doi.org/10.1111/1750-3841.70277

Behnam S, Anvari M, Rezaei M, et al (2015) Effect of nisin as a biopreservative agent on quality and shelf life of vacuum packaged rainbow trout (Oncorhynchus mykiss) stored at 4 °C. J Food Sci Technol 52:2184–2192. https://doi.org/10.1007/s13197-013-1241-2

Bao H, Wang Y, Huang Y, et al (2025) The Beneficial Role of Polysaccharide Hydrocolloids in Meat Products: A Review. Gels 11:55. https://doi.org/10.3390/gels11010055

González-Cuello R, Parada-Castro AL, Ortega-Toro R (2024) Application of a Multi-Component Composite Edible Coating for the Preservation of Strawberry Fruit. J Compos Sci 8:515. https://doi.org/10.3390/jcs8120515

Marine Polysaccharides in Delivery of Bioactive Molecules

Rassoul Kadkhodaee and Sara Keshvari Khojasteh

Abstract Marine-derived polysaccharides have garnered significant interest due to their functional attributes and diverse applications in the culinary, pharmaceutical, food, and biomedical industries. This chapter provides an in-depth review of the structural, physicochemical and the use of most popular marine polysaccharides, including alginate, fucoidan, chitosan, carrageenan, and agar, as natural carriers for the entrapment and delivery of nutraceuticals and bioactive compounds. These biopolymers are valued for their structural versatility, biocompatibility, and ability to form stable matrices, making them ideal candidates for various purposes. Encapsulation plays a vital role in protecting environmentally sensitive bioactive ingredients from volatile losses, oxidative degradation, decomposition under harsh processing conditions, handling, and storage, and interaction with other molecular entities in the surrounding medium, while preserving the color, flavor, texture, and aroma of the matrix in which they are embedded. Additionally, encapsulation can mask the undesirable flavor and odor of the nutraceuticals and facilitate their safe delivery to the targeted sites when ingested orally. Many marine polysaccharides, owing to their gel-forming and emulsifying properties, serve as effective wall materials for encapsulation applications. A wide range of techniques is employed for the encapsulation of bioactive ingredients, with spray drying, freeze-drying, and coacervation being the most commonly utilized methods in the food and pharmaceutical sectors. However, future research is required to focus on the modification of marine polysaccharides and their based-delivery systems, including enzymatic hydrolysis, chemical derivatization, and nanotechnology-based methods, to improve their functional properties and enhance the effectiveness of the corresponding designed delivery matrices.

Keywords Marine polysaccharides · Encapsulation methods · Wall materials · Characterization · Functional properties

---

R. Kadkhodaee (✉) · S. K. Khojasteh
Department of Food Physics, Research Institute of Food Science and Technology (RIFST), Mashhad, Iran
e-mail: r.kadkhodaee@rifst.ac.ir

S. Jana et al. (eds.), *Multifunctional Marine Polysaccharides*,
https://doi.org/10.1007/978-981-95-4126-3_17

1 Introduction

The rise of acute noncommunicable diseases, such as obesity, diabetes, and cardiovascular disorders, due to unhealthy lifestyles and imbalanced diets has heightened public awareness and therefore the demands for nutraceuticals and functional foods is on the rise (Awuchi and Okpala 2022). Naturally occurring bioactive components possess antibacterial, anticancer, antioxidant, and anti-inflammatory properties that can boost the immune system, enhance physiological functions, and prevent a wide variety of illnesses. However, despite their diverse health-promoting benefits, bioactive ingredients are prone to being adversely influenced by environmental conditions and the physicochemical properties of the matrix in which they are incorporated. Additionally, they may also have inherent properties, such as unfavorable flavor and poor solubility. This makes their direct application in foods and other formulations limited and challenging. Therefore, to effectively take advantage of the benefits of bioactive compounds, appropriate encapsulation and delivery systems with high bioavailability are essential (Dong et al. 2021). Maintaining the effectiveness of bioactive compounds and nutraceuticals requires protecting them from environmental agents such as light, pH, temperature, oxygen, and degrading enzymes, as well as the harsh conditions of the digestive tract. The use of encapsulation techniques can be an effective way to protect these substances from decomposition and increase their bioavailability during digestion. Incorporating bioactive compounds into food provides additional health benefits, such as boosting the immune system, preventing metabolic disorders, and reducing the risk of acute physiological diseases, that go beyond just supplying routine nutritional and caloric requirements. This is achieved when the bioactive ingredient is sufficiently absorbed by the gastrointestinal tract, delivered to a the targeted site, and at a reasonable dose (Maleki et al. 2022). A broad range of materials can be utilized to encapsulate bioactive ingredients. Conventional food-grade wall materials are derived from carbohydrates, proteins, and lipids (Alu'datt et al. 2022). Polysaccharides, due to their high modifiability, solubility, and ability to interact through their functional groups, are particularly suitable wall materials for encapsulation purposes (Maleki et al. 2022). Recently, marine polysaccharides have attracted significant interest for the delivery of nutraceuticals and bioactive compounds due to their unique structures and diverse physicochemical properties that enhance their stability and bioavailability (Cotas et al. 2024; Ji et al. 2025; Sepe et al. 2025). Notably, polysaccharides such as alginate, carrageenan, and fucoidan, because of their gelling capabilities, are ideal for delivery applications (Akdaşçi et al. 2025; Bao et al. 2025).

2 Marine Polysaccharides

According to their sources, marine polysaccharides can be classified into three categories: plant, animal, and microbial (Fig. 1). Marine plant polysaccharides are primarily extracted from algae, including alginic acid, agar, and carrageenan. Marine animal polysaccharides are obtained from crustaceans, specifically chitin. Marine microbial polysaccharides are derived from various genera, such as Pseudomonas, Bacillus, Acinetobacter, and Vibrio (Zhang et al. 2025). In the following sections, the main marine polysaccharides will be briefly introduced.

2.1 Algal-Derived Polysaccharides

2.1.1 Alginate

Structure and Functional Features

Alginate is a natural polysaccharide found in the extracellular matrix of brown algae. It has been used for many years as a thickening and gelling agent, and more recently as an encapsulant in culinary, pharmaceutical, and biotechnological applications (Lopez-Sanchez et al. 2022). Alginate is a linear anionic polysaccharide made up of

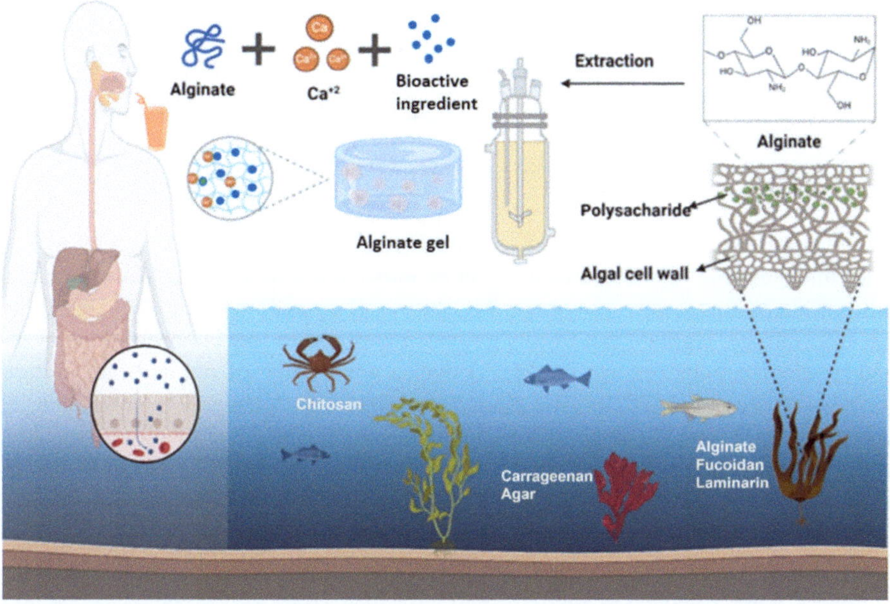

Fig. 1 Schematic representation of the primary sources of marine polysaccharides, with a specific focus on the extraction of alginate and its application as a wall material for encapsulation

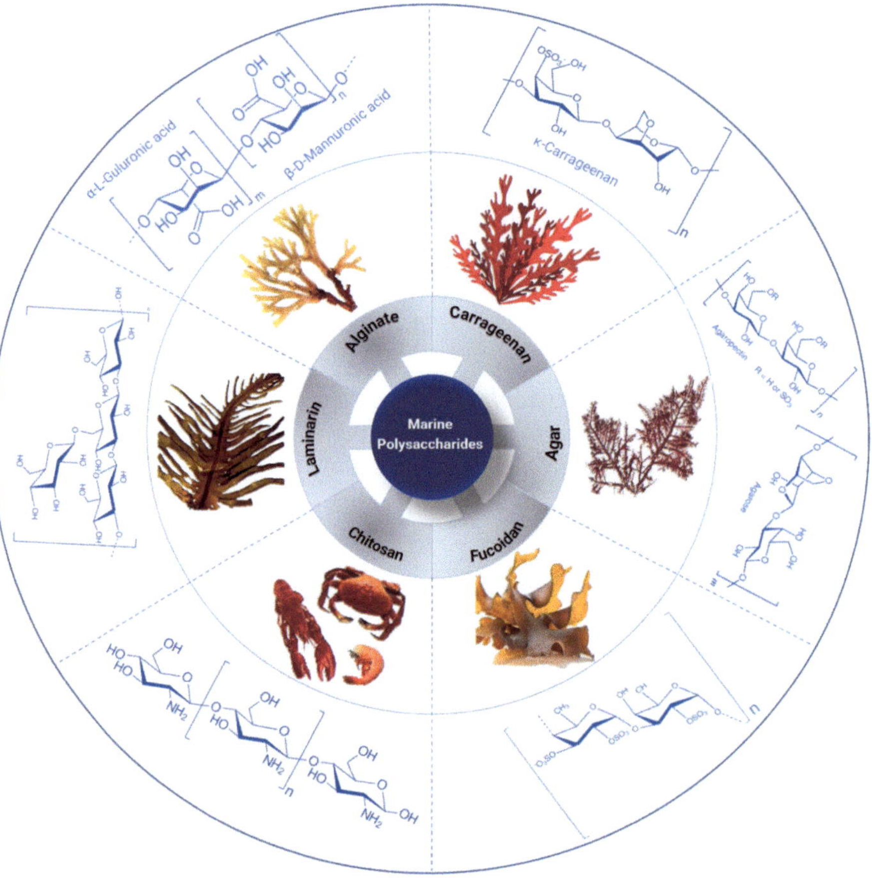

Fig. 2 Chemical structure of marine polysaccharides and their representative sources

β-D-mannuronic acid (M) and α-L-guluronic acid (G) blocks connected by glycosidic linkages (Fig. 2). These chains can be either homo-polymeric M or G blocks only or alternating hetero-polymeric MG blocks (Fernando et al. 2020). Due to its negative charge, alginate can form a gel when exposed to low concentrations of di- and trivalent cations (except for Mg^{2+}) over a wide range of pH and temperature (Lopez-Sanchez et al. 2022). The ability of alginates to form gels is influenced by various intrinsic and extrinsic factors, including the length, composition, sequence, and M/G ratio of the polymer chains, as well as the concentration of cross-linking agent. The strength of the gel is also affected by the level and length of G blocks, which have a higher affinity for cationic cross-linkers compared to M blocks. This allows for the creation of alginate-based delivery systems with different release rates of bioactive ingredients. For example, alginates with a high percentage of M residues or a high M/G ratio tend to produce weaker and more flexible gels and capsules with lower diffusion permeability (Shafiq and Rizvi 2023). On the other hand, alginate with a higher percentage of G blocks results in stiffer stiff hydrogels with wider pores, making it easier for bioactive compounds to diffuse from the polymer network (Okolie et al. 2020). This highlights the importance of the configuration of alginate in the design and development of the alginate-based delivery systems. As a natural and biocompatible polysaccharide, alginate offers many advantages, including high encapsulation efficiency, stability at ambient temperature, and pH-responsive behavior, especially when used in the form of calcium alginate gels. Additionally, the processing of alginate is relatively simple and cost-effective, allowing for the creation of gels with a wide range of mechanical and functional properties (Oroná et al. 2024). The versatility of alginate as a delivery matrix has been well-documented in the encapsulation of various bioactive compounds, such as polyphenols (e.g., apigenin, curcumin, ellagic acid, gallic acid, and quercetin). The use of alginate not only improves the stability of these compounds but also enhances their biological activity (Kučuk et al. 2024).

Modification

A variety of modification strategies have been utilized to improve the functional performance of alginate in delivery systems. Each approach is designed to achieve specific objectives, such as controlled release kinetics, improved stability, and enhanced bioactivity. Currently, the structures and associated properties of various chemically modified alginates have been extensively documented, including acetylated alginate, phosphorylated alginate, sulfated alginate, hydrophobically modified alginate, graft copolymerized alginate, and covalently cross-linked alginate, among others (Li et al. 2021). These modifications expand the physicochemical versatility of alginate and allow for its application in more complex and demanding delivery environments. One method of modifying alginate is through hydrophobization, which involves grafting hydrophobic groups onto its backbone. This enhances the molecular flexibility of alginate by reducing intramolecular hydrogen bonds, thereby altering its functionality. For instance, the reductive amination of oxidized alginate derivative (RAOA) has significant self-assembly characteristics, making it suitable for delivering hydrophobic components (Tosuwan et al. 2024). Additionally, incorporating hydrophobic functional groups is a commonly used strategy to improve the emulsifying capacity of alginate. For example, partial hydrophobic modification using dodecenyl succinic anhydride has been shown to significantly reduce interfacial tension by adsorbing at the oil-water interface and forming an oil-stabilizing layer. This structural modification has been linked to improved encapsulation efficiency, highlighting its potential as an effective bio-based emulsifier (Akshaya and Nathanael 2024). Furthermore, chemical modification with octenyl succinic anhydride (OSA) has been found to enhance the mechanical integrity of alginate beads, resulting in improved encapsulation efficiency and protection of sensitive bioactive compounds (Farahani et al. 2022). Moreover, combining alginate with complementary biopolymers, such as chitosan, has led to the development of hybrid delivery systems that leverage the advantageous properties of each component to achieve superior delivery performance (Wang et al. 2022). These hybrid systems often exhibit modulated mechanical behavior and biodegradation rates, which can be precisely tailored to meet specific release kinetics for diverse applications, including drug delivery and regenerative medicine (Neves et al. 2020).

2.1.2 Carrageenan

Structure and Functional Features

Carrageenan is a sulfated linear polysaccharide primarily extracted from specific species of red seaweeds through a hot alkali treatment. Its structure consists of alternating units of galactose and 3,6-anhydrogalactose, connected via α-1,3- and β-1,4-glycosidic linkages (Fig. 2). Based on their degree of sulfation and the presence or absence of 3,6-anhydrogalactose, carrageenans are classified into six principal types: kappa (κ)-, iota (ι)-, lambda (λ)-, mu (μ)-, nu (ν)-, and theta (θ)-carrageenan, each exhibiting distinct physicochemical and functional properties (Álvarez-Viñas et al. 2021; Pathiraja et al. 2022). The different types of carrageenan have distinct physicochemical properties, such as gelling capacity and solubility. Among them, kappa and iota are the most commonly used for gelation. The gelation process involves a conformational shift from a random coil to a helical shape, which forms a three-dimensional network (Dong et al. 2021; Geonzon et al. 2023). This network not only provides a high water retention but also offers substantial porosity and surface area, which are essential for encapsulating and controlling the release of bioactive and therapeutic agents (Obaidat et al. 2018). The sulfate groups in carrageenan give the polymer a negative charge, allowing for ionic interactions with positively charged drugs. This supports the formation of polyelectrolyte complexes, which can enhance drug loading and modulate release kinetics (Mokhtari et al. 2021). Furthermore, carrageenan has several advantages over other encapsulating materials. For example, κ-carrageenan is more compatible with acidic environments compared to alginate, leading to better protection of encapsulated bioactive components (Feng et al. 2021). On the other hand, the thermoreversible nature of carrageenan gels is unique and cannot be replaced by other polysaccharides. This property is particularly valuable for applications that require temperature-induced sol-gel transition, allowing for easy encapsulation of bioactive compounds under mild conditions and subsequent release under physiological environments (Rode et al. 2018). Additionally, carrageenan-based delivery systems have notable benefits compared to others. Carrageenan can improve the retention and loading efficiency of bioactive ingredients, promote their loading efficiency, and enhance their release rate. It also protects the core substances from enzymatic degradation, improving their stability under digestive conditions and facilitating their delivery to targeted sites (Dong et al. 2021).

Modification

The highly hydrophilic nature of carrageenan poses limitations for its application in delivering hydrophobic compounds, and its intrinsic mechanical strength may be inadequate for certain industrial and biomedical applications. To enhance its utility, carrageenan has been subjected to chemical and ionic modifications (Kumar et al. 2025). Among chemical modifications, carboxymethylation has emerged as a promising approach to tailor carrageenan's pH responsiveness and swelling behavior, enabling targeted delivery within the intestinal tract where pH gradients can be effectively exploited (Leong et al. 2011). Additionally, physicochemical modifications have been integrated into carrageenan-based systems to enhance their bioavailability and molecular interaction capabilities. For instance, ionic cross-linking with monovalent cations can induce a coil-to-helix conformational transition in κ-carrageenan, resulting in modified rheological and mechanical properties. This transition supports the formation of stable hydrogels, suitable for sustained release of bioactive agents (Mahapatra et al. 2023). Furthermore, the incorporation of carrageenan into hybrid systems with other biopolymers such as chitosan or with inorganic components has demonstrated the ability to enhance structural integrity, mechanical strength, and drug loading efficiency (Mokhtari et al. 2021).

2.1.3 Agar

Structure and Functional Features

Agar is a hydrocolloid derived from the cell walls of certain red algae. It is insoluble in cold water but hydrates in boiling water, resulting in a transparent and isotropic solution. When cooled to below 35–45 °C, agar forms strong and stable gels that remain solid up to 80–85 °C (Shah et al. 2024; Zhang et al. 2023). Agar's chemical structure consists of a combination of agaropectin (the non-gelling component) and agarose (the gelling component) (Fig. 2). Agarose is a linear polysaccharide composed of repeating units of D-galactose and 3–6,anhydro-L-galactose, interconnected by alternating α-(1 → 3) and β-(1 → 4) glycosidic linkages. Agaropectin, on the other hand, is marginally branched and sulfated (Mostafavi and Zaeim 2020). It is highly anionic, containing acidic side groups such as sulfate and pyruvate, while agarose is neutral and has longer chains (Junaid et al. 2024; Mostafavi and Zaeim 2020).

Modification

To improve the functional performance of agar and maximize its efficacy as a drug delivery vehicle, it has been structurally modified using various methods. One significant approach is the chemical substitution of functional groups on the agar backbone, particularly the addition of hydrophobic groups like alkyl carbon chains.

This increases steric hindrance in the matrix, resulting in a looser polymeric network that enhances water permeation and strengthens the hydrogel's ability to encapsulate hydrophobic bioactive compounds. One such compound is curcumin, a natural polyphenol known for its anti-inflammatory and anticancer properties, but with limited applications due to its low water solubility and stability. Moreover, esterified agar has shown improved amphiphilicity and structural flexibility, making it suitable for use in various delivery systems such as hydrogels and nanoparticles (Zhang et al. 2023). Esterification of agar with citric acid has also been reported to enhance its functionality by increasing hydrophobicity and emulsion stabilizing properties across a wide pH range. These features improve controlled release behavior and drug loading efficiency by creating hydrophobic cavities that can trap lipophilic molecules (Jiang et al. 2024).

2.1.4 Fucoidan

Structure and Functional Features

Fucoidan is a water-soluble sulfated polysaccharide primarily found in brown algae. It is a complex molecule with a molecular weight ranging from 100 to 1600 kDa (Kraithong et al. 2025; Meng et al. 2025). However, its structure is not been fully understood due to its variability and irregularity. This intriguing polysaccharide is typically classified into two distinct types based on its backbone composition. Type I consists of repeated (1–3)-α-L-fucopyranose residues (Fig. 2), while Type II features a more intricate arrangement of alternating and repeated (1–3)- and (1–4)-α-L-fucopyranose residues. Understanding these distinctions is essential for fully realizing the potential applications of fucoidan (Zhang et al. 2022).

Modification

Although fucoidan is a non-gelling polysaccharide by nature and cannot form gels on its own (Wang et al. 2021), it can be induced to gel under specific conditions or through interactions with other biopolymers or ions, expanding its potential as an encapsulating agent. One mechanism involves the interaction between fucoidan's sulfate groups and divalent cations (e.g., calcium), which promotes ionic cross-linking and the formation of a stable gel network (Wu et al. 2018). Additionally, fucoidan can form gels when combined with other gelling agents such as alginate, carrageenan, or gelatin. In these cases, ionic bonding, hydrogen bonding, and molecular entanglement play essential roles in gel formation, while hydrophobic interactions under certain conditions further enhance the structural integrity of the gel network. Fucoidan has been successfully used in combination with other hydrocolloids or proteins to encapsulate a variety of compounds, including curcumin (Zhang et al. 2021), catechin (Ettoumi et al. 2023), and bacterial strains such as *Lacticaseibacillus* spp. (Lei et al. 2024). Despite its promising functionality, several challenges limit the practical application of fucoidan. One significant limitation is its source variability; the structural and physicochemical properties of fucoidan can differ greatly depending on the species of seaweed and extraction conditions, which can impact reproducibility and functionality (Omuzbuken et al. 2022). Fucoidan may also exhibit unpredictable interactions with other components within encapsulation systems, potentially altering release profiles and reducing the overall efficacy of the encapsulated substances. Additionally, the limited solubility of fucoidan in various solvents can restrict its use in certain formulations. However, with careful formulation strategies, these limitations can be overcome, and the potential of fucoidan as an encapsulating material can be fully realized (Du et al. 2022).

2.1.5 Laminarin

Laminarin, also known as laminaran, was first identified in brown macroalgae. It has a molecular weight (MW) of approximately 5 kDa, which can vary depending on the degree of polymerization. The degree of branching also affects its solubility, with highly branched laminarin being soluble in cold water, while less branched varieties require warm water for solubility (Carrasqueira et al. 2025). The typical structure of laminarin consists of a backbone of β-1,3-glucose and a side chain of β-1,6-glucose (Fig. 2) (Chen et al. 2021). Despite its unique properties, there are relatively few reports on the modification of laminaran due to its poor gelling properties, which present challenges for its modification and application (Zhou and Li 2024).

2.2 Animal-Derived Marine Polysaccharides

2.2.1 Structure of Chitin and Chitosan and Their Functional Features

Chitin, a precursor to chitosan and the second most abundant biopolymer in nature after cellulose, is a linear polysaccharide composed of poly-β-[1,4]-N-acetyl-D-glucosamine units. This eco-friendly polymer can be sourced from various origins, including the exoskeletons of crabs. However, the fully acetylated structure of chitin limits its application due to its high thermochemical stability and poor solubility in both aqueous media and most organic solvents. Chitosan, the N-deacetylated derivative of chitin, is produced through chemical or enzymatic deacetylation and also occurs naturally in the cell walls of certain fungi. It is a linear copolymer composed of alternating hydrophilic D-glucosamine units and residual hydrophobic N-acetyl-D-glucosamine units, as shown in Fig. 2 (El-Araby et al. 2024; Wang et al. 2025). Due to its exceptional biocompatibility, biodegradability, mucoadhesiveness, and unique cationic nature (uncommon among polysaccharides), chitosan plays a crucial role in the food and nutraceutical industries (Sangnim et al. 2023; Wong et al. 2021). It has a wide range of applications, particularly in the production of controlled release systems, and functional food components.

The functional properties of chitosan are largely dependent on its molecular weight and degree of deacetylation (DD), which plays a crucial role in determining its effectiveness in various applications, including biomolecule delivery systems (Famiglietti et al. 2022; Verardi et al. 2023; Zhou et al. 2021). Owing to its positively charged and water-soluble nature, chitosan is able to form electrostatic interactions with negatively charged macromolecules, resulting in the formation of complex nanoparticles. This unique characteristic has been widely utilized in the encapsulation of bioactive compounds (Rajabi et al. 2019).

Modification

Despite its promising characteristics, chitosan has limited capacity to control the release of encapsulated compounds primarily due to its hydrophilic nature and solubility in acidic media. Additionally, its low water solubility under neutral and basic conditions, coupled with inherent mechanical weaknesses, restricts its broader application in drug delivery systems. To address these limitations, chemical modifications at the hydroxyl and free amino groups are often employed to modulate its solubility, stability, and overall functionality for use in pharmaceutical formulations (Desai et al. 2023; George and Abraham 2006). Several modifications have been achieved to improve the drug delivery properties of chitosan. For example, thiolated chitosan is a covalently substituted thiol-bearing moieties on its backbone made by attaching-SH groups to amino groups, primarily at the 2-position of glucosamine subunits (George and Abraham 2006). This derivatization enhances its physicochemical properties, such as mucoadhesiveness and permeation features, making it suitable for peroral drug delivery purposes. Furthermore, the modification of chitosan using anhydrides or long-chain acyl chlorides leads to the formation of hydrophobically modified derivatives, which tend to self-assemble in aqueous media, forming nanoparticles or micelles that serve as promising carriers for drug delivery (Poshina et al. 2025). These structural alterations not only improve chitosan's solubility and stability but also expand its utility for controlled and targeted drug delivery applications (Le Tien et al. 2003). Another effective modification is grafting chitosan with an isocyanate-terminated polyurethane copolymer, which has been shown to significantly improve its physicochemical characteristics, facilitating more controlled release of the core material. The integration of polyurethane into the chitosan matrix has been shown to enhance both its mechanical strength and thermal stability, while also modulating its hydrophilicity and solubility, which are essential parameters for sustained release. The degree of substitution during grafting governs the network structure of the resulting copolymer, influencing its swelling behavior and overall solubility (Kumar et al. 2015).

3 Marine Polysaccharide-Based Delivery Systems for Bioactive Compounds

Bioactive delivery systems are a diverse range of specially designed structures that are typically created through encapsulation, either in solid or liquid form. Encapsulation involves enclosing a core material within a protective matrix to shield it from external factors. Depending on the size of the capsules, this technique is classified as nano- (<0.2 μm), micro- (0.2–5000 μm), or macro- (>5000 μm) encapsulation. Micro- and nano-encapsulation, the most promising of these, are predominantly used in food and nutritional applications. Specifically, encapsulation is utilized for various purposes, such as active packaging, retaining natural flavors, preservatives, and antioxidants, functionalization of agri-food by-products, and enhanced transport and protection of both nutrients and non-nutrient bioactive compounds (Alu'datt et al. 2022).

3.1 Encapsulation Techniques

Marine polysaccharides have gained significant attention as biomaterials that can be tailored for use in various encapsulation methods. The versatile compounds are utilized in advanced applications across the pharmaceutical, nutraceutical, cosmetic, and food sectors, serving as effective encapsulating matrices. They play a crucial role in modulating release kinetics and, importantly, in enhancing the stability of active ingredients (Borgogna et al. 2011). A variety of encapsulation techniques, such as fluid bed coating, extrusion, emulsification, spray chilling, coacervation, spray drying, freeze-drying, and molecular inclusion, are commonly used. The following sections will discuss specific methods that involve marine polysaccharides as encapsulating matrices. The choice of an appropriate encapsulation technique is primarily based on the desired characteristics, including particle uniformity, process scalability, and preservation of the integrity of the encapsulated bioactive compound. Table 1 highlights the most commonly used techniques for encapsulating bioactive ingredients based on marine polysaccharides.

3.2 Spray Drying

Spray drying is a cost-effective method for microencapsulation that is widely used in various industries, including food, pharmaceutical, and agriculture. This process involves converting a concentrated liquid solution or suspension into a powdered product (Sánchez-Osorno et al. 2023; Yan and Kim 2024). The core and wall materials are dispersed in water to create a homogeneous liquid or emulsion, which is then introduced into a hot air stream (100–300 °C). The water evaporates

Table 1 Overview of encapsulation techniques for bioactive compounds and probiotics using marine polysaccharides as wall materials

Encapsulation technique	Wall material	Bioactive ingredient/probiotic	References
Emulsification	Alginate	Cold-pressed grape seed oil	Lević et al. (2024)
Spray drying	Alginate and pectin	Gallic acid	Nájera-Martínez et al. (2023)
Complex coacervation	Hazelnut protein isolate and sodium alginate	Quercetin	Adrar et al. (2024)
Extrusion	Alginate	*Lactobacillus casei*	Dimitrellou et al. (2019)
Freeze drying	Carrageenan/gum tragacanth	Fish oil	Pourashouri et al. (2021)
Freeze drying	κ-carrageenan/sodium alginate	*Bifidobacterium bifidum*	Afzaal et al. (2020)
Complex coacervation	Mung bean protein/ succinylated chitosan	Curcumin	Mirmohammad Meiguni et al. (2022)
Spray drying	Whey protein concentrate/water-soluble chitosan	*Kluyveromycesmarxianus* VM004/peanut skin polyphenolic extract	Centomo et al. (2024)
Emulsification	Chitosan/gum Arabic	Tunisian thyme essential oil	Snoussi et al. (2022)
Complex coacervation	Soybean protein isolate/fucoidan	Curcumin	Fan et al. (2021)
Emulsification	Fucoidan/chitosan	Catechin	Ettoumi et al. (2023)
Complex coacervation	Chitosan/zein/tween-80/fucoidan	*Lacticaseibacillus rhamnosus*	Lei et al. (2024)

quickly from the droplets, resulting in either powder or agglomerated particles, depending on the properties of the input materials and the design and operational parameters of the dryer (Mohammed et al. 2020). This method has been successfully used to encapsulate a variety of bioactive compounds into marine polysaccharide matrices, such as alginate and chitosan, increasing their stability against environmental factors (Centomo et al. 2024; Nájera-Martínez et al. 2023).

3.3 Freeze Drying

Freeze drying, also known as lyophilization, is another encapsulation technique involving the direct phase transition of water from solid to vapor state, resulting in the entrapment of core material within a solid polymeric matrix. This method is commonly used in the food and pharmaceutical industry. The process begins with freezing a dispersion or emulsion of core-wall materials, followed by sublimation of water under reduced pressure conditions. This results in a spongy mass that can be ground into a fine powder. Unlike spray drying, freeze drying does not involve high temperatures, which prevents damage and loss of bioactive compounds during the process (Nowak and Jakubczyk 2020; Pudziuvelyte et al. 2020). Therefore, it is the preferred method for encapsulating heat-sensitive substances and probiotics (Silva-Espinoza et al. 2021). Chitosan and alginate have been successfully used in this method for encapsulating various probiotics (Afzaal et al. 2020) and bioactive compounds (Pourashouri et al. 2021).

3.4 Emulsification

Emulsification is another notable method for encapsulation, in which two immiscible liquids are mixed together and stabilized by emulsifying agents. This results in one liquid being dispersed into the other in the form of fine droplets. Emulsions can be simple, such as oil-in-water (O/W) or water-in-oil (W/O), or multiple, with the droplets of one emulsion dispersed into another continuous phase in the form of either W/O/W or O/W/O. This technique is particularly useful for encapsulating hydrophobic substances within a hydrophilic matrix, or vice versa. Another unique binary system, known as water-in-water (W/W) emulsion, can also be used for encapsulating bioactive ingredients. This type of emulsion is composed of two thermodynamically incompatible polymers, with the core polymer (dispersed phase) selected based on its high partitioning coefficient for the bioactive substance. Emulsification can be achieved by applying high mechanical shear using a variety of commercially available devices, such as rotor-stator, high pressure, or ultrasonic homogenizers (Fernandes et al. 2024; Santosa et al. 2021). The resulting emulsions can then be dehydrated using freeze drying or spray drying, which helps to extend the storage stability of the product and retain the core material. It is important to note that the choice of drying method can affect the characteristics of the final product (Bashir et al. 2024). Marine-derived polysaccharides such as alginate, chitosan, and fucoidan, have been widely used in emulsification-based encapsulation of various bioactive compounds. These polysaccharides have shown good sustained release profiles and have been effective in protecting sensitive substances from degradation (Ettoumi et al. 2023; Snoussi et al. 2022).

3.5 Coacervation

Coacervation is a spontaneous process in which a homogeneous monophasic colloidal solution separates into two distinct phases at a specific pH. One phase is a dense coacervate with a high concentration of colloidal components, while the other is a diluted phase with fewer components (Peng et al. 2024). This method is highly effective for microencapsulation due to its high loading capacity, low temperature requirements, and minimal damage to the core material. It also offers the advantage of tunability for controlled release and does not require specialized equipment, toxic solvents, or excessive agitation. However, the main challenges associated with this technique are difficulty with scale-up and controlling particle size, as coacervates tend to agglomerate (Pudziuvelyte et al. 2022). Marine polysaccharide-based coacervates, such as alginate, fucoidan, and chitosan have been successfully developed for the encapsulation of curcumin (Fan et al. 2021; Mirmohammad Meiguni et al. 2022), quercetin (Adrar et al. 2024), and probiotics (Lei et al. 2024).

3.6 Extrusion

The extrusion method is a process that produces dense microcapsules by extruding immiscible core and wall materials through concentric nozzles. This technique involves coextrusion, where the wall material envelops the core material, resulting in capsules of varying sizes depending on the dimensions of the die used. The solidification of capsules can occur through cooling or in a gelling bath, resulting in larger microcapsules due to aggregation (Al-Hamayda et al. 2023; Choudhury et al. 2021). One of the main advantages of extrusion is its ability to create a solid dense barrier to oxygen, reducing the diffusion of ambient gases through the hydrophilic matrix of the wall material. This is particularly beneficial for protecting oxidation-sensitive molecules that are embedded within the interior of the capsules. However, it should be noted that the cost of extrusion can be twice as high as spray drying due to the need for high pressure to generate the required shear forces (Huang et al. 2023). Marine polysaccharides, such as alginate and chitosan, are commonly used as wall materials in extrusion-based encapsulation, especially for probiotics. These biopolymers have been shown to improve the viability and protection of probiotics in harsh gastrointestinal conditions (Dimitrellou et al. 2019; Lee et al. 2019).

4 Bioactive Compounds

Bioactive compounds and nutraceuticals are a diverse group of naturally occurring molecules found in plants, fungi, microorganisms, and other sources. These substances offer unique health benefits and can help prevent diseases, making them crucial components of both human and animal diets. Based on their structural characteristics, bioactive compounds and nutraceuticals are classified into different categories, such as terpenoids, polyphenols, alkaloids, nitrogen-containing constituents, dietary fibers, peptides, and vitamins. Each of these categories can be further divided into different subcategories. Most bioactive compounds are non-nutrients and are known as secondary metabolites. They are typically produced by plants in response to external stresses and stimuli. However, due to their sensitivity to

Table 2 Delivery systems developed for bioactive materials utilizing marine polysaccharides as wall materials

Wall material	Bioactive component	References
Sodium alginate/ovalbumin	Curcumin	Li et al. (2024a)
κ-Carrageenan	Curcumin	Kadota et al. (2020)
O-Carboxymethyl chitosan/ fucoidan	Curcumin	Huang and Kuo (2016)
Chitosan/tripolyphosphate	Curcumin	Shah et al. (2016)
Laminarin	Curcumin	Ye et al. (2023)
Sodium alginate/ κ-carrageenan	Chlorophyll	Jin et al. (2024)
Calcium alginate/trehalose/ chitosan	Lycopene	Aguirre Calvo and Santagapita (2017)
Alginate	Polyphenols from spirulina sp. LEB-18	Machado et al. (2022)
Agarose/sodium alginate	Lycopene & resveratrol	Li et al. (2024b)
Bovine serum albumin/fucoidan	Curcumin & anthocyanins	Chen et al. (2024a)
Alginate	Betacyanins	Calvo et al. (2018)
Carrageenan/sodium alginate	Probiotic bacteria (*L. acidophilus*)	Afzaal et al. (2019)
Chitosan/poly(vinylalcohol)	*Bifidobacteriumanimalis* subsp. *lactis* Bb12	Mojaveri et al. (2020)
Chitosan	Vitamin A	Mobin et al. (2024)
Sodium alginate	*Cinnamomum zeylanicum* essential oil	Paris et al. (2020)
Agar/alginate/carrageenan	Zataria essential oil	Kavoosi et al. (2018)
Soybean protein isolate/xanthan gum/carrageenan	Vitamin B12 & Vitamin E	Gao et al. (2023)
Calcium alginate	Vitamin B12	Parin (2021)
Chitosan/alginate	Vitamin D	Duysak and Sargin (2024)
Chitosan/sodium tripolyphosphate	Vitamin C	Alishahi et al. (2011)

environmental conditions, such as oxygen, light, and temperature, as well as their likely unpleasant taste and odor, they must be encapsulated before being incorporated into food and drug formulations. Encapsulation is also necessary to improve their bioavailability and achieve sustainable release. Examples of various bioactive ingredients encapsulated using marine polysaccharides are presented in Table 2. In the following sections, the major groups of bioactive compounds will be reviewed and the efforts made to encapsulate them using marine polysaccharides will be outlined.

4.1 Vitamins

Vitamins are essential organic molecules that play a crucial role in the metabolic activities of living organisms. They are involved in energy production, cell repair, and immunological function. These molecules are classified as either water-soluble (C and B) or fat-soluble (A, D, E, and K). However, owing to their high sensitivity and poor stability in harsh environments, innovative delivery methods are needed to maintain their stability and extend their shelf life (Maleki et al. 2022; Rezagholizade-Shirvan et al. 2024). Research has shown that encapsulating vitamins using marine polysaccharides not only protects them from degradation, but also improves their bioavailability and enables their controlled release (Sun et al. 2021). Among these polysaccharides, chitosan stands out due to its excellent film-forming capacity, mucoadhesive properties, and chemical modifiability. In acidic conditions, chitosan's positively charged amino groups easily interact with negatively charged biomolecules, thereby improving stability and enabling sustained release of sensitive vitamins such as vitamin C and vitamin A (Alishahi et al. 2011; Mobin et al. 2024). Moreover, when chitosan is combined with alginate, the resulting polyelectrolyte complexes exhibit enhanced mechanical strength and a modulated release profile, making them effective in encapsulating vitamin D (Duysak and Sargin 2024). Similarly, carrageenan, with its ability to form stable gel networks, has shown promise in encapsulating water-soluble vitamins such as different types of vitamin B. By reducing their volatility and degradation in aqueous environments, carrageenan helps maintain the stability of these vitamins (Gao et al. 2023). Overall, these examples highlight the effectiveness of marine polysaccharide-based delivery systems in enhancing the functional stability and bioefficacy of vitamins.

4.2 Antimicrobials

The use of synthetic chemical preservatives in food has raised concerns about their negative effects on human health, leading to a growing interest in natural alternatives. Essential oils, known for their antimicrobial properties, have been widely used in food systems to prevent microbial spoilage and extend shelf life. However, their effectiveness is often limited due to their low solubility in water and volatility, making them susceptible to heat, light, pressure, and oxygen. To address these challenges, encapsulation has been identified as a promising method to enhance the stability and functionality of essential oils in food matrices (Akbari-Alavijeh et al. 2020; Rezagholizade-Shirvan et al. 2024). It has been shown that alginate can effectively encapsulate essential oils from *Cinnamomum zeylanicum*, due to its gel-forming ability and hydrophilic nature, which allows for the formation of a stable network that traps the essential oil components. This encapsulation matrix enables controlled release and preserves the antimicrobial efficacy of the essential oil. Studies have reported encapsulation efficiencies of over 90%, highlighting the potential of this method for food preservation (Paris et al. 2020). Other marine polysaccharides, such as carrageenan and agar, have also shown promise in encapsulating essential oils. In a comparative study, these biopolymers were used to encapsulate *Zataria multiflora* essential oil into a film matrix. The results showed that all three polysaccharides reduced the volatility of the essential oil, while increasing its stability and bioavailability (Kavoosi et al. 2018).

4.3 Polyphenols

Polyphenols are present in a variety of products, including dark chocolate, olive oil, red wine, almonds, cashew nuts, walnuts, berries, green tea, apples, artichokes, mushrooms, leafy vegetables, and coffee (Zorzi et al. 2020). These compounds are known for their exceptional antioxidant activity, which is attributed to their unique chemical structure. The number and position of hydroxyl groups in their molecules play a crucial role in their antioxidant activity (Santos et al. 2021). Polyphenols can be classified into three categories: phenolic acids, flavonoids, and non-flavonoids. These substances have the ability to neutralize free radicals, which can cause cellular damage and lead to various diseases such as cancer and cardiovascular disorders (Mandal and Domb 2024; Rana et al. 2022; Rathee et al. 2023). Despite their potential health benefits, polyphenols are limited by their chemical instability and sensitivity to environmental factors such as light, temperature, oxygen, alkaline pH, and enzymatic activity. These conditions can induce the degradation of polyphenolic compounds and also affect the sensory properties of food products, particularly their aroma and flavor. To overcome these challenges, encapsulation strategies have been developed to protect and stabilize polyphenols, thereby preserving their bioactivity and functional integrity during processing and storage (Koop et al. 2022). Among these strategies, alginate-based delivery systems have gained significant attention for their ability to improve the bioavailability, ensure targeted delivery, and sustain the release of polyphenolic compounds in both food and biomedical applications (Li et al. 2024b; Machado et al. 2022).

4.4 Probiotics, Prebiotics, and Postbiotics

The human gut microbiota, a complex community of bacteria that resides in the gastrointestinal tract, plays a crucial role in maintaining overall health. Recent research has focused on dietary methods of manipulating this microbiome to promote beneficial strains and improve health, specifically through the use of probiotics, prebiotics, and postbiotics. Each of these components serves a unique function in promoting gut health and preserving microbial balance (Rezagholizade-Shirvan et al. 2024). Probiotics are commonly found in food and beverages, including infant formulas, feed, and nutritional supplements. They have been shown to restore and maintain a healthy gut microbiome, protect against pathogen infections, regulate immune function, and preserve the integrity of the intestinal barrier (Martorell et al. 2021). Marine polysaccharides, such as sodium alginate, carrageenan, and chitosan, have been extensively studied for their ability to encapsulate probiotics, in order to enhance their stability in adverse conditions. It has been shown that alginate and carrageenan capsules effectively maintain the integrity of probiotic cells during storage and simulated gastrointestinal transit, resulting in significantly improved survival rates compared to free cells (Afzaal et al. 2019). Additionally, chitosan's biodegradability, biocompatibility, and acid stability make it an ideal candidate for creating hybrid matrices, such as chitosan/poly (vinyl alcohol), which provide additional thermal and osmotic protection for probiotics (Mojaveri et al. 2020). Overall, these encapsulation strategies effectively mitigate environmental stresses while ensuring targeted delivery and sustained release of probiotics in various food matrices.

4.5 Pigments

Natural food colorants are bioactive compounds extracted from plants, animals, and microorganisms that can be used to add color to food, pharmaceutical, and cosmetic products. As consumers' demand for healthier and more natural ingredients increases, the industry is shifting towards using natural pigments instead of synthetic dyes. This is because natural pigments not only enhance the appearance of the product, but also offer various health benefits such as antibacterial, anti-inflammatory, and antioxidant properties (Rezagholizade-Shirvan et al. 2024). In the following sections, the main categories of natural pigments will be discussed, along with recent attempts to encapsulate them using marine polysaccharides.

4.5.1 Carotenoids

Carotenoids, including beta-carotene, lycopene, lutein, and zeaxanthin, are responsible for the vibrant red, yellow, and orange colors found in many fruits and vegetables. These pigments are powerful antioxidants, and have been linked to reducing the risk of certain cancers and eye diseases. Beta-carotene, which is present in carrots and sweet potatoes, is a precursor to vitamin A and is essential for vision and immune function. Lycopene existing in tomatoes has been documented to lower the risk of prostate cancer and cardiovascular diseases. Lutein and zeaxanthin occurring in green leafy vegetables like spinach and kale are crucial for maintaining eye health and may reduce the risk of age-related macular degeneration (Singh and Omer 2024). To improve the stability and bioavailability of these sensitive compounds, they can be encapsulated using marine polysaccharides, such as alginate. Encapsulating lycopene in alginate-based hydrogel beads allows for controlled release and preserves its functional integrity. The incorporation of chitosan into these beads may improve their structural strength, resulting in improved loading efficiency and thermal stability, making this method highly suitable for nutraceutical applications (Aguirre Calvo and Santagapita 2017).

4.5.2 Chlorophyll

Chlorophyll, a complex green pigment found in plants, algae, and certain bacteria, plays a crucial role in the process of photosynthesis by absorbing light energy and converting it into chemical energy (Martins et al. 2023). The primary sources of chlorophyll include green leafy vegetables, such as spinach and broccoli, and microalgae, like Chlorella and Spirulina (Ferreira et al. 2023; Khairunnisa et al. 2024). Chlorophyll is a group of related tetrapyrrole pigments, with the two main forms being chlorophyll a and chlorophyll b. Chlorophyll a is the primary photosynthetic pigment, while chlorophyll b is an accessory pigment (Roca et al. 2024). Despite its well-documented biological benefits such as antioxidant, anti-inflammatory, and anticancer properties (Martins et al. 2021), the application of chlorophyll in food systems remains limited due to its instability under adverse environmental conditions, including light, heat, and low pH (Chen et al. 2023). This can lead to color changes and loss of the desired green hue in food products (Ferreira et al. 2023). To address these limitations, researchers have explored the use of marine polysaccharides, specifically alginate and carrageenan, to encapsulate chlorophyll. These biopolymers form protective matrices around chlorophyll, improving its stability, color retention, and resistance to photodegradation. When used together, alginate provides biodegradability and efficient gelation, while carrageenan forms heat-stable gels that are ideal for controlled-release applications. The combination of alginate and carrageenan creates a synergistic encapsulation system that greatly enhances the functionality of chlorophyll in both food and pharmaceutical formulations (Jin et al. 2024).

4.5.3 Betalains

Betalains have been extracted from various sources beyond just red beet, such as bougainvillea, amaranth, prickly pear, and dragon fruit. These pigments are divided into two main structural groups: the red-violet betacyanins and the yellow-orange betaxanthins (Flint et al. 2024). Among them, betanin is a prominent red pigment known for its antioxidant, anti-inflammatory, and anticancer activities, attributed to its potent radical-scavenging properties (Zin et al. 2020). However, due to their sensitivity to light, heat, and oxygen, betalains are prone to degradation, posing challenges for their application in food and pharmaceutical formulations. To address this, researchers have focused on encapsulation strategies to enhance their stability and bioavailability (López de Dicastillo et al. 2023). One effective method involves encapsulating beetroot-derived betacyanins in Ca (II)-alginate hydrogel beads via ionotropic gelation. The use of additives such as sucrose can improve encapsulation efficiency, demonstrating the potential of marine-derived alginates as robust carriers for betalain delivery in functional food systems (Calvo et al. 2018).

4.5.4 Curcumin

Turmeric (*Curcuma longa*), which belongs to the Zingiberaceae family of ginger plants, contains curcumin as its primary bioactive compound. This curcuminoid possesses strong anti-inflammatory, antioxidant, and anti-angiogenic properties, making it an effective treatment for endometriosis (Singh et al. 2023). Additionally, curcumin has a strong antioxidant capacity, effectively scavenging free radicals and reactive oxygen species (Sandhiutami et al. 2022). This high antioxidant activity is attributed to the hydrogen-atomic donation function of the curcumin phenol group (Roy and Rhim 2020). However, despite these unique functionalities and biological activities, curcumin is poorly water-soluble, unstable in environmental conditions, and has low bioavailability, hindering its applications. To tackle these issues, various marine polysaccharides with different chemical functionalities have been investigated for encapsulating curcumin (Huang and Kuo 2016; Kadota et al. 2020; Li et al. 2024a; Shah et al. 2016; Ye et al. 2023). Formulations based on carrageenan and fucoidan have been found to provide enhanced protection against thermal and photostability challenges, achieving an excellent curcumin encapsulation efficiency of up to 95.28% with a loading capacity of 4.16% (Chen et al. 2024b).

4.6 Comparative Evaluation of Marine Polysaccharides for Food Bioactive Encapsulation

Marine polysaccharides have unique functionalities that make them ideal wall materials for encapsulating bioactive compounds. Based on their performance and potential industrial applications, alginate is considered the most suitable candidate for encapsulating food bioactive constituents. It undergoes mild calcium-induced gelation at low temperatures, resulting in high encapsulation efficiency and biocompatibility. However, its porous network may cause burst release (Chusak et al. 2025; Li et al. 2021). On the other hand, carrageenan forms thermoreversible, high-viscous gels that enhance the stability of bioactive compounds, although its performance is affected by ionic strength and temperature variations (Pacheco-Quito et al. 2020). Fucoidan, on the other hand, typically tends to create weak gels if used alone, compromising mechanical stability and leading to less controlled release of bioactive compounds. Therefore, fucoidan is often used in co-encapsulation strategies, where its properties are combined with other stronger gelling agents (Haggag et al. 2023). Agar forms firm and thermally stable gels when cooled after being dissolved at high temperatures. The gelation process involves heating near boiling to dissolve agar, followed by cooling, resulting in a rigid gel network. The structure of this gel is influenced by microdomain formation in the range of 55–40 °C (Jung et al. 2023). Agar's rigidity provides excellent stability and protection for encapsulated bioactive components during storage and processing. However, its tight network structure may impede the diffusion of vitamins, potentially delaying their release beyond the desired timeframe. Therefore, agar is most suitable for applications where prolonged retention is acceptable or when used in combination with less rigid polymers to fine-tune release kinetics (Tomadoni et al. 2022). Chitosan offers distinct advantages due to its cationic nature and pH-dependent solubility. Unlike other polysaccharides, chitosan does not primarily rely on thermal gelation but rather on ionic or polyelectrolyte complexation. This allows it to be used as a coating material over other micro/nanocapsules or as a standalone nanoparticle matrix (Călinoiu et al. 2019; Wang et al. 2025). Its ability to form complexes with anionic polymers (such as alginate or carrageenan) has been utilized to improve control over bioactive release, particularly in protecting it from premature degradation in the upper gastrointestinal tract (Wong et al. 2021). However, chitosan's solubility is limited at neutral pH, and its relatively high viscosity may require modification or blending with other polymers to achieve the desired processing characteristics (Desai et al. 2023).

5 Challenges in Marine Polysaccharide-Based Delivery Systems

The use of marine polysaccharides in food delivery systems presents several challenges that can greatly impact their efficiency and application. One major disadvantage is their susceptibility to variations as the molecular weight and structure of these polysaccharides can change depending on the harvesting zone and the season. While industrial refinement can produce high-quality products with consistent functionalities, it also leads to higher production expenses (Sun et al. 2021). This variability poses challenges for their performance in food delivery systems and makes predicting their interactions with bioactive compounds complex (Lukova and Katsarov 2023). Another significant issue is the enzymatic modification of marine polysaccharides. While enzymatic modification can enhance their solubility and bioavailability, uncontrolled degradation/hydrolysis can result in detrimental by-products that adversely affect food quality and safety (Li et al. 2023). Additionally, environmental conditions such as temperature and pH during storage and processing can compromise the functional characteristics and structural integrity of marine polysaccharides (Carrasqueira et al. 2025).

6 Future Directions and Research Trends

Marine polysaccharides offer numerous advantages, including biocompatibility, biodegradability, low immunogenicity, and high natural availability, making them promising materials for encapsulating bioactive ingredients, nutraceuticals, and probiotics. However, their functionality still requires improvement to enhance their efficiency and performance. The presence of multifunctional groups, such as hydroxyl, carboxyl, and amine, on their molecular backbone makes them easily modifiable through chemical, biochemical, or enzymatic methods (Sun et al. 2021). Recent advances in extraction and modification techniques, such as enzymatic hydrolysis, chemical derivatization, and nanotechnology-based approaches, have enabled the development of novel marine polysaccharide-based materials with improved functional properties. Furthermore, their potential applications in biomedicine, food, and pharmaceuticals have driven research into their bioavailability, bioaccessibility, and mechanisms of action. A growing trend is the use of marine polysaccharides in drug delivery systems, tissue engineering, and functional food formulations due to their biocompatibility, biodegradability, and bioactive properties. Additionally, with increasing concerns about environmental sustainability, there is a need for research to explore eco-friendly extraction processes and the valorization of marine biomass to ensure the efficient and responsible utilization of these valuable biopolymers. Future studies will also focus on the interaction of marine polysaccharides with gut microbiota and their role in modulating health benefits, further expanding their applications in nutraceuticals and personalized medicine.

References

Adrar, N., Ceylan, F. D., & Capanoglu, E. (2024). Hazelnut Protein and Sodium Alginate Complex Coacervates: An Effective Tool for the Encapsulation of the Hydrophobic Polyphenol Quercetin. *ACS Omega*, *9*(35), 37243–37252.

Afzaal, M., Saeed, F., Arshad, M. U., Nadeem, M. T., Saeed, M., & Tufail, T. (2019). The effect of encapsulation on the stability of probiotic bacteria in ice cream and simulated gastrointestinal conditions. *Probiotics and Antimicrobial Proteins*, *11*, 1348–1354.

Afzaal, M., Saeed, F., Ateeq, H., Ahmed, A., Ahmad, A., Tufail, T.,…Anjum, F. M. (2020). Encapsulation of Bifidobacterium bifidum by internal gelation method to access the viability in cheddar cheese and under simulated gastrointestinal conditions. *Food Science & Nutrition*, *8*(6), 2739–2747.

Aguirre Calvo, T. R., & Santagapita, P. R. (2017). Encapsulation of a free-solvent extract of lycopene in alginate-Ca (II) beads containing sugars and biopolymers. *Chemical and Biological Technologies in Agriculture*, *4*, 1–8.

Akbari-Alavijeh, S., Shaddel, R., & Jafari, S. M. (2020). Encapsulation of food bioactives and nutraceuticals by various chitosan-based nanocarriers. *Food hydrocolloids*, *105*, 105774.

Akdaşçi, E., Duman, H., Eker, F., Bechelany, M., & Karav, S. (2025). Chitosan and Its Nanoparticles: A Multifaceted Approach to Antibacterial Applications. *Nanomaterials*, *15*(2), 126.

Akshaya, S., & Nathanael, A. J. (2024). A review on hydrophobically associated alginates: approaches and applications. *ACS Omega*, *9*(4), 4246–4262.

Al-Hamayda, A., Abu-Jdayil, B., Ayyash, M., & Tannous, J. (2023). Advances in microencapsulation techniques using Arabic gum: A comprehensive review. *Industrial Crops and Products*, *205*, 117556.

Alishahi, A., Mirvaghefi, A., Tehrani, M., Farahmand, H., Shojaosadati, S., Dorkoosh, F., & Elsabee, M. Z. (2011). Shelf life and delivery enhancement of vitamin C using chitosan nanoparticles. *Food Chemistry*, *126*(3), 935–940.

Alu'datt, M. H., Alrosan, M., Gammoh, S., Tranchant, C. C., Alhamad, M. N., Rababah, T.,…Tan, T.-C. (2022). Encapsulation-based technologies for bioactive compounds and their application in the food industry: A roadmap for food-derived functional and health-promoting ingredients. *Food Bioscience*, *50*, 101971.

Álvarez-Viñas, M., Souto, S., Flórez-Fernández, N., Torres, M. D., Bandín, I., & Domínguez, H. (2021). Antiviral activity of carrageenans and processing implications. *Marine Drugs*, *19*(8), 437.

Awuchi, C. G., & Okpala, C. O. R. (2022). Natural nutraceuticals, especially functional foods, their ma-jor bioactive components, formulation, and health benefits for disease prevention-An overview. *Journal of Food Bioactives*, *19*.

Bao, H., Wang, Y., Huang, Y., Zhang, Y., & Dai, H. (2025). The Beneficial Role of Polysaccharide Hydrocolloids in Meat Products: A Review. *Gels*, *11*(1), 55.

Bashir, I., Wani, S. M., Bhat, A. A., Khan, A. A., Hussain, S. Z., Ganai, S. A., & Anjum, N. (2024). Effect of freeze drying and spray drying on physical properties, morphology and in vitro release kinetics of vitamin D3 nanoparticles. *Powder Technology*, *432*, 119164.

Borgogna, M., Bellich, B., & Cesaro, A. (2011). Marine polysaccharides in microencapsulation and application to aquaculture:"from sea to sea". *Marine Drugs*, *9*(12), 2572–2604.

Călinoiu, L., Ştefănescu, B., Pop, I., Muntean, L., & Vodnar, D. (2019). Chitosan coating applications in probiotic microencapsulation. Coatings 9 (3): 194. In.

Calvo, T. R. A., Perullini, M., & Santagapita, P. R. (2018). Encapsulation of betacyanins and polyphenols extracted from leaves and stems of beetroot in Ca (II)-alginate beads: A structural study. *Journal of Food Engineering*, *235*, 32–40.

Carrasqueira, J., Bernardino, S., Bernardino, R., & Afonso, C. (2025). Marine-Derived Polysaccharides and Their Potential Health Benefits in Nutraceutical Applications. *Marine Drugs*, *23*(2), 1–35.

Centomo, A. M., Diaz Vergara, L. I., Rossi, Y. E., Vanden Braber, N. L., Bodoira, R., Maestri, D., …Montenegro, M. A. (2024). Co-encapsulated of potential probiotic yeast Kluyveromyces marxianus and peanut skin polyphenolic extract as a functional ingredient. *International Journal of Food Science and Technology*, *59*(6), 3918–3928.

Chen, J., Yang, J., Du, H., Aslam, M., Wang, W., Chen, W.,…Liu, X. (2021). Laminarin, a major polysaccharide in stramenopiles. *Marine Drugs*, *19*(10), 576.

Chen, X., Qin, H., Zhai, J. M., Wang, J. H., Zhang, Y. H., Chen, Y.,…Li, H. J. (2024a). Co-encapsulation of curcumin and anthocyanins in bovine serum album–fucoidan nanocomplex with a two-step pH-driven method. *Journal of the Science of Food and Agriculture*, *104*(5), 3100–3112.

Chen, Y., Cai, S., He, N., Huang, X., Hong, Z., He, J.,…Zhang, Y. (2024b). An effective method to prepare curcumin-loaded soy protein isolate nanoparticles co-stabilized by carrageenan and fucoidan. *Pharmaceuticals*, *17*(4), 534.

Chen, Z., Wu, W., Wen, Y., Zhang, L., Wu, Y., Farid, M.S, …Zhao, C. (2023). Recent advances of natural pigments from algae. *Food Production, Processing and Nutrition*, *5*(1), 39.

Choudhury, N., Meghwal, M., & Das, K. (2021). Microencapsulation: An overview on concepts, methods, properties and applications in foods. *Food Frontiers*, *2*(4), 426–442.

Chusak, C., Balmori, V., Kamonsuwan, K., Suklaew, P.O, & Adisakwattana, S. (2025). Enhancing Viability of Lactobacillus rhamnosus GG and Total Polyphenol Content in Fermented Black Goji Berry Beverage Through Calcium–Alginate Encapsulation with Hydrocolloids. *Foods*, *14*(3), 518.

Cotas, J., Lomartire, S., Gonçalves, A. M., & Pereira, L. (2024). From Ocean to Medicine: Harnessing Seaweed's Potential for Drug Development. *International Journal of Molecular Sciences*, *25*(2), 797.

Desai, N., Rana, D., Salave, S., Gupta, R., Patel, P., Karunakaran, B.,…Kommineni, N. (2023). Chitosan: a potential biopolymer in drug delivery and biomedical applications. *Pharmaceutics*, *15*(4), 1313.

Dimitrellou, D., Kandylis, P., Lević, S., Petrović, T., Ivanović, S., Nedović, V., & Kourkoutas, Y. (2019). Encapsulation of Lactobacillus casei ATCC 393 in alginate capsules for probiotic fermented milk production. *Lwt, 116*, 108501.

Dong, Y., Wei, Z., & Xue, C. (2021). Recent advances in carrageenan-based delivery systems for bioactive ingredients: A review. *Trends in Food Science & Technology, 112*, 348–361.

Du, B., Zhao, Q., Cheng, C., Wang, H., Liu, Y., Zhu, F., & Yang, Y. (2022). A critical review on extraction, characteristics, physicochemical activities, potential health benefits, and industrial applications of fucoidan. *EFood, 3*(4), e19.

Duysak, G., & Sargin, I. (2024). ENCAPSULATION OF VITAMIN D IN THE EXINE-ALGINATE-CHITOSAN MICROCAPSULE SYSTEM. *Konya Journal of Engineering Sciences, 12*(1), 192–204.

El-Araby, A., Janati, W., Ullah, R., Ercisli, S., & Errachidi, F. (2024). Chitosan, chitosan derivatives, and chitosan-based nanocomposites: Eco-friendly materials for advanced applications (a review). *Frontiers in Chemistry, 11*, 1327426.

Ettoumi, F.-E., Zhang, R., Xu, Y., Li, L., Huang, H., & Luo, Z. (2023). Synthesis and characterization of fucoidan/chitosan-coated nanoliposomes for enhanced stability and oral bioavailability of hydrophilic catechin and hydrophobic juglone. *Food Chemistry, 423*, 136330.

Famiglietti, M., Savastano, A., Gaglione, R., Arciello, A., Naviglio, D., & Mariniello, L. (2022). Edible films made of dried olive leaf extract and chitosan: Characterization and applications. *Foods, 11*(14), 2078.

Fan, L., Lu, Y., Ouyang, X.-K., & Ling, J. (2021). Development and characterization of soybean protein isolate and fucoidan nanoparticles for curcumin encapsulation. *International journal of biological macromolecules, 169*, 194–205.

Farahani, Z., Mousavi, M., Ardebili, S., & Bakhoda, H. (2022). Modification of sodium alginate by octenyl succinic anhydride to fabricate beads for encapsulating jujube extract. Curr Res Nutr Food Sci 5: 157–166. In.

Feng, T., Wu, K., Xu, J., Hu, Z., & Zhang, X. (2021). Low molecular weight kappa-carrageenan based microspheres for enhancing stability and bioavailability of tea polyphenols. *Processes, 9*(7), 1240.

Fernandes, J. G., Rodrigues, R. C., Pereira, L., Stringheta, P. C., Campelo, P. H., & Martins, E. (2024). Encapsulation of hydrophobic active ingredients in plant proteins: Modulation of interfacial properties and encapsulation efficiency. *Current Opinion in Food Science*, 101170.

Fernando, I. P. S., Lee, W., Han, E. J., & Ahn, G. (2020). Alginate-based nanomaterials: Fabrication techniques, properties, and applications. *Chemical Engineering Journal, 391*, 123823.

Ferreira, A. S., Pereira, L., Canfora, F., Silva, T. H., Coimbra, M. A., & Nunes, C. (2023). Stabilization of Natural Pigments in Ethanolic Solutions for Food Applications: The Case Study of Chlorella vulgaris. *Molecules, 28*(1), 408.

Flint, H. V., Tito, H. A. R., James, R. D., Cucinotta, F., Gibson, E., & Caceda, M. E. Q. (2024). Betanin dye extracted from ayrampo (Opuntia soehrensii) seeds to develop dye-sensitized solar cells. *RSC advances, 14*(14), 9913–9919.

Gao, T., Wu, X., Gao, Y., Teng, F., & Li, Y. (2023). Co-Delivery System of Vitamin B12 and Vitamin E Using a Binary W/O/W Emulsion Based on Soybean Isolate Protein–Xanthan Gum/Carrageenan: Emulsification Properties, Rheological Properties, Structure, Stability, and Digestive Characteristics. *Foods, 12*(23), 4361.

Geonzon, L. C., Hashimoto, K., Oda, T., Matsukawa, S., & Mayumi, K. (2023). Elaborating Spatiotemporal Hierarchical Structure of Carrageenan Gels and Their Mixtures during Sol–Gel Transition. *Macromolecules, 56*(21), 8676–8687.

George, M., & Abraham, T. E. (2006). Polyionic hydrocolloids for the intestinal delivery of protein drugs: alginate and chitosan—a review. *Journal of Controlled Release, 114*(1), 1–14.

Haggag, Y. A., Abd Elrahman, A. A., Ulber, R., & Zayed, A. (2023). Fucoidan in pharmaceutical formulations: a comprehensive review for smart drug delivery systems. *Marine Drugs, 21*(2), 112.

Huang, K., Yuan, Y., & Baojun, X. (2023). A critical review on the microencapsulation of bioactive compounds and their application. *Food reviews international, 39*(5), 2594–2634.

Huang, Y.-C., & Kuo, T.-H. (2016). O-carboxymethyl chitosan/fucoidan nanoparticles increase cellular curcumin uptake. *Food hydrocolloids, 53*, 261–269.

Ji, C., Long, X., Wang, J., Qi, B., Cao, Y., & Hu, X. (2025). Rheological Behavior, Textural Properties, and Antioxidant Activity of Porphyra yezoensis Polysaccharide. *Molecules, 30*(4), 882.

Jiang, F., Xu, X., Xiao, Q., Li, Z., Weng, H., Chen, F., & Xiao, A. (2024). Fabrication, structure, characterization and emulsion application of citrate agar. *International journal of biological macromolecules, 268*, 131451.

Jin, M., Jiang, S., Wang, Y., Wang, Y., Guo, S., Dong, X., & Qi, H. (2024). Formation of chlorophyll–anionic polysaccharide complex coacervates to improve chlorophyll color stability: Thermodynamic and kinetic stability studies. *International journal of biological macromolecules, 275*, 133253.

Junaid, P. M., Dar, A. H., Dash, K. K., Rohilla, S., Islam, R.-U., Shams, R.,…Zaidi, S. (2024). Polysaccharide-based hydrogels for microencapsulation of bioactive compounds: A review. *Journal of Agriculture and Food Research, 15*, 101038.

Jung, H., Geonzon, L. C., Yoon, W. B., & Matsukawa, S. (2023). Change of network structure in agarose solution during gelation studied by multiple particle tracking and NMR measurements. *Food hydrocolloids, 141*, 108740.

Kadota, K., Nogami, S., Uchiyama, H., & Tozuka, Y. (2020). Controlled release behavior of curcumin from kappa-carrageenan gels with flexible texture by the addition of metal chlorides. *Food hydrocolloids, 101*, 105564.

Kavoosi, G., Derakhshan, M., Salehi, M., & Rahmati, L. (2018). Microencapsulation of zataria essential oil in agar, alginate and carrageenan. *Innovative Food Science & Emerging Technologies, 45*, 418–425.

Khairunnisa, K., Hartati, R., & Widowati, I (2024) Chlorophyll Content of Chlorella vulgaris (Beijerinck, 1890) on Different Light Intensity. *Buletin Oseanografi Marina, 13*(1), 107–112.

Koop, B. L., da Silva, M. N., da Silva, F. D., dos Santos Lima, K. T., Soares, L. S., de Andrade, C.J, …Monteiro, A. R. (2022). Flavonoids, anthocyanins, betalains, curcumin, and carotenoids: Sources, classification and enhanced stabilization by encapsulation and adsorption. *Food Research International, 153*, 110929.

Kraithong, S., Theppawong, A., Liu, Y., Sangsawad, P., & Huang, R. (2025). Fucoidan as an Encapsulant material: Applications and advantages in active agents and probiotic encapsulations. *Food Chemistry*, 143570.

Kučuk, N., Primožič, M., Knez, Ž., & Leitgeb, M. (2024). Alginate Beads with Encapsulated Bioactive Substances from Mangifera indica Peels as Promising Peroral Delivery Systems. *Foods, 13*(15), 2404.

Kumar, M. A., Vikas, M., Nitesh, S., Debabrata, D., Sudip, M., Mohan, K., & Pralay, M. (2015). Polyurethane-Grafted Chitosan as New Biomaterials for Controlled Drug Delivery.

Kumar, S., Bhatt, A., & Purohit, P. (2025). Carrageenan Modifications: Improving Biomedical Applications. *Journal of Polymers and the Environment*, 1–22.

Le Tien, C., Lacroix, M., Ispas-Szabo, P., & Mateescu, M.-A. (2003). N-acylated chitosan: hydrophobic matrices for controlled drug release. *Journal of Controlled Release, 93*(1), 1–13.

Lee, Y., Ji, Y. R., Lee, S., Choi, M.-J., & Cho, Y. (2019). Microencapsulation of probiotic Lactobacillus acidophilus KBL409 by extrusion technology to enhance survival under simulated intestinal and freeze-drying conditions.

Lei, Y., Xie, Z., Zhao, A., Colarelli, J., Miller, M. J., & Lee, Y. (2024). Layer-by-layer coating of Lacticaseibacillus rhamnosus GG (LGG) using chitosan and zein/tween-80/fucoidan nanoparticles to enhance LGG's survival under adverse conditions. *Food hydrocolloids, 154*, 110039.

Leong, K. H., Chung, L. Y., Noordin, M. I., Mohamad, K., Nishikawa, M., Onuki, Y.,...Takayama, K. (2011). Carboxymethylation of kappa-carrageenan for intestinal-targeted delivery of bioactive macromolecules. *Carbohydrate Polymers, 83*(4), 1507–1515.
Lević, S. M., Rac, V. A., Rakić, V. M., Salević-Jelić, A. S., Hovjecki, M. R., Malićanin, M. V,... Nedović, V. A. (2024). Cold-Pressed Grape Seed Oil Encapsulation Using a Submerged-Nozzle Dispersion Encapsulation Process. *Processes, 12*(8), 1628.
Li, C., Tang, T., Du, Y., Jiang, L., Yao, Z., Ning, L., & Zhu, B. (2023). Ulvan and Ulva oligosaccharides: a systematic review of structure, preparation, biological activities and applications. *Bioresources and Bioprocessing, 10*(1), 66.
Li, D., Wei, Z., & Xue, C. (2021). Alginate-based delivery systems for food bioactive ingredients: An overview of recent advances and future trends. *Comprehensive reviews in food science and food safety, 20*(6), 5345–5369.
Li, H., Zhao, M., Zhou, S., Zhang, H., Wang, J., Xia, N.,...Tan, G. (2024a). Enhancing encapsulation of curcumin by pH-driven and sodium alginate blending with ovalbumin as a carrier. *Food hydrocolloids, 149*, 109623.
Li, M., Li, X., Ren, H., Shao, W., Wang, C., Huang, Y.,...Yin, M. (2024b). Preparation and characterization of agarose-sodium alginate hydrogel beads for the co-encapsulation of lycopene and resveratrol nanoemulsion. *International journal of biological macromolecules, 277*, 133753.
Lopez-Sanchez, P., Assifaoui, A., Cousin, F., Moser, J., Bonilla, M. R., & Ström, A. (2022). Impact of glucose on the nanostructure and mechanical properties of calcium-alginate hydrogels. *Gels, 8*(2), 71.
López de Dicastillo, C., Velásquez, E., Rojas, A., Garrido, L., Moreno, M. C., Guarda, A., & Galotto, M. J. (2023). Developing Core/Shell Capsules Based on Hydroxypropyl Methylcellulose and Gelatin through Electrodynamic Atomization for Betalain Encapsulation. *Polymers, 15*(2), 361.
Lukova, P., & Katsarov, P. (2023). Contemporary Aspects of Designing Marine Polysaccharide Microparticles as Drug Carriers for Biomedical Application. *Pharmaceutics, 15*(8), 2126.
Machado, A. R., Silva, P. M., Vicente, A. A., Souza-Soares, L. A., Pinheiro, A. C., & Cerqueira, M. A. (2022). Alginate particles for encapsulation of phenolic extract from spirulina sp. LEB-18: physicochemical characterization and assessment of in vitro gastrointestinal behavior. *Polymers, 14*(21), 4759.
Mahapatra, P., Likhith, K., Mateti, T., Changmai, U., Patil, P., NV, A. K.,...Thakur, G. (2023). Physicochemical investigations of nanoemulsified, curcumin-loaded, crosslinked κ-carrageenan hydrogels.
Maleki, G., Woltering, E. J., & Mozafari, M. (2022). Applications of chitosan-based carrier as an encapsulating agent in food industry. *Trends in Food Science & Technology, 120*, 88–99.
Mandal, M., & Domb, A. (2024). Antimicrobial Activities of Natural Bioactive Polyphenols. In (Vol. 192, pp. 193): Pharmaceutics.
Martins, M., Fernandes, A. P., Torres-Acosta, M. A., Collén, P. N., Abreu, M. H., & Ventura, S. P. (2021). Extraction of chlorophyll from wild and farmed Ulva spp. using aqueous solutions of ionic liquids. *Separation and Purification Technology, 254*, 117589.
Martins, T., Barros, A. N., Rosa, E., & Antunes, L. (2023). Enhancing health benefits through chlorophylls and chlorophyll-rich agro-food: A comprehensive review. *Molecules, 28*(14), 5344.
Martorell, P., Alvarez, B., Llopis, S., Navarro, V., Ortiz, P., Gonzalez, N.,...Ramon, D. (2021). Heat-treated Bifidobacterium longum CECT-7347: a whole-cell postbiotic with antioxidant, anti-inflammatory, and gut-barrier protection properties. *Antioxidants, 10*(4), 536.
Meng, W., Zhang, J., Hou, H., Yu, L., & Dong, P. (2025). Exploring the structures and molecular mechanisms of bioactive compounds from marine foods for hyperuricemia prevention: a systematic review. *Critical Reviews in Food Science and Nutrition*, 1–19.
Mirmohammad Meiguni, M. S., Salami, M., Rezaei, K., Ghaffari, S. B., Aliyari, M. A., Emam-Djomeh, Z.,...Gruen, I. (2022). Curcumin-loaded complex coacervate made of mung bean

protein isolate and succinylated chitosan as a novel medium for curcumin encapsulation. *Journal of Food Science*, *87*(11), 4930–4944.

Mobin, L., Diosady, L. L., & Haq, M. A. (2024). Enhancing vitamin A stability using saponin–chitosan polyelectrolytes coating: Optimization, characterization, and controlled release. *Journal of Food Science*, *89*(10), 6268–6282.

Mohammed, N. K., Tan, C. P., Manap, Y. A., Muhialdin, B. J., & Hussin, A. S. M. (2020). Spray drying for the encapsulation of oils—A review. *Molecules*, *25*(17), 3873.

Mojaveri, S. J., Hosseini, S. F., & Gharsallaoui, A. (2020). Viability improvement of Bifidobacterium animalis Bb12 by encapsulation in chitosan/poly (vinyl alcohol) hybrid electrospun fiber mats. *Carbohydrate Polymers*, *241*, 116278.

Mokhtari, H., Tavakoli, S., Safarpour, F., Kharaziha, M., Bakhsheshi-Rad, H. R., Ramakrishna, S., & Berto, F. (2021). Recent advances in chemically-modified and hybrid carrageenan-based platforms for drug delivery, wound healing, and tissue engineering. *Polymers*, *13*(11), 1744.

Mostafavi, F. S., & Zaeim, D. (2020). Agar-based edible films for food packaging applications-A review. *International journal of biological macromolecules*, *159*, 1165–1176.

Nájera-Martínez, E. F., Flores-Contreras, E. A., Araújo, R. G., Iñiguez-Moreno, M., Sosa-Hernández, J. E., Iqbal, H. M.,…Parra-Saldívar, R. (2023). Microencapsulation of gallic acid based on a polymeric and pH-sensitive matrix of pectin/alginate. *Polymers*, *15*(14), 3014.

Neves, M. I., Moroni, L., & Barrias, C. C. (2020). Modulating alginate hydrogels for improved biological performance as cellular 3D microenvironments. *Frontiers in bioengineering and biotechnology*, *8*, 665.

Nowak, D., & Jakubczyk, E. (2020). The freeze-drying of foods—the characteristic of the process course and the effect of its parameters on the physical properties of food materials. Foods 9 (10): 1488. In.

Obaidat, R. M., Alnaief, M., & Mashaqbeh, H. (2018). Investigation of carrageenan aerogel microparticles as a potential drug carrier. *Aaps Pharmscitech*, *19*, 2226–2236.

Okolie, C. L., Mason, B., Mohan, A., Pitts, N., & Udenigwe, C. C. (2020). Extraction technology impacts on the structure-function relationship between sodium alginate extracts and their in vitro prebiotic activity. *Food Bioscience*, *37*, 100672.

Omuzbuken, B., Alyuruk, H., & Kacar, A. (2022). Stimulation of the Biofilm's of a marine bacterium, Pseudoalteromonas agarivorans-by Fucoidan extracted from macroalgae.

Oroná, J. D., Zorrilla, S. E., & Peralta, J. M. (2024). Assessment of calcium alginate gels as wall materials for encapsulation systems. *Journal of the Science of Food and Agriculture*, *104*(4), 2458–2466.

Pacheco-Quito, E.-M., Ruiz-Caro, R., & Veiga, M.-D. (2020). Carrageenan: drug delivery systems and other biomedical applications. *Marine Drugs*, *18*(11), 583.

Parin, F. N. (2021). Retrospective, Perspective and Prospective of B-Complex Vitamins: Encapsulation of Vitamins and Release from Vitamin-Loaded Polymers. In *B-Complex Vitamins-Sources, Intakes and Novel Applications*. IntechOpen.

Paris, M., Ramírez-Corona, N., Palou, E., & López-Malo, A. (2020). Modelling release mechanisms of cinnamon (Cinnamomum zeylanicum) essential oil encapsulated in alginate beads during vapor-phase application. *Journal of Food Engineering*, *282*, 110024.

Pathiraja, D., Cho, J., Stougaard, P., & Choi, I.-G. (2022). Enzymatic Process for the Carrageenolytic Bioconversion of Sulfated Polygalactans into β-Neocarrabiose and 3, 6-Anhydro-d-galactose. *Journal of agricultural and food chemistry*, *71*(1), 635–645.

Peng, Q., Wang, T., Yang, D., Peng, X., Zhang, H., & Zeng, H. (2024). Recent advances in coacervation and underlying noncovalent molecular interaction mechanisms. *Progress in Polymer Science*, 101827.

Poshina, D. N., Rakshina, A. D., & Skorik, Y. A. (2025). Hydrophobic Chitosan Derivatives for Gene and Drug Delivery in Cancer Therapies. *Polysaccharides*, *6*(1), 11.

Pourashouri, P., Shabanpour, B., Heydari, S., & Raeisi, S. (2021). Encapsulation of fish oil by carrageenan and gum tragacanth as wall materials and its application to the enrichment of chicken nuggets. *Lwt*, *137*, 110334.

Pudziuvelyte, L., Marksa, M., Sosnowska, K., Winnicka, K., Morkuniene, R., & Bernatoniene, J. (2020). Freeze-drying technique for microencapsulation of Elsholtzia ciliata ethanolic extract using different coating materials. *Molecules*, *25*(9), 2237.

Pudziuvelyte, L., Siauruseviciute, A., Morkuniene, R., Lazauskas, R., & Bernatoniene, J. (2022). Influence of Technological Factors on the Quality of Chitosan Microcapsules with Boswellia serata L. Essential Oil. *Pharmaceutics*, *14*(6), 1259.

Rajabi, H., Jafari, S. M., Rajabzadeh, G., Sarfarazi, M., & Sedaghati, S. (2019). Chitosan-gum Arabic complex nanocarriers for encapsulation of saffron bioactive components. *Colloids and Surfaces A: Physicochemical and Engineering Aspects*, *578*, 123644.

Rana, A., Samtiya, M., Dhewa, T., Mishra, V., & Aluko, R. E. (2022). Health benefits of polyphenols: A concise review. *Journal of Food Biochemistry*, *46*(10), e14264.

Rathee, P., Sehrawat, R., Rathee, P., Khatkar, A., Akkol, E. K., Khatkar, S.,…Sobarzo-Sánchez, E. (2023). Polyphenols: natural preservatives with promising applications in food, cosmetics and pharma industries; problems and toxicity associated with synthetic preservatives; impact of misleading advertisements; recent trends in preservation and legislation. *Materials*, *16*(13), 4793.

Rezagholizade-Shirvan, A., Soltani, M., Shokri, S., Radfar, R., Arab, M., & Shamloo, E. (2024). Bioactive compound encapsulation: Characteristics, applications in food systems, and implications for human health. *Food Chemistry: X*, 101953.

Roca, M., Chen, K., & Pérez-Gálvez, A. (2024). Chlorophylls. In *Handbook on natural pigments in food and beverages* (pp. 193–226). Elsevier.

Rode, M. P., Batti Angulski, A. B., Gomes, F. A., da Silva, M. M., Jeremias, T. d. S., de Carvalho, R. G.,…Trentin, A. G. (2018). Carrageenan hydrogel as a scaffold for skin-derived multipotent stromal cells delivery. *Journal of Biomaterials Applications*, *33*(3), 422–434.

Roy, S., & Rhim, J.-W. (2020). Curcumin incorporated poly (butylene adipate-co-terephthalate) film with improved water vapor barrier and antioxidant properties. *Materials*, *13*(19), 4369.

Sánchez-Osorno, D. M., López-Jaramillo, M. C., Caicedo Paz, A. V., Villa, A. L., Peresin, M. S., & Martínez-Galán, J. P. (2023). Recent advances in the microencapsulation of essential oils, lipids, and compound lipids through spray drying: A review. *Pharmaceutics*, *15*(5), 1490.

Sandhiutami, N. M. D., Dewi, R. S., Khairani, S., & Putri, R. N. A. (2022). Enhancement of curcumin level and hepatoprotective effect in rats through antioxidant activity following modification into nanosized particles. *Veterinary World*, *15*(9), 2323.

Sangnim, T., Dheer, D., Jangra, N., Huanbutta, K., Puri, V., & Sharma, A. (2023). Chitosan in oral drug delivery formulations: A review. *Pharmaceutics*, *15*(9), 2361.

Santos, S. C., Fortes, G. A., Camargo, L. T., Camargo, A. J., & Ferri, P. H. (2021). Antioxidant effects of polyphenolic compounds and structure-activity relationship predicted by multivariate regression tree. *Lwt*, *137*, 110366.

Santosa, T. P., Cejasb, C. M., & Cunhaa, R. L. (2021). Microfluidics as a platform to assess and induce emulsion destabilization. *Faculdade de Engenharia de Alimentos*, *21*.

Sepe, F., Valentino, A., Marcolongo, L., Petillo, O., Conte, R., Margarucci, S.,…Calarco, A. (2025). Marine-Derived Polysaccharide Hydrogels as Delivery Platforms for Natural Bioactive Compounds. *International Journal of Molecular Sciences*, *26*(2), 764.

Shafiq, S., & Rizvi, Z. F. (2023). Promising substitute of inconsistent algal alginates: exploring the biocompatible properties of di-O-acetylated, poly-L-guluronate-deficient alginate from soil bacterium Pseudomonas aeruginosa CMG1418. *BioTechnologia*, *104*(2), 137.

Shah, B. R., Li, Y., Jin, W., An, Y., He, L., Li, Z.,…Li, B. (2016). Preparation and optimization of Pickering emulsion stabilized by chitosan-tripolyphosphate nanoparticles for curcumin encapsulation. *Food hydrocolloids*, *52*, 369–377.

Shah, M., Hameed, A., Kashif, M., Majeed, N., Muhammad, J., Shah, N.,…Khan, A. (2024). Advances in agar-based composites: a comprehensive review. *Carbohydrate Polymers*, 122619.

Silva-Espinoza, M. A., García-Martínez, E., & Martínez-Navarrete, N. (2021). Protective capacity of gum Arabic, maltodextrin, different starches, and fibers on the bioactive compounds and antioxidant activity of an orange puree (Citrus sinensis (L.) Osbeck) against freeze-drying and in vitro digestion. *Food Chemistry*, *357*, 129724.

Singh, A., & Omer, K. (2024). Recent Advancement in Therapeutic Activity of Carotenoids. In *Dietary Carotenoids-Sources, Properties, and Role in Human Health*. IntechOpen.

Singh, I., Shaw, R., Saha, P., Ojha, K. K., & Chaube, R. (2023). Evaluating the Relative Efficacy of Synthetic and Natural Drugs in Endometriosis Adopting Molecular Modelling Approach. *Journal of Endocrinology and Reproduction*, 279–291.

Snoussi, A., Chouaibi, M., Koubaier, H. B. H., & Bouzouita, N. (2022). Encapsulation of Tunisian thyme essential oil in O/W nanoemulsions: Application for meat preservation. *Meat Science*, *188*, 108785.

Sun, Y., Ma, X., & Hu, H. (2021). Marine polysaccharides as a versatile biomass for the construction of nano drug delivery systems. *Marine Drugs*, *19*(6), 345.

Tomadoni, B., Fabra, M. J., Méndez, D. A., Martínez-Abad, A., & López-Rubio, A. (2022). Electrosprayed agar nanocapsules as edible carriers of bioactive compounds. *Foods*, *11*(14), 2093.

Tosuwan, P., Leese, H. S., & Chuck, C. J. (2024). Developing Hydrophobic Alginate-Amine Derivatives as a Coating for Food Packaging. *ACS Applied Polymer Materials*, *6*(17), 1066–10677.

Verardi, A., Sangiorgio, P., Lopresto, C. G., Casella, P., & Errico, S. (2023). Enhancing carotenoids' efficacy by using chitosan-based delivery systems. *Nutraceuticals*, *3*(3), 451–480.

Wang, N., Tian, J., Wang, L., Song, S., Ai, C., Janaswamy, S., & Wen, C. (2021). Fucoidan hydrogels induced by κ-carrageenan: Rheological, thermal and structural characterization. *International journal of biological macromolecules*, *191*, 514–520.

Wang, X., Gao, S., Yun, S., Zhang, M., Peng, L., Li, Y., & Zhou, Y. (2022). Microencapsulating alginate-based polymers for probiotics delivery systems and their application. *Pharmaceuticals*, *15*(5), 644.

Wang, Z. X., Wang, Y. Z., Chen, X., Wu, A. J., Liu, W., & Li, H. J. (2025). Construction of chitosan hydrochloride-carboxymethyl chitosan nanoparticles using anti-solvent method for the co-delivery of puerarin and resveratrol. *Journal of Food Science*.

Wong, S. K., Lawrencia, D., Supramaniam, J., Goh, B. H., Manickam, S., Wong, T.W.,…Tang, S. Y. (2021). In vitro digestion and swelling kinetics of thymoquinone-loaded pickering emulsions incorporated in alginate-chitosan hydrogel beads. *Frontiers in Nutrition*, *8*, 752207.

Wu, H., Gao, S., Fu, M., Sakurai, T., & Terakawa, S. (2018). Fucoidan inhibits Ca2+ responses induced by a wide spectrum of agonists for G-protein-coupled receptors. *Molecular medicine reports*, *17*(1), 1428–1436.

Yan, C., & Kim, S.-R. (2024). Microencapsulation for pharmaceutical applications: a review. *ACS applied bio materials*, *7*(2), 692–710.

Ye, N., Zhao, P., Ayue, S., Qi, S., Ye, Y., He, H.,…Gao, F. (2023). Folic acid-modified lactoferrin nanoparticles coated with a laminarin layer loaded curcumin with dual-targeting for ulcerative colitis treatment. *International journal of biological macromolecules*, *232*, 123229.

Zhang, H., Jiang, L., Tong, M., Lu, Y., Ouyang, X.-K., & Ling, J. (2021). Encapsulation of curcumin using fucoidan stabilized zein nanoparticles: Preparation, characterization, and in vitro release performance. *Journal of Molecular Liquids*, *329*, 115586.

Zhang, J., Tang, J., Shi, S., Huang, H., Li, Y., Liu, W.,…Wu, C. (2025). Research progress on marine polysaccharide-based Pickering emulsions and their potential applications in the food industry. *Food Research International*, 116073.

Zhang, L., Xiao, Q., Xiao, Z., Zhang, Y., Weng, H., Chen, F., & Xiao, A. (2023). Hydrophobic modified agar: Structural characterization and application in encapsulation and release of curcumin. *Carbohydrate Polymers*, *308*, 120644.

Zhang, X., Wei, Z., & Xue, C. (2022). Physicochemical properties of fucoidan and its applications as building blocks of nutraceutical delivery systems. *Critical Reviews in Food Science and Nutrition*, *62*(32), 8935–8953.

Zhou, D.-Y., Wu, Z.-X., Yin, F.-W., Song, S., Li, A., Zhu, B.-W., & Yu, L.-L. (2021). Chitosan and derivatives: Bioactivities and application in foods. *Annual review of food science and technology*, *12*(1), 407–432.

Zhou, T., & Li, X. (2024). Chemically modified seaweed polysaccharides: Improved functional and biological properties and prospective in food applications. *Comprehensive reviews in food science and food safety*, *23*(4), e13396.

Zin, M. M., Anucha, C. B., & Bánvölgyi, S. (2020). Recovery of phytochemicals via electromagnetic irradiation (microwave-assisted-extraction): Betalain and phenolic compounds in perspective. *Foods*, *9*(7), 918.

Zorzi, M., Gai, F., Medana, C., Aigotti, R., Morello, S., & Peiretti, P. G. (2020). Bioactive compounds and antioxidant capacity of small berries. *Foods*, *9*(5), 623.

Plant-Based Marine Polysaccharides in Food Applications

Basak Ebru Ozcan

Abstract Marine plants such as algae, seagrasses, and mangroves are important because they contain various polysaccharides with biological activities such as anti-inflammatory, antimicrobial, antioxidant, and anticancer, and properties such as multifunctionality, natural abundance, biodegradability, and minimal toxicity. The increase in industrial and dietary use of various plant-based polysaccharides such as alginate, carrageenan, fucoidan, ulvan, and agar, which are found in high amounts in the dry biomass of seaweeds, has a global economic impact. Plant-based marine polysaccharides (PMPs) are intensively used as food additives due to their stabilizing, gelling, thickening, fat replacement, and prebiotic properties in the industry. In addition, PMPs have become popular in the packaging industry as an alternative to plastic packaging materials due to environmental and health concerns, as environmentally friendly, renewable, biodegradable, and nontoxic materials. The high demand for functional foods containing bioactive component-loaded carrier systems has popularized the use of PMPs in encapsulation technology due to their high binding, carrier, and stabilizing properties. Moreover, due to the recent high demand for foods with personalized nutritional values, the use of PMPs as building materials in 3D printing applications has gained importance. In this section, food applications of PMPs are explained in detail.

Keywords Marine polysaccharides · Food packaging · Encapsulation agent · 3D food printing · Fat replacer

1 Introduction

The marine ecosystem is the most comprehensive among other ecosystems in terms of species diversity and rich bioactive components (Karuppan Perumal et al. 2023). Marine polysaccharides are among these bioactive substances that have garnered

B. E. Ozcan (✉)
Department of Food Engineering, Faculty of Engineering, Kirklareli University, Kırklareli, Turkey

S. Jana et al. (eds.), *Multifunctional Marine Polysaccharides*,
https://doi.org/10.1007/978-981-95-4126-3_18

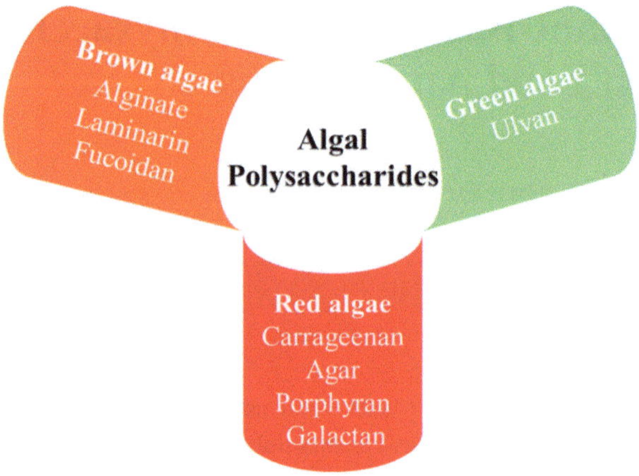

Fig. 1 Algal polysaccharides

interest because of their significance in forming sustainable life and their variety of strong bioactive component classes. Natural polysaccharides and their derivatives, which have various biological features like antioxidant, anti-inflammatory, antibacterial, hypoglycemic, and immunological qualities, are utilized in the food and medical industries today (Jha et al. 2022). Marine plants contain a variety of polysaccharides. Algal polysaccharides (Fig. 1), seagrass polysaccharides, and mangrove polysaccharides are the three main categories into which plant-based marine polysaccharides (PMPs) can be divided according to their sources (Zhang et al. 2025).

Seaweeds are widespread in the marine flora and are remarkable for their diverse biological and physiological properties. Seaweeds are categorized into three primary families according to their pigments: red (*Rhodophyceae*), green (*Chlorophyceae*), and brown (*Phaeophyceae*) (El-Beltagi et al. 2022). Brown seaweeds are the most commercially valuable, comprising two-thirds of the world's macroalgae production (Anjana and Arunkumar 2024).

Seaweeds are a valuable resource for various industries, including cosmetics, pharmaceuticals, and food, as they can produce a variety of bioactive compounds, including polysaccharides, proteins, lipids, and vitamins (Rengasamy et al. 2020). Polysaccharides are generally synthesized by seaweed for energy storage and as fundamental components of the cell (Sarkar et al. 2024). Seaweed polysaccharides have attracted a lot of attention because of their special structural characteristics and multifunctional capabilities (Deniaud-Bouët et al. 2017). These polysaccharides exhibit a number of advantageous properties, including low toxicity, biodegradability, biocompatibility, swelling capacity, and colloidal characteristics, when combined with other bioactive ingredients (Ramadan et al. 2025).

In the food industry, PMPs offer a lot of potential, particularly for the creation of functional health foods. In functional health foods, these polysaccharides offer a range of health advantages, including antiviral, anticancer, and antihypertensive effects, as well as anti-inflammatory, antioxidant, and intestinal environment regulation properties (Zhang et al. 2025). Moreover, PMPs are extensively used in the food industry as a fat replacer, gelling agent, stabilizer, and encapsulation agent (Roy et al. 2024). Moreover, in the packaging industry, there is intense interest in the use of PMPs as food packaging materials. Along with active compounds that can prolong the shelf life of food components, packaging applications have increased demand for premium, environmentally friendly, biodegradable, and natural base materials (Varghese et al. 2020). Furthermore, 3D printing applications are widely used in food science and industry to produce customized foods with specific compositions, forms, textures, and nutritional profiles using hydrocolloids such as PMPs as structural components (Ma et al. 2024). In this chapter, PMPs and their food applications have been discussed.

2 Plant-Based Marine Polysaccharides (PMPs)

Marine plants contain important polysaccharides. Macromolecular carbohydrates that are extracted from marine plants are known as PMPs. Algal, seagrass, and mangrove polysaccharides are the three types of PMPs that are being researched. In this section, PMPs such as alginate, carrageenan, agar, ulvan, porphyran, cellulose, and pectin are discussed.

2.1 Algal Polysaccharides

Seaweeds, multicellular algae rich in proteins, vitamins, minerals, and dietary fiber found in marine waters, are an important component of biomedicine, pharmacology, and especially the food industry (Yuan et al. 2024). Seaweeds are widely used to produce important food polysaccharides such as carrageenan, alginate, and agar, which are used in food products for different purposes.

2.1.1 Alginate

Alginate is an anionic polysaccharide found in the intercellular matrix and cell wall of brown macroalgae. 1,4-linked β-$_{\text{D}}$-mannuronic acid (M) and α-$_{\text{L}}$-guluronic acid (G) residues compose this linear block polymer. Different G/M block ratios and sequences are seen in each natural alginate (Yuan et al. 2024). Alginate containing Na^+, K^+, Li^+ monovalent cations dissolve in water, and when they bind to Ca^{2+}, Mg^{2+}, Ba^{2+} divalent cations, they become gel form (Abka-khajouei et al. 2022).

The most prevalent alginate salt is sodium alginate. It is environmentally friendly, widely accessible, and reasonably priced to create. Numerous alginate-based uses in the food, pharmaceutical, and medical sectors have emerged as a result of this and some other benefits, including biocompatibility, biocompostability, and low toxicity (Sharma et al. 2012).

Alginate is widely utilized in the food sector as a stabilizer and thickener in various products such as beverages, gelatins, ice creams, and dessert goods because of its exceptional stabilizing and thickening qualities (Liu et al. 2019a). In addition, alginate has beneficial health effects as its incorporation into food potentially reduces glycemic response and the risks associated with cardiovascular disease (Brownlee et al. 2005).

2.1.2 Laminarin

Laminarin, also called laminaran, makes up 5–30% of the dry weight of brown algae and is a significant storage carbohydrate (Li et al. 2021). A complex polymer, laminarin, consists of glucose units joined by β-1,3 and β-1,6 glycosidic bonds. In recent years, the use of laminarin in the production of functional food and nutraceutical products as an anti-inflammatory and antioxidant agent has increased (Karuppan Perumal et al. 2023).

2.1.3 Fucoidan

The natural sulfated heteropolysaccharide fucoidan, which makes up 1–5% of the dry weight of brown algae, is present in their cell walls. It is a water-soluble anionic polysaccharide. It is mostly made up of sulfated L-fucose with varying amounts of xylose, mannose, galactose, glucose, and uronic acid (Yuan et al. 2024). Fucoidans have been successfully included in numerous food matrices and are favored in the food industry due to their potential health benefits (Zhao et al. 2018).

2.1.4 Carrageenan

A linear sulfated polymer, carrageenan, is mostly extracted from the intercellular matrix and cell wall of red algae, such as *Eucheuma denticulatum* and *Gelidium amansii* (Yin et al. 2025). It consists of α-D-galactopyranose and β-D-galactopyranose units linked by 1,3 and 1,4 bonds. The ester sulfate content of this anionic polysaccharide, which has an average molecular weight of over 100 kDa, is 15–40% (Cunha and Grenha 2016). The six primary forms of carrageenan are κ-, ι-, λ-, μ-, ν-, and θ-carrageenan. The food and pharmaceutical industries, and bioengineering widely use ι-, κ-, and λ-carrageenans. Carrageenan finds extensive applications in the food industry owing to its significant attributes, including low production costs, non-toxicity, biocompatibility, and minimal immunogenicity (Dong et al. 2021).

2.1.5 Agar

Agar, a structural polysaccharide present in the cell walls of red algae such as carrageenan, comprises two distinct fractions: agarose and agaropectin. Agar is a natural polysaccharide with a linear chain, and the agaropectin fraction consists of short and heterogeneous sulfated chains, while agarose consists of long uncharged chains (Yuan et al. 2024). The disaccharide units of 1,3-linked β-$_D$-galactose (G) and β-1,4-linked 3,6-anhydro-$_L$-galactose (L-G) constitute the basic structure of agarose, whereas agaropectin is a combination of G and L-G with substituted pyruvate and sulfate moieties (Ouyang et al. 2018).

2.1.6 Porphyran

Porphyran is mostly found in the cell wall of *Porphyra*, a red algea, and is one of its primary constituents. Porphyran is mostly made up of alternating 1,4-linked α-$_L$-galactopyranose-6-sulfate and 1,3-linked β-$_D$-galactopyranose. It contains monosaccharides such as xylose, glucose, mannose, and arabinos. Porphyran, which has excellent solubility, bioavailability, and significant biological activities due to its low molecular weight, has application prospects in the food, pharmaceutical, and cosmetic fields (Wang et al. 2023).

2.1.7 Galactan

Sulfated galactans are predominantly produced by red algae and, to a lesser degree, by certain green algae species, especially those of the *Codium* genus (Liu et al. 2019b). The complicated structure of sulfated galactans derived from seaweed is determined by the sulfate location, side chain substitution, linkage, and presence of methyl ester or sugars. Sulfated galactans are added to low-calorie meals and utilized as texturing agents (Budiyanto et al. 2022).

2.1.8 Ulvan

Ulvan is a sulfated hydrophilic polysaccharide and constitutes 9–36% of the dry weight of green algae. The primary sugars include xylose, rhamnose, and uronic acids (glucuronic and iduronic acids (Kidgell et al. 2019). As a fingerprint structure marker, the ulvan backbone is made up of α- and β-(1 → 4) connected sugars with repeating disaccharide units. Ulvan has potential applications in biomaterials science, nutraceuticals, functional foods, and agriculture (Chi et al. 2020).

2.2 *Seagrass Polysaccharides*

Seagrasses constitute a polyphyletic assemblage of angiosperm plants that originated from primitive monocotyledonous terrestrial plants. Seagrasses are an important part of coastal ecosystems worldwide. Seagrass cell walls are mostly made of pectins, cellulose, and hemicelluloses (Pfeifer et al. 2022).

2.2.1 Pectin

Many plant species, including seagrass, contain the carbohydrate pectin. An anionic polymer, pectin is mostly made up of α-1,4 D-galacturonic acid units that are covalently bound together. In the food industry, pectin, traditionally used as a gelling agent, thickener, and stabilizer, has recently begun to replace fat and be used as a functional ingredient that supports health (Ozcan et al. 2024b).

2.2.2 Cellulose

Cellulose is the most abundant cell-wall polysaccharide in seagrasses (Pfeifer et al. 2022). Cellulose is a linear polymer consisting of β-1,4 glycosidic linkages joining D-glucopyranose units. Cellulose has a wide range of food applications due to its excellent properties, such as film-forming ability, foamability, emulsifiability, fat replacement, and health benefits (Ozcan et al. 2024b).

2.2.3 Hemicellulose

Hemicelluloses are heteropolysaccharides consisting of short side chains connected by β-(1 → 4)-glycosidic or β-(1 → 3)-glycosidic bonds (Chockchaisawasdee and Stathopoulos 2022). Hemicelluloses, like celluloses, are considered the main components of cell walls in marine plants (Pfeifer et al. 2022).

2.3 *Mangrove Polysaccharides*

Mangrove plants grow abundantly in coastal areas, estuaries, and backwaters because they require a muddy substrate of varying depth and consistency for their growth (Patra and Thatoi 2011). Mangrove plants also contain cellulose, hemicellulose, and pectin polysaccharides, just as seagrass.

3 Food Applications of Plant-Based Marine Polysaccharides (PMPs)

Natural bioactive compounds and metabolites that are considered safe for human consumption are widely used in many food applications. Appropriate utilization of such compounds has received special attention both for the development of foods and for the potential health benefits of these compounds. Polysaccharides derived from marine plants, which are among the various beneficial bio-components, are widely preferred in the food sector. Numerous recent reports have revealed the potential food applications of polysaccharides from various marine plants. In this section, the applications of different PMPs in the food industry are discussed (Fig. 2).

3.1 *Food Packaging*

Food packaging mitigates the degradation of food quality and spoilage by preserving moisture, preventing oxidation, and averting contamination from bacteria or other pollutants throughout transport and sale, hence ensuring food quality and safety (He et al. 2025). Petroleum-based food packaging materials are widely used in the

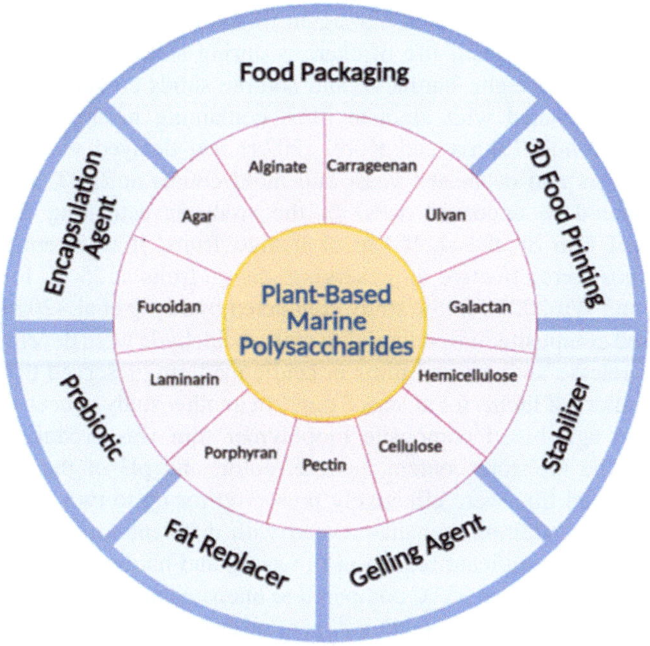

Fig. 2 Food applications of plant-based marine polysaccharides

food packaging sector because they are easy to shape, convenient, and durable (Ozcan et al. 2024b). However, limitations on the biodegradability, recyclability, biocompatibility, and reusability of these packaging materials have caused harmful effects of plastic waste on the environment and human health (Perera et al. 2021). As a result of the increasing concerns about the use of plastic packaging materials, studies on developing food packaging materials with biodegradable polymers are gradually increasing (Gadaleta et al. 2022).

Various polysaccharides obtained from marine plants, such as alginate, carrageenan, agar, and fucoidan, are used as biopolymers in the production of biodegradable food packaging materials to extend food quality and increase microbial safety (Mahmud et al. 2021). These important components significantly increase the mechanical, barrier, and physical properties of biofilms while also imparting strong antioxidant and antibacterial properties to the packaging material (Manikandan and Min 2023). Table 1 provides details on the use of PMPs in food packaging.

Moller et al. (2023) investigated the effectiveness of an allyl isothiocyanate-treated carrageenan/chitosan-based coating against lactic acid bacteria, aerobic bacteria, yeast, and mold at 4 °C for 21 days of storage of chicken breast and reported that the shelf life of the coated chicken breast increased. Fresh beef wrapped with sodium alginate/pectin-based film containing cinnamic acid developed by Tong et al. (2023) showed a significant reduction of 84.09% in bacterial load. Similarly, chitosan/sodium alginate-based films containing pterostilbene-loaded nanoemulsion showed similar results to polyethylene for postharvest shiitake mushroom preservation up to 10 days (Ruchika et al. 2025). The films developed by adding natural wormwood extract as an antimicrobial agent to sodium alginate and starch matrix effectively extended the shelf life of cherries during storage for 15 days at 4 °C, delaying the loss of weight, hardness, and soluble solids content (Li et al. 2025). Fresh mandarins coated with alginate films containing natamycin and vanillin, developed by Konuk Takma and Korel (2024) had delayed weight, color, and softening changes and decreased yeast and mold counts at 25 °C for 21 days of storage compared to uncoated ones. In the study investigating the effects of fucoidan-based film on the shelf life of mango fruits, it was reported that the developed films were effective in preserving mango fruits at 25 °C for 35 days of storage (Xu and Wu 2021). In the study conducted by Liang et al. (2024), fucoidan/chitosan-based composite films containing cinnamaldehyde were developed, and the pH-sensitive release antibacterial films in acidic medium preserved the appearance and quality indices of litchis for at least 8 days. In another study, a beeswax-modified guar gum and agar-based composite biopolymer film was produced for cheese preservation. The moisture content, texture, color, and pH of the cheese coated with the developed film were effectively preserved for up to two months (Pal and Agarwal 2024). In addition, bananas coated with different concentrations of agar suspension showed significant reduction in weight and hardness loss, soluble solid concentration for 15 days at 25 °C compared to uncoated ones (Hussein Ziedan et al. 2018). Moreover, agar films containing Argentine croquette protein isolate and clove essential oil significantly delayed the development of microorganisms that produce H_2S in flounder fillets for 15 days at 5 °C in storage, increasing shelf life (da Rocha

Table 1 Use of plant-based marine polysaccharides (PMPs) in food packaging

PMPs	Other polymers/ Components	Applied food products	Results/Effects	References
Alginate	Pectin, Cinnamic acid, glycerol	Fresh beef	The produced film demonstrated a soil degradability of 43.26% during 15 days. The bacterial load on the meats covered with the film was significantly reduced by 84.09% throughout the experiment	Tong et al. (2023)
Alginate	Natamycin, vanillin, glycerol	Mandarin	The films were delayed weight, color, and softening changes of mandarins and reduced yeast and mold counts during 21 days of storage at 25 °C	Konuk Takma and Korel (2024)
Alginate	Rice straw, hemicellulose, glycerol	Freshly-cut lemon slices	Lemon slices showed a notable increase in antioxidant activity and a significant concentration-dependent decrease in weight loss	Ismail et al. (2024)
Alginate	Gelatin, green tea extract, glycerol	Mushroom	The films prolonged the mushrooms' shelf life up to seven days at 4 °C and successfully maintained their postharvest quality	Shan et al. (2023)
Alginate	Gelatin, clove essential oil, Nanoclay, glycerol	Cheddar cheese	At 4 °C storage, the film preserved the weight, pH, appearance and microbiological growth values of the cheese and extended its shelf life by 15 days	Perera et al. (2023)
Carrageenan	Chitosan, allyl isothiocyanate	Chicken breast	A carrageenan/chitosan coating treated with allyl isothiocyanate extended the shelf life of chicken breast stored at 4 °C for 21 days	Moller et al. (2023)
Carrageenan	Cinnamon essential oil, glycerol	Pork meat	The films retarded the growth of lactic acid and H_2S-producing bacteria in pork meat and reduced the level of lipid oxidation. After 7 days of storage at 4 °C, the meat still had an attractive, bright red color	He and Wang (2022)
Carrageenan	Olive leaf extract, glycerol	Lamb meat	Thanks to the antimicrobial capacity of the film, the number of psychrophiles decreased fivefold during the storage of lamb meat compared to samples packed with control and commercial films	Martiny et al. (2020)

(continued)

Table 1 (continued)

PMPs	Other polymers/ Components	Applied food products	Results/Effects	References
Agar	–	Banana	Bananas coated with agar suspension showed significant reduction in incidence and severity of postharvest diseases	Hussein Ziedan et al. (2018)
Agar	Gelatin, Natamycin, glycerol	Strawberry	Strawberries covered with film containing natamycin had significantly reduced fungal colony counts compared to uncoated strawberries. Film-packaged strawberries showed lower water loss rate during storage at 4 °C (1.43%) and 20 °C (7.66%)	Wang et al. (2022)
Agar	Clove essential oil, argentine croaker protein isolate, glycerol	Flounder fillets	The films significantly retarded the growth of H_2S-producing microorganisms in halibut fillets during 15 days of storage at 5 °C	da Rocha et al. (2018)
Fucoidan	–	Mango	Fucoidan coatings inhibited respiration, nutrient, and weight loss of mango fruits and protected fruits from biological damage during storage at room temperature	Xu and Wu (2021)
Fucoidan	Chitosan, Cinnamaldehyde, glycerol	Litchi	The developed films retained the appearance and quality parameters of litchis for at least 8 days	Liang et al. (2024)

et al. 2018). In ginger essential oil-loaded chitosan/porphyran-based films developed by Al-Harrasi et al. (2022), it was observed that the presence of porphyran significantly increased the antioxidant effects of the films.

3.2 *Encapsulation Agent*

Encapsulation is described as the process of enveloping one substance (active agent) within another substance (wall material). The encapsulation technique in the food sector can be utilized for several purposes. Enhancing the transport of bioactive substances, including vitamins, minerals, antioxidants, and living cells into food can be accomplished through encapsulation (Alu'datt et al. 2022). Encapsulation technology widely uses food biopolymers as coating materials. Among these biopolymers, polysaccharides have the potential to be a good encapsulating material because of their many benefits, including their ability to gel, bind, and stabilize emulsions (Rehman et al. 2019). Nowadays, in many studies, polysaccharides from marine plants, such as sodium alginate (Faidi et al. 2019), carrageenan (Alavi et al. 2023), and agar, were successfully used as wall materials in encapsulation technology. Table 2 provides details on the food products enriched with encapsulated bioactive compounds by different PMPs.

In the study conducted by Ozcan et al. (2024a), alginate-carrageenan emulgel beads containing purple basil leaf extract were used in the production of gelatin-based jelly candy. Jelly candies enriched with extract-loaded beads exhibited higher hardness, cohesiveness, elasticity, and chewiness compared to samples containing free extract. In addition, the bitter taste was masked by the encapsulation of the free extract, resulting in the highest sensory acceptance scores for candies containing beads. In another study, betalain-rich *Opuntia-ficus-indica* fruit extract was encapsulated using calcium alginate using ionic gelation, and the capsules were added to gummy candies as a model food system. The stability of the betalain color in the capsules added to the gummy candies resulted in the candies having a vibrant red-purple color (Otálora et al. 2019). Teymuri-Yeghaneh et al. (2025) used alginate capsules containing cardamom and garlic essential oils-loaded β-cyclodextrin in yogurt production and found that the capsules increased the shelf life of yogurt compared to free essential oils, and maintained the sensory and antibacterial properties. In another study where yogurt was selected as a model food, black carrot anthocyanins were encapsulated with the ionic gelation technique using pectin/alginate, and the anthocyanin protection reached up to 62%, and antioxidant capacity reached up to 55.6% in yogurt samples fortified with capsules (Tavlasoglu et al. 2022). In another study, functional bread with garlic oil-loaded alginate microcapsules showed lower hardness values as compared to the control bread with no microcapsules. Also, no change in the cohesiveness and springiness was observed in all fortified bread throughout the 7-day storage period (Narsaiah et al. 2019). Moreover, curcumin-loaded Pickering emulsion containing alginate beads was added to milk, apple juice, yogurt, and mineral water as a model food application, and the beads maintained their physical stability for 28 days of storage in food systems (Aw et al. 2023).

3.3 3D Food Printing

3D food printing is a cutting-edge processing technology that employs computer-generated digital models. The advancement of 3D food printing technology has accelerated in recent years due to its various benefits, including reduced production prices, the capability to fabricate intricate structures, and diminished manufacturing time (Wedamulla et al. 2025). The development of novel foods with complex shapes, unique textures, and enhanced nutritional value is made possible via 3D food printing. Furthermore, this technology enables customized food design that

Table 2 Food products enriched with encapsulated bioactive compounds by different plant-based marine polysaccharides (PMPs)

PMPs	Bioactive compounds	Other polymers	Encapsulation technique	Food products	Main findings	References
Alginate	Betalain	–	Ionic gelation	Gummy candy	The stability of the color of the betalain encapsulated in alginate capsules resulted in a vibrant red-purple color of the candies to which they were added.	Otálora et al. (2019)
Alginate	Cinnamaldehyde	–	Electrospraying	Mongolian cheese	The microcapsules showed inhibitory effects on microorganism growth during the storage of Mongolian cheese.	Cao et al. (2024)
Alginate	Garlic and cardamom essential oils	β-cyclodextrin	Ionic gelation	Yogurt	The shelf life of yogurt increased, and sensory and antibacterial properties were preserved for 21 days of storage.	Teymuri-Yeghaneh et al. (2025)
Alginate	Black carrot anthocyanins	Pectin	Ionic gelation	Yogurt	In yogurt samples fortified with capsules, anthocyanin protection reached up to 62%, and antioxidant capacity reached up to 55.6%.	Tavlasoglu et al. (2022)
Alginate	Garlic oil	–	Air atomization	Bread	Fortified bread with microcapsules showed lower hardness values as compared to the control bread with no microcapsules.	Narsaiah et al. (2019)
Alginate	Curcumin	Cellulose nanocrystal	Ionic gelation	Milk, apple juice, yogurt, mineral water	Following a 28-day storage period in food systems, the beads demonstrated excellent physical stability.	Aw et al. (2023)
Carrageenan	Ferulic acid	Ovalbumin	Pickering emulsion	Bread	While the color characteristics of the bread did not change, the hardness and chewiness decreased during storage.	Su et al. (2023)
Alginate, carrageenan	Purple basil leaf extract (anthocyanins)	–	Hybrid system (double emulsion and ionic gelation)	Jelly candy	Jelly candies enriched with encapsulated extract received the highest sensory acceptance scores.	Ozcan et al. (2024a)
Carrageenan	Fish oil	Tragacanth gum	Freeze drying	Chicken nugget	Fish oil encapsulation enhanced the enriched nuggets' oxidative storage life and sensory qualities while also protecting against lipid and protein oxidation.	Pourashouri et al. (2021)

appeals to particular groups and individualized nutrition. For a variety of 3D food printing applications, extrusion, binder injection, and inkjet printing technologies have generally been investigated (Wang et al. 2024a). Materials used in 3D food printing can be categorized as carbohydrate-based, protein-based, or fat-based (Wedamulla et al. 2025). Polysaccharides, including PMPs such as κ-carrageenan and alginate, are used in 3D food printing formulations to modify material properties.

Liu et al. (2024) developed a 3D printable curcumin-loaded Pickering emulsion gel stabilized by pea protein isolate/κ-carrageenan complex. According to 3D printing tests, Pickering emulsion gel with more than 0.3% κ-carrageenan concentration exhibited smooth extrusion ability and effectively maintained the desired shape structure. In another study, compound diets based on the nutritional needs of older adults were 3D printed using κ-carrageenan and inulin, and κ-carrageenan was found to increase the hardness, flexibility, and chewability of the developed product (Yu et al. 2025). In the study conducted by Ma et al. (2024), Pickering emulsions stabilized with sodium alginate and pea protein isolate were used in 3D food printing, and the shapes printed with the emulsions maintained their structural integrity for up to 24 hours. In the application of extrusion-based 3D printing to create new shapes from mashed potatoes, it has been reported that 0.5–1.5% alginate and 0.5–1% agar concentrations provide the best printing ability and product stability (Dankar et al. 2018).

3.4 *Food Additive*

Polysaccharides have always attracted great attention in the food industry as additives to enhance the texture, flavor, character, appearance, and nutritional value of foods due to their non-toxicity, wide availability, reproducibility, and health-promoting benefits (Wang et al. 2024b). PMPs are widely preferred as additives in the food industry due to their prebiotic, emulsifying, fat-replacing, and gelling properties.

3.4.1 Prebiotic

Prebiotics are compounds that are resistant to being hydrolyzed by human digestive enzymes. When they enter the colon, intestinal microbes ferment them, enabling beneficial bacteria to proliferate and transform them into metabolites that improve health (Gonçalves et al. 2023). The increasing knowledge about the crucial role of gut microbiota in human health and disease has heightened the significance of prebiotics, owing to their capacity to enhance health and address diseases by modulating gut microbiota (Ji et al. 2023). For this purpose, the use of polysaccharides, including PMPs, with prebiotic properties, in the production of functional foods has become more widespread day by day. Many previous studies have reported that PMPs such as laminaran, porphyran, and agar have prebiotic properties (Seong et al. 2019; Ajanth Praveen et al. 2019; Chamidah and Awaludin Prihanto 2016).

Shalaby (2019) produced yogurt using different percentages of ulvan polysaccharide as a prebiotic ingredient. According to the results, it was seen that yogurt with good chemical and physical properties could be produced by adding 1–2% ulvan polysaccharide, but adding a high percentage of ulvan (4%) caused delayed fermentation and weak texture in yogurt. In the study where 100% wheat flour was used as a control, white breads containing 4% carrageenan were produced. The presence of carrageenan improved the hydration properties of the flour and decreased the bread volume and hardness (Raman et al. 2019).

3.4.2 Gelling Agent

The regenerative nature, cost-effectiveness, biocompatibility, and biodegradability of food gels may render them superior to synthetic alternatives (Ozcan et al. 2024b). Gel formation can efficiently alter the texture and structure of food, giving it a sticky and appropriate taste in addition to enhancing its ability to hold water, thicken, and connect particles (Wang et al. 2024b). Polysaccharides such as alginate, carrageenan, and agar are used to enhance the viscosity, gelatinization, and other qualities of jellies, jams, yogurts, and ice creams because of their gel-forming capabilities (Naqash et al. 2017).

de Avelar and Efraim (2020) evaluated the cold-setting potential of alginate in the production of jelly candies. Compared to jelly candy obtained with only pectin (6.2 N), pectin jellies containing alginate showed a higher hardness value (16.2 N) and an opaque and lighter color. In addition, alginate as a gelling agent significantly affected the physicochemical parameters of the confectionery. Another study reported that when sodium alginate was added to milk and butter and then added to the dry ingredients, the moistened sodium alginate gel in the milk formed a superior mixture in terms of strong emulsion boundaries and small ice crystals and air cells (Goraya et al. 2021). Song et al. (2022) developed vegan gummy candies using different polymers (konjac glucomannan, xanthan gum, carboxymethylcellulose sodium, pectin, locust bean gum) with κ-carrageenan as a gelling agent, and κ-carrageenan improved the texture and water retention of the gummy candies. Similarly, Nguyen et al. (2024) developed gummy candies using gelatin and agar and reported that 0.5% agar supplementation had a significant effect on the structure of the product.

3.4.3 Stabilizer

In recent years, the use of biopolymers as food-grade stabilizers without health concerns to create edible emulsions and expand their applications in food systems has become the subject of increasing research (Shao et al. 2020). Among these natural biopolymers are plant-based polysaccharides, which have excellent biological qualities and low processing costs, making them appropriate for use as stabilizers in food emulsions. These factors make plant polysaccharides—including PMPs—excellent emulsion stabilizers, and they are frequently utilized for making emulsions for use in food applications (Pogorelova and Sarnitskaya 2024).

Seo and Oh (2022) used κ-carrageenan/milk protein isolate conjugate as a stabilizer in ice cream production and reported that the conjugate increased the physical properties of ice cream. Similarly, in another study, a stabilizer mixture containing different concentrations of κ-carrageenan was used to reduce hardness, control overrun, and improve overall sensory qualities in ice cream production, and the addition of κ-carrageenan resulted in a significant increase in overrun and a decrease in hardness. Additionally, the samples were accepted by the panelists as a result of sensory analysis (Roy et al. 2024). In a study conducted by Ketut Budaraga et al. (2024), it was investigated how the presence of alginate as a stabilizer in pumpkin ice cream affected the quality of ice cream. According to the findings of the study, the addition of sodium alginate significantly changed the amount of water, protein, fat, antioxidant activity, overflow, and melting time. Moreover, the mixture of sodium alginate and κ-carrageenan used as a stabilizer in the production of Spirulina ice cream improved the texture quality of ice cream (Farhah and Ekantari 2020). Furthermore, λ- and κ-carrageenans obtained from *Halymenia* sp. and *Kappaphycus alvarezii* were used in bread production, and it was reported that the bread volume increased and the texture and structure of the bread crumbs improved (Widyastuti et al. 2021).

3.4.4 Fat Replacer

Numerous chronic illnesses, including atherosclerosis, diabetes, cardiovascular disease, cancer, and high blood pressure, are linked to high-fat consumption (Bourouis et al. 2023). Recently, as a result of the increasing interest of consumers in low-fat products, efforts to produce healthier products in the food industry have also increased. As a result, there has been an increase in the use of polysaccharides as fat replacers in low-fat foods due to their ability to maintain similar technological functions and sensory properties similar to animal fat or seed oil (Ozcan et al. 2024b). The primary way that polysaccharides substitute fat is by stabilizing huge volumes of water in a gel-like matrix, which results in a fluidity and creaminess that is comparable to fat (Bourouis et al. 2023). In recent years, studies on the use of PMPs as fat replacers in food products have increased.

Öztürk-Kerimoğlu (2021) used a gel system consisting of pea protein isolate and agar agar as a fat replacer in model meat emulsions and observed that lightness and yellowness increased and redness decreased in the developed meats. Also, the use of κ-carrageenan/monoglyceride-based bigels in cookies resulted in a significant decrease in the fat content and hardness of the cookies (Sharifi et al. 2025). Moreover, another study found that the presence of sodium alginate influenced the rate of protein release and the disintegration of the cheese matrix when it was used to substitute fat in Cheddar cheese (Sharma Khanal et al. 2020). Furthermore, in previous studies, κ-carrageenan was used as a fat replacer in different food products such as dairy desserts (Bayarri et al. 2010), yogurt (Nguyen et al. 2017).

4 Conclusions

Many polysaccharides found in marine plants originate from mangroves, seagrass, and algae. Because of their many biological qualities, including immunological, hypoglycemic, antibacterial, anti-inflammatory, and antioxidant, these natural polysaccharides are used extensively in many industries today. The food industry uses a variety of polysaccharides derived from seaweeds, including ulvan, carrageenan, agar, and alginate. Today, the increase in the use of algae polysaccharides in the food industry, especially in food industry, has a global economic impact. PMPs, which are widely used as stabilizers, gelling agents, fat substitutes, and prebiotics in the food industry, are preferred due to their gelling, binding, and stabilizing abilities, especially as wall materials in the encapsulation of bioactive components. In addition, the increasing demand for biodegradable, environmentally friendly packaging materials as a result of concerns brought by plastic packaging has increased the use of PMPs in food packaging applications. Moreover, as a result of the advancement of 3D printing technology, the intense demand for foods with low production costs, desired textures, and customized nutritional values has increased the use of PMPs as building materials in 3D food printing formulas. In summary, PMPs are natural materials of great importance used in food applications as additives, packaging materials, encapsulation agents, and 3D food printing materials, and will continue to be highly important materials in the future.

References

Abka-khajouei R, Tounsi L, Shahabi N, Patel AK, Abdelkafi S, Michaud P (2022) Structures, Properties and Applications of Alginates. Mar Drugs 20

Ajanth Praveen M, Karthika Parvathy KR, Jayabalan R, Balasubramanian P (2019) Dietary fiber from Indian edible seaweeds and its in-vitro prebiotic effect on the gut microbiota. Food Hydrocoll 96:343–353. https://doi.org/10.1016/j.foodhyd.2019.05.031

Alavi N, Golmakani MT, Hosseini SMH, Niakousari M, Moosavi-Nasab M (2023) Enhancing phycocyanin solubility via complexation with fucoidan or κ-carrageenan and improving phycocyanin color stability by encapsulation in alginate-pregelatinized corn starch composite gel beads. Int J Biol Macromol 242. https://doi.org/10.1016/j.ijbiomac.2023.124762

Al-Harrasi A, Bhtaia S, Al-Azri MS, Makeen HA, Albratty M, Alhazmi HA, Mohan S, Sharma A, Behl T (2022) Development and Characterization of Chitosan and Porphyran Based Composite Edible Films Containing Ginger Essential Oil. Polymers (Basel) 14(9). https://doi.org/10.3390/polym14091782

Alu'datt MH, Alrosan M, Gammoh S, Tranchant CC, Alhamad MN, Rababah T, Zghoul R, Alzoubi H, Ghatasheh S, Ghozlan K, Tan TC (2022) Encapsulation-based technologies for bioactive compounds and their application in the food industry: A roadmap for food-derived functional and health-promoting ingredients. Food Biosci 50

Anjana K, Arunkumar K (2024) Brown algae biomass for fucoxanthin, fucoidan and alginate; update review on structure, biosynthesis, biological activities and extraction valorisation. Int J Biol Macromol 280

Aw YZ, Lim HP, Low LE, Goh BH, Chan ES, Tey BT (2023) Pickering emulsion hydrogel beads for curcumin encapsulation and food application. J Food Eng 350. https://doi.org/10.1016/j.jfoodeng.2023.111501

Bayarri S, Chuliá I, Costell E (2010) Comparing λ-carrageenan and an inulin blend as fat replacers in carboxymethyl cellulose dairy desserts. Rheological and sensory aspects. Food Hydrocoll 24(6–7):578–587. https://doi.org/10.1016/j.foodhyd.2010.02.004

Bourouis I, Pang Z, Liu X (2023) Recent advances on uses of protein and/or polysaccharide as fat replacers: Textural and tribological perspectives: A review. J Agric Food Res 11. https://doi.org/10.1016/j.jafr.2023.100519

Brownlee IA, Allen A, Pearson JP, Dettmar PW, Havler ME, Atherton MR, Onsøyen E (2005) Alginate as a source of dietary fiber. Crit Rev Food Sci Nutr 45(6):497–510. https://doi.org/10.1080/10408390500285673

Budiyanto F, Ghandourah MA, Bawakid NO, Alorfi HS, Abdel-Lateff A, Alarif WM (2022) Threat and gain: The metabolites of the red algae genus Acanthophora. Algal Res 65

Cao M, Zheng Y, Zhou R, Ma M (2024) Optimization and characterization of alginate/cinnamaldehyde electrosprayed microcapsule and its application to mongolian cheese preservation. Int J Biol Macromol 283. https://doi.org/10.1016/j.ijbiomac.2024.136865

Chamidah A, Awaludin Prihanto A (2016) Prebiotics Activity of Laminaran Derived from Sargassum Crassifolium

Chi Y, Li H, Wang P, Du C, Ye H, Zuo S, Guan H, Wang P (2020) Structural characterization of ulvan extracted from Ulva clathrata assisted by an ulvan lyase. Carbohydr Polym 229. https://doi.org/10.1016/j.carbpol.2019.115497

Chockchaisawasdee S, Stathopoulos CE (2022) Functional Oligosaccharides Derived from Fruit-and-Vegetable By-Products and Wastes. Horticulturae 8

Cunha L, Grenha A (2016) Sulfated seaweed polysaccharides as multifunctional materials in drug delivery applications. Mar Drugs 14

da Rocha M, Alemán A, Romani VP, López-Caballero ME, Gómez-Guillén MC, Montero P, Prentice C (2018) Effects of agar films incorporated with fish protein hydrolysate or clove essential oil on flounder (Paralichthys orbignyanus) fillets shelf-life. Food Hydrocoll 81:351–363. https://doi.org/10.1016/j.foodhyd.2018.03.017

Dankar I, Pujolà M, El Omar F, Sepulcre F, Haddarah A (2018) Impact of Mechanical and Microstructural Properties of Potato Puree-Food Additive Complexes on Extrusion-Based 3D Printing. Food Bioproc Tech 11(11):2021–2031. https://doi.org/10.1007/s11947-018-2159-5

de Avelar MHM, Efraim P (2020) Alginate/pectin cold-set gelation as a potential sustainable method for jelly candy production. LWT 123. https://doi.org/10.1016/j.lwt.2020.109119

Deniaud-Bouët E, Hardouin K, Potin P, Kloareg B, Hervé C (2017) A review about brown algal cell walls and fucose-containing sulfated polysaccharides: Cell wall context, biomedical properties and key research challenges. Carbohydr Polym 175:395–408

Dong Y, Wei Z, Xue C (2021) Recent advances in carrageenan-based delivery systems for bioactive ingredients: A review. Trends Food Sci Technol 112:348–361

El-Beltagi HS, Mohamed AA, Mohamed HI, Ramadan KMA, Barqawi AA, Mansour AT (2022) Phytochemical and Potential Properties of Seaweeds and Their Recent Applications: A Review. Mar Drugs 20

Faidi A, Lassoued MA, Becheikh MEH, Touati M, Stumbé JF, Farhat F (2019) Application of sodium alginate extracted from a Tunisian brown algae Padina pavonica for essential oil encapsulation: Microspheres preparation, characterization and in vitro release study. Int J Biol Macromol 136:386–394. https://doi.org/10.1016/j.ijbiomac.2019.06.023

Farhah AN, Ekantari N (2020) Combination of Sodium Alginate and Kappa-Carrageenan Increases Texture Stability of Spirulina platensis Ice Cream. In: E3S Web of Conferences. EDP Sciences

Gadaleta G, De Gisi S, Picuno C, Heerenklage J, Cafiero L, Oliviero M, Notarnicola M, Kuchta K, Sorrentino A (2022) The influence of bio-plastics for food packaging on combined anaerobic digestion and composting treatment of organic municipal waste. Waste Management 144:87–97. https://doi.org/10.1016/j.wasman.2022.03.014

Gonçalves DA, González A, Roupar D, Teixeira JA, Nobre C (2023) How prebiotics have been produced from agro-industrial waste: An overview of the enzymatic technologies applied and the models used to validate their health claims. Trends Food Sci Technol 135:74–92

Goraya RK, Singla M, Bajwa U, Kaur A, Pathania S (2021) Impact of sodium alginate gelling and ingredient amalgamating order on ingredient interactions and structural stability of ice cream. LWT 147. https://doi.org/10.1016/j.lwt.2021.111558

He B, Gao Y, Lou W, Wang J, Xin S, Ma K, Li L (2025) Biodegradable food packaging films: Material source, mechanical and water vapor barrier properties, and improvement strategies—A comprehensive review. Food Research International 211

He S, Wang Y (2022) Antimicrobial and Antioxidant Effects of Kappa-Carrageenan Coatings Enriched with Cinnamon Essential Oil in Pork Meat. Foods 11(18). https://doi.org/10.3390/foods11182885

Hussein Ziedan ES, El Zahaby HM, Maswada HF, El Rafh Zoeir EHA (2018) Agar-agar a promising edible coating agent for management of postharvest diseases and improving banana fruit quality. J Plant Prot Res 58(3). https://doi.org/10.24425/122938

Ismail SA, Abozed SS, Taie HAA, Hassan AA (2024) Preservation of freshly-cut lemon slices using alginate-based coating functionalized with antioxidant enzymatically hydrolyzed rice straw-hemicellulose. Sci Rep 14(1). https://doi.org/10.1038/s41598-024-77670-6

Jha N, Madasamy S, Prasad P, Lakra AK, Tilwani YM, Arul V (2022) Physico-chemical and functional characterization of polysaccharide purified from mangrove Rhizophora mucronata leaves having potent biological activity. South African Journal of Botany 147:659–669. https://doi.org/10.1016/j.sajb.2022.02.036

Ji J, Jin W, Liu SJ, Jiao Z, Li X (2023) Probiotics, prebiotics, and postbiotics in health and disease. MedComm (Beijing) 4

Karuppan Perumal MK, Gandhi D, Rajasekaran MBS, Kudiyarasu S, Renuka RR, Julius A, Samrot AV, Lakshmi Narayanan A (2023) Inhibition of angiogenesis using laminarin a natural polysaccharide from brown seaweeds—A review. Biocatal Agric Biotechnol 54

Ketut Budaraga I, Hermalena L, Aisyah S (2024) Alginate Addition from Sargassum Seaweed (Sargassum sp.) on Pumpkin Ice Cream (Cucurbita Moschata Durch.) Characteristics

Kidgell JT, Magnusson M, de Nys R, Glasson CRK (2019) Ulvan: A systematic review of extraction, composition and function. Algal Res 39

Konuk Takma D, Korel F (2024) Enhancement of Post-harvest Quality of Fresh Mandarins with Alginate-Based Edible Coating Containing Natamycin and Vanillin. Applied Fruit Science. https://doi.org/10.1007/s10341-024-01141-5

Li Y, Li M, Teng R, Wang S, Liu Z, Wu S, Zhou T, Wang T, Ruan W (2025) Preparation and characterization of sodium alginate/starch/wormwood extract composite film and its application in cherry preservation. Journal of Food Measurement and Characterization. https://doi.org/10.1007/s11694-025-03189-7

Li Y, Zheng Y, Zhang Y, Yang Y, Wang P, Imre B, Wong ACY, Hsieh YSY, Wang D (2021) Brown algae carbohydrates: Structures, pharmaceutical properties, and research challenges. Mar Drugs 19

Liang F, Liu C, Geng J, Chen N, Lai W, Mo H, Liu K (2024) Chitosan–fucoidan encapsulating cinnamaldehyde composite coating films: Preparation, pH-responsive release, antibacterial activity and preservation for litchi. Carbohydr Polym 333. https://doi.org/10.1016/j.carbpol.2024.121968

Liu J, Yang S, Li X, Yan Q, Reaney MJT, Jiang Z (2019a) Alginate Oligosaccharides: Production, Biological Activities, and Potential Applications. Compr Rev Food Sci Food Saf 18:1859–1881

Liu Z, Gao T, Yang Y, Meng F, Zhan F, Jiang Q, Sun X (2019b) Anti-Cancer Activity of Porphyran and Carrageenan from Red Seaweeds. Molecules 24

Liu Z, Ha S, Guo C, Xu D, Hu L, Li H, Hati S, Mo H (2024) 3D printing of curcumin enriched Pickering emulsion gel stablized by pea protein-carrageenan complexes. Food Hydrocoll 146. https://doi.org/10.1016/j.foodhyd.2023.109170

Ma C, Yan J, Li W, Wang Y, McClements DJ, Liu X, Liu F (2024) Enhanced printability of food-grade edible inks: Emulsions formulated with modified pea protein and sodium alginate. Food Hydrocoll 152. https://doi.org/10.1016/j.foodhyd.2024.109946

Mahmud N, Islam J, Tahergorabi R (2021) Marine biopolymers: Applications in food packaging. Processes 9

Manikandan V, Min SC (2023) Biofabrication of carbon quantum dots and their food packaging applications: a review. Food Sci Biotechnol 32:1159–1171

Martiny TR, Raghavan V, de Moraes CC, da Rosa GS, Dotto GL (2020) Bio-based active packaging: Carrageenan film with olive leaf extract for lamb meat preservation. Foods 9(12). https://doi.org/10.3390/foods9121759

Moller A, Leone C, Kataria J, Sidhu G, Rama EN, Kroft B, Thippareddi H, Singh M (2023) Effect of a carrageenan/chitosan coating with allyl isothiocyanate on microbial spoilage and quality of chicken breast. Poult Sci 102(3). https://doi.org/10.1016/j.psj.2022.102442

Naqash F, Masoodi FA, Rather SA, Wani SM, Gani A (2017) Emerging concepts in the nutraceutical and functional properties of pectin—A Review. Carbohydr Polym 168:227–239

Narsaiah K, Sharma M, Sridhar K, Dikkala P (2019) Garlic Oil Nanoemulsions Hybridized in Calcium Alginate Microcapsules for Functional Bread. Agricultural Research 8(3):356–363. https://doi.org/10.1007/s40003-018-0363-1

Nguyen PTM, Kravchuk O, Bhandari B, Prakash S (2017) Effect of different hydrocolloids on texture, rheology, tribology and sensory perception of texture and mouthfeel of low-fat pot-set yoghurt. Food Hydrocoll 72:90–104. https://doi.org/10.1016/j.foodhyd.2017.05.035

Nguyen TBK, Cao HKN, Nguyen TDLH, Doan TPD, Phan TD, Le MT, Dong TAD (2024) Improvement of gummy candy structure by gelling ingredients and cooling temperature. Vietnam Journal of Chemistry. https://doi.org/10.1002/vjch.202400211

Otálora MC, de Jesús Barbosa H, Perilla JE, Osorio C, Nazareno MA (2019) Encapsulated betalains (Opuntia ficus-indica) as natural colorants. Case study: Gummy candies. LWT 103:222–227. https://doi.org/10.1016/j.lwt.2018.12.074

Ouyang QQ, Hu Z, Li SD, Quan WY, Wen LL, Yang ZM, Li PW (2018) Thermal degradation of agar: Mechanism and toxicity of products. Food Chem 264:277–283. https://doi.org/10.1016/j.foodchem.2018.04.098

Ozcan BE, Karakas CY, Karadag A (2024a) Application of purple basil leaf anthocyanins-loaded alginate-carrageenan emulgel beads in gelatin-based jelly candies. Int J Biol Macromol 277. https://doi.org/10.1016/j.ijbiomac.2024.134547

Ozcan BE, Tetik N, Aloglu HS (2024b) Polysaccharides from fruit and vegetable wastes and their food applications: A review. Int J Biol Macromol 276

Öztürk-Kerimoğlu B (2021) A promising strategy for designing reduced-fat model meat emulsions by utilization of pea protein-agar agar gel complex. Food Structure 29. https://doi.org/10.1016/j.foostr.2021.100205

Pal N, Agarwal M (2024) Development and characterization of eco-friendly guar gum-agar-beeswax-based active packaging film for cheese preservation. Int J Biol Macromol 277. https://doi.org/10.1016/j.ijbiomac.2024.134333

Patra JK, Thatoi HN (2011) Metabolic diversity and bioactivity screening of mangrove plants: A review. Acta Physiol Plant 33:1051–1061

Perera KY, Jaiswal AK, Jaiswal S (2023) Extending cheese shelf-life using eco-friendly sodium alginate-gelatin films reinforced with nanoclay. Food Biosci 56. https://doi.org/10.1016/j.fbio.2023.103304

Perera KY, Sharma S, Pradhan D, Jaiswal AK, Jaiswal S (2021) Seaweed polysaccharide in food contact materials (Active packaging, intelligent packaging, edible films, and coatings). Foods 10

Pfeifer L, van Erven G, Sinclair EA, Duarte CM, Kabel MA, Classen B (2022) Profiling the cell walls of seagrasses from A (Amphibolis) to Z (Zostera). BMC Plant Biol 22(1). https://doi.org/10.1186/s12870-022-03447-6

Pogorelova NA, Sarnitskaya NA (2024) Polysaccharides as food system stabilizers. In: BIO Web of Conferences. EDP Sciences

Pourashouri P, Shabanpour B, Heydari S, Raeisi S (2021) Encapsulation of fish oil by carrageenan and gum tragacanth as wall materials and its application to the enrichment of chicken nuggets. LWT 137. https://doi.org/10.1016/j.lwt.2020.110334

Ramadan NE, Youssef FR, Alshishtawy AAK, Elshikh FM, Newir O, Abdelazeem SH, Ma'ruf NK, Shouman H, Ali SS, El-Sheekh MM (2025) Marine algal polysaccharides for drug delivery applications: A review. Int J Biol Macromol 295

Raman M, Dinakaran A, Ravindran A, Sankar TV, Gopal TKS (2019) Dietary Supplementation of κ-Carrageenan to Improve the Physio-Chemical and Functional Properties of White Bread. Food Nutr Sci 10(08):997–1010. https://doi.org/10.4236/fns.2019.108071

Rehman A, Ahmad T, Aadil RM, Spotti MJ, Bakry AM, Khan IM, Zhao L, Riaz T, Tong Q (2019) Pectin polymers as wall materials for the nano-encapsulation of bioactive compounds. Trends Food Sci Technol 90:35–46

Rengasamy KR, Mahomoodally MF, Aumeeruddy MZ, Zengin G, Xiao J, Kim DH (2020) Bioactive compounds in seaweeds: An overview of their biological properties and safety. Food and Chemical Toxicology 135. https://doi.org/10.1016/j.fct.2019.111013

Roy S, Hussain SA, Prasad WG, Khetra Y (2024) Effect of kappa-carrageenan inclusion in the stabilizer blend on rheology, texture, and physical properties of high protein ice cream. Int Dairy J 159. https://doi.org/10.1016/j.idairyj.2024.106052

Ruchika, Sharma SK, Kumar R, Yadav SK, Saneja A (2025) Development of a multifunctional and sustainable pterostilbene nanoemulsion incorporated chitosan-alginate food packaging film for shiitake mushroom preservation. Int J Biol Macromol 293. https://doi.org/10.1016/j.ijbiomac.2024.139241

Sarkar P, Bandyopadhyay TK, Gopikrishna K, Nath Tiwari O, Bhunia B, Muthuraj M (2024) Algal carbohydrates: Sources, biosynthetic pathway, production, and applications. Bioresour Technol 413

Seo CW, Oh NS (2022) Functional application of Maillard conjugate derived from a κ-carrageenan/milk protein isolate mixture as a stabilizer in ice cream. LWT 161. https://doi.org/10.1016/j.lwt.2022.113406

Seong H, Bae JH, Seo JS, Kim SA, Kim TJ, Han NS (2019) Comparative analysis of prebiotic effects of seaweed polysaccharides laminaran, porphyran, and ulvan using in vitro human fecal fermentation. J Funct Foods 57:408–416. https://doi.org/10.1016/j.jff.2019.04.014

Shalaby S (2019) Potential Using of Ulvan Polysaccharide from Ulva lactuca as a Prebiotic in Synbiotic Yogurt Production. J Prob Health 7:1. https://doi.org/10.4172/2329-8901.100208

Shan P, Wang K, Yu F, Yi L, Sun L, Li H (2023) Gelatin/sodium alginate multilayer composite film crosslinked with green tea extract for active food packaging application. Colloids Surf A Physicochem Eng Asp 662. https://doi.org/10.1016/j.colsurfa.2023.131013

Shao P, Feng J, Sun P, Xiang N, Lu B, Qiu D (2020) Recent advances in improving stability of food emulsion by plant polysaccharides. Food Research International 137

Sharifi M, Ghiasi F, Zare M, Hedayati S, Abbasi A (2025) Production of bigel based on κ-carrageenan and monoglyceride for potential application as a shortening replacer in cookie. Food Hydrocoll 164. https://doi.org/10.1016/j.foodhyd.2025.111160

Sharma Khanal BK, Bhandari B, Prakash S, Bansal N (2020) Simulated oral processing, in vitro digestibility and sensory perception of low fat Cheddar cheese containing sodium alginate. J Food Eng 270. https://doi.org/10.1016/j.jfoodeng.2019.109749

Sharma S, Sanpui P, Chattopadhyay A, Ghosh SS (2012) Fabrication of antibacterial silver nanoparticle - Sodium alginate-chitosan composite films. RSC Adv 2(13):5837–5843. https://doi.org/10.1039/c2ra00006g

Song X, Chiou B Sen, Xia Y, Chen M, Liu F, Zhong F (2022) The improvement of texture properties and storage stability for kappa carrageenan in developing vegan gummy candies. J Sci Food Agric 102(9):3693–3702. https://doi.org/10.1002/jsfa.11716

Su T, Zhang E, Yang Y, Zheng T, Xin T, Dong L, Huang F, Su D (2023) Utilization of ovalbumin-ferulic acid-carrageenan Pickering emulsion in baked bread for butter reduction: Bread microstructural properties and quality. LWT 185. https://doi.org/10.1016/j.lwt.2023.115124

Tavlasoglu M, Ozkan G, Capanoglu E (2022) Entrapment of Black Carrot Anthocyanins by Ionic Gelation: Preparation, Characterization, and Application as a Natural Colorant in Yoghurt. ACS Omega 7(36):32481–32488. https://doi.org/10.1021/acsomega.2c03962

Teymuri-Yeghaneh M, Salarbashi D, Derakhshankhah H, Jaymand M (2025) Yogurt enrichment with sulfated alginate microcapsules containing garlic- and cardamom essential oils-loaded β-cyclodextrin: Investigating physicochemical and biological properties. Carbohydrate Polymer Technologies and Applications 9. https://doi.org/10.1016/j.carpta.2025.100694

Tong WY, Ahmad Rafiee AR, Leong CR, Tan WN, Dailin DJ, Almarhoon ZM, Shelkh M, Nawaz A, Chuah LF (2023) Development of sodium alginate-pectin biodegradable active food packaging film containing cinnamic acid. Chemosphere 336. https://doi.org/10.1016/j.chemosphere.2023.139212

Varghese SA, Siengchin S, Parameswaranpillai J (2020) Essential oils as antimicrobial agents in biopolymer-based food packaging - A comprehensive review. Food Biosci 38. https://doi.org/10.1016/j.fbio.2020.100785

Wang H, Zhu B, Yao Z (2023) Porphyran, porphyran oligosaccharides and porphyranase: Source, structure, preparation methods and applications. Algal Res 73

Wang J, Jiang Q, Huang Z, Muhammad AH, Gharsallaoui A, Cai M, Yang K, Sun P (2024a) Rheological and mechanical behavior of soy protein-polysaccharide composite paste for extrusion-based 3D food printing: Effects of type and concentration of polysaccharides. Food Hydrocoll 153. https://doi.org/10.1016/j.foodhyd.2024.109942

Wang XH, Song XJ, Zhang DJ, Li ZJ, Wang HJ (2022) Preparation and characterization of natamycin-incorporated agar film and its application on preservation of strawberries. Food Packag Shelf Life 32. https://doi.org/10.1016/j.fpsl.2022.100863

Wang Z, Wang L, Yu X, Wang X, Zheng Y, Hu X, Zhang P, Sun Q, Wang Q, Li N (2024b) Effect of polysaccharide addition on food physical properties: A review. Food Chem 431

Wedamulla NE, Choi Y-J, Zhang Q, Kim E-K (2025) Use of food by-products to design 3D food printing inks: Potential of bioactives extraction and encapsulated 3D food printing ink formulation. Food Research International 213:116376. https://doi.org/10.1016/j.foodres.2025.116376

Widyastuti S, Rien Handayani B, Werdiningsih W, Devi Ariyana M, Rahayu N Special Issue 2, 2021 for ICST2017

Xu B, Wu S (2021) Preservation of mango fruit quality using fucoidan coatings. LWT 143. https://doi.org/10.1016/j.lwt.2021.111150

Yin X, Geng X, Li W, Che T, Yan L, Yuan B, Qin S (2025) Advance of the application of seaweed polysaccharides on antitumor drug delivery systems. Int J Pharm 675

Yu X, Li C, Zhou M, Prakash S, Dong X (2025) Improved the quality of dietary for older with dysphagia by κ-carrageenan/inulin: Textural, rheological, oral process and 3D printing properties. Food Research International 202. https://doi.org/10.1016/j.foodres.2025.115683

Yuan M, Wang J, Geng L, Wu N, Yang Y, Zhang Q (2024) A review: Structure, bioactivity and potential application of algal polysaccharides in skin aging care and therapy. Int J Biol Macromol 272

Zhang J, Tang J, Shi S, Huang H, Li Y, Liu W, Shi J, Tong C, Pang J, Wu C (2025) Research progress on marine polysaccharide-based Pickering emulsions and their potential applications in the food industry. Food Research International 208

Zhao Y, Du W, Koe B, Connolley T, Irvine S, Allan PK, Schlepütz CM, Zhang W, Wang F, Eskin DG, Mi J (2018) 3D characterisation of the Fe-rich intermetallic phases in recycled Al alloys by synchrotron X-ray microtomography and skeletonisation. Scr Mater 146:321–326. https://doi.org/10.1016/j.scriptamat.2017.12.010

Animal-Based Marine Polysaccharides in Food Packaging

Bandana Padhan, Susrishta Mukherjee, Bidisha Ray, Samridhi Bhattacharjee, Rishita Rakshit, and Joyjyoti Das

Abstract Growing environmental concerns over synthetic plastic waste have intensified the search for sustainable, biodegradable alternatives, particularly in the food packaging sector. Animal-based marine polysaccharides, primarily derived from crustaceans and marine organisms offer a promising, eco-friendly solution. Key polysaccharides such as chitin and its deacetylated derivative, chitosan, are extracted predominantly from shrimp and crab shells, which are otherwise seafood processing waste. These biopolymers possess excellent film-forming, biodegradable, antioxidant, and antimicrobial properties, making them ideal candidates for active and intelligent food packaging. Chitosan, in particular, has garnered attention for its ability to inhibit a wide range of spoilage and pathogenic microorganisms due to its positive charge, which interacts with negatively charged microbial membranes. Other marine-derived polysaccharides like gelatin, glycosaminoglycans, and hyaluronic acid further enhance film properties by improving mechanical strength, flexibility, and water vapor permeability. Their application not only prolongs shelf life and preserves food quality but also promotes circular bioeconomy by converting marine waste into value-added products. However, challenges such as poor mechanical stability under humid conditions, high production costs, and limited scalability remain significant barriers to commercial adoption. Ongoing research focuses on blending marine polysaccharides with other natural polymers, nanoparticles, or essential oils to enhance their functionality. This review highlights the potential of animal-based marine polysaccharides in transforming the food packaging industry by offering renewable, safe, and sustainable packaging alternatives that align with global environmental goals.

Keywords Animal-based polysaccharides · Marine biopolymers · Food packaging · Biodegradable films · Active packaging · Antimicrobial properties

---

B. Padhan · S. Mukherjee · B. Ray · S. Bhattacharjee · R. Rakshit · J. Das (✉)
Department of Biotechnology, School of Life Science & Biotechnology, Adamas University, Kolkata, West Bengal, India
e-mail: joyjyoti1.das@adamasuniversity.ac.in

S. Jana et al. (eds.), *Multifunctional Marine Polysaccharides*,
https://doi.org/10.1007/978-981-95-4126-3_19

1 Introduction

Food quality, safety, shelf life, and marketing messages are all impacted by packaging, which is a crucial component of the food business. Conventional food packaging protects food from harm and allows food items to be stored until they are eaten. In addition to promoting marketing, packaging displays logos and nutritional data (Yan et al. 2022). In comparison to other produced materials, traditional packaging materials are obtained from an abundant supply of natural materials, are easy to handle, and have no costs or environmental pollution related to their processing or technology (Ezeudu et al. 2021). Plastic films have been used for decades as a barrier to protect food from dust, dirt particles, heat, moisture, and bacteria. They have been the most popular option for food packaging applications because of their low weight, simplicity of production, and affordability. Because of their superior performance features, robust molecular networks, and ease of manufacture, polyethylene (PE), polypropylene (PP), polyvinyl chloride (PVC), polyethylene-co-vinyl acetate (EVA), and polyethylene terephthalate (PET) have also been used (Yan et al. 2022). Because glass is nonreactive and impermeable, it has been used for millennia as a traditional food packing material to protect food quality and avoid contamination. It is perfect for long-term food storage because of its many benefits, which include superior recyclability, chemical stability, and resistance to temperature changes (Emblem and Emblem 2012).

However, these materials damage the environment, creating an urgent demand for alternative biodegradable fibers (Siciliano et al. 2024). Because of their persistence in ecosystems and role in pollution, nonbiodegradable food packaging materials including plastic, glass, and metals present serious environmental problems. A significant amount of food-related waste is made up of plastic packaging, which degrades very slowly and accumulates as microplastic in soil and water, harming both marine and terrestrial life (Hopewell et al. 2009). Despite being recyclable, the energy-intensive manufacture and recycling procedures of glass result in a large carbon footprint. During extraction and production, metal packaging, such as cans of aluminium and tin, contribute to greenhouse gas emissions and resource depletion. These issues are made worse by inadequate infrastructure for recycling and disposal, which increases environmental pollution and landfill overflow. (Jambeck et al. 2015). Consequently, replacing these materials with biodegradable packaging materials, such as biopolymers, is one of the best ways to address this issue (Panou and Karabagias 2023).

Biopolymers are a safe and sustainable substitute for nonbiodegradable plastic polymers. They are made from food, plants, and agricultural waste (Siciliano et al. 2024). Bio-based materials have several uses, especially in food packing, food coating, and food and encapsulating edible films. Widespread use of biopolymers in food packaging can lead to sustainable resource exploitation, less plastic waste, and decreased greenhouse gas emissions (Ncube et al. 2020). Polysaccharides including cellulose, starch, chitosan, alginate, agar, guar gum, carrageenan, and pectin are widely found in nature. They typically consist of one or more alternating monosaccharide types, such as glucose, fructose, mannose, and galactose, in linear or branched chains. In addition to their great accessibility, cheap cost, biodegradability, and compostability, many polysaccharides have good film-forming qualities, making them attractive options for usage in more environmental-friendly food packaging systems (Nilsen-Nygaard et al. 2021).

Among the biopolymers derived from marine animal polysaccharides are the vital active substances present in microbes, plants, and animals. These substances have a variety of biological functions, such as anti-diabetic, anti-obesity, anti-enteritis, antioxidant, and anticoagulant qualities. They have been isolated from a number of marine sources, including *Rhopilemaesculentum*, *Halaelurusburgeri*, *Raja pulchra*, *Scylla tranquebarica*, and *Thunnusthynnus* (Guan et al. 2024). Because of their solubility in aqueous solvents and extraction media, and important biological characteristics like their antibacterial, adhesive, biocompatible, biodegradable, and anti-inflammatory qualities, they have been widely used in food packaging (Cardoso et al. 2016). Polysaccharides, such as glycosaminoglycans (GAGs) and polymers generated from chitin, are abundant in marine species. A linear polymer produced from chitin, chitosan finds extensive usage in biomedical applications as scaffolds, membranes, films, beads, nanoparticles, and capsules for tissue engineering and regenerative medicine. A significant part of the extracellular matrix, hyaluronans are linear glycosaminoglycans with antibacterial and anti-inflammatory qualities. The pharmaceutical industry has utilized chondroitin sulfates, a sulfated glycosaminoglycan with anticoagulant qualities, as an active ingredient in anticoagulant medications, as a supplement to prevent arthritis, and as hydrogels for the regeneration of cartilage tissue. Heparin may be replaced by dermatan sulfate, a glycosaminoglycan that was isolated from ray skin and possesses anticoagulant and antithrombotic qualities. Because of its anti-adhesive qualities, keratan sulfate inhibits axon development and lowers the immunological response in conditions like osteoarthritis. Microbiology and food industries employ agarose, a marine biomaterial that resembles carrageenan in structure, as a gel for culture media. Specifically, hydrogels for the release of bioactive substances are linked to its use in biological applications (Cardoso et al. 2016).

Animal-based marine polysaccharides offer biodegradable, antimicrobial, and oxygen-barrier properties, making them sustainable alternatives to synthetic food packaging. Their ability to extend shelf life and reduce plastic waste has driven significant interest in eco-friendly packaging solutions (Priyadarshi and Rhim 2020). Food packaging materials employ cellulose, a plentiful renewable polymer, because of its ability to withstand fat and gas. It may be produced by microbes and separated from plant-based materials such as wood, cotton, and hemp. Plant-based glucans called starches have strong tensile strength and oxygen barrier qualities, although plasticizer can lessen their brittleness (Panou and Karabagias 2023). Chitosans, a diverse class of cationic polysaccharides, have low gas permeability and strong mechanical qualities, their high water vapor permeability restricts their use. Positively charged chitosan and negatively charged microbial cell membranes are thought to interact electrostatically to provide chitosan's antibacterial effects (Nilsen-Nygaard et al. 2021). Gelatin's capacity to form films makes it a popular ingredient (Yan et al. 2022). Fruits and vegetables with high respiratory activity and oxidation sensitivity can be packaged with starch because of its superior barrier qualities, high biodegradability, and biocompatibility (Panou and Karabagias 2023). Because of their high gelling, thickening, stabilizing, protective coating, and fat-substituting properties, carrageenans—natural linear sulfated polysaccharides derived from red edible seaweeds—are utilized in the food business. They provide a range of biological functions and are nontoxic, biocompatible, and biodegradable. A peptide with strong elastic properties, gelatin is created when collagen is partially hydrolyzed. It may be used to create gels, stabilizers, and emulsifiers. Although gelatin-based films have excellent mechanical and functional qualities, functional nanoparticles and additives can help them with their low water barrier qualities (Panou and Karabagias 2023).

The growing demand for sustainable food packaging has led to extensive research on biodegradable alternatives, with marine polysaccharides emerging as promising candidates. This chapter explores the unique properties and applications of polysaccharides derived from marine animals such as chitin, chitosan, and hyaluronic acid. Traditional food packaging materials, primarily petroleum-based plastics, pose significant environmental threats, necessitating the development of biodegradable solutions. Marine polysaccharides offer excellent barrier properties, antimicrobial activity, and biodegradability, making them ideal for food preservation. This chapter comprehensively covers the different animal-based marine polysaccharides, their properties, and applications in active and intelligent packaging. It also addresses technical and regulatory challenges, environmental implications, and future innovations in sustainable packaging. By providing a thorough analysis of these biopolymers, the chapter aims to bridge the gap between material science advancements and practical implementation in food safety and sustainability. Animal-based marine polysaccharides like chitin, chitosan, and hyaluronic acid (shown in Fig. 1) exhibit excellent film-forming, antimicrobial, and biodegradable properties, making them ideal for sustainable food packaging (Velhal et al. 2024). Their oxygen and moisture barrier properties help in extending food shelf life and reducing microbial contamination. Chitosan-based films, in particular, have shown promising results in active packaging due to their natural antimicrobial effects. However, challenges such as scalability, cost, and regulatory approval need to be addressed for widespread commercial applications (Xie et al. 2024).

2 Chitin

Chitin represents a transformative solution for sustainable food packaging, offering a marine-derived biopolymer that addresses the global plastic pollution crisis. Its exceptional mechanical properties coupled with environmental sustainability position it as a leading candidate for next-generation packaging materials (Bose et al. 2021; Yu et al. 2020). The urgent need to tackle plastic pollution has intensified efforts to find sustainable packaging alternatives, especially as millions of tons of

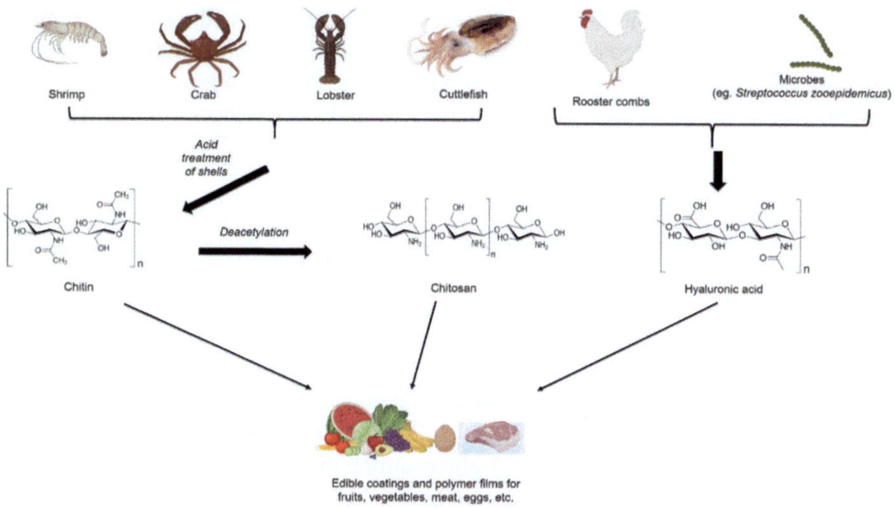

Fig. 1 Various animal-based marine polysaccharides used for food packaging. (Created in Biorender.com)

plastic waste enter oceans annually and petroleum-based plastics persist for centuries. The packaging industry is therefore under increasing pressure to adopt eco-friendly solutions, and chitin is particularly promising due to its abundance, multifunctionality, and biodegradability. A key advantage of chitin lies in its dual environmental benefit: it offers a biodegradable alternative to conventional plastics while also converting seafood industry waste into valuable materials. This waste-to-resource approach exemplifies circular economy principles crucial for sustainable industrial practices. Globally, the seafood sector generates approximately 2.9 million tons of shell waste annually, an abundant but underutilized resource for biopolymer production (Novak et al. 2020; Santos et al. 2020).

2.1 Sources & Extraction Process of Chitin

Chitin's abundant and accessible sources enhance its attractiveness for sustainable packaging applications. Unlike many bio-based materials requiring dedicated agricultural inputs, chitin is obtained predominantly as a by-product of existing marine and seafood industries—providing economic and environmental benefits through resource valorization (Chakravarty and Edwards 2022; Santos et al. 2020; Uranga et al. 2021). The primary sources of chitin are marine organisms such as shellfish, with seafood processing generating significant chitin-rich waste suitable for extraction into packaging materials via established chemical methods. This approach also mitigates environmental challenges associated with seafood waste disposal (Tan et al. 2020). Chemical extraction commonly involves three main steps:

deproteinization using alkaline solutions, demineralization with acids to remove calcium carbonate, and discoloration. These processes yield chitin that retains desirable structural properties for packaging applications. Emerging greener extraction methods, such as microbial fermentation and deep eutectic solvents, offer environmentally friendly alternatives that may improve scalability and purity.

2.2 Chemical & Physical Properties of Chitin

Understanding chitin's molecular structure and physical properties is fundamental to appreciating its packaging potential. Chitin's molecular composition provides a blend of durability, chemical resistance, and mechanical strength necessary for protective food packaging (Hou et al. 2021). Chitin is a linear polysaccharide made of β-(1 → 4)-linked N-acetyl-D-glucosamine units. Structurally akin to cellulose, it differs by possessing acetamido groups that confer high crystallinity and water insolubility. The polymer chains form strong hydrogen bonds, creating a tough, chemically resilient material. This molecular architecture underpins chitin's natural structural role in marine exoskeletons and correlates with its functional advantages in packaging, such as mechanical robustness and resistance to degradation (Moussian 2019). Chitin's versatility enables its use in diverse food packaging applications, ranging from simple protective films to sophisticated active packaging systems. These materials inherently meet essential packaging criteria: shielding food from environmental factors, preserving quality, prolonging shelf life, and ensuring consumer safety.

2.3 Food Packaging Applications of Chitin

Chitin is commonly used to produce thin, transparent films that can directly contact food products. These films provide effective mechanical protection and maintain product visibility, which is crucial for consumer acceptance. Moreover, chitin's natural antimicrobial properties help inhibit the growth of spoilage microorganisms and pathogens, enhancing the safety of perishable foods like fruits, vegetables, meat, and seafood. Beyond traditional uses, chitin's unique physical and biological properties support development of advanced packaging technologies (Cazón and Vázquez 2019). This includes active packaging systems that not only protect but also extend shelf life by actively inhibiting microbial growth and oxidation. Some chitin-based films incorporate bioactive agents, nanofillers, or natural extracts to provide additional antimicrobial, antioxidant, and UV-protective functions. Furthermore, chitin films can be engineered as intelligent packaging that delivers real-time quality monitoring offering visual indicators of freshness or spoilage, thereby improving supply chain transparency and consumer trust (Flórez et al. 2022; Khan et al. 2024).

3 Chitosan

Chitosan is a linear polysaccharide predominantly found in the crustacean and arthropod exoskeleton, which was initially discovered in 1884. It is generated through deacetylation of chitin (poly (β-(1 → 4)-N-acetyl-glucosamine)) as depicted schematically in Fig. 2. The difference between chitin and chitosan lies in the degree of acetylation, which is defined as the ratio of the two types of residues (Barbosa et al. 2019). The level of acetylation and position of acetyl groups along the chains control the physical properties of chitosan. With a pKa close to 6, the accessibility of amine groups makes it neutral at alkaline pH values and cationic at acidic ones. The cationic nature of chitosan and high charge density in solution, responsible for pH responsiveness and mucoadhesive properties, ensures its interesting characteristics (Saneja et al. 2016). In addition to being nontoxic, biocompatible, and biodegradable polysaccharides, chitosan and its derivatives have antibacterial, antifungal, and metal-chelating qualities. Furthermore, chitosan has been studied for usage primarily

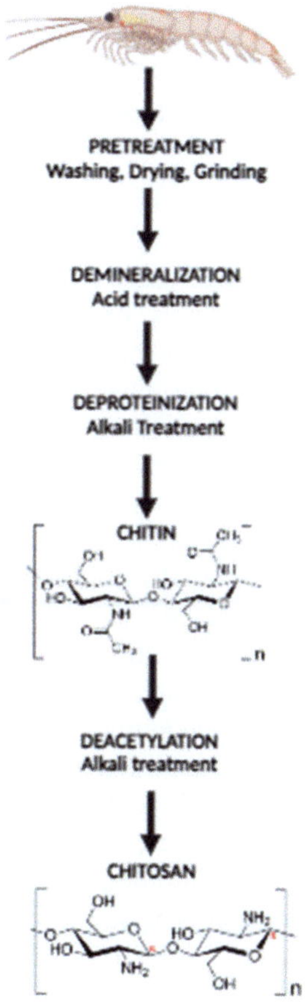

Fig. 2 Extraction process of chitosan

in the food, healthcare, and chemical industries due to its exceptional film-forming qualities (Bakshi et al. 2020).

3.1 Chemical Properties of Chitosan

Various parameters like temperature, pH, degree of acetylation, polymer molecular weight, and polymer crystallinity influence the extent of solubility of chitosan. Homogeneous deacetylation (alkali treatment, 0 °C) of chitin enables polymers to become soluble in acetic acid water solutions with the lowest value of degree of deacetylation as 28%; no such value is ever reached when this occurs through heterogeneous deacetylation (alkali treatment, elevated temperature). Further, the samples are also water-soluble with a degree of deacetylation of 49%. The occurrence of this result can be accounted for on the basis that homogenous deacetylation alters the polymer's crystalline structure and the number of units of glucosamine (Sogias et al. 2010).

3.2 Chitosan-Based Films and Edible Coatings in Food Preservation

Chitosan, a biodegradable polysaccharide, has emerged as a versatile material for food packaging due to its antimicrobial, antioxidant, and barrier properties. These properties can be further enhanced with natural additives such as plant extracts, essential oils, or nanoparticles. The effectiveness of chitosan-based materials has been widely demonstrated across a range of food products, improving shelf life, sensory attributes, and microbial safety. Chitosan-based food packaging films have been shown to effectively extend the shelf life of various food products by utilizing their antimicrobial, antioxidant, and barrier properties, often enhanced through the incorporation of natural additives.

Javdani et al. (2025) developed a sustainable biopolymer film using chitosan and polyvinyl alcohol, enriched with anthocyanins from *Echiumamoenum* and carbon dots derived from onion peel. The resulting film demonstrated enhanced mechanical properties, strong antibacterial activity against *Staphylococcus aureus* and *Escherichia coli*, potent antioxidant capacity, and a high colorimetric response (80.2%) to ammonia vapor. Notably, the film effectively detected red meat spoilage via visible color change and extended shelf life to 19 days at 4 °C, positioning it as a promising intelligent and active packaging material for food monitoring. In a study by Mora-Sánchez et al. (2023), edible films containing chitosan, glycerol, citric acid, and lemon-onion extract were evaluated for their ability to preserve fresh guacamole stored at 4 °C and 20 °C for 28 days. Among the tested formulations, film comprising of 2% chitosan, 1% glycerol, 1.5% citric acid, and 2% lemon-onion extract showed most effectively delayed browning, preserved antioxidant activity, and maintained low microbial counts. The film also demonstrated excellent consumer acceptance, highlighting its potential for extending shelf life in fresh produce. Ribeiro et al. (2023) analyzed ethanol extracts of *Persea americana* pulp using GC-MS and incorporated them into alginate and chitosan-based edible coatings for minimally processed Fuji apples. Alginate coatings outperformed chitosan by significantly reducing enzymatic browning, improving visual quality, and extending shelf life up to 15 days. Sensory evaluations favored the alginate-based coatings with avocado extract, confirming their applicability in fresh-cut fruit preservation. Roy et al. (2024) examined the effectiveness of *aloe vera*, tulsi extract, and their combination (ALTE) as edible coatings for tomatoes stored at ~26 °C for 25 days. Coatings, particularly AL and ALTE, significantly reduced weight loss, delayed ripening, and lowered disease incidence. AL coating retained higher phenolic levels and delayed the accumulation of lycopene and β-carotene, while ALTE showed the best disease control, reducing incidence to 31% compared to 100% in uncoated controls. Ali et al. (2024) used a layer-by-layer (LBL) approach with chitosan (CH) and carboxymethyl cellulose to coat mangoes stored at 15 °C for 20 days. This LBL system reduced weight loss, ethylene and CO_2 emissions, decay, and enzymatic activity associated with ripening. Antioxidant enzyme activities were enhanced, resulting in delayed ripening and superior maintenance of firmness, chlorophyll content, and acidity, suggesting the potential of CH-CMC coatings for postharvest quality retention.

Pang et al. (2024) assessed poly(ethylene-co-vinyl acetate) (EVA) films and chitosan (CTS) coatings in maintaining mango quality at 20 °C. Both treatments improved antioxidant enzyme activity, reduced Polyphenol oxidase (PPO) activity, suppressed ethylene biosynthesis genes (ETR1, ETR2, ERS2), and minimized decay and weight loss. EVA films outperformed CTS coatings in extending mango shelf life, indicating their industrial relevance. Parvin et al. (2023) tested chitosan coatings (750, 1000, and 1500 ppm) on mangoes under ambient and refrigerated conditions. The 1000 ppm CTS coating combined with refrigeration (4 °C) and zip-bag packaging yielded the best results by minimizing microbial counts and maintaining key nutritional attributes such as vitamin C, sugar, and protein content. The results support the commercial viability of chitosan-based coatings. Shah and Hashmi (2020) evaluated 1% CTS and CTS combined with aloe vera gel (AVG) in prolonging mango shelf life at 12 ± 1 °C and 25 ± 1 °C. The CTS + AVG treatment was more effective in reducing decay, respiration, ethylene production, and weight loss. It also preserved quality parameters including acidity, firmness, and ascorbic acid content, supporting the combined coating's potential for commercial postharvest use. Bazaraa et al. (2025) examined six coating formulations on refrigerated chicken fillets and identified a chitosan-based mix (T6) containing a bacteriocin-producing fusant, EDTA, and sodium acetate as the most effective. T6 significantly reduced lipid oxidation (TBA: 1.25 vs. 4.77 in control), improved film barrier properties, and extended microbial shelf life by over 31 days. Sensory attributes also improved, highlighting its potential in fresh poultry preservation. Musalem et al. (2024) investigated chitosan nanoparticles (CHN) loaded with ginger essential oil (GEO) for coating chicken fillets stored at 4 °C. The 1% GEO-loaded CHN treatment (NCHGO 1%) provided synergistic effects by reducing protein and fat degradation, improving sensory characteristics, and inhibiting microbial growth, extending shelf life from 4 to 28 days. Karimnezhad et al. (2019) used chitosan coatings incorporated with 1% and 2% oregano essential oil (OEO) on chicken fillets stored at 4 °C. The 2% OEO chitosan film showed the greatest antimicrobial activity, reducing bacteria populations by up to 3.53 log CFU/g, and demonstrated enhanced shelf life and food safety. Mehdizadeh and Mojaddar Langroodi (2019) evaluated the synergistic effects of chitosan (CH) with propolis extract (PE) and *Zataria multiflora* essential oil (ZEO) on poultry meat stored at 4 °C. CH-PE-ZEO coatings effectively reduced spoilage markers (TVB-N, TBARS, pH), microbial counts, and retained sensory quality. The optimal combination of 1% PE and either 0.5% or 1% ZEO significantly extended shelf life.

López-Patiño et al. (2021) addressed the strong flavor limitations of propolis by testing ethanol-free and honeydew-supplemented variants on beef. These modified propolis extracts preserved antimicrobial efficacy, delayed pH and redness loss, and improved sensory acceptance, with ethanol-free propolis delivering the highest microbial inhibition.

Jonaidi Jafari et al. (2018) examined 2% chitosan coatings combined with 1% and 2% ethanolic propolis extract on chicken fillets stored at 4 °C. The treatments significantly inhibited bacterial growth and delayed chemical spoilage (TVB-N, TBARS, peroxide values). Sensory evaluations confirmed better overall quality and acceptance, supporting the use of these coatings for shelf life extension. Sabaghi et al. (2015) studied chitosan coatings with green tea extract (GTE) on walnut kernels over 18 weeks. The 10 g/L chitosan coating effectively suppressed lipid oxidation and completely prevented fungal growth. While higher GTE levels reduced sensory acceptance, the Chi10-GTE5 formulation balanced preservation with consumer acceptability. Rezaiyan Attar et al. (2023) investigated walnut kernel preservation using 1% chitosan with thyme essential oil (TEO) at 500 and 1000 $\mu L\ L^{-1}$ under various packaging methods. Active packaging with TEO–chitosan treatments showed the best results in lightness, oxidation prevention, and mold control over 120 days at 4 °C, highlighting the importance of combining coatings with smart packaging systems for optimal shelf life extension. Table 1 summarizes recent applications of chitosan-based materials in food preservation.

4 Hyaluronic Acid

Hyaluronic acid (HA) is a naturally occurring glycosaminoglycan and mucopolysaccharide found in all living organisms, primarily in the extracellular and pericellular matrix. Structurally, it is a linear polyanion composed of repeating disaccharide units [(1 → 3)-β-dGlcNAc-(1 → 4)-β-d-GlcA-] and possesses unique physicochemical properties, including high water retention capacity, film-forming ability, and biocompatibility. Its hydrophilic nature allows it to absorb and retain

Table 1 Recent applications of chitosan-based materials in food preservation

Food product	Chitosan-based material	Effects	Shelf life extended	References
Guacamole	Chitosan film + lemon-onion extract	Delayed enzymatic browning, maintained antioxidant capacity, limited microbial growth	Up to 28 days	Mora-Sánchez et al. (2023)
Guacamole	Chitosan, glycerol, citric acid, lemon-onion extract (EF1)	Minimal color change, strong antioxidant retention, low microbial counts	Up to 28 days	Mora-Sánchez et al. (2023)
Fuji apples	Chitosan/alginate coating with avocado ethanol extract	Inhibited browning, extended freshness	Up to 15 days	Ribeiro et al. (2023)
Tomatoes	Chitosan + aloe vera + tulsi extract	Reduced weight loss, delayed ripening, lower disease incidence	Up to 25 days	Roy et al. (2024)
Mangoes	Chitosan-CMC layer-by-layer coating	Reduced respiration and ethylene, enhanced antioxidants, delayed ripening	Up to 20 days	Ali et al. (2024)
Mangoes	Chitosan coating and EVA film	Suppressed ethylene, delayed aging and spoilage, preserved antioxidant enzymes	Not specified	Pang et al. (2024)
Mangoes	Chitosan (1000 ppm) + refrigeration + zip bag	Reduced weight loss, preserved vitamin C, sugars, protein, microbial control	Not specified	Parvin et al. (2023)
Mangoes	1% chitosan + aloe vera gel	Reduced decay, weight loss, ethylene; enhanced antioxidant activity	Up to 28 + 5 days	Shah and Hashmi (2020)
Chicken fillet	Chitosan + bacteriocin-producing fusant + EDTA + sodium acetate	Reduced lipid oxidation, microbial growth, extended shelf life, high sensory score	Over 31 days	Bazaraa et al. (2025)
Chicken fillet	Chitosan nanoparticles with 1% ginger essential oil	Inhibited spoilage microbes, reduced degradation, enhanced sensory quality	Up to 28 days	Musalem et al. (2024)

(continued)

Table 1 (continued)

Food product	Chitosan-based material	Effects	Shelf life extended	References
Chicken fillet	Chitosan +2% oregano essential oil	Inhibited aerobic, coliform, psychrotrophic bacteria	Up to 12 days	Karimnezhad et al. (2019)
Chicken fillet	Chitosan +1% propolis extract +1% Zataria multiflora essential oil	Lower microbial counts, better pH, TBARS, sensory quality	Up to 16 days	Mehdizadeh and Mojaddar Langroodi (2019)
Minced beef	Chitosan + ethanolic propolis extract	Reduced oxidation, inhibited microbial growth	~14 days	Jonaidi Jafari et al. (2018)
Beef	Modified propolis extract (with honeydew or ethanol-free)	Reduced microbial growth, improved pH, color, and sensory scores	Not specified	López-Patiño et al. (2021)

large amounts of water, making it ideal for preserving perishable foods like fruits, vegetables, and meats (Necas et al. Necas et al. 2008). Because of its viscoelastic qualities, HA can be used to make biodegradable films that have antibacterial activity and protect against environmental influences, hence lowering the incidence of foodborne infections. Used in active and intelligent packaging, as well as in smart systems to detect rotting and guarantee food safety, it is an environmentally benign substitute for petroleum-based plastics. Future studies will concentrate on using nanotechnology and biopolymer changes to optimize HA-based packaging (Cheng et al. 2023).

4.1 Sources of Marine-Derived Hyaluronic Acid

The exploration of marine organisms as alternative sources for hyaluronic acid (HA) production has gained momentum in recent years, motivated by the high costs, ethical concerns, and limited sustainability associated with conventional sources such as rooster combs and microbial fermentation using commercial media. Various marine species, including fish viscera, jellyfish, stingrays, bivalves, blue-fin tuna, etc. have been investigated for their potential to yield high-quality HA. A study explored *Acromitus flagellates*, a jellyfish species, as a novel source of HA, capitalizing on the environmental issue posed by jellyfish population booms (Raj et al. 2025). Similarly, Sadhasivam et al. (2013) isolated HA from the liver of the stingray *Aetobatusnarinari*, a previously untapped resource. Furthermore, a comparative study on two marine bivalves, *Mytilusgalloprovincialis* (Mediterranean mussel) and *Crassostrea gigas* (Pacific oyster), demonstrated their viability as sustainable HA sources for biomedical applications.

Another study focused on the extraction and characterization of hyaluronic acid (HA) from the vitreous humor of bluefin tuna, aiming to explore its antioxidant and pharmacological properties. The extracted HA exhibited a high uronic acid content (55.8%) and a molecular weight of 888 kDa. It demonstrated significant antioxidant activity and showed promising anti-inflammatory and analgesic effects in various experimental models. The findings suggest that the by-products of bluefin tuna, particularly its eyeballs, can serve as a valuable source of bioactive compounds with potential applications in biomedical and pharmaceutical fields (Elhiss et al. 2024).

4.2 Chemical and Functional Properties of Hyaluronic Acid

Hyaluronic acid (HA) is a homogeneous unbranched glycosaminoglycan (GAG) composed of repeating disaccharide units arranged in a linear fashion, specifically β1–3-D-N-acetyl glucosamine and β1–4-D-glucuronic acid. It has a constant chemical structure characterized by variations in molecular size, which can significantly influence its biochemical properties and functionality. HA displays two functional groups, carboxyl and hydroxyl, that are often subjected to chemical modifications, leading to derivatives with altered physical and chemical properties. These modifications can enhance interactions with biologically active molecules, affect solubility, and prolong in vivo residence time. HA's molecular weight influences its biological activity, with higher molecular weight forms exhibiting different interactions and functions in biological systems, including roles in the extracellular matrix (ECM) and cellular responses (Al-Khateeb and Prpic 2019). HA can modulate viscosity and its viscoelastic behavior which makes it suitable for packaging applications where elasticity and resistance to physical stress are required. It helps films withstand handling and environmental changes without compromising integrity. HA also functions as an emulsifier and stabilizer, allowing for uniform dispersion of lipids or bioactive compounds within film matrices, which improves barrier functionality and durability. Its role in reducing water vapor transmission further enhances the protective properties of the films, extending the shelf life of perishable goods.

Hence, the chemical and physical characteristics of HA, rooted in its molecular architecture, make it an ideal candidate for sustainable, edible, and functional food packaging. Its incorporation improves not only the mechanical and barrier properties of the films but also supports broader goals in food preservation and eco-friendly material development.

The structural integrity and molecular weight of HA directly influence its physiological functionality and suitability for various applications. HA extracted from *A. flagellates* jellyfish, as characterized by Raj et al. (2025), exhibited hygroscopic, fine-textured, off-white characteristics with superior water-retention ability—surpassing glycerol for up to four hours. FTIR and UV-Vis spectral analyses confirmed the molecular structure of HA, while SDS-PAGE validated its high purity, revealing no residual protein contamination.

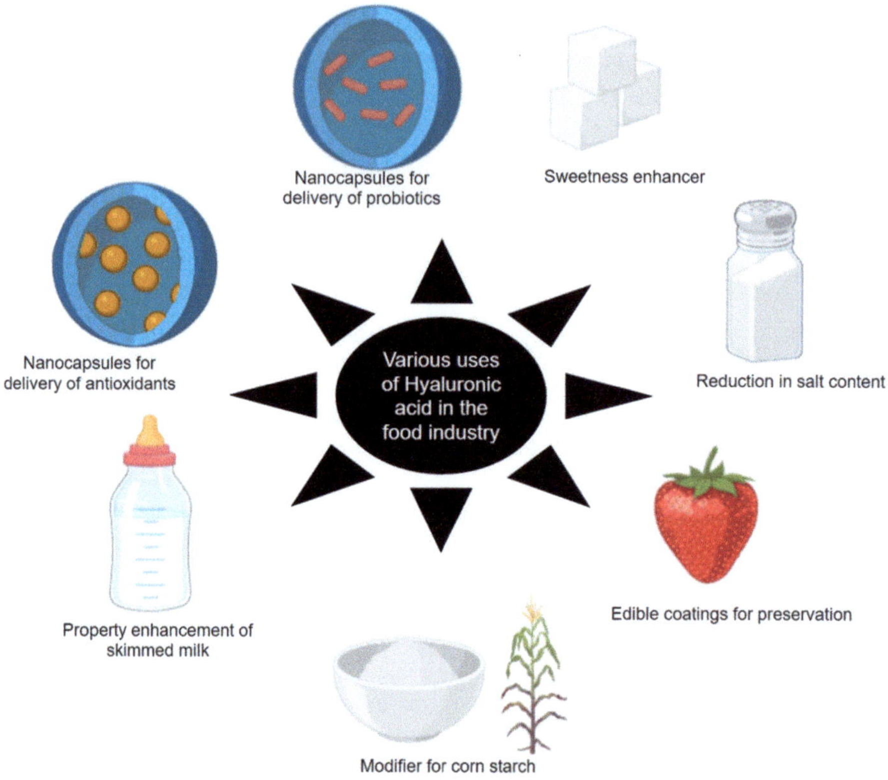

Fig. 3 Different uses of hyaluronic acid in the food industry. (Created in Biorender.com)

In a more chemically intensive study, Sadhasivam et al. (2013) reported the isolation of high molecular weight HA (13.65 MDa) from stingray liver. The composition revealed substantial uronic acid (43.7%) and N-acetyl glucosamine (50.5%) content; hallmark constituents of HA's disaccharide repeat units. Bivalve-derived HA also demonstrated excellent structural and biochemical characteristics. Both mussel- and oyster-sourced HA exhibited strong free radical scavenging activity, aligning with the growing interest in antioxidant-rich biomaterials for cosmeceutical applications (Bouriga et al. 2022). The various reported uses of HA in the food industry is schematically represented in Fig. 3.

4.3 Extraction and Modification Techniques of Hyaluronic Acid

In contrast, direct extraction from marine tissues has been seen in studies involving jellyfish, stingrays, and bivalves, typically includes tissue homogenization, enzymatic or chemical hydrolysis, followed by alcohol precipitation and chromatographic purification. Sadhasivam et al. (2013) applied multiple analytical techniques post-extraction to ensure molecular specificity and purity of HA, while Raj et al. (2025) emphasized the importance of spectroscopic methods in verifying the absence of protein contamination and confirming the characteristic vibrational bands of HA. Hyaluronic acid (HA) was extracted from the vitreous humor of bluefin tuna by solubilizing the humor in deionized water, followed by dialysis against sodium chloride to remove residual cetylpyridinium chloride (CPC) and subsequently against distilled water to eliminate salts. The solution was then neutralized and freeze-dried to obtain HVHA (Hyaluronic Acid extracted from the Vitreous Humor).

The most effective extraction methods for aquatic polysaccharides include hot water extraction, alkaline extraction, ultrasound-assisted extraction, microwave-assisted extraction, and enzyme-assisted extraction. Hot water extraction is simple and cost-effective, suitable for various species, but primarily targets extracellular polysaccharides. Alkaline extraction enhances solubility and can break down cellular structures for higher yields. Ultrasound-assisted extraction improves extraction rates by disrupting cell walls but requires careful parameter control to prevent polysaccharide degradation. Microwave-assisted extraction offers rapid heating and shortened extraction times, yet needs strict power management to avoid damage. Enzyme-assisted extraction effectively increases yield and purity and is often combined with other methods. Joint extraction techniques that leverage multiple methods are increasingly favored for optimizing both efficiency and purity of the extracted polysaccharides, making them promising options for commercial applications (Xiong et al. 2020).

4.4 Applications of Hyaluronic Acid in Food Packaging

Hyaluronic acid (HA) exhibits exceptional moisture-retention capabilities due to its hydrophilic nature and large molecular size, enabling it to form gel-like networks that hold water effectively. This makes HA an ideal component in food packaging films, helping maintain food texture, flavor, and extend shelf life. The research highlights HA's role as a film-former, emulsifier, and stabilizer, improving packaging integrity and product quality. Studies confirm that high-molecular-weight HA enhances moisture retention and supports sustainable, bio-based packaging solutions aimed at reducing spoilage and promoting food safety (Al-Khateeb and Prpic 2019).

Hyaluronic acid (HA) plays a crucial role in advanced food packaging by serving as a biocompatible, biodegradable, and moisture-retentive material ideal for forming hydrogel-based systems. In a study, HA was chemically modified with dopamine (DA-HA) to enhance its adhesive properties through catechol functional groups, allowing strong attachment to packaging surfaces. When cross-linked with 3-carboxyphenylboronic acid-grafted chitosan, it formed a CO_2-responsive hydrogel matrix capable of responding to changes in the packaging environment caused by microbial activity. This hydrogel system not only provided visual freshness indication through pH-sensitive dyes but also enabled the controlled, stimuli-responsive release of eugenol, an antimicrobial agent. Thus, HA contributed significantly to the development of multifunctional, intelligent packaging materials that can extend shelf life and improve food safety (Du et al. 2024).

Al-Hilifi et al. (2024) worked on developing hyaluronic acid (HA)-based edible coatings by combining HA with chitosan and gelatin to extend the shelf life and preserve the quality of strawberries. HA was extracted from local potatoes and blended in varying ratios with the other biopolymers to form composite coatings (e.g., 5CS:2G:3HA). These coatings were then applied to fresh strawberries and evaluated over a 15-day refrigerated storage period. The results showed that the addition of HA significantly improved the coatings' effectiveness, especially in terms of moisture retention, which led to reduced weight loss in strawberries. Coatings with higher HA concentrations better maintained pH and titratable acidity, indicating slower degradation and spoilage. Moreover, HA helped preserve key antioxidant compounds such as ascorbic acid and total phenolic content, and enhanced DPPH radical scavenging activity, reflecting stronger antioxidant defense. Microscopic and thermal analyses confirmed the structural compatibility and stability of the HA-chitosan-gelatin coatings. Visually, strawberries coated with HA-based films showed minimal signs of decay or mold, unlike uncoated controls which deteriorated significantly by Day 9. Overall, the study demonstrates that HA enhances the functional and protective properties of edible coatings, offering a natural, bioactive, and sustainable approach to food packaging and postharvest preservation. Zhou et al. (2024) developed a natural, multifunctional fruit preservation coating by incorporating a cinnamaldehyde and 2-hydroxypropyl-β-cyclodextrin (HP-β-CD) inclusion complex into hyaluronic acid. This approach overcomes CIN's volatility and strong aroma, enabling slow, sustained release. The HA/CIN@HP-β-CD coating showed strong antimicrobial and antioxidant properties, universal surface adhesion, and no toxicity. Applied to bananas and fresh-cut apples, it effectively maintained color, reduced weight loss, inhibited microbial growth, and significantly extended freshness, demonstrating strong potential for natural fruit preservation. Fan et al. (2023) investigated the hyaluronic acid (HA)-based composite films incorporating curcumin and cellulose nanofibers (CNF) for egg preservation. Curcumin enhanced antimicrobial activity, while CNF improved film viscosity, permeability, and strength. In a 56-day storage test at 25 °C and 70% humidity, the optimal film (0.5% HA, 0.025% curcumin and CNF, 2 min coating) reduced egg weight loss to 13.88% and maintained a Haugh unit of 52.08, surpassing control values by Day 35 and extending shelf life by at least 14 days. This highlights the film's potential for postharvest food preservation. Table 2 summarizes recent studies on hyaluronic acid-based materials used in food preservation, demonstrating their effects on shelf-life extension across various food products.

Table 2 Applications of hyaluronic acid-based materials in food preservation, highlighting the shelf-life extension across different food products

Food product	Hyaluronic-based material	Effects	Shelf life extended	References
General fresh produce	Dopamine-modified HA + boronic acid-grafted chitosan hydrogel	Intelligent response to spoilage, antimicrobial release, visual indicator	Enhanced freshness	Du et al. (2024)
Bananas, fresh-cut apples	HA + CIN@HP-β-CD (cinnamaldehyde complex)	Sustained CIN release, reduced microbial growth, preserved color	Significantly extended	Zhou et al. (2024)
Strawberries	HA + chitosan + gelatin (e.g., 5CS:2G:3HA)	Reduced weight loss, retained pH, antioxidant preservation, delayed spoilage	Up to 15 days	Al-Hilifi et al. (2024)
Eggs	HA + curcumin + cellulose nanofiber (0.5% HA, 0.025% CUR/CNF)	Improved antimicrobial activity, better film strength, less weight loss	+14 days vs control	Fan et al. (2023)

4.5 Physical and Mechanical Properties of Hyaluronic Acid

The chemical structure of hyaluronic acid (HA) confers distinctive physicochemical characteristics that render it a highly useful biopolymer in the design of functional food packaging materials. Chemically, HA is a linear glycosaminoglycan with alternating D-glucuronic acid and N-acetyl-D-glucosamine units, linked through β-1,4 and β-1,3 glycosidic bonds. This arrangement facilitates broad hydrogen bonding, both among HA chains and between HA and water molecules, leading to the formation of rigid, gel-like networks with high affinity for water (Hryshchenko and Starovoitova 2024). These properties are critical for packaging applications, where moisture management and film integrity directly impact the preservation of food quality.

From the standpoint of film formation, HA's hydrophilicity and high molecular weight allow it to form flexible, smooth, and continuous films. The polymer's water retention property helps impart its cohesive quality, which is able to produce a uniform matrix with low surface roughness—a critical property for food-contact surfaces that need to be both visually and tactilely uniform (Sionkowska et al. 2020). Atomic force microscopy (AFM) and surface energy measurements in recent research have established that HA-integrated films have lower roughness values and improved wettability than films prepared from conventional polymers (Bai et al. 2015) . These enhancements of film texture and surface properties are crucial to achieving efficient barrier properties, especially protection against environmental influences such as oxygen and moisture. Another prominent strength of HA is its role in mechanical strength and flexibility. HA increases the tensile strength and elastic response of the formed films when it is combined with other biopolymers like collagen or chitosan. This can be attributed mainly to its viscoelasticity, which enables HA to deform and absorb mechanical stress without fracturing—characteristics that are critical in food packaging systems where products need to withstand handling, transportation, and storage (Kweon and Han 2023). Additionally, incorporation of HA in polymer matrices enhances the uniformity of film thickness, further aiding mechanical stability and tear resistance under stress. HA-containing films also exhibit greatly improved barrier properties because of its water-binding functional groups, e.g., hydroxyl and carboxylate moieties. These functional groups bind with water molecules to create a dense matrix that hinders water vapor transmission. This role is especially important in packaging fresh fruits and moisture-sensitive foods since it ensures the internal humidity of the packaging system, minimizes weight loss, and prevents microbial spoilage (Zhou et al. 2024). Studies have demonstrated that higher concentrations of HA in film formulations correlate with improved water vapor barrier efficiency, leading to extended shelf life and preservation of food quality (Fan et al. 2023).

Beyond moisture control, HA also exhibits emulsifying and stabilizing properties, allowing it to effectively incorporate and distribute lipid-based or bioactive components within the film matrix. This results in structurally stable films with enhanced cohesion and barrier performance, particularly useful for active packaging systems that aim to deliver antioxidants or antimicrobials directly to the food surface (Bai et al. 2015; Zhou et al. 2024). Such applications are becoming increasingly relevant as the industry moves toward smart packaging technologies that do more than passively contain food—they actively preserve and enhance its quality.

All these properties combined facilitate the production of biodegradable, edible, and multifunctional packaging films that meet current requirements for sustainability, safety, and food quality maintenance. HA's combined film-forming, flexibility, barrier effectiveness, and bioactivity place it as a key material in driving next-generation food packaging systems forward.

5 Conclusion and Future Prospects

Overall, marine polysaccharides of animal origin offer a very promising new direction for the development of biodegradable food packaging. Chitosan is the most versatile and successful substitute among the rest. Chitosan, predominantly obtained from crustacean exoskeletons like shrimp and crabs, is special due to its robust natural antibacterial and antifungal properties, biodegradability, and remarkable film-forming capacity, attributes that are all crucial in enhancing food preservation. Chitosan films can function independently or easily be enhanced with bioactive additives to produce active or smart packaging, unlike chitin and hyaluronic acid, which often needs to be mixed with other polymers to possess adequate mechanical and barrier properties.

In addition, chitosan is an extremely useful packaging material because it is biocompatible and adaptable with numerous food types, such as fresh fruit, dairy products, and meat. Advances in processing technology and composite formulation, along with increased academic and industry interest, will likely make chitosan-based films a leading contender in the shift towards greener, functional food packaging. The application of chitosan and other marine polysaccharides to food packaging would also seem to have a promising future based on the strong support of environmental programs and the increasing demand from the public for alternatives to plastic. These biopolymers that are predominantly from fish waste and crustacean shells possess unique advantages such as the ability to form films, biodegradability, and inherent antibacterial properties. These materials are also being explored for their ability to enhance food safety and shelf life as well as their environmental benefits as the food industry shifts towards more sustainable alternatives to synthetic plastics. For instance, incorporation of natural antioxidants or nanoparticles into chitosan film can improve its mechanical strength, barrier properties, and antibacterial properties so that it can be applied to more types of foods.

In addition, it is expected that improvements in the extraction and purification techniques would make such biopolymers more economically viable by making their production scalable and cheaper. Strategies towards circular economy, such as utilizing the seafood industry waste streams as raw materials, also align with worldwide sustainability goals and give marine by-products more economic value. Regulatory support and increasing consumer recognition of plastic pollution will help promote the use of packaging composed of marine polysaccharides.

Resolution of current challenges of moisture sensitivity, mechanical performance, and standardization will require continued multidisciplinary investigation supported by industrial collaborations. Ultimately, these materials hold potential as innovative solutions for sustainable food packaging systems, enabling the development of a food supply system that is more sustainable and resilient.

References

Al-Hilifi, S. A., Al-Ali, R. M., Dinh, L. N. M., Yao, Y., & Agarwal, V. (2024). Development of hyaluronic acid based polysaccharide-protein composite edible coatings for preservation of strawberry fruit. *International Journal of Biological Macromolecules*, *259*, 128932. https://doi.org/10.1016/j.ijbiomac.2023.128932

Ali, S., Ishtiaq, S., Nawaz, A., Naz, S., Ejaz, S., Haider, M. W., Shah, A. A., Ali, M. M., & Javad, S. (2024). Layer by layer application of chitosan and carboxymethyl cellulose coatings delays ripening of mango fruit by suppressing cell wall polysaccharides disassembly. *International Journal of Biological Macromolecules*, *256*, 128429. https://doi.org/10.1016/j.ijbiomac.2023.128429

Al-Khateeb, R., & Prpic, J. (2019). Hyaluronic Acid: The Reason for Its Variety of Physiological and Biochemical Functional Properties. *Applied Clinical Research, Clinical Trials and Regulatory Affairs*, *6*(2), 112–159. https://doi.org/10.2174/2213476X06666190405094637

Bai, H., Sun, Y., Xu, J., Dong, W., & Liu, X. (2015). Rheological and structural characterization of HA/PVA-SbQ composites film-forming solutions and resulting films as affected by UV irradiation time. *Carbohydrate Polymers*, *115*, 422–431. https://doi.org/10.1016/j.carbpol.2014.08.103

Bakshi, P. S., Selvakumar, D., Kadirvelu, K., & Kumar, N. S. (2020). Chitosan as an environment friendly biomaterial—a review on recent modifications and applications. *International Journal of Biological Macromolecules*, *150*, 1072–1083. https://doi.org/10.1016/j.ijbiomac.2019.10.113

Barbosa, A. I., Coutinho, A. J., Costa Lima, S. A., & Reis, S. (2019). Marine Polysaccharides in Pharmaceutical Applications: Fucoidan and Chitosan as Key Players in the Drug Delivery Match Field. *Marine Drugs*, *17*(12), 654. https://doi.org/10.3390/md17120654

Bazaraa, W. A., Khattab, A. E.-N. A., Osman, E. M., & Ali, M. R. (2025). Extension of chicken fillets shelf life using genetically improved probiotic strain and chitosan. *Food Control*, *168*, 110827. https://doi.org/10.1016/j.foodcont.2024.110827

Bose, I., Singh, R., Negi, P., & Singh, Y. (2021). Chitin as bio-based nanomaterial in packaging: A review. *Materials Today: Proceedings*, *46*, 11254–11257. https://doi.org/10.1016/j.matpr.2021.02.656

Bouriga, N., Mili, S., Bahri, W. R., Jammeli, B., Ben-Attia, M., Quignard, J.-P., & Trabelsi, M. (2022). Skin Wound Healing Potential and Antioxidant Effect of Hyaluronic Acid Extracted from Mytilus galloprovincialis and Crassostrea gigas. *Pharmaceutical Chemistry Journal*, *56*(3), 381–386. https://doi.org/10.1007/s11094-022-02647-6

Cardoso, M., Costa, R., & Mano, J. (2016). Marine Origin Polysaccharides in Drug Delivery Systems. *Marine Drugs*, *14*(2), 34. https://doi.org/10.3390/md14020034

Cazón, P., & Vázquez, M. (2019). Applications of Chitosan as Food Packaging Materials. In G. Crini & E. Lichtfouse (Eds.), *Sustainable Agriculture Reviews 36: Chitin and Chitosan: Applications in Food, Agriculture, Pharmacy, Medicine and Wastewater Treatment* (pp. 81–123). Springer International Publishing. https://doi.org/10.1007/978-3-030-16581-9_3

Chakravarty, J., & Edwards, T. A. (2022). Innovation from waste with biomass-derived chitin and chitosan as green and sustainable polymer: A review. *Energy Nexus*, *8*, 100149. https://doi.org/10.1016/j.nexus.2022.100149

Cheng, Q., Liu, C., Zhao, J., Li, W., Guo, F., Qin, J., & Wang, Y. (2023). Unlocking the potential of hyaluronic acid: Exploring its physicochemical properties, modification, and role in food applications. *Trends in Food Science & Technology*, *142*, 104218. https://doi.org/10.1016/j.tifs.2023.104218

Du, H., Liu, X., Sun, X., An, H., Li, Y., Zhu, Z., & Wen, Y. (2024). CO2-responsive multifunctional label based on chitosan and hyaluronic acid for visualizing and maintaining postharvest freshness. *Food Hydrocolloids*, *157*, 110438. https://doi.org/10.1016/j.foodhyd.2024.110438

Elhiss, S., Hamdi, A., Chahed, L., Boisson-Vidal, C., Majdoub, H., Bouchemal, N., Laschet, J., Kraiem, J., Le Cerf, D., Maaroufi, R. M., Chaubet, F., & Ben Mansour, M. (2024). Hyaluronic acid from bluefin tuna by-product: Structural analysis and pharmacological activities. *International Journal of Biological Macromolecules*, *264*, 130424. https://doi.org/10.1016/j.ijbiomac.2024.130424

Emblem, A., & Emblem, H. (Eds.). (2012). *Packaging technology: Fundamentals, materials and processes*. Woodhead Publishing.

Ezeudu, O. B., Agunwamba, J. C., Ezeudu, T. S., Ugochukwu, U. C., & Ezeasor, I. C. (2021). Natural leaf-type as food packaging material for traditional food in Nigeria: Sustainability aspects and theoretical circular economy solutions. *Environmental Science and Pollution Research*, *28*(7), 8833–8843. https://doi.org/10.1007/s11356-020-11268-z

Fan, Z., Hao, Y., Wang, Y., Hu, X., & Li, T. (2023). Characterisation of hyaluronic acid-curcumin-cellulose nanofibre composite film and application in egg preservation. *International Journal of Food Science & Technology*, *58*(12), 6263–6271. https://doi.org/10.1111/ijfs.16729

Flórez, M., Guerra-Rodríguez, E., Cazón, P., & Vázquez, M. (2022). Chitosan for food packaging: Recent advances in active and intelligent films. *Food Hydrocolloids*, *124*, 107328. https://doi.org/10.1016/j.foodhyd.2021.107328

Guan, X., Wang, F., Zhou, B., Sang, X., & Zhao, Q. (2024). The nutritional function of active polysaccharides from marine animals: A review. *Food Bioscience*, *58*, 103693. https://doi.org/10.1016/j.fbio.2024.103693

Hopewell, J., Dvorak, R., & Kosior, E. (2009). Plastics recycling: Challenges and opportunities. *Philosophical Transactions of the Royal Society B: Biological Sciences*, *364*(1526), 2115–2126. https://doi.org/10.1098/rstb.2008.0311

Hou, J., Aydemir, B. E., & Dumanli, A. G. (2021). Understanding the structural diversity of chitins as a versatile biomaterial. *Philosophical Transactions of the Royal Society A: Mathematical, Physical and Engineering Sciences*, *379*(2206), 20200331. https://doi.org/10.1098/rsta.2020.0331

Hryshchenko, M., & Starovoitova, S. (2024). From production to regulation: The comprehensive role of hyaluronic acid in the food and cosmetic industry. *Ukrainian Food Journal*, *13*(3), 476–506. https://doi.org/10.24263/2304-974X-2024-13-3-5

Jambeck, J. R., Geyer, R., Wilcox, C., Siegler, T. R., Perryman, M., Andrady, A., Narayan, R., & Law, K. L. (2015). Plastic waste inputs from land into the ocean. *Science*, *347*(6223), 768–771. https://doi.org/10.1126/science.1260352

Javdani, H., Abedi-Firoozjah, R., Beikzadeh, S., Bahramian, B., Ebrahimi, A., Ehsani, A., & Tavassoli, M. (2025). Application of Chitosan/Polyvinyl Alcohol-Based Functional Films Integrated with Anthocyanins from Echium amoenum and Carbon Dots Derived from Onion Peel for Tracking Freshness and Increasing the Shelf Life of Red Meat Sample. *Food and Bioprocess Technology*, 1–24. https://doi.org/10.1007/s11947-025-03900-y

Jonaidi Jafari, N., Kargozari, M., Ranjbar, R., Rostami, H., & Hamedi, H. (2018). The effect of chitosan coating incorporated with ethanolic extract of propolis on the quality of refrigerated chicken fillet. *Journal of Food Processing and Preservation*, *42*(1), e13336. https://doi.org/10.1111/jfpp.13336

Karimnezhad, F., Razavilar, V., Anvar, A., Dashtgol, S., & Pilehvar Zavareh, A. (2019). Combined Effect of chitosan-Based Edible Film Containing Oregano Essential Oil on the Shelf-Life Extension of Fresh Chicken Meat. *Journal of Nutrition and Food Security*, *4*(4), 236–242. https://doi.org/10.18502/jnfs.v4i4.1720

Khan, A., Riahi, Z., Kim, J. T., & Rhim, J. W. (2024). Chitosan/gelatin-based multifunctional films integrated with sulfur-functionalized chitin for active packaging applications. *Food Hydrocolloids*, *149*(109537). https://doi.org/10.1016/j.foodhyd.2023.109537

Kweon, D.-K., & Han, J.-A. (2023). Development of hyaluronic acid-based edible film for alleviating dry mouth. *Food Science and Human Wellness*, *12*(2), 371–377. https://doi.org/10.1016/j.fshw.2022.07.039

López-Patiño, C. L., Arroqui, C., Horvitz, S., & Vírseda, P. (2021). Strategies to Enhance Propolis Ethanolic Extract's Flavor for its Use as a Natural Preservative in Beef. *Current Research in Nutrition and Food Science Journal*, *9*(2), 521–532. https://www.foodandnutritionjournal.org/volume9number2/strategies-to-enhance-propolis-ethanolic-extracts-flavor-for-its-use-as-a-natural-preservative-in-beef/

Mehdizadeh, T., & Mojaddar Langroodi, A. (2019). Chitosan coatings incorporated with propolis extract and *Zataria multiflora* Boiss oil for active packaging of chicken breast meat. *International Journal of Biological Macromolecules*, *141*, 401–409. https://doi.org/10.1016/j.ijbiomac.2019.08.267

Mora-Sánchez, M., Hernández-Carranza, P., Ramírez-López, C., Ruiz-López, I. I., & Ochoa-Velasco, C. E. (2023). Developing active chitosan-based edible film for extending the shelf life of guacamole. *Frontiers in Sustainable Food Systems*, *7*, 1254337. https://doi.org/10.3389/fsufs.2023.1254337

Moussian, B. (2019). Chitin: Structure, Chemistry and Biology. *Advances in Experimental Medicine and Biology*, *1142*, 5–18. https://doi.org/10.1007/978-981-13-7318-3_2

Musalem, S., Hamdy, M. M., Mashaly, M. M., Kamoun, E. A., & Malak, N. M. L. (2024). Extending the shelf-life of refrigerated chicken fillets by using polymeric coating layer composed of ginger Zingiber officinale essential oil loaded-chitosan nanoparticles. *Journal of Umm Al-Qura University for Applied Sciences*. https://doi.org/10.1007/s43994-024-00172-8

Ncube, L. K., Ude, A. U., Ogunmuyiwa, E. N., Zulkifli, R., & Beas, I. N. (2020). Environmental Impact of Food Packaging Materials: A Review of Contemporary Development from Conventional Plastics to Polylactic Acid Based Materials. *Materials, 13*(21), 4994. https://doi.org/10.3390/ma13214994

Necas, J., Bartosikova, L., Brauner, P., & Kolar, J. (2008). Hyaluronic acid (hyaluronan): A review. *Veterinární Medicína, 53*(8), 397–411. https://doi.org/10.17221/1930-VETMED

Nilsen-Nygaard, J., Fernández, E. N., Radusin, T., Rotabakk, B. T., Sarfraz, J., Sharmin, N., Sivertsvik, M., Sone, I., & Pettersen, M. K. (2021). Current status of biobased and biodegradable food packaging materials: Impact on food quality and effect of innovative processing technologies. *Comprehensive Reviews in Food Science and Food Safety, 20*(2), 1333–1380. https://doi.org/10.1111/1541-4337.12715

Novak, U., Bajić, M., Kõrge, K., Oberlintner, A., Murn, J., Lokar, K., Triler, K. V., & Likozar, B. (2020). From waste/residual marine biomass to active biopolymer-based packaging film materials for food industry applications—a review. *Physical Sciences Reviews, 5*(3). https://doi.org/10.1515/psr-2019-0099

Pang, X., Huang, Y., Xiao, N., Wang, Q., Feng, B., & Ali Shad, M. (2024). Effect of EVA film and chitosan coating on quality and physicochemical characteristics of mango fruit during postharvest storage. *Food Chemistry: X, 21*, 101169. https://doi.org/10.1016/j.fochx.2024.101169

Panou, A., & Karabagias, I. (2023). Biodegradable Packaging Materials for Foods Preservation: Sources, Advantages, Limitations, and Future Perspectives. *Coatings, 13*(7), 1176. https://doi.org/10.3390/coatings13071176

Parvin, N., Rahman, A., Roy, J., Rashid, M. H., Paul, N. C., Mahamud, Md. A., Imran, S., Sakil, Md. A., Uddin, F. M. J., Molla, Md. E., Khan, M. A., Kabir, Md. H., & Kader, Md. A. (2023). Chitosan Coating Improves Postharvest Shelf-Life of Mango (Mangifera indica L.). *Horticulturae, 9*(1), 64. https://doi.org/10.3390/horticulturae9010064

Priyadarshi, R., & Rhim, J.-W. (2020). Chitosan-based biodegradable functional films for food packaging applications. *Innovative Food Science & Emerging Technologies, 62*, 102346. https://doi.org/10.1016/j.ifset.2020.102346

Raj, R., Sreelakshmi K. R., Minimol V. A., George Ninan, & Asha K.K. (2025). Jelly fish, *Acromitus flagellates* as a Potential Source of Hyaluronic Acid for Cosmetic Applications: Jelly fish as a Potential Source of Hyaluronic Acid. *Fishery Technology, 62*(1). https://doi.org/10.56093/ft.v62i1.154443

Rezaiyan Attar, F., Sedaghat, N., Pasban, A., Yeganehzad, S., & Hesarinejad, M. A. (2023). Modified atmosphere packaging with chitosan coating to prevent deterioration of fresh in-hull Badami's pistachio fruit. *Chemical and Biological Technologies in Agriculture, 10*(1), 16. https://doi.org/10.1186/s40538-023-00393-9

Ribeiro, A. A. P., Sanfelice, R. C., Malpass, G. R. P., Okura, M. H., Malpass, A. C. G.(2023). Shelf life and sensory analysis comparison of alginate and chitosan edible coating incorporating avocado extract applied to minimally processed apples. *Food Materials Research, 3*(1), Article FMR-2023-0026. https://doi.org/10.48130/FMR-2023-0026

Roy, J., Islam, Md. N., Yasmin, S., & Mahomud, Md. S. (2024). Improvement of quality and shelf-life of tomatoes with *Aloe vera* coatings enriched with tulsi extract. *Applied Food Research, 4*(2), 100449. https://doi.org/10.1016/j.afres.2024.100449

Sabaghi, M., Maghsoudlou, Y., Khomeiri, M., & Ziaiifar, A. M. (2015). Active edible coating from chitosan incorporating green tea extract as an antioxidant and antifungal on fresh walnut kernel. *Postharvest Biology and Technology, 110*, 224–228. https://doi.org/10.1016/j.postharvbio.2015.08.025

Sadhasivam, G., Muthuvel, A., Pachaiyappan, A., & Thangavel, B. (2013). Isolation and characterization of hyaluronic acid from the liver of marine stingray Aetobatus narinari. *International*

Journal of Biological Macromolecules, *54*, 84–89. https://doi.org/10.1016/j.ijbiomac.2012.11.028

Saneja, A., Nehate, C., Alam, N., & Gupta, P. N. (2016). Recent Advances in Chitosan-Based Nanomedicines for Cancer Chemotherapy. In P. K. Dutta (Ed.), *Chitin and Chitosan for Regenerative Medicine* (pp. 229–259). Springer India. https://doi.org/10.1007/978-81-322-2511-9_9

Santos, V. P., Marques, N. S. S., Maia, P. C. S. V., de Lima, M. A. B., Franco, L. de O., & de Campos-Takaki, G. M. (2020). Seafood Waste as Attractive Source of Chitin and Chitosan Production and Their Applications. *International Journal of Molecular Sciences*, *21*(12), 4290. https://doi.org/10.3390/ijms21124290

Shah, S., & Hashmi, M. S. (2020). Chitosan–aloe vera gel coating delays postharvest decay of mango fruit. *Horticulture, Environment, and Biotechnology*, *61*(2), 279–289. https://doi.org/10.1007/s13580-019-00224-7

Siciliano, S., Lopresto, C. G., & Lamonaca, F. (2024). From traditional packaging to smart bio-packaging for food safety: A review. *Euro-Mediterranean Journal for Environmental Integration*, *9*(4), 1971–1986. https://doi.org/10.1007/s41207-024-00627-8

Sionkowska, A., Michalska-Sionkowska, M., & Walczak, M. (2020). Preparation and characterization of collagen/hyaluronic acid/chitosan film crosslinked with dialdehyde starch. *International Journal of Biological Macromolecules*, *149*, 290–295. https://doi.org/10.1016/j.ijbiomac.2020.01.262

Sogias, I. A., Khutoryanskiy, V. V., & Williams, A. C. (2010). Exploring the Factors Affecting the Solubility of Chitosan in Water. *Macromolecular Chemistry and Physics*, *211*(4), 426–433. https://doi.org/10.1002/macp.200900385

Tan, Y. N., Lee, P. P., & Chen, W. N. (2020). Microbial extraction of chitin from seafood waste using sugars derived from fruit waste-stream. *AMB Express*, *10*(1), 17. https://doi.org/10.1186/s13568-020-0954-7

Uranga, J., Zarandona, I., Andonegi, M., Guerrero, P., & de la Caba, K. (2021). Biopolymers Derived from Marine Sources for Food Packaging Applications. In *Sustainable Food Packaging Technology* (pp. 35–56). John Wiley & Sons, Ltd. https://doi.org/10.1002/9783527820078.ch2

Velhal, M., Dave, M., Sun, E., Holla, S., & Liang, H. (2024). Plant and animal-based bioderived materials: A review of their antimicrobial mechanisms and applications. *Materials Today Sustainability*, *27*, 100885. https://doi.org/10.1016/j.mtsust.2024.100885

Xie, C., Lee, Z. J., Ye, S., Barrow, C. J., Dunshea, F. R., & Suleria, H. A. R. (2024). A Review on Seaweeds and Seaweed-Derived Polysaccharides: Nutrition, Chemistry, Bioactivities, and Applications. *Food Reviews International*, *40*(5), 1312–1347. https://doi.org/10.1080/87559129.2023.2212055

Xiong, Q., Song, Z., Hu, W., Liang, J., Jing, Y., He, L., Huang, S., Wang, X., Hou, S., Xu, T., Chen, J., Zhang, D., Shi, Y., Li, H., & Li, S. (2020). Methods of extraction, separation, purification, structural characterization for polysaccharides from aquatic animals and their major pharmacological activities. *Critical Reviews in Food Science and Nutrition*, *60*(1), 48–63. https://doi.org/10.1080/10408398.2018.1512472

Yan, M. R., Hsieh, S., & Ricacho, N. (2022). Innovative Food Packaging, Food Quality and Safety, and Consumer Perspectives. *Processes*, *10*(4), 747. https://doi.org/10.3390/pr10040747

Yu, Z., Ji, Y., Bourg, V., Bilgen, M., & Meredith, J. C. (2020). Chitin- and cellulose-based sustainable barrier materials: A review. *Emergent Materials*, *3*(6), 919–936. https://doi.org/10.1007/s42247-020-00147-5

Zhou, C., Li, L., Li, D., Zhang, R., Hu, S., Zhong, K., & Yan, B. (2024). Hyaluronic acid-based multifunctional bio-active coating integrated with cinnamaldehyde/hydroxypropyl-β-cyclodextrin inclusion complex for fruit preservation. *International Journal of Biological Macromolecules*, *271*, 132605. https://doi.org/10.1016/j.ijbiomac.2024.132605

Marine-Based Polysaccharides in Food: Safety and Regulation

Pottabathula Shyam Sundar, Veerachamy Alagarsamy, Subhash Chandra Bose, Arehalli S. Manjappa, Sunil T. Galatage, Potti Lakshmanarao, Kaipu Malli Karjun, and Viswas Raja Solomon

Abstract Marine-derived polysaccharides such as alginate, carrageenan, chitin, fucoidan, ulvan, and floridean starch play a significant role in the global food industry due to their diverse functional attributes, including gelling, thickening, stabilizing, and potential health benefits. This chapter provides a comprehensive overview of the regulatory frameworks governing the use of these polysaccharides in major international regions, including the United States, the European Union, Japan, China, South Korea, Australia/New Zealand, India, and Canada. It highlights important regulatory classifications such as "Generally Recognized as Safe" (GRAS) designations, assessments of acceptable daily intake (ADI), and recent updates from authorities like the FDA, EFSA, MHLW, FSANZ, and Codex Alimentarius. The chapter also examines safety profiles based on toxicological data, historical dietary usage, and contemporary risk assessments, with a particular emphasis on vulnerable groups, such as infants. Additionally, emerging polysaccharides, such as fucoidan and ulvan, are discussed in light of increasing regulatory attention and their growing significance in the functional food market. By integrating current scientific evidence with regulatory perspectives, this chapter provides insights for researchers, food developers, and regulatory professionals involved in the application and oversight of marine-based polysaccharides in food systems.

P. S. Sundar (✉)
Department of Pharmaceutical Chemistry, Vasantidevi Patil Institute of Pharmacy, Kodoli, Maharashtra, India

V. Alagarsamy · V. R. Solomon (✉)
Department of Medicinal Chemistry, MNR College of Pharmacy, Sangareddy, Telangana, India

S. C. Bose
Department of Pharmaceutics, MNR College of Pharmacy, Sangareddy, Telangana, India

A. S. Manjappa · S. T. Galatage · P. Lakshmanarao
Department of Pharmaceutics, Vasantidevi Patil Institute of Pharmacy, Kodoli, Maharashtra, India

K. M. Karjun
Department of Pharmacology, Vasantidevi Patil Institute of Pharmacy, Kodoli, Maharashtra, India

S. Jana et al. (eds.), *Multifunctional Marine Polysaccharides*,
https://doi.org/10.1007/978-981-95-4126-3_20

Keywords Marine polysaccharides · Alginate · Carrageenan · Safety · Regulatory approval · Food products

1 Introduction

The pool of marine polysaccharides available for food applications has expanded remarkably in recent years, incorporating novel sources from plants and microbes that differ from traditional options. Following thorough evaluations that adhere to established standards, polysaccharides are increasingly utilized across the food, pharmaceutical, and cosmeceutical sectors. Regulatory entities such as the Joint FAO/WHO Expert Committee on Food Additives (JECFA), the US Food and Drug Administration (FDA), and the European Food Safety Authority (EFSA) recognize and permit specific polysaccharides for use as food additives, ensuring their safety and efficacy according to the guidelines outlined in CODEX.

Food additive means any substance not normally consumed as a food by itself and not normally used as a typical ingredient of the food, whether or not it has nutritive value, the intentional addition of which to food for a technological (including organoleptic) purpose in the manufacture, processing, preparation, treatment, packing, packaging, transport or holding of such food results, or may be reasonably expected to result (directly or indirectly), in it or its by-products becoming a component of or otherwise affecting the characteristics of such foods. The term does not include contaminants or substances added to food for the purpose of maintaining or improving its nutritional qualities (FAO 2023).

The Acceptable Daily Intake (ADI) is an estimate by JECFA of the amount of a food additive, expressed on a body weight basis, that can be ingested daily over a lifetime without appreciable health risk (International Labour Organization 1987).

Acceptable Daily Intake "Not Specified" (NS) (FAO 2016) is a term applicable to a food substance of very low toxicity for which, on the basis of the available data (chemical, biochemical, toxicological, and other), the total dietary intake of the substance, arising from its use at the levels necessary to achieve the desired effect and from its acceptable background levels in food, does not, in the opinion of JECFA, represent a hazard to health.

Maximum use level of an additive is the highest concentration of the additive determined to be functionally effective in a food or food category and agreed to be safe by the Codex Alimentarius Commission. It is generally expressed as mg additive/kg of food.

Food additives can be derived from plants, animals or minerals, or they can be chemically synthesized. There are several thousand food additives used, all of which are designed to do a specific job. This chapter only discusses the polysaccharide food additives derived from marine sources.

Safety assessments: Food additives are assessed for potential harmful effects on human health before they are approved for use. Authoritative bodies at the national, regional, and international levels are responsible for evaluating the safety of food additives. The Joint FAO/WHO Expert Committee on Food Additives (JECFA) is the international body responsible for evaluating the safety of food additives for use in foods that are traded internationally.

1.1 Evaluating the Health Risk of Food Additives

WHO, in cooperation with the Food and Agriculture Organization of the United Nations (FAO), is responsible for assessing the risks to human health from food additives. Risk assessments of food additives are conducted by an independent, international expert scientific group—the Joint FAO/WHO Expert Committee on Food Additives (JECFA). Only food additives that have undergone a JECFA safety assessment and are found not to present an appreciable health risk to consumers can be used internationally. This applies whether food additives come from natural sources or are synthetic. National authorities, either based on the JECFA assessment or a national assessment, can then authorize the use of food additives at specified levels for specific foods. JECFA evaluations are based on scientific reviews of all available biochemical, toxicological, and other relevant data on a given additive. Mandatory tests in animals, research studies, and observations in humans are also considered. The toxicological tests required by JECFA include acute, short-term, and long-term studies that determine how the food additive is absorbed, distributed, and excreted, as well as the possible harmful effects of the additive or its by-products at certain exposure levels.

1.2 International Standards for the Safe Use of Food Additives

The safety assessments completed by JECFA are used by the joint intergovernmental food standard-setting body of FAO and WHO, the Codex Alimentarius Commission, to establish levels for maximum use of additives in food and drinks. Codex standards serve as the reference for national standards in consumer protection and for international trade in food, ensuring that consumers everywhere can be confident that the food they eat meets the agreed-upon standards for safety and quality, regardless of its origin. Once a food additive has been deemed safe for use by JECFA and maximum use levels have been established in the Codex General Standard for Food Additives, national food regulations must be implemented to permit the actual use of the food additive. The Codex Alimentarius Commission also establishes standards and guidelines on food labelling. These standards are implemented in most countries, and food manufacturers are required to disclose the presence of additives in their products. In the European Union, for example, there is legislation governing the labelling of food additives according to a set of

Table 1 Regulatory authorities of different countries

Region	Regulatory authorities
United states	Food and drug administration—FDA
European Union	European food safety authority—EFSA
Japan	Ministry of health, labour welfare—MHLW
China	China food and drug administration—CFDA
South Korea	Korea Food and Drug Administration—KFDA
India	Food safety and Standards Authority of India—FSSAI
Brazil	Brazilian National Health Surveillance—ANVISA
Australia/NZ	Food Standards Australia New Zealand—FSANZ

pre-defined E-numbers. People with allergies or sensitivities to certain food additives should carefully check labels.

Food additives used in accordance with this standard should be of high-quality food grade. They should, at all times, conform to the applicable Specifications of Identity and Purity recommended by the Codex Alimentarius Commission (FAO 2016) or, in the absence of such specifications, to appropriate specifications developed by responsible national or international bodies. In terms of safety, food-grade quality is achieved by conformance of additives to their specifications as a whole (not merely with individual criteria) and through their production, storage, transport, and handling in accordance with GMP (Good Manufacturing Practice).

WHO encourages national authorities to monitor and ensure that food additives in food and drinks produced in their countries comply with permitted uses, conditions, and legislation. National authorities should oversee the food business, which bears the primary responsibility for ensuring that the use of food additives is safe and complies with relevant legislation. Different countries have their own regulatory authorities to regulate marine polysaccharides in food products, ensuring their safety and quality, in collaboration with the Joint FAO/WHO Expert Committee on Food Additives (JECFA). The Codex Alimentarius Commission sets international standards for food additives (Table 1).

1.3 Good Manufacturing Practice (GMP)

All food additives subject to the provisions of this Standard shall be used under conditions of good manufacturing practice (FAO 2023), which include the following:

(a) The quantity of the additive added to food shall be limited to the lowest possible level necessary to accomplish its desired effect.
(b) The quantity of the additive that becomes a component of food as a result of its use in the manufacturing, processing, or packaging of a food and which is not intended to accomplish any physical, or other technical effect in the food itself, is reduced to the extent reasonably possible.

(c) The additive is of appropriate food-grade quality and is prepared and handled in the same way as a food ingredient.

***Food Additives with an ADI of "Not Specified"*:** When an additive has been allocated an ADI "not specified" (International Labour Organization 1987), it could, in principle, be allowed for use in foods in general with no limitation other than in accordance with Good Manufacturing Practices (GMP). It should, however, be borne in mind that ADI not specified does not mean that unlimited intake is acceptable.

***Food Additives Evaluated as "Acceptable" for Certain Purposes*:** In some cases, JECFA has been unable to allocate an ADI but found a specific use of a substance acceptable. In such cases, the additive in question should only be authorized in accordance with the conditions specified. In the event of any other reported uses, CCFA should request that JECFA re-evaluate the additive in question in light of the new information on its uses.

The General Standard for Food Additives (GSFA) is the single authoritative reference point for food additives. The "Codex General Standard for Food Additives" (GSFA, Codex STAN 192-1995) sets forth the conditions under which permitted food additives may be used in all foods, whether or not they have previously been standardized by Codex, available at the Codex General Standard for Food Additives (GSFA) online database.

2 Alginic Acid and Alginate

Alginic acid and alginate, derived from brown seaweeds, are widely used in the food industry as thickeners, gelling agents, and stabilizers. Alginate, a copolymer of mannuronic and guluronic acids, has a long history of safe consumption, supported by toxicological data and regulatory approvals. However, their food safety is governed by region-specific standards that address purity, intake levels, and potential contaminants.

2.1 Safety and Regulatory Framework of Alginic Acid and Alginatein Global Food Systems

2.1.1 Safety

Oral LD_{50} in rats exceeds 11,000 mg/kg, indicating extremely low toxicity. No adverse effects are observed at doses up to 5000 mg/kg (Krishna et al. 2022). Thirteen-week studies in rats at 5% dietary agar (w/w) report no toxicological concerns, with a NOAEL of 2500 mg/kg/day. Agar is safe at typical levels (e.g., 0.5–2 g/day in gelatin substitutes), with mild laxative effects at higher doses (>5 g/

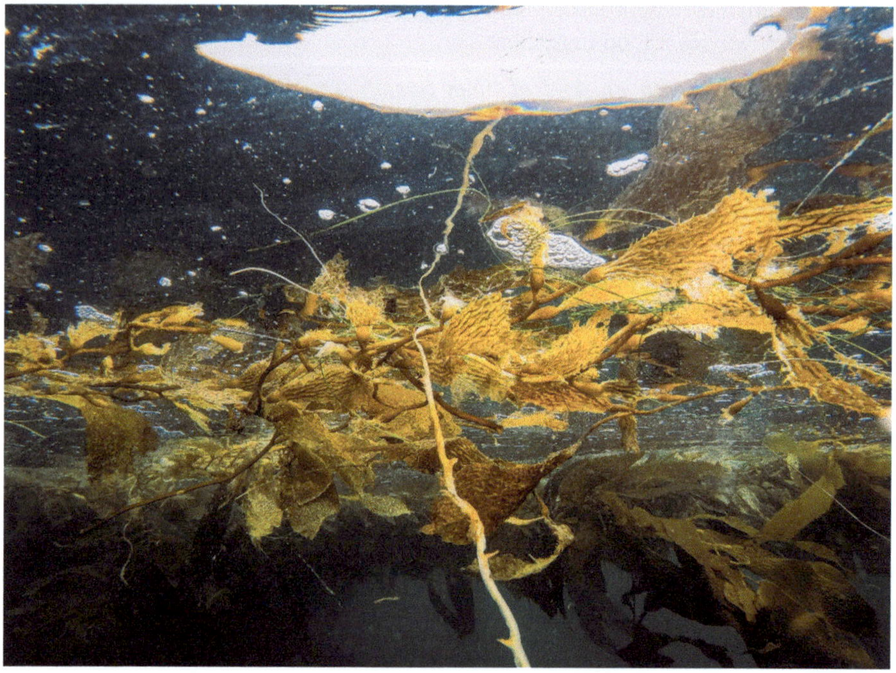

Fig. 1 Brown seaweed: a source of alginic acid and alginate. (Source-Photo by Kindel Media: Photo by Kindel Media: https://www.pexels.com/photo/yellow-aquatic-plants-in-close-up-photography-8849650/)

day) due to its indigestible nature (Rychen et al. 2017). Like alginate, agar poses no allergenic risk; however, impurities in crude preparations could irritate if not properly refined. Both alginate and agar may contain heavy metals (e.g., lead, arsenic) or microbial contaminants if sourced from polluted waters, necessitating strict purity standards (e.g., lead <10 ppm) (Fig. 1).

2.1.2 Regulatory Framework of Alginic Acid and Alginatein Global Food Systems

Alginate and agar, both derived from marine algae, are widely utilized in food processing for their gelling, stabilizing, and thickening properties. Their regulatory acceptance across major jurisdictions reflects a consistent safety profile, supported by traditional dietary use and contemporary toxicological evaluations.

In the United States, the Food and Drug Administration (FDA) classifies sodium alginate (21 CFR § 184.1724) and propylene glycol alginate (21 CFR § 184.1721) as Generally Recognized as Safe (GRAS) (Michel & Macfarlane 1996) (Caliceti et al. 2002). These designations permit unrestricted use under good manufacturing practices, with no specific upper intake limit. Notably, a 2023 GRAS Notice (GRN

No. 1023) expanded the use of alginates to include applications in plant-based meat alternatives, reinforcing their technological versatility. Likewise, agar is designated as GRAS under 21 CFR § 184.1115. Its safety is further ensured through compliance with defined purity specifications, such as arsenic content below 3 ppm. In practice, alginate and agar are typically used at concentrations ranging from 0.1% to 1% (w/w), with levels substantially below thresholds associated with adverse effects. Within the European Union, the European Food Safety Authority (EFSA) authorizes alginates (E 400–E 404) under Regulation (EC) No. 1333/2008. These additives are assigned an Acceptable Daily Intake (ADI) of "not specified," reflecting their low toxicological concern. A 2022 EFSA re-evaluation confirmed the safety of alginates, including their use in infant formulas (Shaikh et al. 2023) (*EU Rules - European Commission* n.d.) (Younes et al. 2017). Similarly, agar (E 406) retains an ADI of "not specified," supported by both EFSA and Joint FAO/WHO Expert Committee on Food Additives (JECFA) assessments. Both categories are permitted at quantum satis levels, provided they meet strict impurity limits, such as lead concentrations below 5 ppm. In Japan, the Ministry of Health, Labour and Welfare (MHLW) permits the use of alginate and agar as food additives under the Food Sanitation Act (*News Japan Amends the Positive List of Food Contact Materials: Ad* n.d.). The long-standing cultural consumption of seaweed, particularly in traditional products such as kanten (agar-based desserts), supports its continued use. Japanese standards align closely with those set by JECFA, and typical use levels range from 0.1% to 2% (w/w), depending on the application.

Similarly, in China, the National Food Safety Standards (GB 2760) include alginate and agar as approved food additives (*Navigating the Regulatory Pathways and Requirements of Wound Dressing Products - Gsap* n.d.). A 2023 regulatory update emphasized the need for source traceability, ensuring purity and environmental sustainability. Standard usage concentrations typically range from 0.1% to 1% (w/w), while regulatory controls address heavy metal contamination (e.g., lead <5 ppm) and microbiological quality to ensure public health safety. In South Korea, the Ministry of Food and Drug Safety (MFDS) authorizes alginate and agar for food applications. Regulatory guidelines recommend usage levels between 0.1% and 1%, consistent with traditional consumption data from seaweed-based foods (*FSSAI* n.d.). These approvals strongly align with international safety evaluations. In Australia and New Zealand, Food Standards Australia New Zealand (FSANZ) lists alginate (Additive No. A-5) and agar (Additive No. A-1) under Standard 1.3.1. These additives are permitted without a defined ADI, which is consistent with their demonstrated safety and low toxicity profiles. Under quantum satis principles, approval is granted, indicating usage levels sufficient to achieve the intended effect without exceeding safe thresholds. Brazil: ANVISA regulates alginate and agar in food and health products, with a 2023 update expanding the use of agar in cosmetics (*Additives | Food Standards Australia New Zealand* n.d.). In India, the Food Safety and Standards Authority of India (FSSAI) regulates alginate and agar under the Food Safety and Standards Act, 2006, and the Food Safety and Standards Regulations, 2011. Usage levels typically range from 0.1% to 2% (w/w), and associated purity requirements align with Codex Alimentarius specifications, ensuring global consistency. The Codex Alimentarius establishes global benchmarks (e.g., INS 400–404 for alginate, INS 406 for agar), influencing national regulations. JECFA's safety evaluations (e.g., 2016 for alginate, 2018 for agar) reinforce their acceptance, with ongoing reviews of novel forms like alginate oligosaccharides (Tables 2, 3, and 4).

3 Agar

3.1 Safety and Regulatory Framework of Agarin Global Food Systems

Agar, derived from brown and red seaweeds, is widely used in the food industry as a thickener, gelling agent, and stabilizer. Agar (E 406) is authorized as a food additive in the European Union (EU) in accordance with Annex II to Regulation (EC) No 1333/2008 on food additives. Specific purity criteria for agar (E 406) have been defined in Commission Regulation (EU) No. 231/2012. In the EU, agar (E 406) has been evaluated by the Scientific Committee for Food (SCF) in 1989 (SCF 1989) and by the Joint FAO/WHO Expert Committee on Food Additives (JECFA) in 1974 (JECFA 1974). The SCF did not consider it necessary to specify an acceptable daily intake (ADI); consequently, it allocated to agar a not unspecified ADI. JECFA considered very few data (two animal studies and one human study) to conclude a *non-limited* ADI. Agar is extracted from certain strains of marine algae of the families Gelidiaceae and Gracilariaceae and relevant red algae of the class Rhodophyceae (Commission Regulation (EU) No 231/2012). Due to its polysaccharidic nature, agar can serve as a substrate for microbiological contamination during storage. The latter has been recently demonstrated by the mycotoxin contaminations of gums (Zhang et al. 2014). Degradation of agar has been investigated in an in vitro human model. This study demonstrated that agar would be partially fermented during its passage through the large intestine by the action of the intestinal tract microflora. The rate of hydrolysis in the human gastrointestinal tract is unknown; however, the Panel considered that agar is unlikely to be absorbed unchanged and that the limited extent of agar fermentation would lead to the production of short-chain fatty acids (SCFA). Based on the available knowledge on the role of SCFA as end products of the fermentation of dietary fibers by the anaerobic intestinal microflora (Topping and Clifton 2001; Den Besten et al. 2013), the Panel considered that their potential formation as fermentation products from agar does not raise any concerns. According to the conceptual framework for the risk assessment of certain food additives re-evaluated under Commission Regulation (EU) No. 257/2010 (EFSA ANS Panel 2014) and given that, the acute toxicity of agar in mice, rats and rabbits is low, there is no concern with respect to the genotoxicity of agar (E 406); no carcinogenic effects were reported in carcinogenicity studies in mice and rats at the doses of 4500 mg/kg bw per day and 2500 mg/kg

Table 2 Alginic acid and alginate permitted for use under specified conditions in certain food categories or individual food items according to Codex GSFA

Food category number	Food category	Maximum level	Notes	Year adopted
01.2.1.1	Fermented milks (plain), not heat-treated after fermentation	GMP	234, 235, & 634	2024
01.2.1.2	Fermented milks (plain), heat-treated after fermentation	GMP	234	2013
01.4.1	Pasteurized cream (plain)	GMP	XS288	2013
01.4.2	Sterilized and UHT creams, whipping and whipped creams, and reduced fat creams (plain)	GMP		2013
04.1.1.2	Surface-treated fresh fruit	GMP	454	2021
04.2.2.7	Fermented vegetable (including mushrooms and fungi, roots and tubers, pulses and legumes, and aloe vera) and seaweed products, excluding fermented soybean products of food categories 06.8.6, 06.8.7, 12.9.1, 12.9.2.1, and 12.9.2.3	GMP	XS294	2023
06.4.1	Fresh pastas and noodles and like products	GMP	211	2014
06.4.2	Dried pastas and noodles and like products	GMP	256	2014
09.2.1	Frozen fish, fish fillets, and fish products, including mollusks, crustaceans, and echinoderms	GMP	16, XS36, XS92, XS95, XS165, XS190, XS191, XS292, XS312, & XS315	2017
09.2.2	Frozen battered fish, fish fillets, and fish products, including mollusks, crustaceans, and echinoderms	GMP	41 & 332	2015
09.2.3	Frozen minced and creamed fish products, including mollusks, crustaceans, and echinoderms	GMP		2015
09.2.4.1	Cooked fish and fish products	GMP	325	2015
09.2.4.2	Cooked mollusks, crustaceans, and echinoderms	GMP	16	2015
09.2.4.3	Fried fish and fish products, including mollusks, crustaceans, and echinoderms	GMP	41 & 332	2015
09.2.5	Smoked, dried, fermented, and/or salted fish and fish products, including mollusks, crustaceans, and echinoderms	GMP	300, 332, XS167, XS189, XS222, XS236, XS244, & XS311	2018

(continued)

Table 2 (continued)

Food category number	Food category	Maximum level	Notes	Year adopted
11.4	Other sugars and syrups (e.g., xylose, maple syrup, sugar toppings)	GMP	258	2014
12.1.2	Salt substitutes	GMP		2014
01.2.1.1	Fermented milks (plain), not heat-treated after fermentation	GMP	234, 235, & 634	2024
01.2.1.2	Fermented milks (plain), heat-treated after fermentation	GMP	234	2013
01.4.1	Pasteurized cream (plain)	GMP	XS288	2013
01.4.2	Sterilized and UHT creams, whipping and whipped creams, and reduced fat creams (plain)	GMP		2013
04.1.1.2	Surface-treated fresh fruit	GMP	454	2021
04.2.2.7	Fermented vegetable (including mushrooms and fungi, roots and tubers, pulses and legumes, and aloe vera) and seaweed products, excluding fermented soybean products of food categories 06.8.6, 06.8.7, 12.9.1, 12.9.2.1, and 12.9.2.3	GMP	XS294	2023
06.4.1	Fresh pastas and noodles and like products	GMP	211	2014
06.4.2	Dried pastas and noodles and like products	GMP	256	2014
09.2.1	Frozen fish, fish fillets, and fish products, including mollusks, crustaceans, and echinoderms	GMP	16, XS36, XS92, XS95, XS165, XS190, XS191, XS292, XS312, & XS315	2017
09.2.2	Frozen battered fish, fish fillets, and fish products, including mollusks, crustaceans, and echinoderms	GMP	41 & 332	2015
09.2.3	Frozen minced and creamed fish products, including mollusks, crustaceans, and echinoderms	GMP		2015
09.2.4.1	Cooked fish and fish products	GMP	325	2015
09.2.4.2	Cooked mollusks, crustaceans, and echinoderms	GMP	16	2015
09.2.4.3	Fried fish and fish products, including mollusks, crustaceans, and echinoderms	GMP	41 & 332	2015

(continued)

Table 2 (continued)

Food category number	Food category	Maximum level	Notes	Year adopted
09.2.5	Smoked, dried, fermented, and/or salted fish and fish products, including mollusks, crustaceans, and echinoderms	GMP	300, 332, XS167, XS189, XS222, XS236, XS244, & XS311	2018
11.4	Other sugars and syrups (e.g., xylose, maple syrup, sugar toppings)	GMP	258	2014
14.1.5	Coffee, coffee substitutes, tea, herbal infusions, and other hot cereal and grain beverages, excluding cocoa	GMP	160	2014

Table 3 Food safety regulations for alginic acid and alginate by region

Region	Regulatory body	Status	Maximum use level	Safety standards
United states	FDA	GRAS (21 CFR 184)	0.1–1% (w/w)	Heavy metals <10 ppm, NOAEL 1000 mg/kg/day (alginate)
European Union	EFSA/EC	E400–E404, E406 (Reg. 1333/2008)	Quantum satis	Lead <5 ppm, ADI "not specified"
Japan	MHLW	Food additives (food sanitation act)	0.1–2% (w/w)	Historical use, no specific limits
China	CFDA (GB 2760)	Food Additives (2023 update)	0.1–1% (w/w)	Traceability, lead <5 ppm
South Korea	MFDS	Food additives	0.1–1% (w/w)	Traditional use, purity standards
Australia/ NZ	FSANZ	Standard 1.3.1 (A-5, A-1)	Quantum satis	No ADI, general safety
India	FSSAI	(2011) regulations	0.1–2% (w/w)	Codex-aligned, lead <10 ppm

Table 4 Recent food safety updates (2020–2025)

Region	Update	Date	Impact
United States	GRN No. 1023: Alginate in plant-based meat alternatives 17 (Caliceti et al. 2002)	2023	Expands applications, supports dietary trends
European Union	EFSA reaffirmed alginate safety in infant formulas	2022	Enhances trust in use for sensitive populations
China	GB 2760 updated with seaweed traceability for alginate	2023	Improves purity, reduces contamination risks

bw per day, respectively, the highest doses tested; oral intake of agar (4500 mg/person corresponding to 64 mg/kg bw per day) was tolerated in humans for 12 weeks without noticeable side effects. The Panel concluded that there is no need for a numerical ADI for agar and that there are no safety concerns for the general population at the refined exposure assessment for the reported uses of agar as a food additive (Tables 5 and 6).

4 Carrageenan

Carrageenan is a common food additive extracted from red seaweed. Incorporation of carrageenan into the batter improves the raw material's viscosity, suspension characteristics, and emulsifying capacity, in addition to enhancing the refrigerated shelf life of the coated products (Fig. 2).

4.1 Safety and Regulatory Framework of Carrageenanin Global Food Systems

Carrageenan's regulatory status and safety profile vary globally due to differences in its perceived risks, historical use, and scientific interpretations. While its high-molecular-weight, food-grade form is widely accepted as safe, controversy persists over degraded carrageenan (poligeenan) and its potential inflammatory effects, which influence regulations. The acceptable daily intake for carrageenans is 75 mg/kg body weight (bw), meaning a daily dose of 3.75 g is safe for a 50 kg person. However, according to EFSA panels, the estimated exposure to carrageenans is 10 g/day, or 200 mg/kg bw per day for a 50 kg adult.

4.1.1 Safety

Carrageenan is a food additive included in Table 3, and as such, may be used in the following foods under the conditions of good manufacturing practices (GMPs) as outlined in the Preamble of the Codex GSFA. Carrageenan is acceptable in foods conforming to the following commodity standards: CS 96-1981, CS 97-1981, CS 105-1981, CS 70-1981 (for use in packing media only), CS 94-1981 (for use in packing media only), CS 119-1981 (for use in packing media only), CS 249-2006, CS 221-2001, CS 250-2006, CS 252-2006, CS 273-1968, CS 275-1973, CS 253-2006 (see functional class table and footnote), CS 262-2006 (for use in cheese mass only), CS 281-1971, CS 282-1971.

Oral LD50 in rats exceeds 5000 mg/kg, indicating low acute toxicity. No mortality or systemic effects are observed at high doses (OECD/OCDE 1987)

Table 5 Agar permitted for use under specified conditions in certain food categories or individual food items according to Codex GSFA

Food category number	Food category	Maximum level	Notes	Year adopted
01.2.1.1	Fermented milks (plain), not heat-treated after fermentation	GMP	234 & 235	2015
01.2.1.2	Fermented milks (plain), heat-treated after fermentation	GMP	234	2015
01.2.2	Renneted milk (plain)	GMP	2015	
01.4.1	Pasteurized cream (plain)	GMP	XS288	2013
01.4.2	Sterilized and UHT creams, whipping and whipped creams	GMP	2013 and reduced fat creams (plain)	
04.1.1.2	Surface-treated fresh fruit	GMP	453 & 454	2021
04.2.1.2	Surface-treated fresh vegetables (including mushrooms and fungi, roots and tubers, pulses and legumes, and aloe vera), seaweeds, and nuts and seeds	GMP	455 & 456	2021
06.4.1	Fresh pastas and noodles and like products	GMP	211	2014
06.4.2	Dried pastas and noodles and like products	GMP	256	2014
08.1.1	Fresh meat, poultry, and game, whole pieces or cuts	GMP	16 & 326	2015
08.1.2	Fresh meat, poultry, and game, comminuted	GMP	281	2015
09.2.1	Frozen fish, fish fillets, and fish products, including mollusks, crustaceans, and echinoderms	GMP	3, 53, XS36, XS92, XS95, XS165, XS190, XS191, XS292, XS312, & XS315	2017
09.2.2	Frozen battered fish, fish fillets, and fish products, including mollusks, crustaceans, and echinoderms	GMP	XS166	2017
09.2.3	Frozen minced and creamed fish products, including mollusks, crustaceans, and echinoderms	GMP		2014
09.2.4.1	Cooked fish and fish products	GMP	241	2015
09.2.4.2	Cooked mollusks, crustaceans, and echinoderms	GMP	241	2015
09.2.4.3	Fried fish and fish products, including mollusks, crustaceans, and echinoderms	GMP	41 & 325	2015
09.2.5	Smoked, dried, fermented, and/or salted fish and fish products, including mollusks, crustaceans, and echinoderms	GMP	300, XS167, XS189, XS222, XS236, XS244, & XS311	2018

(continued)

Table 5 (continued)

Food category number	Food category	Maximum level	Notes	Year adopted
10.2.1	Liquid egg products	GMP	2014	
10.2.2	Frozen egg products	GMP	2014	
11.4	Other sugars and syrups (e.g., xylose, maple syrup, sugar	GMP	258	2014 toppings)
12.1.2	Salt substitutes	GMP	2014	
01.2.1.1	Fermented milks (plain), not heat-treated after fermentation	GMP	234 & 235	2015
01.2.1.2	Fermented milks (plain), heat-treated after fermentation	GMP	234	2015
01.2.2	Renneted milk (plain)	GMP	2015	
01.4.1	Pasteurized cream (plain)	GMP	XS288	2013

Table 6 Recent food safety updates (2020–2025)

Region	Update	Date	Impact
European Union	EFSA reaffirmed agar safety in infant formulas	2022	Enhances trust in use for sensitive populations
China	GB 2760 updated with seaweed traceability for agar	2023	Improves purity, reduces contamination risks
South Korea	MFDS expanded agar use in functional foods 35 (*FSSAI* n.d.)	2024	Broadens market, aligns with health trends

(Cohen & Ito 2002). Ninety-day studies in rats and monkeys at dietary levels of 1–5% (up to 2500 mg/kg/day) showed no significant adverse effects on organ function or histopathology (Younes et al. 2018). The NOAEL is typically 1000–2500 mg/kg/day. Typical intake (20–200 mg/kg/day) is well-tolerated, with no evidence of absorption or metabolism in the gut. Mild gastrointestinal discomfort (e.g., bloating) may occur at high doses (>5 g/day), attributed to its indigestible nature (David et al. 2018). Multiple studies (e.g., JECFA 2015) find no genotoxic or carcinogenic effects in food-grade carrageenan, distinguishing it from poligeenan.

Degraded Carrageenan (Poligeenan)

Poligeenan (molecular weight < 50 kDa), produced by acid hydrolysis, induces inflammation and ulceration in animal models (e.g., guinea pigs, rats) at 0.5–2% dietary levels. It is not used in food and is structurally distinct from food-grade carrageenan (200–800 kDa) (Tobacman 2001) (Table 7).

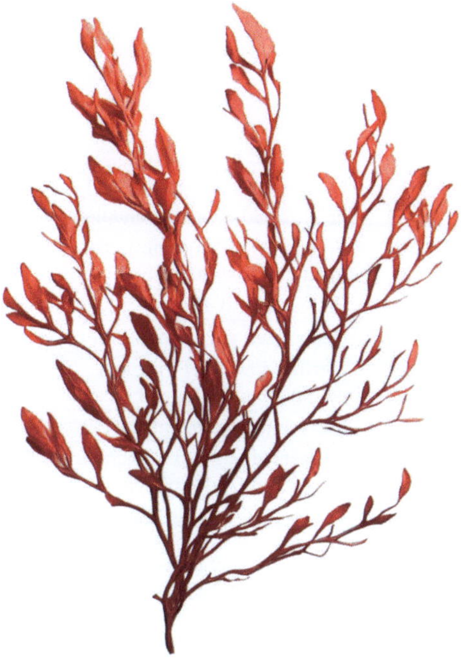

Fig. 2 Carrageenan from red seaweed. (Designed by Freepik, https://www.freepik.com/free-psd/vibrant-red-seaweed-branch-closeup_405497165.htm#fromView=search&page=1&position=1&uuid=0102e2c2-2493-4f0f-9e45-595dd76185d4&query=red+seaweed)

4.1.2 Regulatory Status of Carrageenan Across Global Jurisdictions

Although its regulatory status varies globally, it is widely accepted under food safety frameworks, with distinctions often based on specific applications such as infant nutrition or organic labeling. In the United States, the Food and Drug Administration (FDA) has classified carrageenan as Generally Recognized as Safe (GRAS) under 21 CFR § 172.620 since 1973. This designation permits its use in food products without a defined intake limit, provided compliance with good manufacturing practices (GMPs) is maintained. Notably, a 2022 FDA review reaffirmed the safety of carrageenan for adult consumption. However, its use in infant formula remains under regulatory scrutiny due to concerns over potential gastrointestinal effects. Furthermore 2018, the National Organic Standards Board (NOSB) removed carrageenan from the National List of permitted organic additives, citing public concern over potential pro-inflammatory effects. However, this decision was precautionary rather than data-driven (*Organic Board: Carrageenan Shouldn't Be in Organic Food, No Decision Now on Hydroponics | Food Dive* n.d.) (*ECFR:: 21 CFR 172.620 — Carrageenan* n.d.) (*ECFR:: 21 CFR 172.620 — Carrageenan* n.d.).

Similarly, in the European Union, carrageenan (E 407) and processed *Eucheuma* seaweed (E 407a) are authorized under Regulation (EC) No. 1333/2008. The European Food Safety Authority (EFSA) assigns an Acceptable Daily Intake (ADI) of "not specified," reflecting a generally low toxicological concern. Nonetheless, a 2018 EFSA re-evaluation proposed a conservative exposure threshold of

Table 7 Carrageenan permitted for use under specified conditions in certain food categories or individual food items according to Codex GSFA

Food category number	Food category	Maximum level	Notes	Year adopted
01.1.2	Other fluid milk (plain)	GMP	407 & 438	2019
01.2.1.1	Fermented milks (plain), not heat-treated after fermentation	GMP	234 & 235	2015
01.2.1.2	Fermented milks (plain), heat-treated after fermentation	GMP	234	2015
01.2.2	Renneted milk (plain)	GMP	2015	
01.4.1	Pasteurized cream (plain)	GMP	XS288	2013
01.4.2	Sterilized and UHT creams, whipping and whipped creams	GMP	2013 and reduced fat creams (plain)	
04.1.1.2	Surface-treated fresh fruit	GMP	454	2021
04.2.2.7	Fermented vegetable (including mushrooms and fungi, roots and tubers, pulses and legumes, and aloe vera) and seaweed products, excluding fermented soybean products of food categories 06.8.6, 06.8.7, 12.9.1, 12.9.2.1, and 12.9.2.3	GMP	XS294	2023
06.4.1	Fresh pastas and noodles and like products	GMP	211	2014
06.4.2	Dried pastas and noodles and like products	GMP	256	2014
08.1.1	Fresh meat, poultry, and game, whole pieces or cuts	GMP	16 & 326	2015
08.1.2	Fresh meat, poultry, and game, comminuted	GMP	281	2015
09.2.1	Frozen fish, fish fillets, and fish products, including mollusks, crustaceans, and echinoderms	GMP	332, 391, XS36, XS92, XS95, XS190, XS191, XS292, XS312, & XS315	2017
09.2.2	Frozen battered fish, fish fillets, and fish products	GMP	177 & 332	2015
09.2.3	Frozen minced and creamed fish products, including mollusks, crustaceans, and echinoderms	GMP		2014
09.2.4.1	Cooked fish and fish products	GMP	16 & 325	2015
09.2.4.2	Cooked mollusks, crustaceans, and echinoderms	GMP	16 & 325	2015
09.2.4.3	Fried fish and fish products, including mollusks, crustaceans, and echinoderms	GMP	41, 325, & 332	2015
09.2.5	Smoked, dried, fermented, and/or salted fish and fish	GMP		2018

(continued)

Table 7 (continued)

Food category number	Food category	Maximum level	Notes	Year adopted
	products, including mollusks, crustaceans, and echinoderms		300, 332, XS167, XS189, XS222, XS236, XS244, & XS311	
10.2.1	Liquid egg products	GMP	2014	10.2.1
10.2.2	Frozen egg products	GMP	2014	10.2.2
11.4	Other sugars and syrups (e.g., xylose, maple syrup, sugar	GMP	258	2014 toppings)
12.1.2	Salt substitutes	GMP		2014
13.1.1	Infant formulae	300 mg/kg	381, 584, & 551	2023
13.1.2	Follow-up formulae	300 mg/kg	151, 328, 329, 381, & 551	2023
13.1.3	Formulae for special medical purposes for infants	1000 mg/kg	381, 584, & 551	2023
14.1.5	Coffee, coffee substitutes, tea, herbal infusions, and other hot cereal and grain beverages, excluding cocoa	GMP	160	2014

75 mg/kg body weight/day and prohibited its use in infant formula as a precautionary measure. Although EFSA found no definitive evidence of adverse effects from food-grade carrageenan, it recommended further research on its digestion and systemic absorption (Younes et al. 2018) (*EU Rules - European Commission* n.d.) (Younes et al. 2018). The Ministry of Health, Labour and Welfare (MHLW) permits carrageenan as a food additive under the Food Sanitation Act in Japan (*Food Additives| Ministry of Health, Labour and Welfare|厚生労働省* n.d.). While no specific intake limit is imposed, carrageenan is typically used at concentrations ranging from 0.1% to 1% (w/w). This regulatory stance is supported by a long history of dietary seaweed consumption, with no safety concerns reported at conventional dietary levels. Likewise, carrageenan is permitted under China's National Food Safety Standards (GB 2760) (*CFSA Officially Implements the Standard for the Use of Food Additives (GB 2760–2024) — Food Compliance International* n.d.). A 2023 update emphasized the importance of traceability and purity, including compliance with heavy metal limits (e.g., lead <5 ppm). These measures are particularly relevant given the increasing use of carrageenan in dairy and processed meat products, necessitating strict quality control. In South Korea (*Ministry of Food and Drug Safety > Our Works > Bio&Cosmetics > Approval Process > Biological Products | Ministry of Food and Drug Safety* n.d.), the Ministry of Food and Drug Safety (MFDS) approves carrageenan for food use, with typical inclusion levels ranging from 0.1% to 1% (w/w). Approval is underpinned by traditional consumption patterns of seaweed-derived ingredients, which support its general safety. Carrageenan is authorized by Food Standards Australia New Zealand (FSANZ) under Standard 1.3.1 in Australia and New Zealand (*Additives | Food Standards Australia*

Table 8 Regulatory oversight for carrageenan by region

Region	Regulatory body	Status	Maximum use level	Safety standards
United states	FDA	GRAS (21 CFR 172.620)	GMP	No ADI, not in organic foods (2018)
European Union	EFSA/EC	E407, E407a (Reg. 1333/2008)	75 mg/kg/day (2018)	No infant formula, lead <5 ppm
Japan	MHLW	Food additive (food sanitation act)	0.1–1% (w/w)	Historical use, no specific limit
China	CFDA (GB 2760)	Food Additive (2023 update)	0.1–1% (w/w)	Traceability, lead <5 ppm
South Korea	MFDS	Food additive	0.1–1% (w/w)	Traditional use, purity standards
Australia/NZ	FSANZ	Standard 1.3.1	Quantum satis	No ADI, general safety
Canada	Health Canada	Food additive	GMP	No infant formula, safe for adults

New Zealand n.d.). The additive is permitted at "quantum satis" levels, meaning it can be used as needed to achieve the desired technological effect, provided overall safety is ensured. In Canada, Health Canada has approved carrageenan for use in food products. At the international level, the Joint FAO/WHO Expert Committee on Food Additives (JECFA) has assigned carrageenan an ADI of "not specified," reaffirming its low toxicity at typical consumption levels. A 2014 JECFA evaluation further supported its safety at concentrations up to 1000 mg/L in infant formula for special medical purposes. Moreover, JECFA mandates specific purity criteria, including a minimum viscosity (e.g., >5 cP at 1.5% concentration), to ensure consistent quality and functional performance across global markets (Younes et al. 2018) (Tables 8, 9, 10, and 11).

5 Fucoidan

Fucoidan, a sulfated polysaccharide extracted from brown seaweeds such as *Fucus vesiculosus*, *Undaria pinnatifida*, and *Cladosiphon okamuranus*, has gained prominence as a functional food ingredient due to its reported bioactivities (e.g., anti-inflammatory, antioxidant, and immunomodulatory effects). Its safety for dietary use is well-supported by toxicological studies, but regulatory acceptance varies globally due to differences in historical consumption, purity standards, and intended applications. Fucoidan's sulfate content and molecular weight differ by species and extraction method, affecting bioavailability and safety.

Table 9 Recent regulatory updates (2020–2025)

Region	Update	Date	Impact
United states	FDA reaffirmed carrageenan safety in adult foods, scrutiny for infants 19 (*ECFR:: 21 CFR 172.620 — Carrageenan* n.d.)	2022	Maintains GRAS status, limits organic use
European Union	EFSA review set 75 mg/kg/day safe intake, banned in infant formula (Younes et al. 2018)	2018 (ongoing)	Precautionary approach calls for digestion studies
China	GB 2760 updated with traceability requirements (*CFSA Officially Implements the Standard for the Use of Food Additives (GB 2760–2024) — Food Compliance International* n.d.)	2023	Enhances quality control, supports market growth
Canada	Health Canada confirmed safety for general use, not infant formula (*Oriental Foods Distributor Recalls Two Jelly Cup Products Because of a Choking Hazard ǀ Food Standards Agency* n.d.)	2021	Aligns with EU precautionary stance

Table 10 Regulatory oversight by application and region

Region	Food/Dietary supplements
United states	FDA (GRAS, 250 mg/day, 2019)
European Union	EFSA (novel food, 250 mg/day)
Japan	MHLW (food sanitation act)
China	GB 2760 (2023 traceability)
South Korea	MFDS (supplements, 2022)
Australia	TGA (listed medicines)
Canada	Health Canada (NHPs)

Table 11 Recent regulatory updates (2020–2025)

Region	Update	Date	Impact
United States	Radiolabeled fucoidan safety studies for imaging 28 (Costa et al. 2022)	2023	Advances pharmaceutical potential, pending NDA
European Union	Review of *Cladosiphon okamuranus* fucoidan as a novel food 35 (Tsai et al. 2017)	2024	May expand approved sources, diversify market
Japan	Expanded fucoidan use in oral health products 40 (*EU MDR: Assessing the Impact on Biocompatibility Testing* n.d.)	2022	Broadens functional food applications
China	GB 2760 traceability requirement for fucoidan 42 (*News Japan Amends the Positive List of Food Contact Materials: Ad* n.d.)	2023	Enhances quality control, supports sustainable sourcing
South Korea	MFDS-approved fucoidan scaffolds as biomaterials 45 (*China: Usage Standard for Food Additives Finalized ǀ USDA Foreign Agricultural Service* n.d.-a)	2022	Opens biomedical innovation, e.g., tissue engineering

5.1 *Safety and Regulatory Landscape of Fucoidan: Global Perspectives*

5.1.1 Safety

Oral LD50 values in rats exceed 2000 mg/kg body weight, with no mortality or significant adverse effects observed (Fitton et al. 2015). Studies (e.g., Marinova 2019) report no organ damage at doses up to 1000 mg/kg. Ninety-day feeding studies in rodents at 300–1000 mg/kg/day show no histopathological changes, hematological abnormalities, or metabolic disruptions (Panggabean et al. 2022; Thomas & Rengasamy 2008). Clinical studies (e.g., 250 mg/day for 12 weeks) have demonstrated no adverse effects on the liver, kidney, or gastrointestinal function of healthy adults (Flórez-Fernández et al. 2023). Mild bloating is occasionally reported at higher doses (>500 mg/day), likely due to its fiber-like properties. Fucoidan itself is not allergenic, as seaweed allergies are typically protein-mediated. However, contamination with algal proteins or heavy metals (e.g., arsenic, lead) from polluted waters requires strict quality control (Zhao et al. 2021).

High sulfate content may affect mineral absorption (e.g., calcium, iron) at excessive doses, though this is negligible at approved levels (e.g., 250 mg/day).

5.1.2 Regulatory Framework of Agarin Global Food Systems

Fucoidan is a class of sulfated polysaccharides predominantly derived from brown seaweeds such as *Undaria pinnatifida*, *Fucus vesiculosus*, and *Cladosiphon okamuranus*. Its regulatory status varies significantly across jurisdictions due to its structural heterogeneity, broad application spectrum—including food supplements, pharmaceuticals, and cosmetics—and the absence of a universally accepted definition or specification standard. Despite this complexity, fucoidan has demonstrated a favorable safety profile, with no significant toxicity reported in either human or animal studies at typical dietary exposure levels (e.g., up to 250 mg/day). Regulatory frameworks governing fucoidan generally emphasize source material, extraction method, compositional purity, and intended use. The Food and Drug Administration (FDA) has granted Generally Recognized as Safe (GRAS) status to specific fucoidan extracts in the United States. Notably, fucoidans derived from *Undaria pinnatifida* and *Fucus vesiculosus* (Maritech by Marinova) received GRAS (Generally Recognized as Safe) notification in 2019, authorizing their use at levels up to 250 mg/day in conventional food products, including beverages and dietary supplements (Sicherer 1999). This designation followed comprehensive toxicological evaluations and safety dossier submissions, establishing a no-observed-adverse-effect level (NOAEL) (Rajauria et al. 2023). The GRAS approval includes specifications on purity criteria—such as heavy metals content (<10 ppm)—and explicitly excludes uncharacterized or mixed-source extracts (Wang et al. 2023). In the European Union, fucoidan from *Undaria pinnatifida* and *Fucus vesiculosus* was authorized as a novel food under Commission Implementing Regulation (EU) 2017/2470 (Shikov et al. 2020). The European Food Safety Authority (EFSA) assessed these extracts as substantially equivalent to their source seaweeds and identified no evidence of genotoxicity, mutagenicity, or allergenicity (Mensah et al. 2023). A NOAEL of 300 mg/kg body weight/day was established based on animal data, supporting a human intake of up to 250 mg/day. Regulatory approval in the EU also emphasizes consistent compositional characterization and product traceability. In Japan, the Ministry of Health, Labour and Welfare (MHLW) classifies fucoidan as a safe food ingredient under the Food Sanitation Act (*GRAS Notices* n.d.-a). It is supported by its longstanding consumption in traditional diets rich in seaweeds such as *mozuku* and *wakame*. While no explicit intake limit has been formalized, commercial products typically recommend a daily intake ranging from 100 to 300 mg. The absence of reported adverse effects at these levels reinforces its historical safety record. China includes fucoidan in its National Food Safety Standards (GB 2760), permitting its use as a food additive (*GRAS Notices* n.d.-a). A 2023 regulatory update mandates the traceability of source species and requires adherence to strict contaminant limits, including lead concentrations below 5 ppm and compliance with microbiological criteria. Dietary supplements containing fucoidan typically incorporate 100–250 mg/day, consistent with safety data and market norms. In South Korea, the Ministry of Food and Drug Safety (MFDS) has approved fucoidan for use in dietary supplements (US Food and Drug Administration 2022). Typical recommended intake levels range between 100 and 300 mg/day, grounded in traditional seaweed consumption and modern safety assessments of *Undaria*-derived extracts. Australia regulates fucoidan under two parallel frameworks: The Therapeutic Goods Administration (TGA) includes it in complementary medicines as per the Therapeutic Goods Act. At the same time, Food Standards Australia New Zealand (FSANZ) permits its use in seaweed-derived foods without a specific maximum limit, provided general safety conditions are met (*Implementing Regulation - 2017/2470 - EN - EUR-Lex* n.d.). In Canada, fucoidan is permitted in natural health products (NHPs) under Health Canada's regulatory framework. Product approvals are species-specific (e.g., *Fucus vesiculosus*), with intake recommendations not exceeding 250 mg/day based on safety evaluations conducted during product licensing. At the international level, the Codex Alimentarius (Ottawa n.d.) does not currently define standards specific to fucoidan; however, it provides general guidelines for seaweed-derived polysaccharides, which indirectly influence national regulatory standards. The Joint FAO/WHO Expert Committee on Food Additives (JECFA) has supported the safety of seaweed polysaccharides. However, no International Numbering System (INS) code has been assigned to fucoidan due to its compositional variability.

6 Chitin and Chitosan

Chitin and its derivative chitosan are marine polysaccharides. Chitin, a β-1,4-linked N-acetylglucosamine polymer, and its deacetylated derivative chitosan, extracted primarily from crustacean shells (e.g., shrimp, crab), are versatile marine polysaccharides with applications across food, biomedical, and agricultural sectors. Chitin is the second most common polysaccharide in nature, following cellulose. These biopolymers have gained significant attention in recent decades due to their biocompatibility, biodegradability, and versatile applications in industries ranging from biomedicine and pharmaceuticals to food preservation and agriculture (No et al. 2007). However, the widespread adoption of chitin and chitosan necessitates a thorough understanding of their safety profiles and the regulatory frameworks governing their use (Fig. 3).

Chitosan is utilized in the food industry as a food preservative, a fat-binding agent, and an edible film. Studies showing no adverse effects at intakes up to 3 g/day in humans have affirmed its safety as a dietary supplement. However, long-term consumption studies are limited, and potential interactions with gut microbiota warrant further investigation.

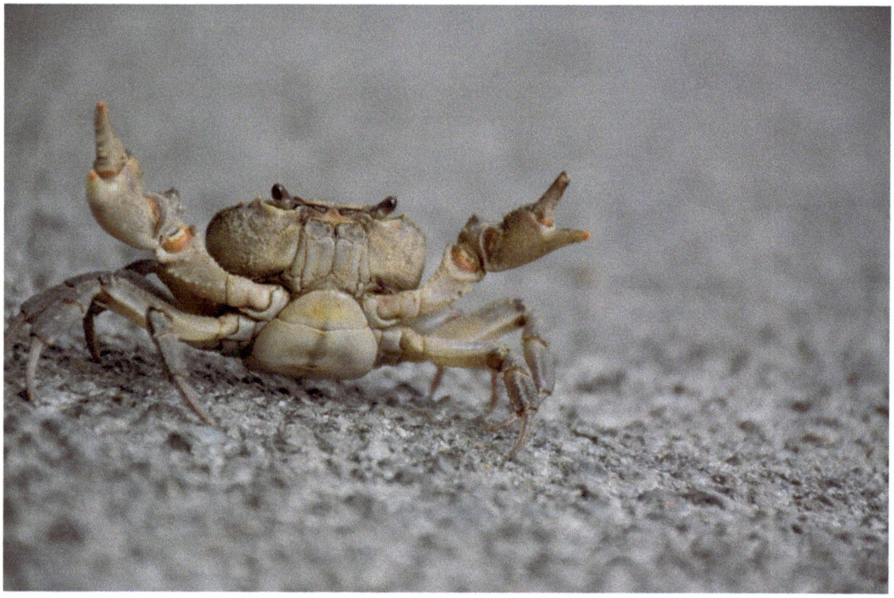

Fig. 3 Crustaceans as a source of chitin and chitosan. (Photo by Tamara Rajkovic: https://www.pexels.com/photo/crab-on-ground-20190879/)

6.1 *Safety and Regulatory Status of Chitin and Chitosan in Global Jurisdictions*

6.1.1 Safety

Chitin and chitosan are generally considered safe (GRAS) for many applications due to their natural origin and biodegradable nature. Toxicological studies have consistently demonstrated low acute toxicity in mammalian models (Lagarto et al. 2015) (*Chitin and Chitosan as Novel Biotechnological Materials - Hirano - 1999 - Polymer International - Wiley Online Library* n.d.). Limited direct consumption data of chitin exist due to its use primarily as a chitosan precursor, but no adverse effects are reported from incidental intake (e.g., via shellfish) (Lagarto et al. 2015). Dietary intake of Chitosanat 1–3 g/day (e.g., as a fat-binding supplement) is well-tolerated, though mild gastrointestinal effects (e.g., bloating) may occur at >5 g/day due to its cationic nature(Jull et al. 2008). Chitosan from crustacean sources raises shellfish allergy concerns (Standards Agency 2021), but purified forms (<0.1% residual protein) show no significant reactions in clinical trials 9. Fungal chitosan avoids this risk entirely (Muzzarelli 2010). Crustacean-derived chitosan requires stringent purification to minimize shellfish allergen risks, driving interest in fungal alternatives. Higher Degree of Deacetylation (DD) (>80%) increases chitosan's solubility and bioactivity, but may enhance mild mucosal irritation. Low MW (<50 kDa) chitosan is more bioavailable and cleared faster, while high MW (>200 kDa) may persist longer in tissues (Zakaria et al. 2012). Heavy metals (e.g., lead <10 ppm) and endotoxins from marine sources require strict controls (Xia et al. 2011).

6.1.2 Regulatory Framework of Chitin and Chitosanin Global Food Systems

Chitosan has achieved regulatory recognition in multiple countries, with permitted applications and usage level variations. Chitosan is classified as Generally Recognized as Safe (GRAS) for specified applications in the United States. For example, fungal-derived chitosan was affirmed as GRAS under GRN No. 397 (2011) for dietary supplements at intake levels ranging from 0.5 to 1 g/day (Chen et al. 2014). A subsequent GRAS notification submitted in 2024 expanded chitosan's approval to include its use in edible coatings (*GRAS Notices* n.d.-a). Within the European Union, the European Food Safety Authority (EFSA) authorizes the use of chitosan as a food contact material under Regulation (EU) No 10/2011, and as a processing aid (*Federal Register: Pesticides; Proposal To Add Chitosan to the List of Active Ingredients Permitted in Exempted Minimum Risk Pesticide Products; Notice of Data Availability on Chitosan and Chitosan Salts* n.d.) (Flórez et al. 2022). Fungal chitosan-glucan has been evaluated as a novel food, with an assessment completed in 2010 (Scientific Opinion on the Safety of 'Chitin-Glucan' as a Novel Food

Ingredient 2010); however, no Acceptable Daily Intake (ADI) has been established. In Japan, the Ministry of Health, Labour and Welfare (MHLW) permits chitosan as a functional food ingredient, particularly in glucosamine-based supplements. Due to its extensive consumption history, no specific intake limit has been designated.

China permits the use of chitosan under the National Food Safety Standard GB 2760, with the most recent revision in 2023. Usage is typically regulated within 0.1–1% (w/w), and traceability documentation is required to ensure quality and compliance. In South Korea, the Ministry of Food and Drug Safety (MFDS) authorizes the use of chitosan in both dietary supplements and medical biomaterials (*Welcome to the Ministry of Food and Drug Safety | Ministry of Food and Drug Safety* n.d.-a). Notably, chitosan-based scaffolds received approval in 2022 for specific biomedical applications. India's Food Safety and Standards Authority of India (FSSAI) includes chitosan in its list of permitted food additives (*FSSAI* n.d.). At the same time, the Central Drugs Standard Control Organization (CDSCO) oversees its use in pharmaceutical and medical contexts. In Brazil, the National Health Surveillance Agency (ANVISA) governs the use of chitosan in food and medical products (Rezaiyan Attar et al. 2023). In contrast, the Ministry of Agriculture, Livestock and Food Supply (MAPA) approved its application in agricultural products in a 2023 update.

Internationally, the regulatory framework is further guided by voluntary standards developed by bodies such as the Codex Alimentarius and the International Organization for Standardization (ISO). Standards such as ISO 22000 (food safety management systems) and ISO 13485 (quality management systems for medical devices) are particularly relevant for chitosan and chitin manufacturers aiming to align with global compliance requirements (Tables 12 and 13).

Chitin and chitosan offer remarkable potential across multiple industries, underpinned by their inherent safety and eco-friendly properties. Toxicological and environmental data confirm their low risk, although allergenicity and processing-related concerns necessitate ongoing vigilance. Regulatory frameworks in major markets provide robust oversight; yet, global harmonization remains a goal.

Table 12 Regulations and regions of chitin and chitosan marine polysaccharides

Region	Food/Dietary supplements
United states	FDA (GRAS, DSHEA)
European Union	EFSA (Reg. 10/2011, 2015/2283)
Japan	MHLW, food chemical research foundation
China	CFDA (food safety laws)
South Korea	KFDA (novel food approval)
India	FSSAI (food additives)
Brazil	ANVISA (food safety)

Table 13 Recent regulatory updates (2020–2025)

Region	Update	Date	Impact
United states	EPA added chitosan to the minimum risk pesticide list (40 CFR 152.25(f))	2022	Expands use in agriculture without registration, reduces regulatory burden (*GRAS Notices* n.d.-b)
European Union	EFSA assessed fungal chitosan safety for food contact	2023	Supports sustainable sourcing, may lead to broader approval
South Korea	Approval of insect-derived chitin as novel food	2021	Opens alternative sources, aligns with global sustainability trends (*Welcome to the Ministry of Food and Drug Safety* ǀ *Ministry of Food and Drug Safety* n.d.-a)
Japan	Expanded chitosan use in water treatment under MHLW	2023	Reinforces Japan's leadership in chitosan applications (Coja et al. 2025)
China	NMPA streamlined approval for chitosan-based wound dressings	2024	Accelerates market entry for medical products (Ahmed & Ahmad 2015)

7 Emerging Seaweed-Derived Polysaccharides in Food Applications

In addition to the widely studied seaweed polysaccharides such as carrageenan, alginate, and agar, several other marine-derived polysaccharides have shown promising potential in food applications. Turbellarian, ulvan, and floridean starch are particularly interesting due to their unique functional properties and versatility in food systems (Hettle et al. 2022).

Furcellaran, structurally similar to κ-carrageenan, can form thermally reversible aqueous gels. Its gelation behavior is influenced by the presence of specific cations—such as potassium (K^+), ammonium (NH_4^+), and cesium (Cs^+)—which promote gel formation, while sodium ions (Na^+) act as inhibitors. Additionally, the presence of sugars can modulate the texture of furcellaran gels, shifting them from brittle to more elastic forms. Importantly, furcellaran gels remain stable under acidic conditions, making them suitable for low-pH applications. This polysaccharide is commonly incorporated into puddings, cake fillings, icings, and marmalades. Notably, furcellaran offers a competitive advantage over pectin, which can form stable gels at sugar concentrations below 50–60%. Beyond confectionery applications, furcellaran is also used in processed meat products, including meat spreads, pastes, and pastry fillings, serving as a functional texturiser (Belitz et al. 2004).

While furcellaran finds utility in food products, other seaweed polysaccharides, such as fucoidans and laminarins, are primarily valued for their health-related bioactivities rather than for direct food applications. Fucoidans, for instance, exhibit a broad range of biofunctional properties, including anti-inflammatory, anti-angiogenic, anticoagulant, and anti-adhesive effects. Emerging evidence further supports their potential antitumor (Pradhan et al. 2023), antimutagenic, anticomplementary, immunomodulatory (Pradhan et al. 2023), hypoglycemic, antiviral (Hans et al. 2020), hypolipidemic, and anti-inflammatory activities (Venugopal 2011). These bioactivities position fucoidans as attractive candidates for use in functional foods and nutraceuticals.

Ulvan, another noteworthy polysaccharide extracted from Ulva species (commonly known as sea lettuce), has garnered attention for its structural uniqueness and potential dietary benefits (Pari et al. 2025; Reisky et al. 2019; Tziveleka et al. 2019). Unlike many other dietary fibers, ulvan is resistant to fermentation by colonic bacteria (Bai & Tuvikene 2021), which limits its breakdown in the large intestine. As a result, ulvan functions effectively as a bulking agent with minimal impact on nutrient metabolism, thereby supporting gastrointestinal health (Pradhan et al. 2023).

Furthermore, floridean starch, a reserve carbohydrate found in red seaweeds, exhibits functional characteristics that make it suitable for various modern food applications. Following repeated freeze–thaw cycles, floridean starch exhibits a low gelatinization temperature, low viscosity, high clarity, and minimal retrogradation. These attributes make it particularly well-suited for instant noodles and deep-frozen food products, where stability and texture are critical (Venugopal 2011; Yu et al. 2002).

The **safety and regulations** of **turbellarian**, **ulvan**, and **floridean** marine polysaccharides worldwide, with a focus on their toxicological profiles, current regulatory statuses, and recent developments as of April 8, 2025. In this context, "turbellarian" appears to be a misnomer or typo, referring to a class of flatworms (Turbellaria) rather than a polysaccharide. **Ulvan** is a sulfated polysaccharide derived from green algae (e.g., *Ulva* spp.), which has been widely studied for its bioactivity and potential applications in food and biomedical fields (Tran et al. 2023; Li et al. 2023). **Floridean starch** is a storage polysaccharide in red algae, structurally similar to amylopectin but lacking amylose, and is less common in regulatory contexts due to its limited commercial use. Assuming **fucoidan** (a sulfated polysaccharide from brown algae) as a substitute based on common marine polysaccharide discussions, unless corrected.

7.1 Safety and Regulations of Ulvan, Floridean Starch, and Turbellaria

7.1.1 Safety

Ulvan

Oral LD50 in rats exceeds 5000 mg/kg, indicating low acute toxicity. Studies show no systemic effects due to poor absorption (insoluble in the upper GI tract) (OECD/OCDE 1987). Ninety-day rat studies at 1000 mg/kg/day report no significant adverse effects; NOAEL ≥1000 mg/kg/day (Qi et al. 2013). Mild GI effects (e.g., bloating) noted at higher doses (>5 g/day) due to fermentation in the colon. Ulvan, a polysaccharide from green seaweed, is generally safe when used as a fiber supplement at low concentrations (0.1–1% w/w) in food. However, excessive intake might increase H2S production by gut bacteria, potentially impacting colon health. Ulvan is not known to cause allergic reactions and is distinct from shellfish allergens (Mo'o et al. 2020).

Floridean Starch

No specific LD50 data due to limited testing, but analogous to starch ($LD_{50} > 5000$ mg/kg), suggesting low toxicity (OECD TG420 2001). Limited studies; presumed safe based on similarity to dietary starch. No adverse effects expected at typical intake levels (e.g., <1 g/day from red algae consumption). Historically, it has been consumed in small amounts in seaweed-based diets (e.g., Asia), with no reported toxicity. Fully digestible by amylases into glucose. None were identified; they lack sulfated groups or proteins linked to allergies.

Turbellarian

Oral LD50 in rats >2000 mg/kg; no mortality or significant effects at high doses. Ninety-day studies at 1000 mg/kg/day show no organ toxicity; NOAEL ≥1000 mg/kg/day (OECD/OCDE 1987). Higher doses (>2 g/day) may cause transient diarrhea or anticoagulant effects due to sulfate content. Safe at 0.1–3 g/day in supplements (e.g., for immune support), though anticoagulant properties warrant caution in bleeding-risk populations. Low risk; no direct allergenic proteins, though brown algae allergies are rare and unrelated to fucoidan. All three may contain heavy metals (e.g., lead <10 ppm) or microbial impurities from marine sources, necessitating purity standards.

7.2 *Safety and Regulatory Framework of Ulvan, Floridean Starch, and Turbellaria in Global Food Systems*

Ulvan is a sulfated polysaccharide primarily derived from green seaweeds of the *Ulva* genus. In the United States, Ulvan does not currently hold an independent Generally Recognized as Safe (GRAS) designation; however, it is permitted as a component of *Ulva* spp. (commonly referred to as kelp) under 21 CFR 172.365 (*Generally Recognized as Safe (GRAS) | FDA* n.d.). Notably, a 2023 petition proposed GRAS status for fungal-derived chitosan-glucan analogs, potentially setting a regulatory precedent for ulvan applications in the U.S. market (Gotteland et al. 2020). Within the European Union, *Ulva* spp. are authorized as a novel food under Regulation (EU) 2015/2283, with ulvan recognized as a dietary fiber component (European Parliament and Council of the European Union 2015). Due to its low toxicity profile, no specific acceptable daily intake (ADI) has been established.

Additionally, ulvan is permitted for use in food contact materials as specified under Regulation (EU) No 10/2011. The Ministry of Health, Labour and Welfare (MHLW) allows the use of *Ulva* spp. in Japan (*Ministry of Health, Labour and Welfare: Food with Health Claims, Food for Special Dietary Uses, and Nutrition Labeling* n.d.). In food products, ulvan is considered a natural and unregulated constituent. In China (*China: Usage Standard for Food Additives Finalized | USDA Foreign Agricultural Service* n.d.-b), the national food safety standard GB 2760 (2023 update) permits the use of *Ulva* extracts, including ulvan, at concentrations ranging from 0.1% to 1% (w/w), provided that traceability protocols are maintained. Other regulatory authorities, including the Ministry of Food and Drug Safety (MFDS) in South Korea (*Welcome to the Ministry of Food and Drug Safety | Ministry of Food and Drug Safety* n.d.-b), Food Standards Australia New Zealand (FSANZ) (*Novel Foods | Food Standards Australia New Zealand* n.d.), and the Food Safety and Standards Authority of India (FSSAI), allow the use of seaweed-derived polysaccharides under general food safety provisions (*FSSAI* n.d.). However, no specific quantitative limits are currently assigned to Ulvan.

Floridean starch, a reserve polysaccharide found in red algae such as *Porphyra* and *Gelidium*, falls under broad regulatory frameworks similarly. It is not individually regulated in the United States. Still, it is implicitly covered under the GRAS status for red algae-derived food ingredients (21 CFR 184.1121) (*Generally Recognized as Safe (GRAS) | FDA* n.d.). The European Union classifies red algae as novel foods following Regulation (EU) 2015/2283, with floridean starch considered a minor, unregulated constituent deemed safe under existing approvals (*Regulation (EU) 2015/2283 of the European Parliament and of the Council on Novel Foods, Amending Regulation (EU) No. 1169/2011 of the European Parliament and of the Council and Repealing Regulation (EC) No. 258/97 of the European Parliament and of the Council and Commission Regulation (EC) No. 1852/2001. | FAOLEX* n.d.). In Japan, the MHLW permits the use of red algae (e.g., nori) in food, and floridean starch is presumed safe as a naturally occurring carbohydrate (*List of Approved Products | Pharmaceuticals and Medical Devices Agency* n.d.). China's GB 2760 includes red algae in its positive list of food ingredients, although floridean starch is not explicitly regulated (National Health and Family Planning Committee of China 2015). In other jurisdictions, such as South Korea and India (Pokhrel 2024), the use of seaweed in traditional diets supports the implicit approval of floridean starch, with no specific restrictions due to its starch-like composition and long-standing consumption history (Xu et al. 2022) (Tables 14 and 15).

8 Conclusion

Marine-derived polysaccharides continue to play an increasingly important role in modern food systems, offering multifunctional benefits ranging from textural enhancement to bioactive health effects. Regulatory frameworks across major global markets, such as those established by the FDA, EFSA, MHLW, MFDS, FSANZ,

Table 14 Regulatory oversight by region

Region	Ulvan	Floridean starch	Turbellarian
United states	FDA: *Ulva* spp. (21 CFR 172.365)	FDA: Red algae GRAS (21 CFR 184.1121)	FDA: GRAS (GRN 661, 2016)
European Union	EFSA: Novel food, no ADI	EFSA: Red algae novel food	EFSA: Novel food, 250 mg/day
Japan	MHLW: *Ulva* spp. food-safe	MHLW: Red algae food-safe	MHLW: Functional food, GMP
China	GB 2760: 0.1–1% (2023 update)	GB 2760: Red algae permitted	GB 2760: Brown algae extracts
South Korea	MFDS: Seaweed-derived safe	MFDS: Red algae safe	MFDS: Supplements, 0.1–1 g/day
Australia/ NZ	FSANZ: General seaweed safety	FSANZ: Red algae safe	FSANZ: Supplements, no ADI
India	FSSAI: Seaweed additives	FSSAI: Red algae permitted	FSSAI: General seaweed safety

Table 15 Recent regulatory updates (2020–2025)

Region	Polysaccharide	Update	Date	Impact
United States	Ulvan	Proposal for GRAS status of analogs (*Infant Formula Guidance Documents & Regulatory Information* I *FDA* n.d.)	2023	Potential food use expansion
European Union	Ulvan	EFSA: Novel food (100 mg/day) (Pari et al. 2025)	2022	Supports the supplement market
China	Ulvan	GB 2760 traceability update (*Welcome to the Ministry of Food and Drug Safety* I *Ministry of Food and Drug Safety* n.d.-b)	2023	Enhances quality control

FSSAI, and Codex Alimentarius, provide the foundation for the safe incorporation of marine polysaccharides into a wide range of food products. While well-established polysaccharides, such as alginate, carrageenan, and agar, are widely recognized as safe under various national and international standards, emerging compounds like fucoidan, ulvan, and floridean starch are gaining attention due to expanding scientific evidence supporting their functional and nutritional value. Although different countries have their own regulations, they often follow similar basic rules, such as setting limits on impurities, evaluating safe intake levels, and considering traditional food use. Regular monitoring, updated safety reviews, and improved testing methods are crucial for maintaining consumer safety, particularly for vulnerable groups such as infants and individuals with special dietary needs.

In the future, growing interest in natural ingredients, sustainable sources, and new functional foods is likely to lead to updates in regulations and improved international coordination. As research on new marine polysaccharides continues, strong cooperation between industry, researchers, and regulators will be essential to ensure these materials are used safely and effectively in food products.

References

Additives | Food Standards Australia New Zealand. (n.d.). Retrieved April 11, 2025, from https://www.foodstandards.gov.au/consumer/additives/additiveoverview

Ahmed, S., & Ahmad, M. (2015). Chitosan Based Dressings for Wound Care. *Immunochemistry & Immunopathology*, *01*(02), 1–6. https://doi.org/10.4172/2469-9756.1000106

Bai, R. G., & Tuvikene, R. (2021). Potential Antiviral Properties of Industrially Important Marine Algal Polysaccharides and Their Significance in Fighting a Future Viral Pandemic. *Viruses*, *13*(9), 1817. https://doi.org/10.3390/V13091817

Caliceti, M., Argese, E., Sfriso, A., & Pavoni, B. (2002). Heavy metal contamination in the seaweeds of the Venice lagoon. *Chemosphere*, *47*(4), 443–454. https://doi.org/10.1016/S0045-6535(01)00292-2

CFSA officially implements the standard for the use of food additives (GB 2760-2024) — Food Compliance International. (n.d.). Retrieved April 13, 2025, from https://foodcomplianceinternational.com/industry-insight/news/5218-cfsa-officially-implements-the-standard-for-the-use-of-food-additives-gb-2760-2024

Chen, Y., Zhu, X., Yang, Y., Han, D., Jin, J., & Xie, S. (2014). Effect of dietary chitosan on growth performance, haematology, immune response, intestine morphology, intestine microbiota and disease resistance in gibel carp (Carassius auratus gibelio). *Aquaculture Nutrition*, *20*(5), 532–546. https://doi.org/10.1111/ANU.12106

China: Usage Standard for Food Additives Finalized | USDA Foreign Agricultural Service. (n.d.-a). Retrieved April 11, 2025, from https://www.fas.usda.gov/data/china-usage-standard-food-additives-finalized

China: Usage Standard for Food Additives Finalized | USDA Foreign Agricultural Service. (n.d.-b). Retrieved April 12, 2025, from https://www.fas.usda.gov/data/china-usage-standard-food-additives-finalized

Chitin and chitosan as novel biotechnological materials - Hirano - 1999 - Polymer International - Wiley Online Library. (n.d.). Retrieved April 10, 2025, from https://scijournals.onlinelibrary.wiley.com/doi/10.1002/(SICI)1097-0126(199908)48:8%3C732::AID-PI211%3E3.0.CO;2-U

Cohen, S. M., & Ito, N. (2002). A Critical Review of the Toxicological Effects of Carrageenan and Processed Eucheuma Seaweed on the Gastrointestinal Tract. *Critical Reviews in Toxicology*, *32*(5), 413–444. https://doi.org/10.1080/20024091064282

Coja, T., Adriaanse, P., Choi, J., Finizio, A., Giraudo, M., Kuhl, T., Metruccio, F., McVey, E., Paparella, M., Pieper, S., Scanziani, E., Teodorovic, I., Van der Brink, P., Wilks, M., Marinovich, M., Ferilli, F., Gobbi, A., Panzarea, M., Vianello, G., & Lava, R. (2025). Statement concerning the review of the approval of the basic substances chitosan and chitosan hydrochloride when used in plant protection. *EFSA Journal*, *23*(4). https://doi.org/10.2903/J.EFSA.2025.9318

Costa, B., Corrêa, L. B., Silva, P. M. R.E., Jannini de Sá, Y. A. P., Guimarães, F. V., Alencar, L. M. R., Simões, R. L., Helal-Neto, E., Ricci-Junior, E., Muller de Oliveira Henriques, M. das G., Rosas, E. C., & Santos-Oliveira, R. (2022). Using pure Fucoidan and radiolabeled Fucoidan (99mTc-Fucoidan) as a new agent for inflammation diagnosis and therapy. *Food Hydrocolloids for Health*, *2*, 100049. https://doi.org/10.1016/J.FHFH.2021.100049

David, S., Shani Levi, C., Fahoum, L., Ungar, Y., Meyron-Holtz, E. G., Shpigelman, A., & Lesmes, U. (2018). Revisiting the carrageenan controversy: Do we really understand the digestive fate and safety of carrageenan in our foods? *Food and Function*, *9*(3), 1344–1352. https://doi.org/10.1039/C7FO01721A

eCFR: 21 CFR 172.620 -- Carrageenan. (n.d.). Retrieved April 13, 2025, from https://www.ecfr.gov/current/title-21/chapter-I/subchapter-B/part-172/subpart-G/section-172.620

EU MDR: Assessing the impact on biocompatibility testing. (n.d.). Retrieved April 14, 2025, from https://informaconnect.com/medical-device-regulation-biocompatibility-testing/

EU Rules - European Commission. (n.d.). Retrieved April 13, 2025, from https://food.ec.europa.eu/food-safety/food-improvement-agents/additives/eu-rules_en

FAO, and W. (2016). *Codex Alimentarius International Food Standards*. *4*(1), 1–23.

FAO, and W. (2023). Codex Alimentarius Commission Procedural Manual. *Codex Alimentarius Commission Procedural Manual*. https://doi.org/10.4060/CC5042EN

Federal Register: Pesticides; Proposal To Add Chitosan to the List of Active Ingredients Permitted in Exempted Minimum Risk Pesticide Products; Notice of Data Availability on Chitosan and Chitosan Salts. (n.d.). Retrieved April 10, 2025, from https://www.federalregister.gov/documents/2022/05/06/2022-09731/pesticides-proposal-to-add-chitosan-to-the-list-of-active-ingredients-permitted-in-exempted-minimum

Fitton, J. H., Stringer, D. N., & Karpiniec, S. S. (2015). Therapies from Fucoidan: An Update. *Marine Drugs 2015, Vol. 13, Pages 5920-5946*, *13*(9), 5920–5946. https://doi.org/10.3390/MD13095920

Flórez-Fernández, N., Pontes, J. F., Guerreiro, F., Afonso, I. T., Lollo, G., Torres, M. D., Domínguez, H., Costa, A. M. R. da, & Grenha, A. (2023). Fucoidan from Fucus vesiculosus: Evaluation of the Impact of the Sulphate Content on Nanoparticle Production and Cell Toxicity. *Marine Drugs*, *21*(2). https://doi.org/10.3390/MD21020115

Flórez, M., Guerra-Rodríguez, E., Cazón, P., & Vázquez, M. (2022). Chitosan for food packaging: Recent advances in active and intelligent films. *Food Hydrocolloids*, *124*, 107328. https://doi.org/10.1016/J.FOODHYD.2021.107328

Food Additives|Ministry of Health, Labour and Welfare|厚生労働省. (n.d.). Retrieved April 13, 2025, from https://www.mhlw.go.jp/stf/seisakunitsuite/bunya/kenkou_iryou/shokuhin/syokuten/index_00012.html

FSSAI. (n.d.). Retrieved April 11, 2025, from https://www.fssai.gov.in/cms/food-safety-and-standards-regulations.php

Generally Recognized as Safe (GRAS) | FDA. (n.d.). Retrieved April 14, 2025, from https://www.fda.gov/food/food-ingredients-packaging/generally-recognized-safe-gras

Gotteland, M., Riveros, K., Gasaly, N., Carcamo, C., Magne, F., Liabeuf, G., Beattie, A., & Rosenfeld, S. (2020). The Pros and Cons of Using Algal Polysaccharides as Prebiotics. *Frontiers in Nutrition*, *7*, 571548. https://doi.org/10.3389/FNUT.2020.00163/BIBTEX

GRAS Notices. (n.d.-a). Retrieved April 10, 2025, from https://www.hfpappexternal.fda.gov/scripts/fdcc/index.cfm?set=grasnotices&id=397

GRAS Notices. (n.d.-b).

Hans, N., Malik, A., & Naik, S. (2020). Antiviral activity of sulfated polysaccharides from marine algae and its application in combating COVID-19: Mini review. *Bioresource Technology Reports*, *13*, 100623. https://doi.org/10.1016/J.BITEB.2020.100623

Hettle, A. G., Vickers, C. J., & Boraston, A. B. (2022). Sulfatases: Critical Enzymes for Algal Polysaccharide Processing. *Frontiers in Plant Science*, *13*. https://doi.org/10.3389/FPLS.2022.837636

Implementing regulation - 2017/2470 - EN - EUR-Lex. (n.d.). Retrieved April 14, 2025, from https://eur-lex.europa.eu/eli/reg_impl/2017/2470/oj/eng

Infant Formula Guidance Documents & Regulatory Information | FDA. (n.d.). Retrieved April 14, 2025, from https://www.fda.gov/food/guidance-documents-regulatory-information-topic-food-and-dietary-supplements/infant-formula-guidance-documents-regulatory-information

International Labour Organization. (1987). *Environmental Health Criteria 70 PRINCIPLES FOR THE SAFETY ASSESSMENT OF FOOD ADDITIVES*. https://iris.who.int/handle/10665/37578

Jull, A. B., Ni Mhurchu, C., Bennett, D. A., Dunshea-Mooij, C. A. E., & Rodgers, A. (2008). Chitosan for overweight or obesity. *Cochrane Database of Systematic Reviews*, *3*. https://doi.org/10.1002/14651858.CD003892.PUB3/INFORMATION/EN

Krishna, P. S. R., Jayaraman, A., Nayak, A. D., & Baidya, M. (2022). Toxicological Evaluation of Alginic Acid, a Polysaccharide Isolated from *Turbinaria conoides* (J. Agardh) Kutzing on Wistar Albino Rats. *Toxicology International*, *29*(3), 363–377. https://doi.org/10.18311/TI/2022/V29I3/29301

Lagarto, A., Merino, N., Valdes, O., Dominguez, J., Spencer, E., de la Paz, N., & Aparicio, G. (2015). Safety evaluation of chitosan and chitosan acid salts from Panurilus argus lobster.

International Journal of Biological Macromolecules, *72*, 1343–1350. https://doi.org/10.1016/J.IJBIOMAC.2014.10.030

Li, C., Tang, T., Du, Y., Jiang, L., Yao, Z., Ning, L., & Zhu, B. (2023). Ulvan and Ulva oligosaccharides: a systematic review of structure, preparation, biological activities and applications. *Bioresources and Bioprocessing 2023 10:1*, *10*(1), 1–17. https://doi.org/10.1186/S40643-023-00690-Z

List of Approved Products | Pharmaceuticals and Medical Devices Agency. (n.d.). Retrieved April 14, 2025, from https://www.pmda.go.jp/english/review-services/reviews/approved-information/drugs/0002.html

Mensah, E. O., Kanwugu, O. N., Panda, P. K., & Adadi, P. (2023). Marine fucoidans: Structural, extraction, biological activities and their applications in the food industry. *Food Hydrocolloids*, *142*, 108784. https://doi.org/10.1016/J.FOODHYD.2023.108784

Michel, C., & Macfarlane, G. T. (1996). Digestive fates of soluble polysaccharides from marine macroalgae: involvement of the colonic microflora and physiological consequences for the host. *Journal of Applied Bacteriology*, *80*(4), 349–369. https://doi.org/10.1111/J.1365-2672.1996.TB03230.X

Ministry of Food and Drug Safety>Our Works>Bio&Cosmetics>Approval Process>Biological Products | Ministry of Food and Drug Safety. (n.d.). Retrieved April 13, 2025, from https://www.mfds.go.kr/eng/wpge/m_22/de011012l001.do

Ministry of Health, Labour and Welfare: Food with Health Claims, Food for Special Dietary Uses, and Nutrition Labeling. (n.d.). Retrieved April 11, 2025, from https://www.mhlw.go.jp/english/topics/foodsafety/fhc/

Mo'o, F. R. C., Wilar, G., Devkota, H. P., & Wathoni, N. (2020). Ulvan, a Polysaccharide from Macroalga Ulva sp.: A Review of Chemistry, Biological Activities and Potential for Food and Biomedical Applications. *Applied Sciences 2020, Vol. 10, Page 5488*, *10*(16), 5488. https://doi.org/10.3390/APP10165488

Muzzarelli, R. A. A. (2010). Chitins and Chitosans as Immunoadjuvants and Non-Allergenic Drug Carriers. *Marine Drugs 2010, Vol. 8, Pages 292-312*, *8*(2), 292–312. https://doi.org/10.3390/MD8020292

National Health and Family Planning Committee of China. (2015). China - Peoples Republic of Chinese Standards for Food Additives - GB2760-2015. *Gain Report*, *15013*(1). https://apps.fas.usda.gov/newgainapi/api/report/downloadreportbyfilename?filename=Standard for Food Additive Use - GB2760-2015_Beijing_China - Peoples Republic of_4-28-2015.pdf

Navigating the Regulatory Pathways and Requirements of Wound Dressing Products - Gsap. (n.d.). Retrieved April 12, 2025, from https://gsap.co.il/wound-dressing-products-regulation/

News Japan amends the positive list of Food Contact Materials: Ad. (n.d.). Retrieved April 13, 2025, from https://gpcgateway.com/common/news_details/MTczNA/MTI/

No, H. K., Meyers, S. P., Prinyawiwatkul, W., & Xu, Z. (2007). Applications of Chitosan for Improvement of Quality and Shelf Life of Foods: A Review. *Journal of Food Science*, *72*(5), R87–R100. https://doi.org/10.1111/J.1750-3841.2007.00383.X

Novel foods | Food Standards Australia New Zealand. (n.d.). Retrieved April 14, 2025, from https://www.foodstandards.gov.au/business/novel

OECD/OCDE. (1987). OECD Test Guideline 401 - Acute Oral Toxicity (1987 - Rescinded 2002). *OECD Guideline for Testing of Chemicals*, *50*, 1–6.

OECD TG420. (2001). Acute Oral Toxicity—Fixed Dose Procedure. *OECD Guideline For Testing Of Chemicals*, *December*, 1–14.

Organic board: Carrageenan shouldn't be in organic food, no decision now on hydroponics | Food Dive. (n.d.). Retrieved April 13, 2025, from https://www.fooddive.com/news/carrageenan-hydroponic-organic-nosb/430735/

Oriental Foods Distributor recalls two jelly cup products because of a choking hazard | Food Standards Agency. (n.d.). Retrieved April 13, 2025, from https://www.food.gov.uk/news-alerts/alert/fsa-prin-25-2023

Ottawa, C. (n.d.). *Agenda Item 4 CX/FL 16/43/4 JOINT FAO/WHO FOOD STANDARDS PROGRAMME CODEX COMMITTEE ON FOOD LABELLING Forty-third Session PROPOSED DRAFT REVISION OF THE GUIDELINES FOR THE PRODUCTION, PROCESSING, LABELLING AND MARKETING OF ORGANICALLY PRODUCED FOODS: ORGANIC AQUACULTURE (Comments at Step 3).*

Panggabean, J. A., Adiguna, S. P., Rahmawati, S. I., Ahmadi, P., Zainuddin, E. N., Bayu, A., & Putra, M. Y. (2022). Antiviral Activities of Algal-Based Sulfated Polysaccharides. *Molecules 2022, Vol. 27, Page 1178*, *27*(4), 1178. https://doi.org/10.3390/MOLECULES27041178

Pari, R. F., Uju, U., Hardiningtyas, S. D., Ramadhan, W., Wakabayashi, R., Goto, M., & Kamiya, N. (2025). Ulva Seaweed-Derived Ulvan: A Promising Marine Polysaccharide as a Sustainable Resource for Biomaterial Design. *Marine Drugs 2025, Vol. 23, Page 56*, *23*(2), 56. https://doi.org/10.3390/MD23020056

Pokhrel, S. (2024). Food Safety and Standards (Foods for Infant Nutrition) Regulations, 2020. *Αγαπη*, *15*(1), 37–48.

Pradhan, B., Bhuyan, P. P., & Ki, J. S. (2023). Immunomodulatory, Antioxidant, Anticancer, and Pharmacokinetic Activity of Ulvan, a Seaweed-Derived Sulfated Polysaccharide: An Updated Comprehensive Review. *Marine Drugs 2023, Vol. 21, Page 300*, *21*(5), 300. https://doi.org/10.3390/MD21050300

Qi, H., Liu, X., Wang, K., Liu, D., Huang, L., Liu, S., & Zhang, Q. (2013). Subchronic toxicity study of ulvan from Ulva pertusa (Chlorophyta) in Wistar rats. *Food and Chemical Toxicology*, *62*, 573–578. https://doi.org/10.1016/J.FCT.2013.09.022

Rajauria, G., Ravindran, R., Garcia-Vaquero, M., Rai, D. K., Sweeney, T., & O'Doherty, J. (2023). Purification and Molecular Characterization of Fucoidan Isolated from Ascophyllum nodosum Brown Seaweed Grown in Ireland. *Marine Drugs 2023, Vol. 21, Page 315*, *21*(5), 315. https://doi.org/10.3390/MD21050315

Regulation (EU) 2015/2283 of the European Parliament and of the Council on novel foods, amending Regulation (EU) No. 1169/2011 of the European Parliament and of the Council and repealing Regulation (EC) No. 258/97 of the European Parliament and of the Council and Commission Regulation (EC) No. 1852/2001. | FAOLEX. (n.d.). Retrieved April 14, 2025, from https://www.fao.org/faolex/results/details/en/c/LEX-FAOC151053/

Reisky, L., Préchoux, A., Zühlke, M. K., Bäumgen, M., Robb, C. S., Gerlach, N., Roret, T., Stanetty, C., Larocque, R., Michel, G., Song, T., Markert, S., Unfried, F., Mihovilovic, M. D., Trautwein-Schult, A., Becher, D., Schweder, T., Bornscheuer, U. T., & Hehemann, J. H. (2019). A marine bacterial enzymatic cascade degrades the algal polysaccharide ulvan. *Nature Chemical Biology 2019 15:8*, *15*(8), 803–812. https://doi.org/10.1038/s41589-019-0311-9

Rezaiyan Attar, F., Sedaghat, N., Pasban, A., Yeganehzad, S., & Hesarinejad, M. A. (2023). Modified atmosphere packaging with chitosan coating to prevent deterioration of fresh in-hull Badami's pistachio fruit. *Chemical and Biological Technologies in Agriculture 2023 10:1*, *10*(1), 1–18. https://doi.org/10.1186/S40538-023-00393-9

Rychen, G., Aquilina, G., Azimonti, G., Bampidis, V., Bastos, M. de L., Bories, G., Chesson, A., Cocconcelli, P. S., Flachowsky, G., Kolar, B., Kouba, M., López-Alonso, M., López Puente, S., Mantovani, A., Mayo, B., Ramos, F., Saarela, M., Villa, R. E., Wallace, R. J., … Gropp, J. (2017). Safety and efficacy of sodium and potassium alginate for pets, other non food-producing animals and fish. *EFSA Journal*, *15*(7), e04945. https://doi.org/10.2903/J.EFSA.2017.4945

Scientific Opinion on the safety of 'Chitin-glucan' as a Novel Food ingredient. (2010). *EFSA Journal*, *8*(7). https://doi.org/10.2903/J.EFSA.2010.1687

Shaikh, M. A. J., Gupta, G., Afzal, O., Gupta, M. M., Goyal, A., Altamimi, A. S. A., Alzarea, S. I., Almalki, W. H., Kazmi, I., Negi, P., Singh, S. K., & Dua, K. (2023). Sodium alginate-based drug delivery for diabetes management: A review. *International Journal of Biological Macromolecules*, *236*, 123986. https://doi.org/10.1016/J.IJBIOMAC.2023.123986

Shikov, A. N., Flisyuk, E. V., Obluchinskaya, E. D., & Pozharitskaya, O. N. (2020). Pharmacokinetics of Marine-Derived Drugs. *Marine Drugs 2020, Vol. 18, Page 557*, *18*(11), 557. https://doi.org/10.3390/MD18110557

Sicherer, S. H. (1999). Food allergy: When and how to perform oral food challenges. *Pediatric Allergy and Immunology*, *10*(4), 226–234. https://doi.org/10.1034/J.1399-3038.1999.00040.X

Standards Agency, F. (2021). *COMMITTEE ON TOXICITY OF CHEMICALS IN FOOD, CONSUMER PRODUCTS AND THE ENVIRONMENT Additional information requested by the Committee on allergenicity of chitin and chitosan based BBFCMs Background*. https://www.cfsanappsexternal.fda.gov/scripts/fdcc/?set=GRASNotices&id=73&sort=GRN_No&o

The European Parliament and the Council of the European Union. (2015). Regulation (EU) 2015/2283 of the European Parliament and of the Council, of 25 November 2015. *Official Journal of the European Union*, *2015*(258), 1–22.

Thomas, P. G., & Rengasamy, R. (2008). Toxicological Evaluation of Fucoidan from Cladosiphon okamuranus. *Https://Home.Liebertpub.Com/Jmf*, *11*(4), 638–642. https://doi.org/10.1089/JMF.2007.0127

Tobacman, J. K. (2001). Review of harmful gastrointestinal effects of carrageenan in animal experiments. *Environmental Health Perspectives*, *109*(10), 983–994. https://doi.org/10.1289/EHP.01109983

Tran, V. H. N., Mikkelsen, M. D., Truong, H. B., Vo, H. N. M., Pham, T. D., Cao, H. T. T., Nguyen, T. T., Meyer, A. S., Thanh, T. T. T., & Van, T. T. T. (2023). Structural Characterization and Cytotoxic Activity Evaluation of Ulvan Polysaccharides Extracted from the Green Algae Ulva papenfussii. *Marine Drugs*, *21*(11), 556. https://doi.org/10.3390/MD21110556/S1

Tsai, H. L., Tai, C. J., Huang, C. W., Chang, F. R., & Wang, J. Y. (2017). Efficacy of Low-Molecular-Weight Fucoidan as a Supplemental Therapy in Metastatic Colorectal Cancer Patients: A Double-Blind Randomized Controlled Trial. *Marine Drugs 2017, Vol. 15, Page 122*, *15*(4), 122. https://doi.org/10.3390/MD15040122

Tziveleka, L. A., Ioannou, E., & Roussis, V. (2019). Ulvan, a bioactive marine sulphated polysaccharide as a key constituent of hybrid biomaterials: A review. *Carbohydrate Polymers*, *218*, 355–370. https://doi.org/10.1016/J.CARBPOL.2019.04.074

US Food and Drug Administration. (2022). FDA Executive Summary Prepared for the Meeting of the General and Plastic Surgery Devices Panel of the Medical Devices Advisory Committee - Classification of Topical Hemostatic Wound Dressings . https://www.fda.gov/media/162540/download.

Wang, S., Tian, Z. Bin, Chen, J. W., Cong, P. S., Ding, X. L., Zhang, C. P., Yin, X. Y., Yang, L., Jing, X., Mao, T., Li, X. Y., Sun, Z. Y., Jiang, J. J., & Yu, Y. N. (2023). Effect of fucoidan on gut microbiota and its clinical efficacy in Helicobacter pylori eradication: A randomized controlled trial. *Journal of Digestive Diseases*, *24*(8–9), 461–471. https://doi.org/10.1111/1751-2980.13215

Welcome to the Ministry of Food and Drug Safety | Ministry of Food and Drug Safety. (n.d.-a). Retrieved April 11, 2025, from https://www.mfds.go.kr/eng/index.do

Welcome to the Ministry of Food and Drug Safety | Ministry of Food and Drug Safety. (n.d.-b). Retrieved April 14, 2025, from https://www.mfds.go.kr/eng/index.do

Xia, W., Liu, P., Zhang, J., & Chen, J. (2011). Biological activities of chitosan and chitooligosaccharides. *Food Hydrocolloids*, *25*(2), 170–179. https://doi.org/10.1016/J.FOODHYD.2010.03.003

Xu, S., Wu, Q., He, B., Rao, J., Chow, D. H. K., Xu, J., Wang, X., Sun, Y., Ning, C., & Dai, K. (2022). Interactive effects of cerium and copper to tune the microstructure of silicocarnotite bioceramics towards enhanced bioactivity and good biosafety. *Biomaterials*, *288*, 121751. https://doi.org/10.1016/J.BIOMATERIALS.2022.121751

Younes, M., Aggett, P., Aguilar, F., Crebelli, R., Filipič, M., Frutos, M. J., Galtier, P., Gott, D., Gundert-Remy, U., Kuhnle, G. G., Lambré, C., Leblanc, J. C., Lillegaard, I. T., Moldeus, P., Mortensen, A., Oskarsson, A., Stankovic, I., Waalkens-Berendsen, I., Woutersen, R. A., … Dusemund, B. (2017). Re-evaluation of alginic acid and its sodium, potassium, ammonium and calcium salts (E 400–E 404) as food additives. *EFSA Journal, 15*(11), e05049. https://doi.org/10.2903/J.EFSA.2017.5049

Younes, M., Aggett, P., Aguilar, F., Crebelli, R., Filipič, M., Frutos, M. J., Galtier, P., Gott, D., Gundert-Remy, U., Kuhnle, G. G., Lambré, C., Leblanc, J. C., Lillegaard, I. T., Moldeus, P., Mortensen, A., Oskarsson, A., Stankovic, I., Waalkens-Berendsen, I., Woutersen, R. A., … Dusemund, B. (2018). Re-evaluation of carrageenan (E 407) and processed Eucheuma seaweed (E 407a) as food additives. *EFSA Journal, 16*(4), e05238. https://doi.org/10.2903/J.EFSA.2018.5238

Zakaria, Z., Izzah, Z., Jawaid, M., & Hassan, A. (2012). Chitosan deacetylation. *BioResources, 7*(4).

Zhao, M., Garcia-Vaquero, M., Przyborska, J., Sivagnanam, S. P., & Tiwari, B. (2021). The development of analytical methods for the purity determination of fucoidan extracted from brown seaweed species. *International Journal of Biological Macromolecules, 173*, 90–98. https://doi.org/10.1016/J.IJBIOMAC.2021.01.083

MIX
Papier aus verantwortungsvollen Quellen
Paper from responsible sources
FSC® C105338

If you have any concerns about our products,
you can contact us on
ProductSafety@springernature.com

In case Publisher is established outside the EU,
the EU authorized representative is:
Springer Nature Customer Service Center GmbH
Europaplatz 3, 69115 Heidelberg, Germany

Printed by Libri Plureos GmbH
in Hamburg, Germany